CLINICAL REASONING
FOR
MANUAL THERAPISTS

For Butterworth Heinemann:

Senior Commissioning Editor: Heidi Allen
Associate Editor: Robert Edwards
Project Manager: Samantha Ross
Designer: George Ajayi
Illustration Manager: Bruce Hogarth

CLINICAL REASONING
FOR
MANUAL THERAPISTS

Mark A. Jones BSc (Psych), PT, Grad Dip Advan Manip Ther, MAppSc

*Senior Lecturer, Director, Master of Musculoskeletal and Sports Physiotherapy,
Physiotherapy International Coordinator, School of Health Sciences,
University of South Australia, South Australia, Australia*

AND

Darren A. Rivett BAppSc (Phty), Grad Dip Manip Ther, MAppSc (Manip Phty), PhD

*Associate Professor, Program Convenor and Head,
Discipline of Physiotherapy, School of Health Sciences,
Faculty of Health, The University of Newcastle, New South Wales, Australia*

Foreword by

Lance Twomey BAppSc (WAIT), BSc (Hons), PhD (W. Aust) TTC, MADA

Vice Chanceller, Curtis University of Technology, Perth, Australia

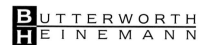
BUTTERWORTH
HEINEMANN

EDINBURGH LONDON NEW YORK OXFORD PHILADELPHIA ST LOUIS SYDNEY TORONTO 2004

BUTTERWORTH-HEINEMANN
An imprint of Elsevier Science Limited

First published 2004

ISBN 0 7506 3906 7

British Library Cataloguing in Publication Data
A catalogue record for this book is available from the British Library

Library of Congress Cataloging in Publication Data
A catalog record for this book is available from the Library of Congress

Notice
Medical knowledge is constantly changing. Standard safety precautions must be
followed, but as new research and clinical experience broaden our knowledge,
changes in treatment and drug therapy may become necessary or appropriate.
Readers are advised to check the most current product information provided by
the manufacturer of each drug to be administered to verify the recommended dose,
the method and duration of administration, and contraindications. It is the
responsibility of the practitioner, relying on experience and knowledge of the
patient, to determine dosages and the best treatment for each individual patient.
Neither the publisher nor the editors assume any liability for any injury and/or
damage to persons or property arising from this publication.

                                                                    The Publisher

Where illustrations have been borrowed from other sources every effort has been
made to contact the copyright owners to get their permission. However, should any
copyright owner come forward and claim that permission was not granted for use
of their material, we will arrange for acknowledgement to be made.

 ELSEVIER SCIENCE your source for books,
journals and multimedia
in the health sciences
www.elsevierhealth.com

The
publisher's
policy is to use
paper manufactured
from sustainable forests

Printed in China

Contents

List of contributors

Mark Bookhout PT, MS
President, Physical Therapy Orthopaedic
Specialists, Inc, Minneapolis & Adjunct Associate
Professor, Department of Physical Medicine and
Rehabilitation, Michigan State University
College of Osteopathic Medicine, East Lansing,
Michigan, USA

David Butler MAppSc
Director, Neuro Orthopaedic Institute and
Lecturer, University of South Australia,
Adelaide, Australia

Helen Clare PT, GradDipManipTher, MAppSc, DipMDeT
International Director of Education,
McKenzie Institute International, Wellington,
Australia

Brian Egloff MS, MPT
Uniformed Services University, Bethesda
MD, USA

Richard E. Erhard DC, PT
Assistant Professor, Department of Physical Therapy,
University of Pittsburgh and Head of Physical
Therapy and Chiropractic Services, University of
Pittsburgh Medical Centre, Pittsburgh, USA

Louis Gifford MAppSc, BSc, FCSP
Private Practitioner, Falmouth Physiotherapy
Clinic, Kestrel, Swanpool, Falmouth,
Cornwall, UK

Toby Hall MSc, PostGradDipManipTher
Adjunct Senior Teaching Fellow, School of
Physiotherapy, Curtin University of Technology,
Perth, Western Australia

Joy Higgs PhD, MHPEd, GradDipPhty, BSc
Faculty of Health Sciences, University of Sydney,
Sydney, Australia

Paul Hodges PhD, BPhty(Hons)
Associate Professor, Department of Physiotherapy,
University of Queensland, Brisbane,
Australia

Gary Hunt PT, DPT, MA, OCS, CPed
Associate Professor, Franklin Pierce College
Physical Therapy Program, Concord,
New Hampshire; Senior Physical Therapist,
Outpatient Physical Therapy Clinic, Cox Health
Systems, Springfield, Missouri, USA

Mark A. Jones BSc(Psych), PT, GradDipAdvanManipTher,
MAppSc
Senior Lecturer, Director, Master of
Musculoskeletal and Sports Physiotherapy,
Physiotherapy International Coordinator,
School of Health Sciences,
University of South Australia,
Adelaide, Australia

Gwendolen Jull MPhty, PhD, FACP
Associate Professor, Department of Physiotherapy,
University of Queensland, Brisbane,
Australia

Freddy Kaltenborn PT, ProfDrhc(USA)
Scheidegg, Germany

Diane Lee BSR, FCAMT
Clinical Director,
Delta Orthopaedic Physiotherapy Clinic,
Delta, BC, Canada

Mary Magarey DipTechPhysioGrad, DipAdvancedManipTherapy, PhD
Senior Lecturer, School of Health Sciences, University of South Australia, Adelaide, Australia

David Magee BPT, PhD
Professor, Department of Physical Therapy, Faculty of Rehabilitation Medicine, University of Alberta, Edmonton, AB, Canada

Geoffrey Maitland MBE, AUA, FCSP, FACP, MAppSc(Hons)
Glenside, South Australia 5065, Australia

Jenny McConnell BAppSc, MbiomedE
Mosman, NSW, Australia

Robin McKenzie CNZM, OBE, FCSP, FNZSP, DipMT, DipMDT
The Mckenzie Institute International, Waikanae, New Zealand

Jan Mens MD, PhD
Department of Rehabilitation Medicine, Faculty of Medicine and Health Sciences, Erasmus MC, Rotterdam, The Netherlands

Brian Mulligan FNZSP(Hon), DipMT
Private Practitioner and Lecturer, Wellington, New Zealand

Stanley Paris PT, PhD, FAPTA
President, University of St. Augustine, Florida, USA

Erl Pettman PT, FCAMT
Owner, McCallum Physiotherapy Clinic, Abbotsford, BC, Canada; Clinical Instructor, DSc PT Program at Andrews University, Berrien Springs, Michigan, USA

Robert Pfund PT, OMT, MAppSc
Private Practitioner and Instructor for Orthopaedic Manual Therapy, Physiotherapy Fetzer and Pfund, Kempten, Germany

Darren A. Rivett BAppSc (Phty), GradDipManipTher, MAppSc(ManipPhty), PhD
Associate Professor, Program Convenor and Head, Discipline of Physiotherapy, School of Health Sciences, Faculty of Health, The University of Newcastle, New South Wales, Australia

Mariano Rocabado DPT
Full Professor, School of Dentistry, University of Chile and Director Physical Therapy and Physical Medical Rehabilitation, INTEGRAMEDICA, Santiago, Chile

Shirley Sahrmann PT, PhD, FAPTA
Professor, Physical Therapy, Neurology, Cell Biology and Physiology, Director, Program in Movement Science and Associate Director, Program in Physical Therapy, Washington University School of Medicine, St. Louis, USA

Tom Arild Torstensen BSc(Hons), PT, CandScient(Advanced MSc)
Specialist in Manipulative Therapy MNFF, Norway

Patricia Trott MSc(Anat), GradDipAdvManTher, FACP
Associate Professor, School of Health Sciences, University of South Australia, Adelaide, Australia

Lance Twomey BAppSc(WAIT), BSc(Hons), PhD(W.Aust), TTC, MADA
Vice Chancellor, Curtis University of Technology, Perth, Australia

John van der Meij PTMT
Private Practitioner Manual Therapy and Clinical Consultant Trilemma, Senior Lecturer in Pain Science and Applied Neuro Science, School for Higher Education Leiden, Leiden, The Netherlands

Andry Vleeming PT, PhD
Clinical Anatomist, Spine and Joint Center, Rotterdam, The Netherlands

Richard Walsh DHSc, BSc(Med)(Hons), DipPhys
Physiotherapy Demonstrator, Department of Anatomy and Structural Biology, University of Otago, Dunedin, New Zealand

Peter E. Wells BA, FCSP, DipTP, MMACP, SRP
Private Practitioner, Postgraduate Teacher, The Physiotherapy Centre, Fulham, London, UK

Israel Zvulun BPT, MAppSc, MIPTS, MMPA
Private Practitioner and Clinical Consultant, Freelance Lecturer in Postgraduate Musculoskeletal Physiotherapy and Head of Clinical Education and Research Unit, Rabin Medical Centre, Golda Campus, Petah, Tikvah, Israel

Foreword

To place this book's emphasis appropriately on sound clinical reasoning within the framework of manual therapy, it is necessary to appreciate the evolution of manual therapy as a discipline in its own right. From tentative beginnings, it has advanced significantly since the 1960s. Initially it focussed on skill acquisition and the careful but prescriptive application of passive movement techniques to vertebral and peripheral joints. The earliest courses in manual therapy concentrated on joint structure, biomechanics, pathology, diagnosis and physical treatment in a mechanistic way, seeking simple cause and effect relationships between a patient's symptoms and signs and their physical treatment protocols.

Present day manual therapy practice and education owes a great deal to the vision and efforts of individual pioneering therapists. A considerable body of work has gradually been developed based on relevant literature from the fields of orthodox medicine, osteopathy, bone-setting and chiropractic. It has been further promoted by personal contact between key international practitioners. In addition, a substantial amount of work has been published, short courses have been developed and tertiary programmes introduced.

Manual therapy has been predominantly a highly individual and structured approach to patient examination and treatment by (largely passive) movement. Historically, it has focussed on the careful evaluation and assessment of a patient, followed by the application of a specific joint movement procedure and the subsequent reassessment of the patient to evaluate the success or otherwise of the procedure. Depending on the feedback, the therapist either continued with more of the same manual procedure or else changed to another technique. Such a method is truly patient centred given that the therapist's actions and treatment protocol are always guided by the patient's responses. This approach to the treatment of joint pain and impairment, along with an extensive repertoire of sophisticated manual skills, remain at the very heart of manual therapy.

Manual therapists are basically problem solvers. They are approached on a daily basis by individuals seeking assistance in the management of their body pain or their activity/participation restrictions. Therefore, contemporary therapists need not only excellent skills in physical assessment and treatment but also first class communication and management skills. They need also to understand legal and ethical issues, to be aware and have knowledge of potential behavioural and psychological issues, to be prepared to work as part of a larger health-care team and to know when to refer patients on and involve other disciplines within the team. Manual therapists have necessarily become more holistic in their care, with a related shift toward greater active management and patient participation.

Clinical reasoning is both collaborative and reflective. The therapist works with the patient and with other disciplines as part of a health-care delivery model. Even manual therapists in sole practices need to be a part of an extended multidisciplinary health network if a patient is to be provided with the most appropriate and timely treatment and advice, pertinent to their particular clinical condition. This approach requires adequate time for reflection and consultation, so as to provide a reasoned and specific response to the patient's problem.

Mark Jones and Darren Rivett have provided in this book an excellent overview of the issues central to clinical reasoning in manual therapy and a wide-ranging selection of case studies from many parts of the world. In addition, Joy Higgs has contributed a key chapter on educational theory and principles relating to learning clinical reasoning. In this chapter readers are taken through the relevant educational theory underpinning the teaching and learning (formal or self-directed) of clinical reasoning. Importantly, this same theory will also assist practising clinicians in their patient management. As Jones and Rivett point out in Chapter 1, teaching is a fundamental component of manual therapy treatment, yet manual therapists traditionally have not received formal training in education/learning theory and the associated teaching strategies. Finally, Jones and Rivett provide a chapter of practical suggestions on how readers can develop their clinical reasoning skills. To this end, the chapter links the clinical reasoning theory and the learning theory from the earlier chapters and encourages the reader to apply this knowledge in assessing the provided case studies and in their everyday clinical practice.

In the past, manual therapy has relied as much on charismatic leadership as it has on objective evidence. For the discipline to continue to progress in this new millennium, it is essential for it to be based on strong research, critical in its scrutiny of evidence provided and reflective in the way in which the various treatment hypotheses and protocols are introduced and evaluated. This will proceed in an environment where professionals are under closer examination than ever before, where patients demand both higher levels of communication with their therapist and involvement in their own treatment, where the ethical relationship between therapist and patient becomes a significant factor, and where the likelihood of adverse publicity remains a potent force in the equation. Skilled clinical reasoning will be critical to the clinician's ability to practise autonomously yet collaboratively, to generate and apply new knowledge and to continue their life-long learning.

Manual therapy will only flourish as a viable discipline through the 21st century if it learns from good basic and applied research and adapts appropriately to the new knowledge available. The case study approach to knowledge acquisition has always been an important factor in professions as diverse as medicine, business and education. It is very pleasing to note the global spread of the case studies in this volume and the ways in which they reinforce the basic tenets of clinical reasoning. This superb book takes the reader down the path of knowledge and reflection to provide better treatment options for all.

Lance Twomey

Preface

This book aims to promote the development of clinical reasoning skills, thinking or decision-making skills, in practitioners and students of manual therapy. For the purposes of this book, we consider a manual therapist to be a health-care practitioner who regularly deals with the problems that are attributed to disorders of the neuromusculoskeletal system. The original professional training of the manual therapist, whether it be in physiotherapy, chiropractic, osteopathy, medicine or another profession, is not important because the clinical reasoning process is universal. As the term implies, manual therapists work to a large degree with their hands, although this should not be seen to limit the role of the manual therapist to techniques such as manipulation, mobilization or soft tissue procedures, or to suggest that the patient's role is merely that of a passive recipient of the therapist's healing hands. Indeed, manual therapists utilize a broad range of hands-off physical and communicative (e.g. teaching) management approaches, and all manual therapy practice requires active patient participation and collaborative decision making. Manual therapists are now more than ever required to account for their clinical decisions against a background of competing demands such as evidence-based practice, funding limitations, legal and ethical issues, and the information explosion in health care; this all makes an increasingly difficult task. As such, this is not a textbook of quick-fix techniques, but rather a self-help book for the motivated practitioner or student seeking to progress along the road to clinical expertise by improving their skills in clinical reasoning.

The core of this book is the 23 detailed case reports in Section 2, which have been contributed by renowned and expert manual therapists from all over the world. We would like to express our sincere gratitude to the case contributors, first for their enthusiasm for this innovative project and, secondly and especially, for their patience as the individual cases were developed and the associated clinical reasoning painstakingly made explicit. Special thanks are also due to Professor Joy Higgs for her important and insightful contribution with Chapter 25.

Finally, we wish to acknowledge the unwavering encouragement and support of Helen and Jannine.

We hope that this book will be of value to manual therapy clinicians, students and teachers and will help to promote the role of clinical reasoning as the common foundation of all forms of manual therapy practice.

M. A. Jones
Adelaide, Australia, 2004
D. A. Rivett
Newcastle, Australia, 2004

Introduction

Manual therapy expertise is multidimensional, incorporating a combination of innate and learned characteristics including intellectual aptitude, personality (e.g. curiosity, empathy, humility), knowledge organization, plus communication, manual and thinking skills. Experts are often considered to be 'good thinkers', but traditionally our academic and continuing education manual therapy programmes have given little formal attention specifically to assessing and teaching thinking skills. It is common for people to question the need to address thinking skills formally, since all of us interpret, judge relevance, hypothesize, extrapolate, test hypotheses, prioritize, weigh evidence, draw conclusions, devise arguments, plan, monitor the effects of our efforts, and engage in numerous other activities that fall in the domain of clinical reasoning anyway, despite possibly never having received focussed instruction in thinking processes. However, this is not to say that we do these things well in all circumstances or that we are unable to learn to do them better.

It is often assumed that the thinking process will improve as students/clinicians acquire the necessary knowledge base and practise applying this knowledge in clinical situations. While this can be true and our manual therapy programmes have obviously produced many good thinkers, many poor thinkers have also come out of this traditional educational system. Weaker students and clinicians often lack key aspects of skilled clinical reasoning, which limits their ability to acquire knowledge through their education, or they acquire the knowledge but have great difficulty in applying this knowledge in a clinical context. Stronger students and clinicians seem to possess good thinking skills already, so when equipped with further knowledge they tend to excel. Or do they? Do we take our strong students and clinicians as far as they are capable? And does this apply to you? Often an individual may have very good logical thinking skills while lacking the creative and lateral thinking abilities required to advance their profession.

Closely associated with the content that is taught in our manual therapy courses are the beliefs we foster. For example, many students and beginning practitioners of manual therapy will adopt an allegiance to a particular clinical approach. This in itself is probably healthy, as a student who has acquired a systematic approach to assessment and management is well equipped to integrate additional philosophies and techniques, providing the necessary open mindedness is there at the outset. Unfortunately, however, political divisions between different manual therapy approaches, and even within some approaches, have held many clinicians back from learning anything more than what their own approach offers. Reflection is not openly promoted and hence students and clinicians historically have not been encouraged to explore and challenge their own beliefs.

Reflective scepticism means not taking for granted any position, policy or justification simply because it has been presented by a source of authority. Many of our earlier beliefs, rules or strategies in manual therapy were formulated on the basis of empirical observations in the clinic and attempts to fit existing biomedical theory to those clinical observations. In contrast, with the increased focus on evidence-based practice, there are growing pressures from both within and outside the profession for greater accountability and substantiation of clinical efficacy. This, combined with the push for manual therapists to adopt the broader biopsychosocial model of health and disability, has contributed to the current state of manual therapy education. Contemporary manual therapy education, while acknowledging its roots, has moved forward to a biopsychosocial, reasoning and evidence-based system. Importantly, this evidence includes both propositional knowledge derived from research and well-tested, practice-generated professional craft knowledge.

The influences of evidence-based practice, biopsychosocial models of health, and clinical reasoning theory have provided an exciting bridge between different approaches to manual therapy. The clinical reasoning process itself, as outlined in Chapter 1, should be fundamental to all approaches of manual therapy. Skilled clinical reasoning is essential for the application of both research-based and experience-based evidence. As such, if all students and clinicians could learn their respective approaches to manual therapy with specific attention to the cognitive skills of reasoning, including being reflectively critical of the assumptions that underlie their own beliefs and open minded to modification of their current views, then the diversity within manual therapy could better contribute to advancement in the assessment and management of patients' problems.

While clinical reasoning has always been implicitly taught in manual therapy education, it has only been since the 1990s that clinical reasoning theory and learning activities have been more explicitly integrated into manual therapy curricula. The text by Higgs and Jones (2000; Clinical Reasoning in the Health Professions), now in its second edition, has provided health science educators with a rich resource of clinical reasoning theory linked to education theory. However, what has been lacking is a practical resource for manual therapy clinicians and students who wish to reflect and improve on their own clinical reasoning. Clinical Reasoning for Manual Therapists has been written specifically for that purpose. This text will also provide manual therapy educators with a valuable bank of patient cases that can be utilized in learning activities designed to facilitate students' clinical reasoning.

Outline of the book

The book commences with a theory chapter (Chapter 1) on clinical reasoning covering both basic and contemporary clinical reasoning theory. It is hoped that readers will read this chapter prior to progressing to the case studies, as the clinical reasoning questions posed to the case contributors and the clinical reasoning commentary that follows their answers draw on this theory. Section 2 (Chapters 2–24) is a compilation

of patient cases contributed by expert manual therapists from around the globe. Experts were selected based on their status in the manual therapy world, as established through their clinical excellence, research, publications and teaching profile. An attempt was made to have different 'approaches' of manual therapy represented, as well as a wide array of patient problems from the more straightforward to the more complex. Case contributors were simply requested to submit a real patient case, including their full examination and management through to the point of closure. Following that, clinical reasoning questions were devised by the editors to extract each clinician's evolving thoughts throughout their own case. Our clinical reasoning commentary was then added with the aim of highlighting examples of clinical reasoning theory in practice. We have not attempted to critique the clinicians' reasoning; rather we merely hope to assist readers' understanding of clinical reasoning theory by pointing out specific examples as they emerged through the unfolding cases reports.

To maximize what can be gained from reviewing these cases, our suggestion is to read through the case and reasoning questions and attempt to formulate your own answer before reading the clinician's answer. Most questions relate to hypotheses formulated on the basis of the information presented to that point. Occasionally, clinicians are asked to extrapolate on their own philosophy or specific assessment and management procedures used. Where the answers differ from what you might have answered, take the opportunity to stop and reflect on the basis for your opinion. Reasoning is not an exact science and the analysis of what are often complex, multifactorial patient presentations cannot be reduced to simple correct versus incorrect interpretations. For these cases to achieve their full educational potential, readers must attempt to reason through each case themselves and then openly reflect on and critique the reasoning expressed, the evidence substantiating judgments made and, importantly, your own reasoning, regardless of whether you agree or disagree with that put forward by the expert clinician.

In order to achieve our aim of providing a resource that will assist students and clinicians to improve their clinical reasoning, it was essential to include a chapter on educational theory and principles related to learning clinical reasoning. Chapter 25 by Joy Higgs provides this background. While the relevance of this chapter to manual therapy educators (including clinical supervisors) is obvious, the theory and principles discussed are equally essential to practising clinicians. Teaching is a central component of manual therapy practice, and patient learning (e.g. altered patient understanding/beliefs, feelings and health behaviours) is a primary outcome sought from collaborative reasoning. As very few manual therapists have received any formal schooling in education or learning theory, this chapter is vital to be able to promote effectively change in your students, your patients and yourself.

Lastly, Chapter 26 has been written to assist those clinicians and students who wish to continue to improve their clinical reasoning and for educators of manual therapy who desire to enhance the development of such skills in their students. We view clinical reasoning as an essential competency in manual therapy and, like any competency, skill is only acquired through continued practice, reflection, feedback and then further practice. In this chapter, following a discussion on the development of clinical expertise and common clinical reasoning errors, we provide a variety of suggestions for learning activities that can be used to further practice and develop your clinical reasoning skills (or that of students). Some of these activities involve using the patient cases found in Section 2, as previously discussed, while others utilize

alternative but readily accessible resources. There are learning activities that can be undertaken alone by the individual clinician, activities that involve a colleague or mentor and ones that can be undertaken within the small group situation. The continual process of learning clinical reasoning in both real life and simulated clinical experiences is discussed in depth and made practical. Examples of high-technology learning activities (e.g. commercially available interactive computer programmes) and low-technology learning activities (e.g. the use of a reflective diary) are given and their 'pros and cons' debated. Indeed, there is a learning experience suitable for every therapist or student, no matter what their stage of education, learning style or available resources.

We expect that this book will be of benefit for students studying manual therapy and for the various types of clinician working in this field and will provide a valuable resource for instructors. To make the most of the book, the reader should strive to keep in mind that the learning of clinical reasoning and the development of related thinking skills requires the individual to participate actively in their learning and at all times maintain an open but sceptical mind during this process. Consequently, the acquisition of clinical reasoning skill, and hence expertise in manual therapy, is in your hands.

Reference

Higgs, J. and Jones, M. (eds.) (2000). Clinical Reasoning in the Health Professions, 2nd edn. Oxford: Butterworth-Heinemann.

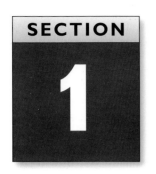

SECTION 1

Principles of clinical reasoning in manual therapy

Introduction to clinical reasoning

Mark A. Jones and Darren A. Rivett

Manual therapists work with a multitude of problem presentations in a variety of clinical practice environments (e.g. outpatient clinics, private practices, hospital or outpatient-based rehabilitation and pain unit teams, sports settings, home care and industrial work sites). The clinical presentations they encounter are, therefore, varied, ranging from discrete well-defined problems amenable to technical solutions to complex, multifactorial problems with uniqueness to the individual that defy the technical rationality of simply applying a 'proven' set course of management. Schön (1987, p. 3) characterizes this continuum of professional practice as existing between the 'high, hard ground of technical rationality' and 'the swampy lowland' where 'messy, confusing problems defy technical solution'. As will be evident in the case studies of this book, manual therapists must, therefore, be able to practise at both ends of the continuum. Manual therapists must have a good biomedical and professional knowledge base as well as advanced technical skills to solve problems of a discrete, well-defined nature. However, to understand and manage successfully the 'swampy lowland' of complex patient problems requires a rich blend of biomedical, psychosocial, professional craft and personal knowledge, together with diagnostic, teaching, negotiating, listening and counselling skills. Contemporary manual therapists must have a high level of knowledge and skills across a comprehensive range of competencies, including assessment, management, communication, documentation, and professional, legal and ethical comportment. Effective performance within and across these competencies requires a broad perspective of what

constitutes health and disability and equally broad skills in both diagnostic and non-diagnostic clinical reasoning.

In this chapter we present a contemporary perspective on clinical reasoning in manual therapy. Clinical reasoning is portrayed as being multidimensional. It is hypothesis oriented, collaborative and reflective. Skilled clinical reasoning contributes to therapists' learning and to the transformation of existing perspectives. A framework that describes the organization of knowledge by manual therapists is proposed together with a model of health and disability/recovery. We consider these will be helpful in promoting a broader perspective on patients' problems and will serve as a reference for exploring the reasoning of individual therapists.

What is clinical reasoning?

Clinical reasoning has been defined as a process in which the therapist, interacting with the patient and significant others (e.g. family and other health-care team members), structures meaning, goals and health management strategies based on clinical data, client choices and professional judgment and knowledge (Higgs and Jones, 2000). It is this thinking and decision making associated with clinical practice that enables therapists to take the best-judged action for individual patients. In this sense, clinical reasoning is the means to 'wise' action (Cervero, 1988; Harris, 1993).

Figure 1.1 depicts the integrated, patient-centred model of collaborative reasoning we hope to promote.

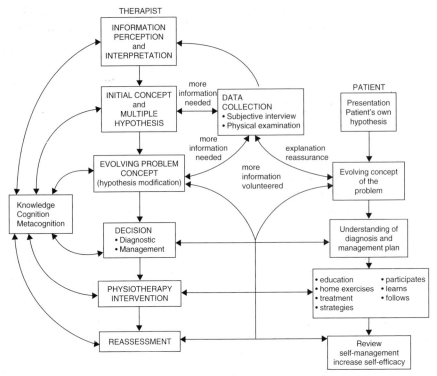

Fig. 1.1 Patient-centred model of clinical reasoning (Edwards and Jones, unpublished assignment).

In this model, clinical reasoning is seen as a process of reflective enquiry comprising three core elements—cognition, metacognition and knowledge—carried out in a collaborative framework with the relevant parties (e.g. the patient, carers, other health-care providers, the workplace and funding bodies) (Edwards and Jones, 1996; Jones et al., 2000).

Numerous variables influence the success of this collaborative therapist–patient reasoning process, including:

■ attributes of the therapist (e.g. breadth, depth and organization of knowledge, familiarity and experience with the type of case being managed, reasoning proficiency, communication and teaching skills, and professional craft skills)

■ attributes of the patient (e.g. needs, beliefs/attitudes and individual physical and psychosocial circumstances, including their capacity and willingness to participate in shared decision making and management)

■ attributes of the environment (e.g. resources, time, funding, and any externally imposed professional or regulatory requirements).

Understanding both the 'problem' and the 'person' determine management

To understand and manage patients and their problems successfully, manual therapists must consider not only the physical diagnostic possibilities (including the structures involved and the associated pathobiology) but also the full range of factors that can contribute to a person's health, particularly the effects these problems may have on patients' lives, and the understanding patients (and significant others) have of these problems and their management. Skilled therapists do this through a process of enquiry/interview, physical and environmental examination and ongoing management, where clues gleaned from the patient's presentation elicit hypotheses regarding the person and their presenting problems (Jones, 1992; Jones et al., 2000; Rivett and Higgs, 1997). Except in very straightforward presentations, when expert clinicians are quickly able to recognize the problem and the solution, these hypotheses then serve to guide further enquiries, assessment and eventually management.

In attempting to understand patients and their problems, manual therapists must be able to think along multiple lines and often think on different levels at the same time.

Hypothesis generation

The clinical reasoning process is hypothesis oriented in that patient data prompt the therapist's consideration of competing interpretations, which are, in turn, clarified and tested through further data collection and reassessment of management interventions (Fig. 1.1). Although many therapists do not realise it, they are generating hypotheses from the opening moments of a patient encounter (Doody and McAteer, 2002; Rivett and Higgs, 1997). That is, initial cues, such as a referral, case notes, observations of the patient in the waiting room, and opening introductions and enquiries with the patient, will evoke a range of initial impressions. While typically not thought of as such, they can be considered hypotheses. These initial hypotheses may be physical, psychological or socially related, with or without a diagnostic implication. They are usually somewhat broad and serve to delineate the boundaries in which the assessment will proceed.

All therapists have an element of routine to their examination. Individual therapists will have identified, through experience, the categories of information which they have found to be particularly useful for understanding and managing patients' problems. For example:

- personal profile including work, family and social circumstances
- site, behaviour and history of symptoms
- psychological/cognitive/affective status, expectations and goals
- general medical status: clinical yellow and red flag screening
- occupational blue flag screening
- socio-occupational black flag screening
- functional and structure-specific tests of the cardiovascular, respiratory and neuromusculoskeletal systems
- ergonomic and environmental analysis, etc.

While a degree of routine commonly exists, the specific enquiries and tests should be tailored to each patient's unique presentation.

Narrative reasoning

Through a process of enquiry, examination and reflective management, the therapist attempts to understand the patient's problem, while at the same time trying to understand the patient's personal story/narrative or the context of the problem beyond the mere chronological sequence of events. Understanding the context, also called 'narrative reasoning' (Christensen et al., 2002; Edwards, 2001; Fleming and Mattingly, 2000; Jones et al., 2000, 2002), requires attempting to understand the patient as a person, including their perspective of the problem, their experiences (e.g. understanding, beliefs, desires, motivations, emotions), the basis of their perspectives and how the problem is affecting their life (i.e. their pain or illness experience). This dimension of reasoning and understanding requires more than a good biomedical knowledge base and technical skills. Successful narrative reasoning, aimed at understanding the person, requires a good organization of biopsychosocial knowledge and the communication skills in order to apply that knowledge successfully. Narrative reasoning also necessitates a level of openness on the part of the therapist, both with respect to accepting the patient's story and with awareness of their own personal perspectives, and even biases, on matters such as chronic disability and pain, compensation cases and cultural issues. Therapists' personal perspectives on such issues will influence their approach (e.g. attitudes, expectations, communication/relationship) to their patients and their problems, with reflection required to recognize, and where necessary alter, inaccurate or unhelpful perspectives.

Patients' understanding/beliefs, attitudes, emotions and expectations represent what Mezirow (1990, 1991) has called their 'meaning perspective' (synonymous with 'frame of reference'). Understanding a patient's meaning perspective is the basis of narrative reasoning. An individual's meaning perspective is acquired and evolves from a combination of personal, societal and cultural experiences, where conscious and unconscious interpretations, attributions and emotions coalesce to make up their views and feelings. Mezirow (1991, p. xiii) states, '...that it is not so much what happens to people but how they interpret and explain what happens to them that determines their actions, their hopes, their contentment and emotional well-being, and their performance'.

In this sense, patients' meaning perspectives create sets of habitual expectations that serve as a (usually tacit) belief system for interpreting and evaluating experiences. In the context of manual therapy, patients' meaning perspectives become filters through which their perceptions and comprehension of any new experience must pass. Therefore, if a patient's meaning perspective is distorted—judged by the therapist to be counterproductive to recovery—such as 'pain equals further damage' or 'the damage I have is permanent and I will not improve further', then their perception (or lack of) and interpretation of new experiences (including the therapist's assessment and management) will also be distorted. In fact, distorted meaning perspectives or beliefs are typically more rigid and less amenable to change (Mezirow, 1991).

Analogous to attempting to identify underlying physical contributing factors to patients' symptomatic structures, it is necessary for manual therapists to delve into the basis of patients' meaning perspectives (i.e. their understanding, emotions, beliefs and attributions) in order to understand these perspectives. Patients' meaning perspectives are reflected in their 'story' or the context in which those views were shaped. While sometimes the information comes forward spontaneously, therapists must be able to listen for and enquire about (i.e. screen) patients' meaning perspectives and their basis, so as to identify patterns of distortion that require attention. While some patients' perspectives will fit recognizable patterns, others will be unique and defy some universal truth of 'normal' or 'unhelpful'. In other words, narrative reasoning decisions cannot be reduced to a correct or incorrect empirical judgment. Rather, therapists' hypotheses regarding patients' meaning perspectives can only be validated through therapist–patient consensus, or what has been labelled communicative (as opposed to procedural) management. As it is beyond the scope of this chapter to cover the full range of psychosocial issues for which therapists should screen, readers are referred to the texts by Butler (2000), Main and Spanswick (2000a), Strong et al. (2002) and Gifford (2000) for more thorough discussions of psychosocial screening.

Diagnostic versus narrative reasoning

A distinction can then be made between understanding and managing the problem to effect change (requiring biomedically driven cause and effect thinking and action: *diagnostic reasoning* and *procedural management*) versus understanding and interacting with the person to effect change (requiring biopsychosocially driven

narrative reasoning and *communicative management*). In reality, a comprehensive diagnosis should encompass what is learned from both the diagnostic reasoning regarding the physical problem and the narrative reasoning regarding the person. All forms of reasoning and management should be carried out collaboratively.

These seemingly different foci of thinking and management (directed to the problem and directed to the person) are not mutually exclusive, as the understanding of one enhances the therapist's understanding of the other. For example, attempting to understand and then attempting to facilitate change in the person (e.g. beliefs, emotions and health behaviours) is aided through a greater insight into the problem. The extent and nature of patients' activity and participation restrictions (World Health Organization, 2001; i.e. physical disabilities and associated handicaps) and impairments forms part of the context in which their psychosocial status must be viewed. A degree of stress and feelings of frustration, anger and even depression may be quite 'normal' in the presence of marked restrictions in activity and participation. Maladaptive thoughts and feelings can also coexist with physical impairment without necessarily driving or being the underlying source of those restrictions.

Similarly, however, understanding a problem and then attempting to facilitate change (e.g. activity restrictions and physical impairments) is aided through greater insight about the person. Patients' feelings, beliefs and health behaviours may be contributory to the recovery or detrimental (i.e. counterproductive to their recovery), and judgments regarding these aspects of the patient require effective interpersonal and enquiry skills, including biopsychosocial knowledge of what to look for, management strategies and referral pathways. Just as activity restrictions (e.g. difficulty climbing stairs) must be considered with respect to any physical impairments that may be present (e.g. mobility and motor control), the patient's feelings, beliefs and health behaviours must also be considered with respect to their experiences and related consequences, which may have contributed to shaping their views and behaviours (Butler, 2000; Gifford, 1998a, 2001, 2002; Main and Booker, 2000; Main and Parker, 2000; Watson, 2000; Watson and Kendall, 2000). Success in promoting change in both the problem and the person necessitates fostering the patient's insight into their own feelings, beliefs and behaviours, including their basis and where change would be beneficial. Reaching this level of mutual understanding requires *collaborative reasoning* or shared decision making between patient and therapist, as well as therapist skills in communicating and teaching. Similarly, as the physical and the psychological are closely linked, both procedural management, consisting of physically oriented active and passive interventions, and communicative management, consisting of education, advice and consensual perspective re-evaluation, will affect the other.

For the purposes of this book, hypothesis-oriented reasoning is defined very broadly as the reflective process of attending to patient information by consciously attempting to relate different features either to recognizable clinical patterns or to new, previously unrecognized patterns unique to the individual. Reflective attention to different patient cues and the subsequent critical search for supporting/confirming cues is put forward as essential to all reasoning processes, including attempting to understand the person and attempting to understand the problem. This cognitive activity of interpreting patient cues with respect to information already obtained represents a form of hypothesis testing and includes attending to and searching for both supporting and negating evidence. As referred to above, while some interpretations can be empirically validated, others will only be validated through therapist–patient consensus of the situation (e.g. patients' beliefs/perspectives and the basis on which they were formed). As the patient's story unfolds, the cumulative information obtained is interpreted for its fit with the broader evidence from available research and the particular patient's presentation, including previously obtained data, hypotheses considered and consensus reached. Even routine enquiries, tests and spontaneous information offered by the patient will be interpreted in the context of initial impressions or hypotheses. In this way, the manual therapist acquires an evolving understanding of the patient and the patient's problem(s). Initial impressions will be modified and new ones considered. The therapist's hypothesis-oriented diagnostic and narrative reasoning continues until sufficient understanding (of the person and the problem) is reached by both therapist and patient to enable joint determination of a plan of management.

The role of re-assessment in reasoning

The clinical reasoning of the therapist and patient continues throughout the ongoing management. In particular, manual therapy intervention (procedural and communicative) serves as another test of the hypotheses formed, consensus made and subsequent chosen course of action. Re-assessment either provides support for these decisions or signals the need for modification (of hypotheses), further perspective discussion (i.e. revisit the previous consensus reached) or further data collection (e.g. additional clinical examination or referral for other health professional consultation). At the micro level, therapists are constantly attending to patient responses (e.g. listening, clarifying, observing, feeling) and using these to build their understanding and guide clinical decisions to modify and improve their interventions. At the macro level, whole treatment sessions or even multiple treatments will be used to test the therapist's and patient's understanding and shared management decisions.

Although this account of management/re-assessment is described within the hypothesis-oriented approach, in reality the reasoning undertaken throughout management cannot be simply reduced to an empirical–analytical approach. The various forms of management (e.g. specific procedures, therapist–patient communication during management and teaching) can be carried out both in an instrumental cause and effect approach, where specified, measurable outcomes are sought, and in a communicative approach, where absolute truths are not available and validation is achieved through therapist–patient common understanding and consensus.

Cognition, featured in the left-hand box in Figure 1.1, is purposeful thought. The cognition underlying clinical reasoning includes the perception of relevant information, specific data interpretations or inductions; drawing inferences and generating hypotheses (deductions) from the synthesis of multiple cues; and testing for competing hypotheses. Higher-order cognition (*metacognition*) in the form of reflective appraisal of one's own thinking and understanding is discussed below under Reasoning as a reflective process.

Pattern recognition

Pattern recognition is a characteristic of all mature thought. In both everyday life and in the realm of manual therapy, knowledge is stored in our memory in chunks or patterns that facilitate more efficient communication and thinking (Anderson, 1990; Ericsson and Smith, 1991; Hayes and Adams, 2000;

Newell and Simon, 1972; Rumelhart and Ortony, 1977; Shön, 1983). These patterns form prototypes of frequently experienced situations that individuals use to recognize and interpret other situations. In manual therapy, patterns exist not only in classic diagnostic syndromes and associated management strategies but also in the pathobiological mechanisms associated with those syndromes and the multitude of environmental, physical, psychological (cognitive and affective), social, behavioural and cultural factors that contribute to the development and maintenance of patients' problems. For example, it is possible to recognize the typical clinical features of a shoulder subacromial impingement problem, as well as different patterns of common anatomical, biomechanical, motor patterning and technique/equipment factors that can contribute to this disorder. Importantly, patients can have the same pathology but quite different contributing factors, necessitating different and very individualized management if success is to be realised and maintained. Manual therapists also must be able to recognize patterns of biomedical factors that contraindicate manual therapy, such as clinical *red flags* (i.e. serious organic pathology) (Roberts, 2000) and biopsychosocial personal, family and work-related factors (*yellow*, *blue* and *black* flags, respectively) that may predispose to chronic pain, prolonged loss of work and serve as potential obstacles to recovery (Kendall et al., 1997; Main and Burton, 2000; Main et al., 2000). These are further discussed below under Prognosis.

Pattern recognition is required to generate hypotheses and hypothesis testing provides the means by which those patterns are refined, proved reliable and new patterns are learned (Barrows and Feltovich, 1987). While expert therapists are able to function largely on pattern recognition, novices who lack sufficient knowledge and experience to recognize clinical patterns will rely on the slower hypothesis testing approach to work through a problem. However, when confronted with a complex, unfamiliar problem, the expert, like the novice, will rely more on the hypothesis-oriented method of clinical reasoning (Barrows and Feltovich, 1987; Patel and Groen, 1991). Narrative reasoning and communicative management are still required to reveal and act on patients' meaning perspectives, regardless of whether pattern recognition or hypothesis testing dominates. Despite pattern recognition being a mode of thinking used by experts in all professions (Schön, 1983), it also represents perhaps the greatest source of errors in our thinking.

Related and other common errors of clinical reasoning are discussed in Chapter 26.

Reasoning as a collaborative process

Successful management of patients' problems requires more than just good diagnostic and manual skills: manual therapists must also be good teachers. In fact, while a certain percentage of patients' problems can be forever resolved through the sole intervention of the therapist's manual techniques, often lasting changes are only effected by understanding the particular determinants of health and behaviour operating and by negotiating changes in the patients' understanding, beliefs/attitudes and behaviours. For example, patients' understanding of their problems has been shown to impact on their self-efficacy, levels of pain tolerance, disability, time off work and eventual outcome (Borkan et al., 1991; Feuerstein and Beattie, 1995; Lackner et al., 1996; Main and Booker, 2000; Main et al., 2000; Malt and Olafson, 1995; Strong, 1995; Watson, 2000).

Manual therapists have generally only learned through personal experience the skills of psychosocial assessment and management (e.g. listening, communicating, negotiating, counselling and motivating) needed to effect positive changes in their patients' health understandings, beliefs and behaviours. While such skills are increasingly being made more explicit in manual therapy curricula, in general these aspects have not historically been given the same attention in terms of theory and application as has clinical reasoning in physical diagnosis and management. Consequently, biopsychosocial knowledge and interpersonal skills are often tacit and underdeveloped in some therapists.

The collaborative nature of the reasoning process is highlighted by the arrows interconnecting the centre and the boxes on the right in Figure 1.1. Whereas the centre boxes feature the therapist's reasoning, the boxes on the right depict the patient's thoughts and understanding. Thus, patients begin their encounter with a manual therapist with their own ideas of and feelings about the nature of their problem(s) and the management they need, as shaped by personal experience and advice from medical practitioners, family and friends. Through a process of evaluating patients' understandings, beliefs and feelings (meaning perspectives), and through the use of explanation, reassurance and shared decision making, the therapist can involve the patient in developing an evolving understanding of the problem and its management. Beliefs and feelings that are counterproductive to a patient's management and recovery, such as excessive fear of movement or pain, can contribute to physical deconditioning, poor compliance with self-management, poor self-efficacy and ultimately a poor outcome (Hill, 1998; Main and Booker, 2000). Patients who have been given an opportunity to share in the decision making have been shown to take greater responsibility for their own management and have a greater likelihood of achieving better outcomes (Bucklew et al., 1994; Burkhardt et al., 1994; Lorig et al., 1999; Niestadt, 1995; Shendell-Falik, 1990). Patient learning is a primary outcome sought from collaborative reasoning (Jones et al., 2000). Rather than being passive recipients of health care, patients construct a new understanding or meaning perspective, one in which they are actively involved in management decisions and share in the responsibility for their health care.

While this discussion has focussed on the collaborative reasoning between therapist and patient, a similar collaborative process should exist between the therapist and carers, as well as with other members of the health-care team and funding bodies. This broader role of the manual therapist in the local and global health-care community as an *interactional professional* is discussed more extensively in Higgs and Hunt (1999a,b).

Reasoning as a reflective process

Learning should be seen as a central outcome of clinical reasoning for both therapist and patient. While all therapists would hopefully see themselves as both teachers and learners, learning theory has traditionally not been a core area of study for manual therapists, apart perhaps from the formal attention to learning theory that accompanies concepts of motor learning. However, given the importance most therapists would acknowledge teaching has in their patient management (Jensen et al., 1999, 2000; Sluijs, 1991), this is an obvious deficiency.

■ Teaching

Teaching is a ubiquitous activity requiring its own focus of reasoning. Edwards (2001) found that expert manual therapists, neurological physiotherapists and domiciliary care physiotherapists skilfully employed such reasoning. It occurs on different levels from the provision of simple advice to motor retraining and explanation directed to changing patients' meaning perspectives. In all situations, the therapist must make judgments concerning the level and amount of teaching that is appropriate for an individual patient and the mode of delivery that is most suitable and likely to be accepted by the patient. For example, expert therapists will often strategically use 'stories' regarding other patients as a means of building rapport, educating and communicating prognostic outcomes (Edwards, 2001). Such real-life scenarios bring credibility to the advice or explanation that they are used to support and can be strategically employed by therapists to strengthen their message.

Learning theory is discussed in Chapter 25, where transformative learning (described by Mezirow (1990) as perspective transformation) is defined as the construction of meaning (i.e. knowledge) from experience. The individual's revised understanding will then guide their future perspectives (understanding, appreciation and behaviour). Facilitating this level of learning necessitates the learner (patient or therapist) engaging in critical reflection. Presuppositions of current beliefs are re-examined, opening the way for new, revised perspectives. Both therapists and patients at times need to reflect critically on the basis of their beliefs, so that distortions in meaning perspectives (beliefs) may be identified and corrected.

■ Learning from reflection

To learn from your own clinical experiences and grow as a therapist requires reasoning that is open minded and reflective. Reflection is an act of cognition that can be used in different ways. In a simplest form, these thoughtful activities represent reflective thought, for example, when the significance of a piece of information is actively considered or when different and sometimes conflicting findings are assessed. However, reflective thinking at a higher level, metacognition, involves thinking about your thinking and the factors that limit it. Metacognition is a well-recognized characteristic of expertise (Alexander and Judy, 1988; Biggs, 1986). Metacognitive reflections may be directed at any of the following:

- the information available (e.g. awareness of the quality and relevance of information obtained)

- the reasoning process (e.g. awareness of specific strategies required to understand the person and the problem and achieve the desired goals)
- the hypotheses formed and decisions reached (e.g. research and experience-based evidence for assessment and management decisions)
- the organization of knowledge (e.g. awareness of one's own knowledge base, personal perspectives, biases and any limitations).

Reflection can occur in what Schön (1983, 1987) has called *reflection-in-action*, where you literally pause during a patient encounter and consider any of these issues, or in hindsight as a *reflection-about-action*. Too often a patient's status changes, for the better or the worse, without the therapist having or taking the time to reflect on the change. In a busy practice, improvement is a godsend as it means the treatment can be repeated with little deliberation. A lack of improvement typically leads to a change in treatment with some consideration of the options available, but often without any serious reflection on prior judgments made and the underlying reasoning that led to the current lack of improvement.

The reflective thinker is sceptical, always questioning the reliability, validity and overall relevance of findings and interpretations, and ever prepared to accept that their own knowledge base may be inadequate. Brookfield (1987, 2000) cites this trait as a key component of all critical thinking, not just clinical reasoning. He stresses the importance of being willing and able to identify and challenge the assumptions that underlie beliefs and actions. Reflecting on the basis of one's preconceptions may include considering such things as what information is relevant; what constitutes a particular diagnostic, psychosocial or behavioural pattern; what evidence (research validated or experience based) exists to support judgments and interventions; and the appropriateness of the model of health and recovery followed.

Awareness of new perspectives

Associated with becoming aware of the assumptions that underlie a belief is the recognition of the context from which those assumptions arose. That is, many of our beliefs are formed from cultural, historical or specific philosophical frames of reference; when these frames of reference are appreciated, a deeper

understanding of the belief itself and a more informed position from which to evaluate the belief can be achieved. A healthy reflective scepticism, where a particular philosophy, position or justification is not taken for granted simply because it has been presented by a source of authority or been unchanged for a long time, is important for skilled clinical reasoning and continued professional growth. This is not to suggest that the only legitimate decisions and actions are those that can be conclusively substantiated by current research, as we hold the view that experience-based non-propositional and personal knowledge, as discussed below, are equally important (Higgs et al., 2001a; Jones and Higgs, 2000). However, it is important to recognize the basis and biases of one's own views and that alternatives exist. This requires looking beyond your own perspectives and contemplating other possibilities, some of which may even be beyond what is empirically known at the present time.

Such open reflection about oneself (by therapists and patients) is no easy task, as Brookfield (2000, p. 63) points out:

> No matter how much we may think we have an accurate sense of our practice, we are stymied by the fact that we are using our own interpretive filters to become aware of our own interpretive filters!... To some extent we are all prisoners trapped within the perceptual frameworks that determine how we view our experiences. A self-confirming cycle often develops whereby our uncritically accepted assumptions shape clinical actions which then serve only to confirm the truth of those assumptions.

Because of this, it is usually difficult to explore your own assumptions effectively. Clinical reasoning in general, and self-reflection in particular, is enhanced when we enlist the help of others. On this basis, Brookfield (2000) describes clinical reasoning as an inherently social process. Peers, teachers and also our patients can be effective critical mirrors, as we can be to our patients, to foster the critical self-reflection necessary to promote change. Brookfield labels the reluctance most of us have for this (i.e. to exposing our reasoning to the critique of others) as 'impostorship': the deep feeling many clinicians have that they do not really understand a problem or how best to manage it and their fear of being 'found out' by the patient and their colleagues. Acknowledging this reality is critical if therapists are seriously trying to improve their own clinical reasoning. Section 3 discusses ways in which this barrier can be broken down and in which critical reflection, and hence transformative learning, can be facilitated.

A key attribute of experts, and a necessary prerequisite to skilled clinical reasoning, is the affective disposition to think in this reflective manner. Such an affective disposition includes inquisitiveness, self-confidence, open mindedness, flexibility, honesty, diligence, reasonableness, empathy and humility (Brookfield, 1987; Ennis, 1987; Fonteyn and Ritter, 2000; Jensen et al., 1999). Clearly critical thinking, as well as being rational, is emotive.

Reasoning requires well-organized knowledge

Research investigating the nature and development of expertise across a range of activities (chess, engineering, mathematics, medicine, physics, statistics) has consistently shown that it is not the command of any generic problem-solving strategies or how much knowledge is possessed that is critical; rather, it is how that knowledge is organized (Allwood and Montgomery, 1982; Arocha et al., 1993; Bloom and Broder, 1950; Bordage and Lemieux, 1991; Boshuizen and Schmidt, 2000; Chi et al., 1981; De Groot, 1965; Patel and Groen, 1986; Patel and Kaufman, 2000; Schmidt and Boshuizen, 1993). As previously discussed, humans store knowledge in chunks or patterns. Therefore, one can think of therapists' organization of knowledge as the breadth and depth of their understandings and beliefs, held together in patterns acquired through both formal academia and personal experience, remembering that diagnostic patterns represent only a fraction of one's knowledge base. In fact, knowledge focussing purely on biomedical, diagnostic pathology is insufficient for full understanding and management of patients' problems. Rather this propositional textbook knowledge must be integrated into a broader organization of non-propositional craft and personal knowledge. Understanding of patients' personal contexts, strategies of reasoning and intervention, and awareness of your own perspective, are important aspects of professional craft and personal knowledge.

It is beyond the scope of this chapter to explore this important topic of knowledge types and knowledge acquisition fully, and readers are referred to the work of Boshuizen and Schmidt (2000), Higgs and Titchen (2000), Higgs et al. (2001b) and Patel and Kaufman (2000) for further discussion of these issues. For the purposes of this book, we will use the broad distinction (proposed by Higgs and Titchen (1995)) of *propositional knowledge* (or 'knowing that'—biomedical and biopsychosocial knowledge ratified by clinical trials and well-founded theories of professional practice) and *non-propositional knowledge*, including *professional craft knowledge* (procedural knowledge or 'knowing how', such as practical skills and strategies of enquiry, reasoning and intervention) and *personal knowledge* (knowledge derived from personal experiences, which shapes your own unique meaning perspectives and influences your interpersonal interactions, personal values and beliefs).

Understanding and successfully managing patients' problems requires a rich organization of all three types of knowledge. Propositional knowledge provides us with theory and levels of substantiation by which the patient's clinical presentation can be considered against research-validated theory and practice. Non-propositional professional craft knowledge allows us the means to use that theory in the clinic while providing additional, often cutting-edge (albeit with unproven generality) clinically derived evidence. Personal knowledge allows a deeper understanding of the clinical problem to be gained within the context of the patient's particular situation and enabling us to practise in a holistic and caring way.

As important as knowledge obviously is to successful clinical reasoning, improving one's organization of knowledge requires a clear understanding of how knowledge is acquired. Glaser (1984, p. 99) states that 'effective thinking is the result of conditionalized knowledge—the knowledge that becomes associated with the conditions and constraints of its use'. That is, knowledge is made particularly meaningful and accessible when it is created or acquired in the context for which it must be used (Cervero, 1988; Rumelhart and Ortony, 1977; Schön, 1983, 1987; Shepard and Jensen, 1990; Tulving and Thomson, 1973). In manual therapy, this means acquiring and constructing links between propositional, professional craft and personal knowledge in the context of real-life patient problems.

This view is consistent with the stage theory of knowledge acquisition and development (Boshuizen and Schmidt, 2000). This proposes that medical students initially function predominantly on biomedically dominated propositional knowledge structures, which gradually become encapsulated into clusters of higher-order concepts (e.g. clinical syndromes). In other words, with clinical experience, textbook knowledge is eventually transposed into clinical patterns anchored within memory through real clinical experiences (Boshuizen and Schmidt, 1992, 2000; Schmidt et al., 1990, 1992). The notion of an 'illness script' is used to depict this higher-order knowledge structure (Feltovich and Barrows, 1984). Illness scripts have three components:

- enabling conditions: conditions or constraints under which a disease or problem occurs, such as personal, social, medical, hereditary and environmental factors
- fault: the pathobiological and psychosocial processes associated with any given disease or disability
- consequences of the fault: signs and symptoms of the particular problem as well as its functional impact on the patient's life.

Even this probably oversimplifies the complexity of a clinician's knowledge organization. Virtually every characteristic of a patient's presentation (enabling conditions, fault and consequences) can be said to exist along a continuum, and judging the relevance of a particular feature often relates to its qualitative characteristics and perceived dominance within the presentation (Bordage and Lemieux, 1986; Bordage and Zacks, 1984). Therefore, in addition to recognizing clinical presentations, therapists must also possess a broader understanding of the determinants of health and recovery.

Patel and Kaufman (2000) challenge the model of knowledge encapsulation put forward by Boshuizen and Schmidt (2000), suggesting it represents an idealized perspective on the integration of basic science in clinical knowledge and argue that biomedical knowledge and clinical knowledge are two separate worlds. They suggest basic science has different significance in different domains, and cite research which has demonstrated that even 'expert' medical clinicians have poorly developed biomedical knowledge. They propose that the key role played by basic science may not be in facilitating clinical reasoning per se but in facilitating explanation and coherent communication. The debate regarding the role of biomedical knowledge is equally important to manual therapy curricula, where some are grounded in promoting clinical decisions on the basis of the patient's presenting signs and symptoms (i.e. impairment based with consideration of but not driven by biomedical factors) while others have pathology and biomedical constructs as the focus of assessment and management.

The mature organism model

We support a model of knowledge organization (and hence curriculum development) that draws on both traditions but is arguably broader in scope. An exciting new model proposed by Gifford (1998b), the *mature organism model* (Fig. 1.2), provides a conceptual framework that we consider will assist therapists to take up this broader perspective. It depicts the interactions of the fundamental pathways (input, processing and output) into and out of the central nervous system (CNS) that are necessary for survival and for the maintenance of health, as well as for the development and continuation of poor health (e.g. pain and disability).

Input mechanisms (i.e. all sensory pathways) sample tissue health and communicate this together with contextual information about the environment, including the immediate environment surrounding an injury and the ongoing environment that makes up a person's pain or illness experience. The brain can then be said to scrutinize (both consciously and unconsciously) incoming information, along with existing engrams of past experiences, for processing to the *output mechanisms* (i.e. somatic motor, autonomic, neuroendocrine, neuroimmune and descending feedback/control systems). Importantly, how the person's health is then manifest via these output mechanisms (behaviourly, cognitively, emotionally and physiologically) depends, in part, on the contextual factors within the person's immediate circumstances, as well as past experiences that have contributed to the person's beliefs, attitudes,

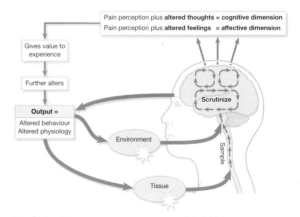

Fig. 1.2 The mature organism model. (With permission from Gifford, L.S. (1998b). Pain, the tissues and the nervous system: a conceptual model. Physiotherapy, 84, 27–36.)

emotions and behaviours. In other words, even given the same extent of tissue injury or illness, no two people will have exactly the same presentation because how they manifest their pain or illness is shaped in part by who they are. Hence, it is inadequate to focus simply on physical diagnosis. Managing patients' problems also requires understanding their unique pain or illness experiences (their understanding, beliefs, feelings, and coping strategies). While all input, processing and output mechanisms will be in operation in any state of ill-health, they will not all necessarily be impaired (i.e. contributing to the problem and/or counterproductive to recovery). Hence, manual therapists must have the necessary knowledge organization and reasoning skills to distinguish between adaptive/ helpful and maladaptive/unhelpful mechanisms and responses. Even those problems that are seen as primarily nociceptive or residing in the tissues can be occurring alongside maladaptive psychological or behavioural 'responses', which provide powerful barriers to active rehabilitation and the restoration of physical confidence. For example, a patient may have a lack of insight into the factors influencing their problem, which can create obstacles to their improvement until addressed through narrative reasoning and communicative management.

At a more physical level, prolonged stress not only can lead to increased levels of tissue sensitivity (i.e. secondary hyperalgesia) but can also predispose to diminished tissue health via associated impairment within the neuroendocrine system (Butler, 2000; Gifford, 1998c; Main et al., 2000; Martin, 1997; Sapolsky, 1998). Here assessment of stress as a contributing factor (along with the associated cognitive, behavioural and emotional effects) is clearly essential to understanding and managing the problem. Based upon this knowledge and reasoning, the clinician is then able to make sound decisions (for and with the client) that relate to assessment of the complete problem, including associated cognitive, behavioural and emotional effects, and appropriate management strategies. Understanding and managing patients' problems requires a broad perspective of the multiple determinants of health and recovery, together with effective reasoning skills to apply that knowledge. The mature organism model was developed to encourage and allow therapists (and patients) to be able to consider openly and without prejudice the multiple factors and multiple levels involved in all pain presentations. It provides a broad conceptual framework from which

any of its elements (e.g. tissue mechanisms, pain mechanisms, effector mechanisms and psychosocial factors) and their respective clinical features or inter-relationships can be explored further (Jones et al., 2002).

Hypothesis categories

From the mature organism model, clinical patterns can be identified within the three categories of pain mechanisms (input, processing and output). Understanding patients' problems requires understanding their unique presentations, including any activity/ participation restrictions, their individual perspectives on their experiences and the physical impairments they may have. This information can then be interpreted with respect to which pain mechanisms are dominant, what structures or tissues sources may be associated with specific physical impairments found, possible contributing factors, precautions, management and prognosis. This can be considered as representing 'categories of hypotheses' (see Table 1.1) that must be appreciated to understand fully patients and their problems and to identify appropriate management strategies. The concept of hypothesis categories was first introduced by Jones (1987), but since then the specific categories considered important to manual therapy practice and the terminology used to describe them has continued to evolve (Butler, 2000; Christensen et al., 2002; Gifford, 1997; Gifford and Butler, 1997; Jones, 1992, 1995; Jones et al., 2000, 2002; World Health Organization, 2001).

These hypotheses should be formulated within broader conceptual models of health and disability, such as the mature organism model (Gifford, 1998a) discussed here. Hypothesis categories can assist therapists to relate the various elements of Gifford's model to the particular types of clinical decision required in contemporary manual therapy.

Activity and participation capability/restriction

Activity restriction refers to difficulties an individual may have in executing activities, where participation restriction refers to problems an individual may have with involvement in life situations. These terms replace the previous terms disability and handicap, respectively, and are also synonymous with the 'dysfunction' hypothesis category, which has been previously used

Table 1.1 Hypothesis categories: categories of judgments that assist in understanding the patient as a person and their problem(s)

- *Activity capability/restriction* (abilities and difficulties an individual may have in executing activities) and *Participation capability/restriction* (abilities and problems an individual may have in involvement in life situations)
- *Patients' perspectives on their experience*
- *Pathobiological mechanisms* (tissue healing mechanisms and pain mechanisms)
- *Physical impairments and associated structure/tissue sources*
- *Contributing factors* to the development and maintenance of the problem
- *Precautions and contraindications* to physical examination and treatment
- *Management and treatment*
- *Prognosis*

(e.g. Gifford and Butler, 1997). The case contributors in Section 2 use all of these terms somewhat interchangeably. Examples of activity restrictions include functional difficulties, such as ascending/descending stairs, walking, lifting, prolonged sitting, etc. Participation restrictions relate to the life involvement consequences of activity restrictions such as restrictions in participation in work or family duties or limitations in sport or leisure participation.

However, the patient's presentation cannot fully be understood by only identifying activity and participation restrictions. Rather, it is equally important for therapists to recognize what their patients can do, that is their activity and participation capabilities. Where restrictions will often correlate with patients' goals, capabilities usually provide the point from where retraining or reactivation must commence. To attend only to restrictions can be discouraging and cognitively behaviourally less effective in changing function and performance. While procedural and communicative management may specifically target identified physical impairments and unhelpful perspectives, respectively, facilitating functional lifestyle improvement requires retraining or recommencement of meaningful activities (physical and social). If patients are only directed to those activities they can no longer perform, the result is often continued unsuccessful performance and failure. Therefore, management of specific physical impairments, such as inadequate motor control, is commenced from postures or activities that

the patient can succeed with. Similarly, general physical and social reactivation commences from what the patient can do and from there aims to increase their activity and participation levels progressively.

Psychosocial factors: patients' perspectives on their experience

Patients' perspectives on their experience are synonymous with other terms used in the literature including their psychosocial status, their cognitive and affective status, their psychological or mental status and, as discussed earlier in this chapter, their pain or illness experience. In reality, when a patient's activity and participation restrictions are identified, consideration should be given to any physical, psychosocial or environmental factors that may be causing or contributing to those restrictions. Hence patients' perspectives is actually a subcategory of 'contributing factors' discussed below. However, patients' perspectives on their experience has been listed as a separate hypothesis category simply to signpost the importance of this area of understanding, which historically was not formally considered by manual therapists.

It is now well recognized that patients' perspectives can be obstacles to their recovery, either as antecedents to their pain states and activity/participation restrictions or as consequences (e.g. Butler, 2000; Gifford, 2000; Main and Booker, 2000; Main and Burton, 2000; Main and Parker, 2000; Main et al., 2000; Unruh and Henriksson, 2002). When attempting to understand the factors that may be causing or contributing to activity/participation restrictions, patients' perspectives (understandings, beliefs, feelings) must be considered and screened for. If a particular perspective has been hypothesized to be potentially relevant as an antecedent to a patient's pain state, the therapist must then, with the patient, endeavour to understand those factors in the patient's life that are responsible for, or have contributed to, the identified perspective. These may include such things as past and present negative personal experiences (e.g. abusive relationships, conflicting or disempowering medical management) that have contributed to shaping the patient's present beliefs, attributions and self-efficacy.

Pathobiological mechanisms

Patients' activity and participation capabilities/restrictions, associated perspectives/psychosocial problems and specific physical impairments are an expression of their pathobiology and life circumstances. This hypothesis category comprises data about tissue and pain mechanisms. It was designed to facilitate reasoning that would include consideration of the mechanisms by which the patient's symptoms and signs are being initiated and/or maintained by the nervous system.

Tissue mechanisms

Tissue mechanisms relate to issues of tissue health and stages of tissue healing. In particular, how well the patient's presentation 'fits' with what would be expected during the corresponding stage of the normal tissue healing process (Gogia, 1992; Hardy, 1989; Vicenzino et al., 2002) is integral in developing a hypothesis of the pain mechanisms at work. For example, an inflammatory presentation in a disorder that has been present for months or years should elicit consideration of other factors (e.g. behavioural, biomechanical, maladaptive central processing) that may be maintaining an inflammatory process or mimicking one through central sensitization.

Pain mechanisms

Pain mechanisms refer to the different input, processing and output mechanisms underlying the patients' activity/participation restrictions, unhelpful perspectives and physical impairments.

Input mechanisms include the sensory and circulatory systems that inform the body about the environment, both internally and externally. Examples of two input pain mechanisms are *nociceptive pain* and *peripheral neurogenic pain* (Butler, 2000; Galea, 2002; Gifford, 1998d; Wright, 2002a). The basic mechanism operating when a high-intensity stimulus, such as a pinprick, activates high-threshold primary afferent nociceptors resulting in pain is well recognized. The same mechanism is in operation with acute injuries, where injury to target tissues, such as ligament, muscle or connective tissue surrounding nerves, will result in nociceptive pain. Peripherally neurogenic pain refers to symptoms that originate from neural tissue outside the dorsal horn or cervicotrigeminal nucleus, such as may occur with spinal nerve root compression or peripheral nerve entrapment. Both nociceptive pain and peripherally evoked neurogenic symptoms have a familiar pattern of presentation, with a predictable stimulus–response relationship, enabling consistent aggravating and easing factors to be quickly identified by patient and therapist.

Processing of input occurs in the CNS, and therapists should be aware of the clinical features indicative of abnormal CNS processing. For example, abnormal processing can occur in patients displaying centrally evoked symptoms (Butler, 2000; Gifford, 1998e; Wright, 2002b), where the pathology lies within the CNS. Here the symptoms provoked from a past target tissue injury can be maintained even after the original injury has healed and the symptoms may no longer behave with stimulus–response predictability. Another example of the clinical relevance of the processing mechanisms is evident when we consider that pain and disability have more than just physical and sensory dimensions (Merskey and Bogduk, 1994). Pain and activity/participation restrictions in all their forms also have affective (e.g. emotional impact such as fear, anxiety and anger) and cognitive (e.g. understanding, beliefs and attributions about the pain or disability) dimensions. Patients' feelings and thoughts about their pain and activity/participation restrictions can significantly contribute to the maintenance of their problems and influence the speed of the recovery (Butler, 2000; Gifford, 1998c; Main and Booker, 2000). While all pain can be exacerbated chemically by emotional and/or general physical stress, in a central pain state both physical and psychosocial stress are thought to be significant contributing factors in maintaining the pain. Hence, a patient's perspectives, including their cognition (e.g. understanding of the problem and intervention required) and affect (e.g. feelings about the problem, management and effects on their life), are important dimensions of all pain states but are particularly significant in central pain.

Ouput mechanisms operate through the motor, autonomic, neuroendocrine and immune systems (Butler, 2000; Gifford, 1998c). The somatic motor mechanism involves altered motor activity (increased or decreased) and movement patterns in response to pathology, but also learning. While painful pathology can inhibit muscle function and lead to altered movement patterns (Hides and Richardson, 2002), many postural and movement abnormalities are associated with problems of motor learning as well as motor control (Shumway-Cook and Woollacott, 2001). These faulty movement patterns may be acquired through habitual postures and activities of life or may develop as a consequence of maintained pain.

The autonomic mechanism is a controversial output system in that features of abnormal sympathetic activity are common in some chronic pain states, although the underlying pathology is still unclear. While the sympathetic nervous system is normally active in all pain states, it can be pathologically active in some. This pathological activity can contribute to disability, impairment and maintained pain (Butler, 2000; Gifford, 1998c; Wright, 2002b).

Other consequences of a stressed system

The neuroendocrine system is responsible for the regulation of metabolism, water and salt balance, blood pressure, response to stress and sexual reproduction. Of these functions, its response to stress is particularly relevant given that many patients have elements of stress that are a predisposing factor to, or the result of, their problems. Like the sympathetic nervous system, the neuroendocrine system is responsive to our thoughts and feelings. Stress, for example, triggers a chain of events from the hypothalamus to the adrenal cortex that enables the appropriate channelling of energy for an individual to escape a perceived threat. However, maintained stress, as is common in so many chronic pain states, can result in maladaptive neuroendocrine activity that is detrimental to tissue health and impedes tissue recovery (Butler, 2000; Gifford, 1998c; Martin, 1997; Sapolsky, 1998).

The neuroimmune system is an output system with close links to the brain, the sympathetic nervous system and the endocrine system. Chronic pain, deconditioning or overconditioning and psychological impairment can interfere with normal immune and healing processes via this system (Butler, 2000; Gifford, 1998c; Mackinnon, 1999; Martin, 1997).

The pathobiological mechanisms hypothesis category is invaluable in focussing thinking to the development of hypotheses about where within the nervous system symptoms are being produced and maintained, and what other systems might be affected. If a patient presents with a 'normal' adaptive pain mechanism, wherein symptoms are the result of pathology of the implicated local tissues, it is appropriate to determine the precise physical impairment/diagnosis and identify a specific site to direct manual treatment. However, when pain symptoms are the result of 'abnormal' maladaptive pain states, resulting from, and maintained by, altered CNS processing, manual therapists must steer away from the sole use of a tissue-based paradigm and instead employ more holistic, less tissue-specific management strategies. While physical impairments may still require attention, these patient presentations critically require promotion of cognitive–behavioural, health/fitness and motor control change through adult/transformative learning. These issues are presented only briefly here; while there are numerous basic pain science papers that support these concepts, readers are referred to the excellent texts by Butler (2000), Gifford (1998f, 2000), Main and Spanswick (2000b) and Strong et al. (2002) for a more thorough review of pain mechanisms and associated strategies of management.

Physical impairments and associated structures/tissue sources

A manual therapy diagnosis should be one that captures the therapist's understanding of the patient and the patient's problem(s). This would include the therapist's judgment regarding each of the hypothesis categories discussed here. In our view, it is not satisfactory simply to identify structures involved, as this alone does not provide sufficient information to understand the problem and its effect on the patient, nor is it sufficient to justify the course of management chosen. The manual therapy diagnosis must include a hierarchy of considerations from the activity/participation restrictions, and any associated unhelpful perspectives or psychosocial problems, to specific physical impairments identified and their associated structure/tissue sources.

Specific physical impairments in a musculoskeletal context are regional neuromusculoskeletal abnormalities detected through the physical examination, such as limited hip active movement, poor transversus abdominis motor control, or excessive glenohumeral joint mobility. The associated structure/tissue sources of physical impairments refers to the actual structure or target tissue from which the symptoms or signs are hypothesized to be emanating, with particular attention (where possible) to the pathology present within that structure. Joints, muscles, ligaments and even nerves are examples of target tissues that can be injured and give rise to pain and physical impairment. Clues to specific physical impairment sources are available from the area, description, behaviour and history of the symptoms. These hypotheses are then tested further in the physical examination, where specific tests of structure and tissue impairment are used.

Interpretations regarding specific sources of the symptoms/impairments must be made with reference to the dominant pain mechanism(s) hypothesized. When nociceptive and peripheral neurogenic mechanisms are dominant, local tissue impairment provides a more accurate reflection of the specific tissues involved. However, care is needed when processing mechanisms are dominant (i.e. maladaptive) as the associated secondary hyperalgesia (CNS-maintained tissue sensitivity) can lead to false-positive clinical findings (e.g. tender tissues, painful movements, etc.), which can then lead to incorrect conclusions regarding the source of the symptoms (Zusman, 1997, 1998). If, in a central pain state, these false positives are interpreted as implicating peripheral target tissues as a local source of symptoms, intervention strategies may then be inappropriately applied to these target tissues, resulting in poor outcomes and possibly even contributing to the maintenance of the problem (Butler, 2000; Watson, 2000).

Attempting to hypothesize about specific structures such as contractile tissues, specific joints or neurogenic pain is important, and sometimes even critical in order to ensure safety (e.g. vertebrobasilar insufficiency, spinal cord pathology or joint instability). However, in reality, it is often not possible to confirm clinically which specific tissues are at fault. Even with the assistance of advanced diagnostic or imaging procedures where pathology can be demonstrated, confirmation of those tissues as being the true source of the symptoms is often impossible. Many degenerative changes evident on the various imaging procedures are asymptomatic and, therefore, may be minimally relevant or even completely unrelated to the patient problem at hand. It is not unusual for even the most skilful and experienced manual therapist to achieve only a relative localization of the source of the symptoms (e.g. lower cervical spine versus local shoulder tissues), even with a detailed evaluation and meticulous reassessment of chosen interventions. Therefore, a balance is required in the specificity of hypotheses generated regarding the source of the symptoms. The therapist must recognize the limitations of such clinical diagnoses and take care to avoid limiting management only to procedures directed to specific tissues. For example, while mobilization or exercise to improve an impairment in active lumbar extension can be substantiated through reassessment of the extension impairment, when the same treatment is only justified

by its potential effect on a specific structure, such as the intervertebral disc, the therapist can easily be misled in attributing the improvement in extension to a change in the disc sensitivity, structure or mechanics. This is, of course, an error of reasoning in that such changes are only inferred.

Of more concern is that solely tissue-based reasoning tends to promote inflexibility of management strategies. Our preference, like others (e.g. Maitland et al., 2001; Sarhmann, 2002), is for therapists to identify potentially relevant impairments and then hypothesize about potential sources of those impairments. Management is then directed to the impairment, although this may include treatment to specific tissues. This relates directly to the value of the disablement model (Guide to Physical Therapy Practice, 2001) and biopsychosocial model (Main and Spanswick, 2000a; Wadell, 1998) of clinical practice, whereby physical treatment is guided by activity/participation restrictions and identified impairments and not solely by diagnostic labels (Maitland et al., 2001). The application of thorough assessment and balanced reasoning, in which identified impairments are considered in conjunction with known and hypothesized pathology, will enable therapists to deliver effective treatments while continuing to improve understanding and to expand and, eventually, validate their clinical impressions.

Contributing factors

Contributing factors are any predisposing or associated factors involved in the development or maintenance of the patient's problem. These factors may be environmental, psychosocial, behavioural, physical/biomechanical and even hereditary. For example, an inflamed subacromial bursa may be the nociceptive source of the patient's symptoms and impaired movements, but commonly either a tight posterior glenohumeral capsule or 'weak' scapular rotator force couples contribute to altered kinematics that predispose the patient to bursal irritation. Similarly, the source of the symptoms may be the CNS and the contributing factors might be the patient's unhelpful perspectives (e.g. understanding, beliefs and feelings), secondary to a combination of conflicting health-professional advice and ineffective coping strategies for a stressful work and family environment. The obvious importance of considering contributing factors relates to management options. Clearly for many nociceptive dominant problems, treatment directed to the actual impairment or source is helpful (e.g. mobilization for a stiff, painful movement or controlled loading of a tendinopathy). In other cases, such as symptomatic hypermobile/unstable spinal or peripheral joints, while some treatment in the form of pain-relieving measures directed to the source of the symptoms may be indicated, the focus of treatment needs to address the contributing factors (e.g. retraining motor control or mobilization of adjacent areas of hypomobility to reduce the load on the symptomatic tissues). Ultimately, it is only through systematic reassessment of the management provided that the optimal balance of treatment directed to sources and contributing factors is determined.

When maladaptive CNS processing is recognized as the dominant pain mechanism, management must be directed to the various patient perspectives, behaviours or physical impairments hypothesized to be contributing to the maintenance of their activity/participation restriction. However it is often difficult to be certain whether an apparent central sensitization is being driven by external contributing factors or whether significant pain and physical impairment may, in fact, be contributing to the patient's stress and psychosocial problems. Again, reassessment is the manual therapist's guide to making this decision. With a true nociceptive problem, the signs and symptoms will improve, and continue to improve, in a predictable manner with time and/or skilled treatment. In contrast, when the patient's symptoms do not improve or maintain improvement from a trial of treatment directed toward a particular impairment or hypothesized nociceptive source, management must be redirected to the different contributing factors hypothesized to be maintaining the central sensitization (Kendall and Watson, 2000).

Precautions and contraindications to physical examination and treatment

Hypotheses regarding precautions and contraindications to physical examination and treatment serve to determine the extent of physical examination that may safely be undertaken and whether physical treatment is contraindicated or limited in any way by safety considerations. Such decisions are determined by consideration of many variables including:

- the dominant pain mechanism
- the patient's perspectives and expectations
- the severity of the disorder

- the irritability of the disorder
- whether the disorder is progressive (and its rate of progression)
- the presence of specific pathology (e.g. rheumatoid arthritis, osteoporosis)
- the stage of healing
- general health
- the suspicion of more sinister pathology (e.g. unexplained weight loss).

If treatment is indicated, the therapist must decide whether any constraints to physical treatment exist (e.g. pain-provoking versus non-provocative treatment techniques and the amount of force that can safely be used). A key examination strategy for identifying potential risk factors is the use of screening questions directed to red flags, or clinical signs and symptoms suggestive of possible serious pathology. *Red flags* exist with respect to serious spinal pathology (Roberts, 2000), vertebrobasilar insufficiency (Barker et al., 2000; Di Fabio, 1999; Rivett, 1997), certain paediatric disorders (e.g. slipped capital femoral epiphysis), and the presence of non-musculoskeletal disorders masquerading as musculoskeletal dysfunction (Boissenault, 1995; Goodman and Snyder, 2000).

Management

Management relates to hypotheses regarding interventions for improving the overall health of the patient, as well as consideration of specific manual therapy measures and techniques. As with all hypothesis categories, management decisions should not be based on any single facet of the patient's presentation. Rather, information gleaned through the history and physical examination, in addition to the patient's response to trial treatments, will collectively determine the pathobiological mechanisms, relevant impairments (and sometimes sources), contributing factors and the need for caution. Management decisions are then guided via the weighting of evidence from each of these other hypothesis categories, with ongoing management informed through the reassessment process.

Prognosis

Estimating patient responses and outcomes is *predictive reasoning* (Edwards, 2001; Jones et al., 2000). Manual therapists must be able to outline possible future scenarios based on consideration of the patient's presentation, responses to management interventions and available evidence (clinically and research based). The likelihood of these scenarios eventuating depends on the nature of the patient's disorder and the patient's ability and willingness to make the necessary changes to those factors contributing to the problem (e.g. physical, lifestyle, personal perspectives/psychosocial). Prognosis should be considered with regard to the patient's broader prospects for recovery and return to function and/or the patient's potential for learning (e.g. changing beliefs and behaviours), which for some may include learning to live and cope with the problem. Like all clinical decision making, prognosis is an inexact science, with both positive and negative prognostic features typically being present in most patient's presentations. Factors that will assist in judging a patient's prognosis include:

- the patient's perspectives and expectations
- the patient's social, occupational and economic status
- the mechanisms of symptoms involved
- the balance of mechanical versus inflammatory components
- the irritability of the disorder
- the degree of damage/impairment
- the length of history and progression of the disorder
- the patient's general health and presence of pre-existing disorders.

Psychosocial risk factors, or yellow flags (e.g. patients' beliefs/coping strategies, distress/illness behaviour, and willingness to change), should be screened for with all patients (Kendall et al., 1997; Main and Burton, 2000; Watson and Kendall, 2000). More recently, Main and colleagues (Main and Burton, 2000; Main et al., 2000) have further delineated the occupational component of the yellow flags into blue and black flags.

Blue flags are derived out of the stress literature. They represent perceived features of work that are generally associated with higher rates of symptoms, ill-health and work loss and which may constitute a major obstacle to the patient's recovery. They are characterized by the following features:

- high demand and low control
- unhelpful management style
- poor social support from colleagues
- perceived time pressure
- lack of job satisfaction.

Interestingly, a person's perception may be more significant than any objective characteristics of the workplace, again highlighting the importance of psychosocial screening in manual therapy assessment.

Black flags include nationally established policy concerning conditions of employment and sickness policy, as well as the specific working conditions of a particular employer:

- national
  - rates of pay
  - negotiated entitlements (benefit system, wage reimbursement)
- employer
  - sickness policy
  - restricted duties policy
  - management style
  - organization size and structure
  - trade union support
- content-specific aspects of work
  - ergonomic (e.g. job heaviness, lifting frequency, postures)
  - temporal characteristics (e.g. number of working hours, shift pattern).

Through the course of the patient examination and ongoing management, screening for red, yellow, blue and black flags, along with the physical examination and response to initial trial treatments, will assist the therapist in formulating a prognosis and determining the appropriate mode of management. Successfully obtaining this breadth and depth of information requires specific enquiries. For example, has the therapist assumed or explicitly explored what the patient wants to do in the future? Further, with consideration of the patient's meaning perspective, is the patient's personal construction of their situation distorting their own view of what the future holds for them and thus distorting their decision making? Therapists must be adept with the various strategies of reasoning (e.g. diagnostic, narrative, collaborative) in order to achieve the necessary level of understanding required to make decisions effectively within each of the different hypothesis categories. The reflective therapist will not only weigh the full spectrum of prognostic variables in judging a patient's prognosis but also critically re-examine the judgment when ongoing reassessment reveals the projected prognosis is not being met.

Often manual therapists' assessment and management decisions require an element of *ethical reasoning*. The scope of ethical decisions facing manual therapists can range from decisions regarding use of potentially aggravating or even life-threatening procedures to decisions of patient autonomy, informed consent, confidentiality, interprofessional relationships, practitioner–client relationship, resource distribution/cost containment and a myriad of day-to-day decisions that underpin quality care. Clinical decisions that are based solely on the therapist's judgment of what is best for the patient are not consistent with ethical decision making. Rather, decisions made for the client must be made with the client. We take the view that, as in other areas of decision making, competent manual therapists should be guided by a combination of community and professional standards (e.g. professional association ethical guidelines) applied in a context-sensitive manner as learned through previous experiences. We are, therefore, in accord with Benner (1991, p. 18) who states, 'Ethics in health care must start with a practice-based understanding of what it is to be a person, what constitutes the relationships among the health care worker, patient, family, and community, and what constitutes care and responsibility toward one another'.

Summary

Manual therapists must work with a multitude of patient and problem presentations, many of which defy simple technical solutions. Contemporary manual therapy requires that therapists not only have a rich organization of clinically relevant biomedical and psychosocial (i.e. biopsychosocial) knowledge but also have skills in diagnostic, narrative, collaborative, prognostic and ethical reasoning. Successful application of that knowledge then requires advanced procedural (e.g. manual techniques and motor control retraining) and communicative (listening, clarifying, explaining, negotiating and counselling) skills. Underpinning all dimensions of clinical reasoning is the ability of therapists to recognize relevant cues (behavioural, psychological, physical, social, cultural, environmental, etc.) and their relationship to other cues, and to test or verify these clinical patterns through further examination and management. In this sense, clinical reasoning in manual therapy is hypothesis oriented.

For all the various strategies manual therapists utilize in their patient management, perhaps the most pervasive are our skills in teaching. Reasoning related to teaching is enhanced when therapists understand concepts and strategies of learning theory, particularly transformative learning, which aims to change individuals' meaning perspectives. How well practitioners learn from the results of their decisions depends on the thoroughness of their deliberations and the time and attention given to their conscious reflection. There are no short cuts to becoming an expert manual therapist. However, it is our view that critical, reflective and collaborative reasoning will improve the breadth and depth of clinical patterns (regarding the person and the problem, including management strategies) that can be recognized and applied. It has been estimated that master chess players have some 50 000 configurations of chess that they can recognize (Posner, 1988). While the breadth of clinical patterns that experts such as those represented in this book possess has not been calculated, it is reasonable to assume their organization of clinically relevant knowledge would be equally staggering. It is our opinion that expertise is not acquired by experience alone. Rather, expertise is developed, in part, through skilled reflective reasoning.

References

Alexander, P.A. and Judy, J.E. (1988). The interaction of domain-specific and strategic knowledge in academic performance. Review of Educational Research, 58, 375–404.

Allwood, C.M. and Montgomery, H. (1982). Detection of errors in statistical problem solving. Scandinavian Journal of Psychology, 23, 131–140.

Anderson, J.R. (1990). Cognitive Psychology and its Implications, 3rd edn. New York: Freeman.

Arocha, J.F., Patel, V.L. and Patel, Y.C. (1993). Hypothesis generation and the coordination of theory and evidence in novice diagnostic reasoning. Medical Decision Making, 13, 198–211.

Barker, S., Kesson, M., Ashmore, J. et al. (2000). Guidance for pre-manipulative testing of the cervical spine. Manual Therapy, 5, 37–40.

Barrows, H.S. and Feltovich, P.J. (1987). The clinical reasoning process. Medical Education, 21, 86–91.

Benner, P. (1991). The role of experience, narrative, and community in skilled ethical comportment. Advances in Nursing Science, 14, 1–21.

Biggs, J.B. (1986). Enhancing learning skills: the role of metacognition. In Student Learning: Research Into Practice—The Marysville Symposium (J.A. Bowden, ed.) pp. 131–148. Melbourne: University of Melbourne: Centre for the Study of Higher Education.

Bloom, B.S. and Broder, L.J. (1950). Problem Solving Processes of College Students, Chicago, IL: University of Chicago Press.

Boissenault, W.G. (1995). Examination in Physical Therapy Practice, Screening for Medical Disease, 2nd edn. New York: Churchill Livingstone.

Bordage, G. and Lemieux, M. (1986). Some cognitive characteristics of medical students with and without diagnostic reasoning difficulties. In Proceedings of the 25th Annual Conference on Research in Medical Education, pp. 185–190. New Orleans.

Bordage, G. and Lemieux, M. (1991). Semantic structures and diagnostic thinking of experts and novices. Academic Medicine, Supplement 66, S70–S72.

Bordage, G. and Zacks, R. (1984). The structure of medical knowledge in the memories of medical students and general practitioners: categories and prototypes. Medical Education, 18, 406–416.

Borkan, J.M., Quirk, M. and Sullivan, M. (1991). Finding meaning after the fall: injury narratives from elderly hip fracture patients. Social Science and Medicine, 33, 947–957.

Boshuizen, H.P.A. and Schmidt, H.G. (1992). On the role of biomedical knowledge in clinical reasoning by experts, intermediates and novices. Cognitive Science, 16, 153–184.

Boshuizen, H.P.A. and Schmidt, H.G. (2000). The development of clinical reasoning expertise. In Clinical Reasoning in the Health Professions, 2nd edn (J. Higgs and M. Jones, eds.) pp. 15–22. Oxford: Butterworth-Heinemann.

Brookfield, S. (1987). Developing Critical Thinkers. San Francisco, CA: Jossey-Bass.

Brookfield, S. (2000). Clinical reasoning and generic thinking skills. In Clinical Reasoning in the Health Professions, 2nd edn (J. Higgs and M. Jones, eds.) pp. 62–77. Oxford: Butterworth-Heinemann.

Bucklew, S.P., Parker, J.C., Keefe, F.J. et al. (1994). Self efficacy and pain behavior among subjects with fibromyalgia. Pain, 59, 377–384.

Burkhardt, C.S., Mannerkorpi, K., Hedenberg, L. and Bjelle, A. (1994). A randomised, controlled trial of education and physical training for women with fibromyalgia. Journal of Rheumatology, 21, 714–720.

Butler, D.S. (2000). The Sensitive Nervous System, pp. 130–151. Adelaide, Australia: Noigroup Press.

Cervero, R.M. (1988). Effective Continuing Education for Professionals. San Francisco, CA: Jossey-Bass.

Chi, M.T.H., Feltovich, P.J. and Glaser, R. (1981). Categorization and representation of physics problems by experts and novices. Cognitive Science, 5, 121–152.

Christensen, N., Jones, M.A. and Carr, J. (2002). Clinical reasoning in orthopedic manual therapy. In Physical Therapy of the Cervical and Thoracic Spine, 3rd edn (R. Grant, ed.) pp. 85–104. New York: Churchill Livingstone.

DeGroot, A.D. (1965). Thought and Choice in Chess. New York: Basic Books.

Di Fabio, R.P. (1999). Manipulation of the cervical spine: risks and benefits. Physical Therapy, 79, 50–65.

Doody, C. and McAteer, M. (2002). Clinical reasoning of expert and novice physiotherapists in an outpatient orthopaedic setting. Physiotherapy, 88, 258–268.

Edwards, I.C. (2001). Clinical Reasoning in Three Different Fields of Physiotherapy: A Qualitative Case Study Approach. Unpublished thesis submitted in partial fulfillment of the PhD in Health Sciences. University of South Australia, Adelaide, Australia.

Edwards, I.C. and Jones, M.A. (1996). Collaborative Reasoning. Unpublished paper submitted in partial fulfilment of the Graduate Diploma in Orthopaedics. University of South Australia, Adelaide, Australia.

Ennis, R.H. (1987). A taxonomy of critical thinking dispositions and abilities. In Teaching Thinking Skills: Theory and Practice (J.B. Baron and R. J. Sternberg, eds.) pp. 9–26. New York: Freeman.

Ericsson, A. and Smith, J. (eds.) (1991). Toward a General Theory of Expertise: Prospects and Limits. New York: Cambridge University Press.

Feltovich, P.J. and Barrows, H.S. (1984). Issues of generality in medical problem solving. In Tutorials in Problem-based Learning: A New Direction in Teaching the Health Professions (H.G. Schmidt and M.L. de Volder, eds.) pp. 128–141. Assen: Van Gorcum.

Feuerstein, M. and Beattie, P. (1995). Biobehavioral factors affecting pain and disability in low back pain: mechanisms and assessment. Physical Therapy, 75, 267–280.

Fleming, M.H. and Mattingly, C. (2000). Action and narrative: two dynamics of clinical reasoning. In Clinical Reasoning in the Health Professions, 2nd edn (J. Higgs and M. Jones, eds.) pp. 54–61. Oxford: Butterworth-Heinemann.

Fonteyn, M.E. and Ritter, B.J. (2000). Clinical reasoning in nursing. In Clinical Reasoning in the Health Professions, 2nd edn (J. Higgs and M. Jones, eds.) pp. 107–116. Oxford: Butterworth-Heinemann.

Galea, M.P. (2002). Neuroanatomy of the nociceptive system. In Pain, A Textbook for Therapists (J. Strong, A.M. Unruh, A. Wright and G.D. Baxter, eds.) pp. 13–41. Edinburgh: Churchill Livingstone.

Gifford, L.S. (1997). Pain. In Rehabilitation of Movement: Theoretical Bases of Clinical Practice (J. Pitt-Brooke, H. Reid, J. Lockwood and K. Kerr, eds.) pp. 196–232. London: Saunders.

Gifford, L.S. (1998a). The mature organism model. In Topical Issues in Pain 1. Whiplash—Science and Management, Fear-avoidance Beliefs and Behaviour (L.S. Gifford, ed.) pp. 45–56. Falmouth, UK: CNS Press.

Gifford, L.S. (1998b). Pain, the tissues and the nervous system: a conceptual model. Physiotherapy, 84, 27–36.

Gifford, L.S. (1998c). Output mechanisms. In Topical Issues in Pain 1. Whiplash—Science and Management, Fear-avoidance Beliefs and Behaviour (L.S. Gifford, ed.) pp. 81–91. Falmouth, UK: CNS Press.

Gifford, L.S. (1998d). Tissue and input related mechanisms. In Topical Issues in Pain 1. Whiplash—Science and Management, Fear-avoidance Beliefs and Behaviour (L.S. Gifford, ed.) pp. 57–65. Falmouth, UK: CNS Press.

Gifford, L.S. (1998e). The 'central' mechanisms. In Topical Issues in Pain 1. Whiplash—Science and Management, Fear-avoidance Beliefs and Behaviour (L.S. Gifford, ed.) pp. 67–80. Falmouth, UK: CNS Press.

Gifford, L.S. (ed.) (1998f). Topical Issues in Pain 1. Whiplash—Science and Management, Fear-avoidance Beliefs and Behaviour. Falmouth, UK: CNS Press.

Gifford, L.S. (ed.) (2000). Topical Issues in Pain 2. Biopsychosocial Assessment, Relationships and Pain. Falmouth, UK: CNS Press.

Gifford, L.S. (2001). Perspectives on the biopsychosocial model—part 1: some issues that need to be accepted? Touch [Journal of the Organisation of Chartered Physiotherapists in Private Practice], 97, 3–9.

Gifford, L.S. (2002). Perspectives on the biopsychosocial model—part 2: the shopping basket approach. Touch [Journal of the Organisation of Chartered Physiotherapists in Private Practice], 99, 11–22.

Gifford, L.S. and Butler, D.S. (1997). The integration of pain sciences into clinical practice. Journal of Hand Therapy, 10, 86–95.

Glaser, R. (1984). Education and thinking: the role of knowledge. American Psychologist, 39, 93–104.

Gogia, P.P. (1992). The biology of wound healing. Ostomy, 38, 12–22.

Goodman, C.C. and Snyder, T.E.K. (2000). Differential Diagnosis in Physical Therapy, 3rd edn. Philadelphia, PA: Saunders.

Guide to Physical Therapist Practice, 2nd edn (2001). Physical Therapy, 81, 9–744.

Hardy, M. (1989). The biology of scar formation. Physical Therapy, 69, 1014–1024.

Harris, I.B. (1993). New expectations for professional competence. In Educating Professionals: Responding to New Expectations for Competence and Accountability (L. Curry and J. Wergin, eds.) pp. 17–52. San Francisco, CA: Jossey-Bass.

Hayes, B. and Adams, R. (2000). Parallels between clinical reasoning and categorization. In Clinical Reasoning in the Health Professions, 2nd edn (J. Higgs and M. Jones, eds.) pp. 45–53. Oxford: Butterworth-Heinemann.

Hides, J. and Richardson, C. (2002). Exercise and pain. In Pain, A Textbook for Therapists (J. Strong, A.M. Unruh, A. Wright and G.D. Baxter, eds.) pp. 245–266. Edinburgh: Churchill Livingstone.

Higgs, J. and Hunt, A. (1999a). Rethinking the beginning practitioner: 'the interactional professional'. In Educating Beginning Practitioners: Challenges for Health Professional Education (J. Higgs and H. Edwards,

eds.) pp. 10–18. Oxford: Butterworth-Heinemann.

Higgs, J. and Hunt, A. (1999b). Redefining the beginning practitioner. Focus on Health Professional Education: A Multidisciplinary Journal, 1, 34–49.

Higgs, J. and Jones, M. (2000). Clinical reasoning in the health professions. In Clinical Reasoning in the Health Professions, 2nd edn (J. Higgs and M. Jones, eds.) pp. 3–14. Oxford: Butterworth-Heinemann.

Higgs, J. and Titchen, A. (1995). Propositional, professional and personal knowledge in clinical reasoning. In Clinical Reasoning in the Health Professions, 2nd edn (J. Higgs and M. Jones, eds.) pp. 129–146. Oxford: Butterworth-Heinemann.

Higgs, J. and Titchen, A. (2000). Knowledge and reasoning. In Clinical Reasoning in the Health Professions, 2nd edn (J. Higgs and M. Jones, eds.) pp. 23–32. Oxford: Butterworth-Heinemann.

Higgs, J., Burn, A. and Jones, M.A. (2001a). Integrating clinical reasoning and evidence-based practice. AACN Clinical Issues: Advanced Practice in Acute and Critical Care—Evidence-based Practice, 12, 482–490.

Higgs, J., Titchen, A. and Neville, V. (2001b). Professional practice and knowledge. In Practice Knowledge and Expertise in the Health Professions (J. Higgs and A. Titchen, eds.) pp. 3–9. Oxford: Butterworth-Heinemann.

Hill, P. (1998). Fear-avoidance theories. In Topical Issues in Pain 1. Whiplash—Science and Management, Fear-avoidance Beliefs and Behaviour (L.S. Gifford, ed.) pp. 159–166. Falmouth, UK: CNS Press.

Jensen, G.M., Gwyer, J., Hack, L.M. et al. (1999). Expertise in Physical Therapy Practice. Boston, MA: Butterworth-Heinemann.

Jensen, G.M., Gwyer, J., Hack, L.M. and Shepard, K.F. (2000). Expert practice in physical therapy. Physical Therapy, 80, 28–52.

Jones, M.A. (1987). The clinical reasoning process in manipulative therapy. In Proceedings of the Fifth Biennial Conference of the Manipulative Therapists Association of Australia (B.A. Dalziel and J.C. Snowsill, eds.) pp. 62–69. Melbourne: Manipulative Therapists Association of Australia.

Jones, M.A. (1992). Clinical reasoning in manual therapy. Physical Therapy, 72, 875–884.

Jones, M.A. (1995). Clinical reasoning and pain. Manual Therapy, 1, 17–24.

Jones, M. and Higgs, J. (2000). Will evidence-based practice take the reasoning out of practice? In Clinical Reasoning in the Health Professions, 2nd edn (J. Higgs and M. Jones, eds.) pp. 307–315. Oxford: Butterworth-Heinemann.

Jones, M., Jensen, G. and Edwards, I. (2000). Clinical reasoning in physiotherapy. In Clinical Reasoning in the Health Professions, 2nd edn (J. Higgs and M. Jones, eds.) pp. 117–127. Oxford: Butterworth-Heinemann.

Jones, M.A., Edwards, I. and Gifford, L. (2002). Conceptual models for implementing biopsychosocial theory in clinical practice. Manual Therapy, 7, 2–9.

Kendall, N.A.S. and Watson, P. (2000). Identifying psychosocial yellow flags and modifying management. In Topical Issues of Pain 2. Biopsychosocial Assessment. Relationships and Pain (L. Gifford, ed.) pp. 131–139. Falmouth, UK: CNS Press.

Kendall, N.A.S., Linton, S.J. and Main, C.J. (1997). Guide to Assessing Psychosocial Yellow Flags in Acute Low Back Pain: Risk Factors for Long Term Disability and Work Loss. Wellington. New Zealand: Accident Rehabilitation and Compensation Insurance Corporation of New Zealand and the National Health Committee.

Lackner, J.M., Caarosella, A.M. and Feuerstein, M. (1996). Pain expectancies, pain and functional self-efficacy expectancies as determinants of disability in patients with chronic low back disorders. Journal of Consulting Clinical Psychology, 64, 212–220.

Lorig, K.R., Sobel, D.S., Stewart, A.L. et al. (1999). Evidence suggesting that a chronic disease self-management program can improve health status while reducing utilization and costs: a randomised trial. Medical Care, 37, 5–14.

Mackinnon, L.T. (1999). Advances in Exercise Immunology. Champaign, France: Human Kinetics.

Main, C.J. and Booker, C.K. (2000). The nature of psychological factors. In Pain Management: An Interdisciplinary

Approach (C.J. Main and C.C. Spanswick, eds.) pp. 19–42. Edinburgh: Churchill Livingstone.

Main, C.J. and Burton, A.K. (2000). Economic and occupational influences on pain and disability. In Pain Management: An Interdisciplinary Approach (C.J. Main and C.C. Spanswick, eds.) pp. 63–87. Edinburgh: Churchill Livingstone.

Main, C.J. and Parker, H. (2000). Social and cultural influences on pain and disability. In Pain Management: An Interdisciplinary Approach (C.J. Main and C.C. Spanswick, eds.) pp. 43–61. Edinburgh: Churchill Livingstone.

Main, C.J. and Spanswick, C.C. (2000a). Models of pain. In Pain Management: An Interdisciplinary Approach (C.J. Main and C.C. Spanswick, eds.) pp. 3–18. Edinburgh: Churchill Livingstone.

Main, C.J. and Spanswick, C.C. (eds.) (2000). Pain Management: An Interdisciplinary Approach. Edinburgh: Churchill Livingstone.

Main, C.J., Spanswick, C.C. and Watson, P. (2000). The nature of disability. In Pain Management: An Interdisciplinary Approach (C.J. Main and C.C. Spanswick, eds.) pp. 89–106. Edinburgh: Churchill Livingstone.

Maitland, G., Hengeveld, E., Banks, K. and English, K. (2001). Maitland's Vertebral Manipulation, 6th edn. Oxford: Butterworth-Heinemann.

Malt, U.F. and Olafson, O.M. (1995). Psychological appraisal and emotional response to physical injury: a clinical, phenomenological study of 109 adults. Psychiatric Medicine, 10, 117–134.

Martin, P. (1997). The Sickening Mind, Brain, Behaviour, Immunity and Disease. London: Harper Collins.

Merskey, H. and Bogduk, N. (1994). Classification of Chronic Pain. Definitions of Chronic Pain Syndromes and Definition of Pain Terms, 2nd edn. Seattle, WA: International Association for the Study of Pain.

Mezirow, J. (1990). Fostering Critical Reflection in Adulthood: A Guide to Transformative and Emancipatory Learning. San Francisco, CA: Jossey-Bass.

Mezirow, J. (1991). Transformative Dimensions of Adult Learning. San Francisco, CA: Jossey-Bass.

Neistadt, M.E. (1995). Methods of assessing clients' priorities: a survey of adult physical dysfunction settings. American Journal of Occupational Therapy, 45, 428–436.

Newell, A. and Simon, H.A. (1972). Human Problem Solving. Englewood Cliffs, NJ: Prentice-Hall.

Patel, V.L. and Groen, G.J. (1986). Knowledge-based solution strategies in medical reasoning. Cognitive Science, 10, 91–116.

Patel, V.L. and Groen, G.J. (1991). The general and specific nature of medical expertise: a critical look. In Toward a General Theory of Expertise: Prospects and Limits (A. Ericsson and J. Smith, eds.) pp. 93–125. New York: Cambridge University Press.

Patel, V.L. and Kaufmann, D.R. (2000). Clinical reasoning and biomedial knowledge: implications for teaching. In Clinical Reasoning in the Health Professions, 2nd edn (J. Higgs and M. Jones, eds.) pp. 33–44. Oxford: Butterworth-Heinemann.

Posner, M.I. (1988). Introduction: what is it to be an expert? In The Nature of Expertise (M.T.H. Chi, R. Glaser and R.J. Farr, eds.) pp. xxix–xxxvi. Hillsdale, NJ: Lawrence Erlbaum.

Rivett, D.A. (1997). Preventing neurovascular complications of cervical spine manipulation. Physical Therapy Reviews, 2, 29–37.

Rivett, D.A. and Higgs, J. (1997). Hypothesis generation in the clinical reasoning behavior of manual therapists. Journal of Physical Therapy Education, 11, 40–45.

Roberts, L. (2000). Flagging the danger signs of low back pain. In Topical Issues of Pain 2. Biopsychosocial Assessment. Relationships and Pain (L. Gifford, ed.) pp. 69–83. Falmouth, UK: CNS Press.

Rumelhart, D.E. and Ortony, E. (1977). The representation of knowledge in memory. In Schooling and the Acquisition of Knowledge (R.C. Anderson, R.J. Spiro and W.E. Montague, eds.) pp. 99–135. Hillsdale, NJ: Lawrence Erlbaum.

Sahrmann, S.A. (2002). Diagnosis and Treatment of Movement Impairment Syndromes. St Louis, MI: Mosby.

Sapolsky, R.M. (1998). Why Zebras Don't get Ulcers. An Updated Guide to Stress, Stress-Related Diseases, and Coping. New York: Freeman.

Schmidt, H.G. and Boshuizen, H.P.A. (1993). On acquiring expertise in medicine. Educational Psychology Review, 5, 205–221.

Schmidt, H.G., Boshuizen, H.P.A. and Norman, G.R. (1992). Reflections on the nature of expertise in medicine. In Deep Models for Medical Knowledge Engineering (E. Keravnou, ed.) pp. 231–248. Amsterdam: Elsevier Science.

Schmidt, H.G., Norman, G.R. and Boshuizen, H.P.A. (1990). A cognitive perspective on medical expertise: theory and implications. Academic Medicine, 65, 611–621.

Schön, D.A. (1983). The Reflective Practitioner: How Professionals Think in Action. London: Temple Smith.

Schön, D.A. (1987). Educating the Reflective Practitioner. San Francisco, CA: Jossey-Bass.

Shendell-Falik, N. (1990). Creating self-care units in the acute care setting: a case study. Patient Education and Counselling, 15, 39–45.

Shepard, K.F. and Jensen, G.M. (1990). Physical therapist curricula for the 1990s: educating the reflective practitioner. Physical Therapy, 70, 566–577.

Shumway-Cook, A. and Woollacott, M.H. (2001). Motor Control: Theory and Practical Applications, 2nd edn. Baltimore, MD: Lippincott, Williams & Wilkins.

Sluijs, E.M. (1991). Patient education in physiotherapy: towards a planned approach. Physiotherapy, 77, 503–508.

Strong, J. (1995). Self-efficacy and the patient with chronic pain. In Moving in on Pain (M. Shacklock, ed.) pp. 97–102. Chatswood: Butterworth-Heinemann.

Strong, J., Unruh, A.M., Wright, A. and Baxter, G.D. (eds.) (2002). Pain, A Textbook for Therapists. Edinburgh: Churchill Livingstone.

Tulving, E. and Thomson, D.M. (1973). Encoding specificity and retrieval processes in episodic memory. Journal of Psychological Review, 80, 352–373.

Unruh, A.M. and Henriksson, C. (2002). Psychological, environmental and behavioural dimensions of the pain experience. In Pain, A Textbook for Therapists (J. Strong, A.M. Unruh, A. Wright, and G.D. Baxter, eds.) pp. 65–80. Edinburgh: Churchill Livingstone.

Vicenzino, B., Souvlis, T. and Wright, A. (2002). Musculoskeletal pain. In Pain, A Textbook for Therapists (J. Strong, A.M. Unruh, A. Wright, and G.D. Baxter, eds.) pp. 327–349. Edinburgh: Churchill Livingstone.

Wadell, G. (1998). The Back Pain Revolution. Edinburgh: Churchill Livingstone.

Watson, P. (2000). Psychosocial predictors of outcome from low back pain. In Topical Issues of Pain 2. Biopsychosocial Assessment. Relationships and Pain (L. Gifford, ed.) pp. 85–109. Falmouth, UK: CNS Press.

Watson, P. and Kendall, N. (2000). Assessing psychosocial yellow flags. In Topical Issues of Pain 2.

Biopsychosocial Assessment. Relationships and Pain (L. Gifford, ed.) pp. 111–129. Falmouth, UK: CNS Press.

World Health Organization (2001). ICF Checklist Version 2.1a, Clinician Form for International Classification of Functioning, Disability and Health. Geneva: WHO. [Available online at http://www.who.int/classification/icf/checklist/icf-checklist.pdf, April 15, 2002.]

Wright, A. (2002a). Neuropathic pain. In Pain, A Textbook for Therapists (J. Strong, A.M. Unruh, A. Wright, and G.D. Baxter, eds.) pp. 351–377. Edinburgh: Churchill Livingstone.

Wright, A. (2002b). Neurophysiology of pain and pain modulation. In Pain,

A Textbook for Therapists (J. Strong, A.M. Unruh, A. Wright, and G.D. Baxter, eds.) pp. 43–64. Edinburgh: Churchill Livingstone.

Zusman, M. (1997). Instigators of activity intolerance. Manual Therapy, 2, 75–86.

Zusman, M. (1998). Structure-oriented beliefs and disability due to back pain. Australian Journal of Physiotherapy, 44, 13–20.

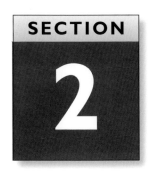

SECTION 2

Clinical reasoning in action: case studies from expert manual therapists

2 Back and bilateral leg pain in a 63-year-old woman

Mark Bookhout

 SUBJECTIVE EXAMINATION

A 63-year-old retired female (Francis) presented to our clinic with a chief complaint of low back pain and bilateral lower extremity pain. She had led an active lifestyle and was happily married, with her husband in good health. She played tennis, travelled and was taking computer classes.

Francis gave a history of low back pain, chronic in nature, resulting from a lifting injury 22 years previously. At the time of her original injury, she was diagnosed by an orthopaedic surgeon as having a herniated lower lumbar disc, but she was unaware of the actual level of herniation. Francis reportedly had been able to self-manage fairly well with intermittent low back pain until her most recent episode, which commenced approximately 4 months before her first consultation with me. At that time, she developed sharp shooting pains into both of her lower extremities without any apparent trauma or predisposing factors that she could recall, other than the fact her symptoms were exacerbated by playing tennis. Francis also noted an increase in her low back pain but reported that her leg pain was more severe and disturbing to her because she had not had any leg symptoms previously. The pain was described as radiating down into the buttocks and the posterior legs as far as the calves and heels, but not into the feet, seemingly following an L5 or S1 dermatomal distribution.

Francis was seen by a physician, who ordered an enhanced computed tomography (CT) scan of the lumbar spine with myelography. The scan revealed central spinal canal stenosis along with multiple level lumbar degenerative disc disease and a grade I spondylolisthesis at L5–S1. Francis then had an epidural steroid injection (4 months ago), which gave her some relief with a notable decrease in pain intensity, but the distribution of the referred pain was unchanged. She reported the pain had been relieved approximately 40–50% by the epidural injection. Subsequently she was placed on an anti-inflammatory medication (nabumetone), which she was still taking when therapy was initiated. Francis reported that the medication helped her quite a lot, decreasing the intensity of her pain by another 20%. She had not received any previous physical therapy treatment for her condition and she was self-referred. A physician had apparently told her that she might be a surgical candidate and her primary goal in seeking physical therapy treatment was to avoid having lumbar spine surgery if at all possible and to be able to continue to play tennis, her main passion in life.

Francis reported that her back pain was aggravated by slow walking, prolonged standing greater than 1 hour, playing tennis and bending slightly forward as in doing her dishes or vacuuming. She reported that her leg pain was specifically accentuated during and after playing tennis, and she could only play 15–20 minutes before noting a significant onset of leg pain. Sleeping was reportedly not a problem and neither was sitting, but lifting heavy loads aggravated her back pain. Coughing and sneezing had no effect on her symptoms. Overall, she rated her level of pain at 4/10 but it could fluctuate from 0/10 on a good day to 5/10 on a bad day.

The medical history was otherwise unremarkable. There was no paraesthesia and no reported subjective numbness. She denied any bowel or bladder problems or any history of trauma. Francis also denied any recent weight gain or loss and her medical history was negative for high blood pressure, tuberculosis, anaemia, cancer, heart problems, depression, thyroid problems, emphysema, hepatitis, asthma, kidney disease or diabetes. She had had one epileptic seizure many years previously and had also been hospitalized for an automobile accident with facial injuries at 17 years of age, but there were no reported residual problems. Francis was particularly distressed about her inability to play tennis without pain and was somewhat fearful of the possibility of lumbar surgery, which she strongly wanted to avoid. There did not appear to be any other significant psychosocial factors.

REASONING DISCUSSION AND CLINICAL REASONING COMMENTARY

1 Please comment on the range of hypotheses you had at this stage regarding possible sources of her symptoms. Which of these did you think was most likely and what was the pattern within the subjective examination that supported this principal hypothesis?

Clinician's answer

I felt that the patient had several possible sources for her symptoms, including central or bilateral lateral foraminal stenosis at L5–S1 (with associated neurogenic claudication), secondary to spondylolisthesis at L5–S1, and/or dynamic instability at L5–S1 secondary to lumbar degenerative disc disease. I also thought that mechanical dysfunction of the lower lumbar facet joints could result in the described pain referral pattern into the lower extremities. I initially believed that the primary source was most likely dynamic lumbar instability at L5–S1 since in her subjective history she reported an accentuation of her symptoms with activity (particularly the leg pain), especially with playing tennis.

2 Did you have any reason at this stage to suspect involvement of 'pathological' central pain mechanisms in her presentation? Please briefly discuss your thoughts on the dominant pain mechanisms you hypothesized were evident from her presentation thus far.

Clinician's answer

After my objective clinical examination in which significant joint restrictions in the lower lumbar facet joints and sacroiliac joint were noted, I felt that her dominant pain mechanism was probably nociceptive arising from faulty and dysfunctional joint mechanics. I did not find evidence to support involvement of any pathological central pain mechanisms or dysfunction within the output systems (i.e. sympathetic, endocrine, immune, motor).

3 Please discuss your reasoning with respect to likely contributing factors to this most recent episode of symptoms.

Clinician's answer

I felt that the most likely contributing factors to this recent episode of symptoms were the patient's age, the likely weakness/ineffectiveness of her core trunk muscular stabilizers and stiffness of the facet joints, all combined with continued activity (i.e. playing tennis on a regular basis) that her spine (structurally and dynamically) was unable to cope with.

4 Were there any features within her subjective examination that signalled the need for caution in your physical examination and treatment?

Clinician's answer

There were no features within the subjective examination that signalled the need for caution or implicated any contraindications to my examination or treatment. Her disorder seemed to present as having a low irritability level with no significant neurological findings and certainly no progressive neurological findings.

Clinical reasoning commentary

The clinician's answers to these questions reflect the breadth of his reasoning through the subjective examination. Importantly, he does not simply accept what the patient spontaneously offers but goes much further by screening for other types of symptom, aggravating factors and general health considerations. Multiple structures are considered as possibly being responsible for the patient's symptoms and these are directly linked to associated structural (e.g. spondylolisthesis) and dynamic (e.g. core trunk muscular stabilizers) contributing factors. Similarly, the clinician's consideration of potential contributing factors is broad in scope, ranging from the patient's age (and associated degenerative state of her spine) to the stability and mobility of her spine. Her lifestyle, in this case her activity level and passion for tennis, are also included, providing a number of options with respect to management and an awareness of the patient's personal goals.

PHYSICAL EXAMINATION

Francis was evaluated from a biomechanical perspective because she was found to be neurologically intact, demonstrating no subjective or objective numbness or sensory deficits and no motor weakness in the lower extremities. Reflexes were not tested. She presented with a mesomorphic body build and was right handed.

Standing

In standing, a hyperlordosis with a palpable step at the L4–L5 segmental level was evident. There was banding of the musculature across the lower lumbar spine and an apparent flattening of the lumbosacral junction. Forward flexion mobility was full range (fingertips touching toes) and without pain provocation, but the standing forward bending test for the sacroiliac joint was positive on the right side. The one-legged stork test, another sacroiliac joint screening test, was also positive on the right side. Both the forward bending test and the one-legged stork test are screening tests for possible involvement of the sacroiliac joint but are non-specific for any particular dysfunction. During the forward bending test, the right posterior superior iliac spine (PSIS) travelled further than the left; with the one-legged stork test on the right side, the right PSIS moved superiorly rather than inferiorly when the patient lifted the right knee up towards the chest. Both of these findings indicated restricted mobility of the right sacroiliac joint (Bourdillion et al., 1992; Greenman, 1996; Isaacs and Bookhout, 2001).

Lumbar side bending range of motion appeared to be within normal limits, both symmetrical and painless, with normal pelvic coupling noted during side bending to either side. The hip drop test, which is a test for side bending of the lower lumbar spine, appeared, however, to be restricted on the right side. The test is performed by having the standing patient bend one knee and allow the pelvis to drop. Thus, if the right knee is bent the pelvis drops on the right side, invoking left side bending at L5–S1. The test can also be used to indicate whether or not the sacral base anteriorly nutates on the side of the hip drop, so the test is not specific for any dysfunction but is again a general screening tool (Isaacs and Bookhout, 2001). Lumbar extension was not pain provocative but was significantly restricted at the lumbosacral junction, with most of the extension movement appearing to occur in the upper lumbar spine.

Sitting

In sitting, the forward bending test appeared to be positive on the right side. With this test, the operator palpates each PSIS with their thumbs and the patient is asked to bend forward. The operator's thumbs follow the PSISs throughout the range of forward bending. In this case, the right PSIS moved superiorly and anteriorly further than the left, indicating restricted joint play motion on the right side. This test is an additional screening test for sacroiliac joint dysfunction but is also non-specific (Bourdillion et al., 1992; Greenman, 1996; Isaacs and Bookhout, 2001). Palpation of the inferior lateral angle (ILA) of the sacrum with the patient in a fully flexed lumbar position revealed asymmetry with the left ILA posterior and inferior. Positional testing of the lumbar spine in full flexion revealed no asymmetry of the transverse processes from approximately L2 to L5, but there was asymmetry at L1, which appeared to be rotated to the right.

Active trunk rotation in sitting appeared to be symmetrical bilaterally with no pain provocation.

Supine

In supine lying, the passive range of motion of the lower extremities revealed a restriction for combined movements of hip flexion, adduction and internal rotation on the right side compared with the left. The patient complained of 'pinching' in the anterior hip and groin on the right side during these combined hip movements. Passive straight leg raising was to 80 degrees bilaterally without pain provocation. Palpation of the pubic symphysis revealed an inferior pube on the right side, with significant tenderness to palpation of the right inguinal ligament. Palpation of the lower abdominal quadrant revealed a marked increase in tone and tenderness of the psoas and iliacus musculature on the right side. Anterior to posterior translation of the innominates revealed a restriction on the right side compared with the left. There was also a loss of anterior to posterior glide of the right hip joint relative to the left joint. Active heel slide in supine lying revealed a significant imbalance in muscle control on the right side versus the left, with Francis unable to maintain a neutral spine on the right side while performing an active right heel slide through full range without the innominate rotating anteriorly. This test is thought to indicate an imbalance between the abdominal and hip flexor musculature, in this case on the right side (Bourdillion et al., 1992; Greenman, 1996; Isaacs and Bookhout, 2001).

Prone

In prone lying, the leg lengths appeared to be symmetrical, as did the ischial tuberosity heights. There was some increase in tension noted on palpation of the right sacrotuberous ligament and there was significant tightness and tenderness noted on palpation of the right long dorsal sacroiliac ligament. The long dorsal sacroiliac ligament is thought to become taut with posterior nutation of the sacral base (Vleeming et al., 1996). Palpation of the ILAs of the sacrum revealed the left ILA to be posterior and inferior. Passive mobility testing of the sacroiliac joints in prone lying indicated a loss of anterior nutational movement of the right sacral base. Positional testing of the lumbar spine in a prone prop position, where the patient supports their head and chin on their hands while propped up on their elbows, revealed that

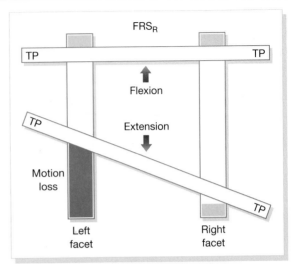

Fig. 2.1 Pictogram illustrating an FRS right, a positional diagnosis for a spinal segment that is held in a flexed, right rotated and right-side bent position. This shows the response of the transverse processes (TP) when there is an inability for the left facet joint to close. Note how the TPs appear asymmetrical (i.e. rotated to the right in extension but not in flexion).

the transverse processes of L5 were asymmetrical, with the right transverse process of L5 being posterior when compared with the left transverse process and the sacral base below. This positional finding is indicative of a loss of the combined movements of extension, left-side bending and left rotation at L5–S1, secondary to the inability to close the left facet joint at L5–S1 (Fig. 2.1). There was also asymmetry of the transverse processes of L4 found with positional testing in prone on elbows. The left transverse process of L4 appeared to be posterior when compared with the right transverse process and L5 below. This positional finding is indicative of an inability to close the right facet joint at L4–L5, with a loss of mobility for the combined movements of extension, right-side bending and right rotation.

Passive accessory intervertebral mobility testing with unilateral posterior to anterior pressures on the right transverse processes from L1 to S1 produced significant local pain at L4 and S1. Positional testing and passive accessory intervertebral mobility testing of the thoracolumbar junction revealed an FRS right (spinal segment that is held in a flexed, right rotated and right-side bent position) at approximately T11–T12, with a loss of the combined movements of extension, left-side bending and left rotation. Active hip extension in prone lying was restricted by over 50%, limited to less than 10 degrees in range bilaterally, with apparent reduction in tone (inhibition) noted on palpation of the gluteus maximus, especially on the right. It was felt that this loss of hip extension was a consequence of tight hip flexors (on the right side greater than the left), in particular the iliopsoas.

REASONING DISCUSSION AND CLINICAL REASONING COMMENTARY

1 Please briefly summarize your reasoning at this point with respect to your hypotheses regarding the principal sources and contributing factors of these symptoms.

Clinician's answer

My initial assessment was that of chronic low back pain and bilateral leg pain initiated by an initial injury 22 years earlier; there was now significant mechanical dysfunction of the lower lumbar facet joints and right sacroiliac joint, along with an L5–S1 grade I spondylolisthesis and lateral spinal stenosis at L5–S1. Francis presented with marked mechanical dysfunction involving the right sacroiliac joint, as well as mechanical dysfunction at L4–L5 and L5–S1, which I felt was responsible for the referred pain following an L5–S1 distribution in her legs. The patient had significant hypertonicity and resultant tightness in the iliopsoas musculature bilaterally, greater on the right side than the left, with limitation of active hip extension mobility, as well as inhibition of gluteus maximus musculature, especially the right. She appeared to have no neurological involvement, although she was not assessed for adverse neural tension signs other than with straight leg raising, which was to 80 degrees and pain-free at the initial visit. There also appeared to be limitations in mobility of the right hip, with loss of the combined movements of hip flexion, adduction and internal rotation, possibly secondary to lumbar and pelvic dysfunction or secondary to a tight posterior right hip capsule.

2 Please elaborate on your analysis of the sacroiliac joint impairment.

Clinician's answer

I felt that sacroiliac joint impairment was evidenced by several key findings during the screening examination. The patient had a positive forward bending test on the right side, both in standing and in sitting, and a positive one-legged stork test on the right side as well.

The patient also had a positive right hip drop test, indicative of impaired coupling at L5–S1 with a loss of left-side bending at L5–S1 and/or a loss of anterior nutational movement of the right sacral base. Palpation of the ILAs, both in forward flexion and in the prone extended position, revealed asymmetry, with the left ILA being posterior and inferior; this is indicative of either a structural anomaly or a sacroiliac dysfunction. Passive mobility testing of the sacroiliac joints revealed a loss of anterior nutation of the right sacral base, confirming a right sacroiliac joint impairment. The patient also had a positive iliac shear test on the right side, demonstrated by a loss of anteroposterior translation of the right innominate. Palpation of the pubic tubercles revealed an inferior pube on the right with tenderness of the right inguinal ligament. Palpation also revealed significant tightness and tenderness of the long dorsal sacroiliac ligament on the right side versus the left. The long dorsal sacroiliac ligament became taut and tender in the presence of a posteriorly nutated sacral base (i.e. loss of anterior nutational movement).

Clinical reasoning commentary

What should be evident throughout the clinician's physical examination and reasoning is the specific nature of his hypothesis testing. That is, hypotheses regarding possible sources and contributing factors formulated during the subjective examination are specifically tested through the physical examination. The physical impairments identified include impairments of spinal, sacroiliac and hip joint mobility, soft tissue/muscle shortening, and increased muscle tone and poor motor control. Nevertheless, the character of the clinician's summary of findings reflects an open mind. Identified impairments are presented as an 'initial assessment', consistent with the subjective presentation. The impairments identified represent treatment options that, through intervention and reassessment, will ultimately establish their relevance.

m Management

I explained my clinical findings to Francis and my recommendations for treatment. She initially understood her treating diagnosis to be mechanical low back pain with an L5–S1 spondylolisthesis and lateral spinal stenosis at L5–S1. I did not feel there were any contraindications to physical therapy intervention and so she was scheduled to see me initially for eight treatment sessions over a 30-day period. Francis and I jointly agreed her goals for treatment would be for her to be able to play tennis without provoking back or leg pain, and to be able to control her symptoms with a home exercise programme and with decreased usage of her pain medication (nabumetone). We also set another functional goal for her, which was to be able to tolerate standing on her feet for prolonged periods of time, up to 1 to 2 hours, without leg pain, such as when window shopping, washing the dishes and hoovering. I anticipated that these functional goals would take approximately 1 month to achieve and that the prognosis for improvement and accomplishment of these goals was good to excellent.

Following the evaluation, treatment was initiated and consisted of muscle energy techniques to treat an FRS right at L5–S1 and an FRS left at L4–L5, so as to restore extension mobility from L4 to S1. For both of these techniques, Francis was treated lying on her side, specifically localizing forces first to L5–S1 and then to L4–L5, with extension from above down and from below up combined with the appropriate side bending and rotation (Fig. 2.2). Francis was asked specifically to work primarily with an active side-bending effort using the leg as a long lever, followed by post-isometric relaxation to increase side bending and extension of the spinal segment. I directly mobilized the sacroiliac joint utilizing a technique to treat a unilateral posteriorly

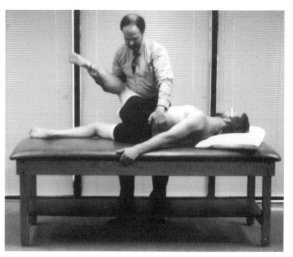

Fig. 2.2 Muscle energy technique for correction of a FRS right (spinal segment that is held in a flexed, right rotated and right-side bent position) at L5–S1.

nutated sacrum on the right to improve anterior nutation of the right sacral base (Bourdillion et al., 1992; Greenman, 1996; Isaacs and Bookhout, 2001). The inferior pube on the right side was also treated with muscle energy techniques, by resisting active hip extension and then upon relaxation correcting the inferior pube by pressing the ischial tuberosity in a superior and medial direction. The reader is referred to Greenman (1996) and Isaacs and Bookhout (2001) for further detail of these techniques. Francis received deep soft tissue mobilization to the iliopsoas musculature, especially on the right side, followed by instruction in kneeling hip flexor stretching and prone transversus abdominis retraining to practise at home. Specifically, I attempted to re-educate and balance the musculature on the right side of the pelvis, based upon her initial inability to perform a supine heel slide on the right side without anteriorly rotating the innominate.

REASONING DISCUSSION AND CLINICAL REASONING COMMENTARY

1 What were the key features in this presentation that you recognized as indicating a good prognosis?

Clinician's answer

I felt Francis had a good prognosis based upon the fact that she had a specific goal in mind for treatment (i.e. returning to playing tennis). She also had good general health habits, appeared to have no psychosocial

factors, and she appeared to have specific mechanical joint restrictions that I felt were directly related to her symptoms and clinical presentation.

2 Mutually agreed formal goal setting is clearly a key feature of your management. Could you briefly highlight your views on the significance of mutual goal setting?

Clinician's answer

I place considerable value on mutual goal setting to establish good communication between myself and the patient. I believe this is an essential component of the first initial visit, to make sure that the patient and I have the same expectations to measure the effectiveness of treatment. If mutual goal setting is not done at the onset of treatment, the patient may have a different goal from that of the therapist, with the patient and therapist measuring the success or failure of treatment from two different perspectives (i.e. the patient's goal is total pain relief while the therapist's goal is increased tolerance for sitting, walking, other activities in daily living). This can create a sense of disappointment over the course of treatment if the patient feels his or her needs are not being met despite 'objective' improvement noted by the treating therapist.

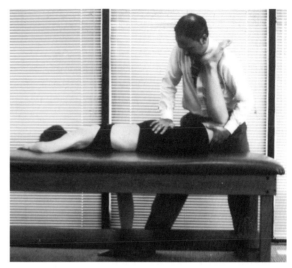

Fig. 2.3   Muscle energy technique for stretching the hip flexors on the left side.

Clinical reasoning commentary

A key dimension of clinical reasoning evident in the clinician's philosophy of management is his collaborative approach with the patient. As discussed in Chapter 1, patients begin their encounter with a manual therapist with their own ideas of and feelings about the nature of their problems and the management they want, as shaped by personal experiences and advice from medical practitioners, family and friends. For some patients, their meaning perspectives (understanding/beliefs, attitudes, emotions and expectations) are distorted and counterproductive to their recovery. Successful patient management is optimized when therapists attend to the patient's perspective and include the patient in the decision making. The clinician's explanation of findings and philosophy of involving the patient in setting treatment goals exemplify this collaborative approach to reasoning.

_m_ | Further management

On a subsequent visit, latissimus dorsi self-stretching was added as Francis appeared to be significantly tight on the right side. The latissimus dorsi was found to be tight by assessing bilateral shoulder flexion in supine lying with the lumbar lordosis eliminated. The latissimus dorsi was stretched using the technique described by Evjenth (Evjenth and Hamberg, 1984) to decrease stress at the lumbosacral junction. After the fifth visit, and approximately 2 weeks into treatment, Francis reported she was able to play tennis without leg pain and had noted a substantial diminution in her need for pain medication, decreasing her dosage by over half. The hips were then treated, utilizing muscle energy techniques to lengthen the iliopsoas, tensor fascia latae and hip external rotator musculature. These muscle groups were stretched in prone lying with the opposite leg off the end of the table and supported on the floor (Fig. 2.3). In addition, the hips were mobilized in a posterior to anterior direction to improve both active and passive hip extension mobility. Piriformis self-stretching in supine lying was added to her home exercise programme, along with gluteus maximus retraining while maintaining a neutral lumbar spine with transversus abdominis activation.

REASONING DISCUSSION AND CLINICAL REASONING COMMENTARY

1 Please discuss briefly your philosophy of reassessment, providing examples of how in this case reassessment was used to determine the effect of any given treatment procedure.

■ Clinician's answer

At each visit, I reassessed the major clinical findings, which included mobility for extension at L4–L5 and L5–S1, as well as mobility of the right sacroiliac joint. I also monitored recruitment of the right gluteus maximus and tranversus abdominis musculature and I reassessed the right hip for combined movements of flexion, adduction and internal rotation. My expectation was to find improvements in joint mobility at L4–L5 and L5–S1, as well as mobility of the right hip and right sacroiliac joint from one treatment session to the next. I attempted to correlate improvements in joint mobility with improvements in functional performance by asking the patient to show active movement (i.e. extend the hip, recheck the forward bending and one-legged stork tests, and recheck the right hip drop test). I feel it is important to show the patient (as well as to remind the patient) of how their original findings have changed, since often a change in movement/mobility, both actively and passively, occurs before the patient's symptoms improve, especially in patients with chronic pain.

2 You have described attempting to re-educate the balance of this patient's lumbopelvic musculature, highlighting examples of training in supine and prone lying. Was it necessary for the patient to progress this retraining to other positions?

■ Clinician's answer

Although not directly discussed in this case, I generally progress patients from non-weight-bearing exercises to weight-bearing exercises and activities, incorporating the patient's exercise programme into functional activities and activities of daily living. I believe this is especially important in retraining muscular control, especially retraining for activities that previously were reported by the patient as pain provoking, in this case rotation in standing (e.g. as in playing tennis).

■ Clinical reasoning commentary

For skilled manual therapists, reassessment is second nature. However, it is important to recognize reassessment as a form of hypothesis testing by which the therapist's understanding of the problem and the person is either supported or not supported, and management continued or altered accordingly. The breadth and specificity of reassessment will vary according to the nature of the problem and the pain mechanism judged to be dominant. In any case, care is needed when hypotheses regarding the 'source' or pathology are tested through reassessment. Clearly an improvement in mobility, muscle control or pain response does not confirm a source or pathology. For that, more sophisticated assessment/reassessment through advanced imaging procedures, electromyography or other medical investigations are needed, many of which themselves have poor predictive validity. We encourage therapists to hypothesize about specific structure/tissue sources and to consider the nature of the pathology, as these deliberations will assist therapists' search for a better understanding of the relationship between pathology, pain and physical impairment. However, to avoid misleading yourself that you have effected a change in the pathology or structure of a specific tissue, it is better to view your treatments, as the clinician has here, as being directed toward a specific impairment (physical or psychological) in order to establish the relevance of the identified impairment to the patient's presentation.

Encouraging patient understanding, which may require modification to their pre-existing perspectives, is an ongoing feature of manual therapy management. Even subtle strategies, as the clinician has alluded to here when pointing out to the patient changes in the impairment, contribute to improved patient understanding. As discussed in Chapter 1, improved understanding fosters greater self-efficacy/responsibility and patient participation in management.

Outcome

Francis received 11 treatments over the course of 2 months. When seen for her last appointment, she reported that she was doing extremely well, was no longer taking any pain medication, and notably had no leg pain complaints even after playing tennis for 1.5 hours. She had intermittent mild low back pain that she reported was not limiting her activities of daily living at all. Francis felt that her exercise programme gave her significant control of her symptoms, and she now rated her low back pain as 2/10 compared with 4/10 initially. Her mechanical findings were reassessed and compared with the initial evaluation. She had regained full and pain-free range of motion of the right hip for flexion, adduction and internal rotation and showed significant improvement in anterior nutational movement of the right sacroiliac joint. Positional and passive mobility testing of the lumbar spine revealed improved mobility at L4–L5, with only slight restriction on the right side at L5, which was treated on her last visit with unilateral posterior to anterior grade IV pressures (Maitland, 1986). She now was better able to recruit the gluteus maximus on the right side during active right hip extension in prone lying, and her hip extension range of motion had notably improved, with the ability to extend the hip 10–15 degrees from the prone lying position bilaterally. Francis was discharged from physical therapy 2 months after initiating treatment and instructed to call should she have any further questions or problems in the future.

References

Bourdillon, J.F., Day, E.A. and Bookhout, M.R. (1992). Spinal Manipulation, 5th edn. Oxford: Butterworth-Heinemann.

Evjenth, O. and Hamberg, J. (1984). Muscle Stretching and Manual Therapy, A Clinical Manual, Vol. 1. Alfta, Sweden: Alfta Rehab.

Greenman, P.E. (1996). Principles of Manual Medicine, 2nd edn. Baltimore, MD: Williams & Wilkins.

Isaacs, E.R. and Bookhout, M.R. (2001). Bourdillon's Spinal Manipulation, 6th edn. Woburn, MA: Butterworth-Heinemann.

Maitland, G.D. (1986). Vertebral Manipulation, 5th edn. London: Butterworth.

Vleeming, A., Pool-Goudzwaard, A.L., Hammudughlu, B. et al. (1996). The function of the long dorsal sacroiliac ligament, its implication for understanding low back pain. Spine, 21, 556–562.

CHAPTER 3

Ongoing low back, leg and thorax troubles, with tennis elbow and headache

David Butler

 SUBJECTIVE EXAMINATION

During my clinical career, I can recall four particular patients who stand out as producing significant changes in my understanding of clinical presentations and my professional direction. The patient described here, with ongoing low back, leg and thorax troubles, plus tennis elbow and headache, is the most recent.

Ruby, a 52-year-old slightly overweight European woman with a sparkle in her eyes was referred via a physician to ascertain the value of continuing physiotherapy treatment for ongoing back pain. I noticed immediately that she had little trouble getting up the two flights of stairs in our practice, and when I introduced myself I had the feeling that she was not too sure about being there.

I asked her an opening question, 'What do you feel is your main problem?', and then she began to talk. I did not have to ask many questions, she only stopped when she wanted to ask a question, and sometimes I just had to nod for her to continue telling her story. I have attempted to group Ruby's story into traditional categories, although the story unfolded as she wanted to tell it.

Ruby said she was 'injured' at work 14 months ago. She was a shop assistant. 'Something definitely went in my low back', she said, 'when I was lifting bundles of clothes onto shelves, nothing much different from what I do normally, but perhaps the bundles were larger.' Prior to this there were just the 'usual aches and pains everyone gets, but I was fit and could

do anything'. Ruby admitted that work was 'a bit stressy' at the time because she worked in a large department store in which there had been some downsizing, and a few of her colleagues around her age had lost their jobs. She was working three half days a week and said that she was just managing, with not much time for anything else. Her goal was to return to her original three full days of work per week.

I asked Ruby to show me where she felt her problems were (Fig. 3.1). She described a wide area of discomfort in her lumbar spine and she ran her hand down her right leg in what looked like a combination of the L4 and L5 dermatomes ('I have done this so many time I think I have rubbed it off', she stated). There, was a small area just right of her lumbosacral segment that she said was particularly tender and which she encouraged me to touch. In addition her whole right foot 'didn't feel right', although there was no paraesthesia or anaesthesia. She had had some diffuse mid-thoracic pain for at least 6 months. 'My shoulder blades make cracking noises too', she added. In addition, Ruby complained of left lateral elbow pain present for 2 months, which she said had been 'dismissed as tennis elbow'. She commented, 'You are the first person to seem interested in my elbow. Most people don't want to know, yet sometimes I think that the elbow can be as bad as the low back.' There were also some headaches and neck pain, but she felt that her lower back was the 'core problem'.

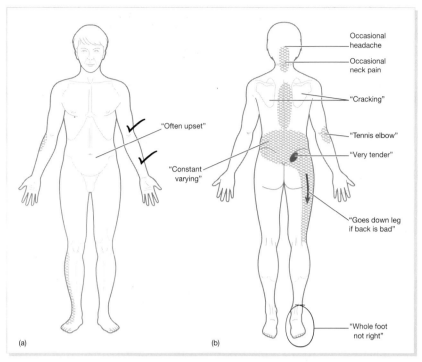

Fig. 3.1 Body chart illustrating the patient's symptoms.

 REASONING DISCUSSION AND CLINICAL REASONING COMMENTARY

1 What were your thoughts at this early stage?

▊ Clinician's answer

My first thought was that Ruby had a pain state from minimal trauma and that there had been plenty of time for the injury to heal. Immediately my thoughts were directed at the possible processes that could be contributing to ongoing sensitivity. My initial thoughts are summarized in the reasoning categories below.

Pathobiological mechanisms

Pathobiological mechanisms are likely to involve multiple processes. Although tissues have had time to heal, they are likely to be unhealthy and there may be significant physical impairment. To explain her pain state, there are hints of peripheral neurogenic (e.g. area of leg pain) and central mechanisms (e.g. spread and persistence of symptoms). There is surely nociceptive (tissue-based) pain, perhaps from combinations of deconditioning, acidosis, neurogenic inflammation, and persistent physical dysfunction. Upregulated nervous systems are likely to involve perturbed output and homeostatic systems, such as the endocrine, autonomic and immune systems.

Sources

If there is impairment with peripheral neurogenic mechanisms, then a reasoned source is the L4 or L5 nerve root. If there is nociceptive impairment, then any of the mobile tissues may potentially be unhealthy and could perhaps be identified on physical examination. The anatomical sources of the central sensitivity are impossible to identify, but descending endogenous pain control pathways, the dorsal horn and multiple brain areas, including sensory, motor, attention, memory and limbic systems, are likely to be involved.

Prognosis

On the 'good' side is her disposition, as indicated by her comment 'its been there only 13 months'. Perhaps some obstacles to recovery are work difficulties and the widespread and worsening nature of her symptoms. I was encouraged at this stage.

Management

Management strategies are likely to involve education regarding the nature of the injury, reasons for pain maintenance and unnecessary fears related to movement. It may involve pacing activities in relation to sensitivity and devising activities that present learnt painful movements to the brain in non-painful ways. It will probably involve active and passive treatment of relevant physical impairments. She will also need to get fitter.

Contributing factors

There are already hints of work-related stress.

2 This lady has quite a diffuse array of symptoms. Can you comment on why you would want to know about all her complaints rather than just her main problem?

■ Clinician's answer

The biological processes behind all the complaints are likely to be the same, but all complaints are needed for a working diagnosis. For example, knowledge of the elbow pain could support a hypothesis of central sensitization or a hypothesis of a generalized inflammatory disorder, or perhaps a local tissue-based pain state from inappropriate use of the part. The big picture is necessary for therapy. For example, it may be the elbow pain that prevents particular activities which may help the low back.

Ruby's main problem(s) may well vary during therapy. This appears to be a clinical feature of central sensitization.

If explanation is hypothesized as a key management tool, she will want all symptoms and features explained. It is important that Ruby knows that the elbow pain, the headaches and the cracking in the thorax are not new problems, but that they are likely to be an expression of one process.

3 Also, you state that she did not have any paraesthesia/anaesthesia, suggesting that you screened for this particular symptom. Could you highlight what sorts of screening questions you would use when the patient does not spontaneously volunteer the information?

■ Clinician's answer

There are many different questions that may need to be asked if the patient is reticent to volunteer information. For example, with respect to other types of symptoms, it may be necessary to ask about pins and needles or whether there are any areas that are numb. Clinicians will need to ensure that the patient's comprehension of 'numb' is the same as theirs. This question is related to the sensory aspects of peripheral neurogenic/central contributions. Asking whether there are areas that 'don't feel the same as before the injury' or which 'don't feel the same as the other side' can also be revealing. Other screening questions, seeking hints of autonomic and motor involvement, include changes in sweating, skin health and feelings of weakness.

■ Clinical reasoning commentary

The breadth and openness of the clinician's 'working diagnosis' is evident. As suggested in Chapter 1, a manual therapy diagnosis should be one that captures the clinician's understanding of the person (i.e. narrative reasoning) and the person's problem(s). This should include, as provided here, the clinician's judgment regarding each of the hypothesis categories. It is not sufficient simply to identify structures involved, as this alone does not provide sufficient information to understand the problem and its effect on the patient, or to justify the course of management chosen. The manual therapy diagnosis must include a hierarchy of considerations, including the activity and participation capabilities/restrictions, the pathobiological mechanisms, patient perceptions of their experience (i.e. psychosocial issues), specific impairments identified and their associated hypothesized sources, and contributing factors.

The clinician's narrative and collaborative reasoning is also evident in this patient-centred interview where he encourages the patient to tell 'her story' in the way 'she wanted to tell it'. This aspect of clinicians' reasoning requires attempting to understand the patient as a person, including their perspective of the problem (e.g. understanding, beliefs, desires, motivations, emotions), the basis of their perspective and how the problem is affecting their life.

Symptom pattern

Ruby felt that there was always some low back pain, although it varied. The leg pain came on when the back pain increased, or if she did a lot of bending. Her few hours at work usually brought it on. This involved some light lifting and general sales. The pains were generally activity related, gardening for instance, but not necessarily. She mentioned that she 'could be watching television and the back and leg might hurt'. Further questioning revealed that sitting was perhaps an aggravating factor and 'staying still could also bring it on'. If she was sitting or doing paperwork while standing at work, she would get uncomfortable and the leg pain would manifest. There were no particular movements that aggravated her symptoms and she said that her spine felt a 'bit stiff'. There were no autonomic or vascular type symptoms. 'I just don't understand it and no-one else seems to either', she complained. The only things that would ease the pain were forgetting about it, time, or sometimes a few gin and tonics would 'take the edge off it or make me forget it'. Listening to music, 'especially Barry Manilow', would also help, but 'none of that heavy rock stuff that my son listens to though'. She was smiling. I asked her about her family. Her husband of many years was supportive and believed she should keep active, and her son was at university and was happy. Her spouse was healthy, although his father had bad back pain, and he had always believed in the value of exercise.

She slept well. She further commented that 'everyone asks me that and they seem surprised when I reply that sleep isn't a problem and once I am in bed I usually sleep very well'.

Activity levels and goals

Ruby's activity levels had altered considerably compared with pre-injury levels. She adored gardening but was frightened about damaging her back any further. She had been warned to stop gardening after the injury and now she 'just potters around' for about half an hour. Walking was restricted to a few times around the block or about 30 minutes. She played no sport, although she had tried tennis with painful results (prior to the accident she played veteran's tournament tennis, golf occasionally and enjoyed working for hours in the garden). Ruby had no specific activity goals but immediately said that she would like to spend more time in the garden as 'it's crying out for attention'. She said spontaneously, 'I feel a bit caged in; I don't know which direction to take. Sometimes I want to fight the pain, but I know from experience that it won't do me any good. My husband avoids the garden and my son is too busy studying.' When pains came on she usually stopped, although she said on some days, 'I just try and forget it and march straight though'. She wanted to return to work, not full-time but about 30 hours per week, just the same as before.

I asked her whether she had developed any new movement habits after the injury. She thought for a moment and said, 'that's interesting'. She explained that she now bent to the right to pick things up and she would squat rather than bend to reach the floor.

Thoughts, beliefs and feelings about the problem

When I asked Ruby what her concept of the problem was, there was silence for a few long seconds. 'Not sure', she said, 'but there is something wrong or out in my back, I know that, maybe a nerve or a disc or something. I don't know why it seems to be spreading and I am getting these new problems. I was worried it was a horrible arthritis like my auntie had, so I was pleased about the blood test (negative, see below). Someone mentioned fibromyalgia once, but not again. The physiotherapist says I have stiff joints and some neural tension. No, I don't really know what has happened to me and I cannot really understand why it does not go away. It would be easier if I had a broken bone. I know that heals and you can show the plaster cast to people.'

Ruby said she had hope that it could be fixed and she thought it would need some exercises and perhaps something 'put back in place'. She wasn't going to give up and thought that there may be surgery that could fix it. The fact that it had been going on for over a year was a big worry, and she added, 'I know the story on back problems isn't too good'. Spontaneously she said, 'I really want to know what is happening in there'. I asked her what it was like when she was angry or stressed and she immediately, almost resignedly,

replied that it was worse, especially if there was leg pain. I told her that that was the case for most pains. She said that she didn't like going out now, and added 'My husband must be getting sick of it—I am not the happy bouncy person I once was'.

REASONING DISCUSSION AND CLINICAL REASONING COMMENTARY

1 Have any patterns (for example, related to pain mechanisms, contributing factors or prognosis) emerged for you from this additional information regarding the symptom pattern?

■ Clinician's answer

While a mechanical pattern has emerged it is not a clear pattern with a closely linked stimulus/response feature. It suggests combinations of primary hyperalgesia (tissue based) and secondary hyperalgesia (central nervous system based). The fact that sitting and standing at work evoked pain suggests that contributing factors such as work-related ergonomic features and job stress may need addressing. Anecdotally, patients with hypothesized central sensitivity can sometimes sleep remarkably well.

2 What is your interpretation of her 'easing factors' (forgetting about the pain, time, alcohol and music)?

■ Clinician's answer

These are frequent characteristics of central sensitization. A small amount of alcohol may be a relaxant through central enhancement of the serotonergic system. The key thing is that these features can be used as part of explaining about what appears to be central sensitivity. It may help to demonstrate to her that focussing on the pain may make it worse, how distractive techniques could be useful, and how she does have some control over the problem. To help to explain increased sensitivity, one could use the example of the more mellow Barry Manilow music being more acceptable than the heavy rock music. This observation could be related to get her to do an

appropriate amount of movement in relation to her sensitivity.

3 Could you comment on your impressions/ hypotheses regarding Ruby's cognitive/affective status (i.e. her perceptions of her experience), specifically with respect to any 'yellow flags' and positive/negative factors in her prognosis for continued pain, disability and likelihood of returning to work?

■ Clinician's answer

The key yellow flags here are:

- a poor explanatory model that has included multiple explanations and the concept of ongoing tissue damage
- the fact that pain is controlling her
- her fear of activity-related damage to a structure
- withdrawal from social interaction.

However it was not all bad. For example, Ruby still had hope, was seeking some self-help via explanation, had a supportive family and appeared likely to accept an active approach to rehabilitation.

■ Clinical reasoning commentary

The concept of hypothesis categories has been put forward in this book as a means by which therapists can organize their knowledge and focus on clinical thinking. However, reasoning regarding the various categories of hypotheses does not occur in any set sequence. Rather, clinical reasoning is a dynamic process and judgments regarding the different hypothesis categories are interlinked. For example, here the clinician describes how the patient's report of 'easing factors' was not only supportive of the pathobiological mechanism of central sensitivity, but also how this same information may also be used in the management strategy of explanation/education.

The key aspect of clinical reasoning evident in the clinician's answer regarding Ruby's cognitive/affective states is his attention to both supporting and negating clues/evidence. While clinical reasoning has a scientific basis, it is not a hard science. Many patient presentations are multifactorial and filled with conflicting evidence. This requires care to avoid premature final judgments and bias, where one or two key features are attended to and conflicting evidence or competing hypotheses are neglected. This is demonstrated in the clinician's predictive reasoning with respect to psychosocial risk factors for chronicity, or yellow flags, where he has identified both supporting and negating evidence.

Questions to identify precautions and red flags

A radiograph taken 3 weeks after the injury showed some degeneration of the lower lumbar spine, most marked at the L4-L5 and L5-S1 levels, and a little worse on the right side. There was minimal encroachment of the intervertebral foramina at these levels. A more recent radiograph was similar. Ruby had been told that there was 'degeneration in the lumbar spine'. A complete blood test revealed no abnormalities. She had been told that they were checking for arthritis and it had been explained that this was normal. A recent computed tomography (CT) scan was also reported as showing 'degeneration in the lower lumbar spine; no nerve compression'. With these results plus my subjective interview, I excluded serious pathology and I again reassured Ruby that 'it sounds promising'.

Ruby had tried a 'cocktail of drugs' over the past year but was currently not taking any medication. She stated that she 'would rather have the pain, than enjoy the little benefit they give, and having to worry about what drugs do to my kidneys'.

Bladder and bowel function she said 'were OK', although there was sometimes pain with her bowel movements. Straining could evoke back and leg pain. She felt that her stomach was much more sensitive than before the injury, when she could eat anything. Other than the pain, Ruby felt in reasonable health, although she admitted to being unfit. She was a non-smoker and there was no impending legal action. 'I have practically given up sex', she added.

REASONING DISCUSSION AND CLINICAL REASONING COMMENTARY

1 What were your thoughts regarding this information?

Clinician's answer

I thought that there was no need to refer her back for further medical assessment and I felt I could reassure her that there was no serious underlying disease process. I also thought it might be worthwhile getting her doctor to reinforce this. In addition, I felt more positive considering her attitude regarding drugs and the lack of impending legal action.

2 Did you think the difficulties with her bowels and the increased sensitivity of her stomach warranted any concern and follow-up investigation?

Clinician's answer

No. My reasoning was that bowel-related pain was mechanical and perhaps related to ongoing nerve root sensitivity as it increased leg pain. At this stage, increased stomach sensitivity could be seen as part of a central sensitivity.

Clinical reasoning commentary

Screening questions serve the purpose of identifying whether other types of symptoms, aggravating or easing factors and, as used here, specific red flags (i.e. symptoms and signs requiring emergency referral to a spinal surgeon and signs and symptoms suggesting possible serious pathology) are present that the patient may not have spontaneously volunteered. Yellow flags (i.e. psychosocial risk factors of chronicity), including blue flags (patient's perception of work) and black flags (actual work characteristics), and symptoms and signs suggestive of a non-musculoskeletal disorder masquerading as musculoskeletal dysfunction should also be routinely screened.

PHYSICAL EXAMINATION

Active movements

I looked at Ruby's general posture and noted a kyphotic thorax and a slight forward head posture. In general, her back looked strong with well-developed musculature. I thought how chronic pain was such that it could be masked and a hidden phenomenon in society. 'Am I looking in the right place?' I thought. She could squat, and there were no great abnormalities detected when I observed her walking. Balance on either leg was not good, especially the right leg, which she could only balance on for a couple of seconds.

Ruby's active lumbar movements seemed reasonable. Lumbar extension looked stiff, particularly in the low lumbar region, and I noted that during extension she shifted to the left, away from the painful lower limb. The movement was restricted but no pain was produced. Lateral flexion to the right seemed a bit more restricted than to the left, particularly in the lower regions. On lumbar flexion, there was a pulling sensation and some diffuse pain across her lumbar spine and buttocks, although she could nearly touch the floor. These symptoms increased when I carefully added cervical flexion.

I looked at thoracic rotation only. There was some stiffness and a little mechanical hyperalgesia in the thorax on rotation to the left. In addition, there was also a cramping feeling in the thorax. Ruby could lift her arms above her head easily and without discomfort. 'That crackling noise should go when you are moving better', I explained. During cervical spine retraction, the thoracic pains were provoked.

Passive movements

I performed a quick palpation examination. There was no excessive warmth in the tissues and I palpated the thorax and lumbar spines both centrally and unilaterally. Ruby was hyperalgesic all along her thorax, especially at the mid-thorax where it felt particularly

stiff to posteroanterior passive accessory intervertebral movements. The lumbar spine was also hyperalgesic, particularly the lower lumbar region and especially on the right side, although I could not detect any localized stiffness. There was also multiple area tenderness when I palpated over the sacrum.

Neurodynamic testing revealed:

- Straight leg raise (SLR) of the left leg was 80 degrees with a pulling feeling behind the knee.
- Right SLR was about 60 degrees with some pulling sensation behind the knee and a 'dragging feeling' in the lumbar spine.
- Passive neck flexion in supine lying produced a very slight pulling feeling in the lumbar spine and a mid-thoracic pain at end of range.
- The slump test was performed actively with some guidance. On initial slump 'nothing' was felt. The addition of neck flexion 'pulled' in the thorax, and left knee extension at minus 10 degrees 'pulled' in the mid-hamstring area. Right knee extension was about minus 20 degrees and evoked symptoms in the back and thorax. There was also a 'vague numbish' feeling in the right foot. All of these symptoms were eased when the cervical spine was extended, even with just upper cervical extension.

Neurological examination

While standing, heel walking revealed some right-sided ankle dorsiflexor weakness, and heel raising also showed some slight right-sided weakness. For both these quick tests, weakness was only evident after five or six repetitions. 'Is it safe to do this?' she asked. 'No problems, you are doing well', I replied.

Her quadriceps reflexes were equal, although somewhat hyper-reflexic. The ankle jerks appeared equal and normal. There was a slight decrease in strength in all right-sided muscle groups below L2. I thought that the L4 muscle test (ankle dorsiflexion) stood out as the weakest. The tendon of the contracted right tibialis anterior muscle was softer to palpation than on the left side. There was hypersensitivity in her posterior right leg to a cursory light touch examination, although this could not be localized to a dermatome. Mild, bilaterally equal ankle clonus was evident. I told her that her 'nerves were firing well'. Pinprick was not performed.

Ruby said that she was a little sore in the back after the examination. I reassured her that this was natural.

Initial assessment

The above subjective and physical examination had taken me about 45 minutes. I told Ruby that I would need to continue the examination and get some more details next time. As she left, I told her that I wanted to achieve four things for her within the next few visits:

1. Explain what I thought was wrong as far as the most current scientific understanding of spinal pain would allow (this would include why the problem was still persisting);

2. Clarify how long it would take to improve and what improvements were possible;
3. Present all the options of what she could do for it.
4. Advise her what physiotherapy could do for the problem. I said that I was sure I could help her and show her how to manage her problem.

She looked at me somewhat quizzically, said 'thanks' and left. I wasn't sure whether she was going to come back.

During the examination, I made notes on what I thought I should specifically attempt to explain to her. These included:

- why the problem had not gone
- the spread of pain
- what the tennis elbow meant
- the cracking noise under the scapula
- why pain came on for no reason
- why there had been various explanations for the problem
- why moods affected the pains
- the radiograph findings.

 REASONING DISCUSSION AND CLINICAL REASONING COMMENTARY

1 Please comment on your thoughts regarding whether your findings on the physical examination fitted with your thoughts following the subjective examination, with respect to pain mechanisms and sources associated with her symptoms and impairments.

Clinician's answer

Yes they fitted. Ruby may have had better general movements than I thought she would, but this is understandable with a hypothesis of central sensitivity. I believe that because I spent a significant amount of time with the subjective evaluation and let her tell her whole story a clinical environment was created which allowed her to move reasonably well.

There is clinical evidence of peripheral tissue involvement (e.g. neurological findings, area of symptoms) and a pattern that, on the basis of modern neurobiology in particular, could be argued as central sensitivity.

2 Many patients expect to receive some 'hands-on' treatment at their first appointment. Could you briefly discuss your views on this and the risk that the patient might not return, as you commented above might be the case with this lady.

Clinician's answer

I believe that it is a myth that this kind of patient desires hands-on treatment at their first visit. Often many patients have had failed hands-on treatment. In this particular case, my reasoned judgment was that her desire for information and support was much stronger than for an instant 'fix it'. If a subjective enquiry reveals that a patient really wants mobilization, traction or ultrasound, then it may be worth giving it to them, so long as the therapist and patient do not fall into the trap of believing that this is the likely sole and necessary treatment.

The danger is that the delivery of such techniques, with possible short-term beneficial results from treatment, may reinforce the notion that tissue damage is the only cause. The patient has to see the place of physical findings in the big picture, as much as clinicians must.

Most patients want a good physical evaluation. There is plenty of useful therapeutic touch in the physical examination. Perhaps we should realise that the physical examination is in fact treatment, and that the patient is consciously and subconsciously learning from your physical examination.

In retrospect, in this particular patient, my fears of her not returning reflected my own insecurities, not hers.

■ Clinical reasoning commentary

As the clinician points out, hands-on treatment is not essential at the first appointment. Management is, however. He rightly argues that a thorough examination should be seen as part of management and that explanation/education is an important, sometimes the most important, aspect of our management. For some patients with complex presentations such as this lady's, allowing time for a more thorough examination and explanation of findings is more appropriate than shortening the examination for the sake of trying to fit in a specific hands-on treatment. But such decisions are not always clear-cut and they must be made collaboratively with the patient.

m Management

■ Appointment 2

Ruby arrived early for the second appointment. She said that she felt quite tired after the previous examination. I quickly went over things that I had forgotten to ask in the first examination or which needed confirmation.

She had received previous treatments. The thorax and lumbar spine had been manipulated many times by various professionals. This would usually give relief, though not always. Hydrotherapy was tried but did not help. She had tried various exercises but found 'when I concentrate on the back, it sometimes gets worse afterwards'.

I rechecked the active movements (no change in pattern observed at first appointment), performed a Babinski examination (negative) and performed a closer palpation of her lumbar spine. The left L4–L5 area was the most tender, although the same generalized tenderness was evident. Both SLRs were similar to Day 1, perhaps a little better. With the right ankle dorsiflexed and inverted, and then the leg raised, there was significantly more hamstring and back pain than on the other side. I checked the slump test in long-sitting. Pain was evoked in the mid-thorax in this position and could be eased by cervical extension and by both left and right knee flexion.

I performed a left upper limb neurodynamic test (Butler, 2000) for the radial nerve. There was a little more sensitivity over the lateral elbow than on the other side, but no apparent tightness or stiffness.

I said that I thought that modern science could provide a reasonable explanation for her problem and that I should go over that first. I also said that there were a few things I could do and that there were many things she could do to help. The interchange below was my attempt to explain the problem:

Clinician I think after listening to your story and examining you, that there has to be some unhealthy, unfit tissues in your lower and middle back. Certainly there are many tender joints and sensitive nerves, and although I haven't tested muscles yet—I will later—they are sure to have lost some of the normal health and vitality they had before your problem began. You probably did strain some joints and muscles in your back a few years ago, as well as probably having some nerve irritation, which caused the leg pain, and these tissues are still a bit sensitive. However, one thing is for sure, over the last year the injured tissues have had every chance to heal and these present pains aren't really serving the original purpose of the pain, which was a warning and a call to action.

Ruby OK, I would like to get things a bit healthier, but how? It just hurts so much. And why doesn't it get better? There has to be something wrong in there. I am not putting it on.

Clinician I know you aren't and we have to answer those important questions. I think I can offer you a good scientifically based explanation of why your back is still so sensitive.

Ruby   I'm all ears.

Clinician   Your once-injured joints, muscles and nerves have had plenty of time to heal. As you know, even a broken bone will heal up nicely in a couple of months. Also, by your decreased activity you have protected yourself, maybe overprotected, from re-injury. But for various reasons, which we'll explore, the tissues are still unhealthy and sensitive. However, they can be made a bit healthier and made to move better, given more blood, and the oil in the joints can be made healthier and slipperier. They are sensitive but they are crying out for movement.

Ruby   OK, but why is it still hurting and shouldn't my attempts to move make me feel better? I always used to feel great after exercise. It's not for the want of trying you know. A couple of times I have said 'stuff it' and gone and exercised and walked lots, but I really pay for it afterwards, sometimes not even sleeping for a couple of nights.

Clinician   Well, it's partly those sensitive unhealthy tissues and getting the right balance for the amount of exercise, but it's probably also because there has been a few sensitivity changes right throughout your nervous system.

Ruby   What on earth do you mean by that?

Clinician   Well, there has been a lot of research into pain mechanisms over the last few years. We now know that when there has been a tissue injury, particularly a painful one such as a joint injury or particularly a nerve compression, and if there has been a bit of stress at the time, that the whole nervous system not only becomes more sensitive, but it can also stay sensitive.

Ruby   Are you inferring that this is all in my head David?

Clinician   Well no, but yes in a way, in a very real way in your nervous system. I have no doubt about the reality of your pains. This is not easy to explain so bear with me. There are some problems in the tissues but we now know that repeated impulses into the nervous system will make it more sensitive, more ready for action. It's a natural thing. It happens in everyone, but for some reason, in some people, these nerves stay sensitive. If this happens, it means that inputs from other parts of the body like the elbow or the thorax can also report pain. Sometimes old pains that you thought

had gone could come back. It is rather like there is an amplifier or a magnifier in your body which makes everything seem worse than it is. Perhaps you could have handled your son's rock music in the past, but now because of your sensitivity being a bit turned up, it is more difficult.

Ruby   Sounds possible. Maybe that music does bug me more these days. And I did have bad elbow pains about 5 years ago. I am not sure about some scientists though. I just want you to know that I am not making this up.

Clinician   I don't think you are making it up and if some colleagues of mine have suggested that, then that is unfortunate and all I can do is apologise. But all pains are real and I am just being a mouthpiece for a lot of recent scientific work. If you want to read about this, I can give you some short articles which I have written.

Ruby   Maybe later, perhaps my husband would be interested. I want to hear more from you.

Clinician   Let me try and express this on a diagram (Fig. 3.2). From my examination, I believe that there are a number of tissues that are sensitive and a bit unhealthy. There are also changes related to sensitivity in the spinal cord. I know that sounds awful but, as I said, it happens to everyone. We are lucky to have this wonderful nervous system that can keep changing its sensitivity depending on how much we need it. I am sure you have heard stories of people who really want to complete a game of sport and during the game they sustain some nasty injury but they can complete the game. We all have the ability to turn the pain system up and down as we need it, and of course some of the changes are automatic. However, sometimes the pain system stays turned up and there is a sort of a magnifier in your system. For example, when I touched your back gently, it hurt. Now there is nothing wrong with your skin otherwise we would see it, but the touch is going into the central nervous system where it is turned into pain. Don't worry, this is very common. We all get it to various degrees and we often see patients where minor inputs such as a collar rubbing on the neck or a little draft seems to cause pain.

Ruby   (After some time looking at the drawing.) So you are saying that the pains I am having are not really the pains I have got.

Clinician   (I was a bit stunned by this response.) Well, yes and no; perhaps more yes. I think that

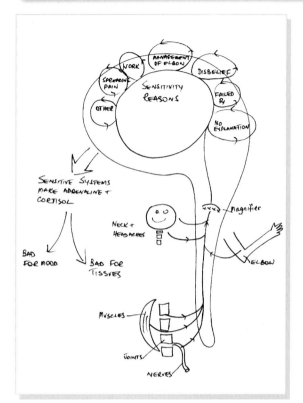

Fig. 3.2   Graphic description of the patient's pain state.

there are some pains coming from the joints, muscles and nerves of the back, but you are right and up to date scientifically if you are thinking that the pains you are experiencing may not be a true reflection of the state of tissue health and healing in the spine. We have to get your whole system less sensitive as well as making those tissues more healthy. Are you OK with all this?

Ruby   Yes I think so, but I want to discuss this with my husband.

Clinician   OK, sure. You can bring him in next visit, if you want. I am going to give you some articles to read and you can give them to him as well.

Ruby   It's comforting to know that I am not alone here. I am looking forward to starting something. What sort of things will I be doing?

Clinician   You have started already. Sometimes when you know a bit about what is going on it takes a bit of sensitivity out of your system already.

Ruby   Yes that's right I am sure, but shouldn't I be given some exercises?

Clinician   Let's call it activity rather than exercise. I had to leave the room for 5 minutes. (When I came back, Ruby looked a little concerned.)

Ruby   I don't really understand it. I can follow your story about impulses making the nervous system sensitive. It sounds sensible, but why me? Why hasn't everyone got chronic pain?

Clinician   Well, there are more people with chronic pain than we ever thought. Approximately one quarter of all Australians have some pain that doesn't go away. In your case, I don't really know for sure, but we can make some educated guesses. First of all, the type of injury is likely to be important. From the sound of it, we can guess that the initial injury may have involved irritation of a nerve. That test when I asked you to slump and lift your legs suggests that there is a bit of irritation or tightness around some nerves, plus there is some minimal weakness and funny feelings in the foot. That's from nerve irritation in the back. If you remember, the test was more sensitive on the right side. There are parts of the nerve close to the spinal cord and near the disc (desk model shown) that keep buzzing for a time after injury. Also, when there is a bit of adrenaline around, which there always is when there is an injury and if you get a bit stressed or upset, it will also make damaged nerves more sensitive. A nerve can be sensitive for quite a while but they nearly always get better, especially if you keep reasonably active and understand what is going on. Secondly, the sensitivity within your nervous system can be increased for a number of reasons. You could think of them as things that are stressing you, some of which you may not be aware of. Now I hardly know you, but just from our two meetings I can see a few reasons for increased sensitivity. For example, with failed treatments and lack of explanation or direction, it is no wonder that you remain sensitive. If you feel as though you have to prove there is something wrong, it naturally only uplifts your sensitivity and this is often the case where there are problems at work. It's a natural survival thing. Walk through the dark and you become more sensitive to the surrounds. This must be related to the fear of not knowing. Your brain in a small way is fearing for your survival so it lifts the sensitivity and makes more stress chemicals like adrenaline and cortisol. We haven't discussed it but it is only natural that you would have some concern for the future. I know you love gardening and perhaps even looking at a garden that needs care is stressful. Work issues are probably stressful. There may be other things in your life that you can think of which may make you a bit sensitive. They may be worth thinking about.

Ruby   Maybe. At the time of the accident I remember being very angry. It was very painful but I don't think they believed me you know. There had been a few women off work and I think they thought we were having a go at the system. It was the same when I had elbow problems 5 years ago. And by the way, have you had a look at the X-rays I brought in?

Clinician   Oh yes, let's look together. There are some changes but they are really just the kisses of time. We all get them and there is nothing to worry about in the bones. Your bones look healthy. An X-ray can't tell much about damaged tissues; sometimes the CT scans can but your CT scan was great. These are typical for someone your age, with or without pain.

Ruby   Well, it's a worry with all that wear and tear, but I follow you.

Clinician   I said during the first visit that I would try and answer four things: what is wrong, how long it will take to get better, what you can do and what I or anyone else can do. Hopefully, I have begun to answer the first. How long it will take to get better is hard to answer, but I am sure that you will be able to function much better once you understand the nature of the pain, that you can edge into it, explore it, even play with it and know it won't harm you. It may never go completely and there will probably be a few flare-ups, but this does not mean your management is failing.

Thirdly, what can you do? From my examination, I believe that you have every reason to remain positive and being positive will help. Simply, positive people make happy healing hormones. We know your nerves are working; we know there is no serious pathology and you are moving quite well. There are a number of things you can do, but it's really all about movement. Edging into pain with less fear is one way, but I think you and I could also come up with a paced exercise programme; that is, a series of activities that you know can hurt but which are performed short of pain. It is teaching your brain that activities that normally hurt don't

have to hurt. When we set an exercise programme, we can make some goals, for example increasing time and activity in the garden. There may always be some pain and you may need to be more active for a while before it settles. For the moment though, try and minimize activities that cause the shooting pain down the leg. I will also discuss other management such as using heat and cold and relaxation.

Fourthly, what can I do? The big picture aims are to get you a bit fitter, and happier to move with greater understanding of your problem. There are some specific exercises I will add, but they can wait until next visit. This will include some general slump exercises to improve flexibility and I think it is worthwhile getting some of the local muscle groups around your low back and the front of your neck more active. I think that in this kind of long-standing problem, there is unlikely to be a single magic click or drug or surgery that can fix it. I will also explain what I am doing to the nurse at your work and I will ring your doctor and send a short report.

▪ Appointment 3

Ruby arrived very early for the appointment. She seemed nervous. 'I don't think I need to come any-more', she said. 'I have been thinking about it all night. For years I have been going to doctors and specialists and therapists and I am sick of it. I really only ever wanted two things. I wanted a good examination and I wanted to know that I could go back and do more gardening and more activity without harming myself. I feel I can do that now. I am just going to slowly work into it a bit more each day. Minor aches and pains, I won't worry about but I will stop at around half an hour and then I will try and increase that the next week, maybe do some digging and planting. That will fit nicely as the days are getting longer now, but I am going to gradually work into more activity, maybe even have a few hits of tennis with my children. I will ring you if I need you and I would be very grateful if you could explain this to the industrial nurse and the doctor. I will increase my time at work. Thank you very much.'

I was very surprised. I thought I had a lot more to offer her, but I felt happy with her responses. I had intended to manage her for approximately 6 weeks, with one visit per week. I had written down my plan for management and it included the following.

- Reassess physical signs including her neurological signs.
- Reassess her hopefully changing beliefs and thoughts about her back, her pain and activity.
- I was going to talk more about movement and the brain, how the brain is hungry for new inputs, how it changes with loss of normal inputs and how physical exercise is as much for the brain as it is for the body. I wanted to keep adding some information each visit.
- Check the need for slump mobilization and spinal exercises. Perhaps treat with some passive as well as active slump mobilization. I may have mobilized or manipulated joint segments eventually, if I felt sure she understood where such a treatment fitted in to the big picture.
- Try and change the maladaptive movement habits. This could begin with the new habit that she had developed to pick thinks up off the floor. Somehow, movements that have been learned to be painful need to be presented to her brain in a non-painful way. This may mean pacing, breaking down movements and using different orders of movement. For instance, there are various different ways of getting up from a chair.

- Introduce and modify a gradual paced programme involving time in the garden. I wanted to establish some base activity levels and then increase these. I would also do this with walking.
- Discuss other coping measures, including some strategies for flare-ups. Strategies could include use of heat, distraction and relaxation exercises: maybe get a dog etc.
- Invite her husband in during one visit for more explanation.
- Initially I thought I could manage her by myself, liaising with the doctor and industrial nurse. If there were no quick beneficial responses I thought that a formal investigation of psychosocial aspects might be relevant, although there were no outstanding contributing factors found in my initial interview.

Perhaps I should have rung Ruby back, but she had said that she would ring me and I respected that. Her doctor told me she was managing better. About 6 months later, her daughter came into the clinic with an injured knee, referred by her mother. 'How's Mum?' I asked. She replied, 'Yeah, not too bad. She's out in the garden a lot, plays a bit of tennis, seems happy at work, still grumbling about her back pain though.'

REASONING DISCUSSION AND CLINICAL REASONING COMMENTARY

1 This patient's perceptions of her experience (i.e. her understanding of her problem and beliefs about what she could do) were obviously in themselves part of the problem and partly holding her back from getting on with the activities she enjoyed. Clearly your management in the form of explanation seems to have contributed significantly to her ability to do more within her pain. It is also evident from your 'plan for management' that in addition to further explanation, you also intended to incorporate treatment aimed at addressing some of her general and specific physical impairments (e.g. fitness, neural mobility). With the increased understanding of chronic pain there is sometimes the implication that the physical signs/impairments identified in an examination are not relevant (i.e. false-positive findings

caused by a secondary hyperalgesia or allodynia). Specific physical treatment for a patient with chronic pain is discouraged by some and has been suggested may even constitute overservicing while further contributing to the patient's reliance on a passive solution. Could you share your views on how to determine the extent that any physical impairment, such as of neural mobility or muscle control in this particular case, might still be contributing to a patient's pain and disability and the process you follow to determine their significance?

■ Clinician's answer

If I thought that physical signs were not relevant in chronic pain, then I would not have spent the time performing such a detailed physical evaluation.

In addition, I am not aware of any 'authority' who would disregard the management of relevant physical impairment in acute or chronic pain. The key is the word 'relevant'. A simple way to answer the question of relevance of specific physical impairment is to ask, 'is this a physical sign that needs to be altered to make the patient function better?' In addition, some knowledge of the neurobiology of pain can help.

Modern neurobiological science makes it clear that many of the physical signs that well-meaning manual therapists in the past have collected are not just indications of processes in the tissue that are presumed to be tested. They are a representation of tissue factors and nervous system factors. Nervous system factors include the representation and meaning of that particular examination technique at that time and in that space. This does mean that false-positive findings must occur. With Ruby, my judgment would be that the slump responses were a combination of tissue factors and an upregulated central nervous system. Hence a relevance judgment requires an understanding of neurobiology and pathobiology. This knowledge is often lacking in manual therapy.

Specific physical impairment does not have to be treated by specific physical techniques. Our physical techniques are just one tool, which in the case of this patient I may have employed. Specific physical impairment may also improve with better understanding, reduction of fear, touch, better general physical health, and return to activity.

2 At the start of this case, you note that this patient was one of four from your career that 'stand out as signifying changes in my understanding of clinical presentations and my professional direction'. Could you comment what was it about this patient that made such an impression on you?

Clinician's answer

It was the third day when Ruby said she did not need to come back. It was a powerful moment as we just looked at each for a period of time not saying anything. I think we were experiencing similar feelings: she some form of awakening and a realisation of the meaning of pain, while I was still awestruck by the power of taking the messages of pain science to patients.

Clinical reasoning commentary

On completion of the patient initial examination, whether achieved in the first appointment or over several, the manual therapist should have identified specific hypotheses in each of the hypothesis categories (see Ch. 1). Collectively, these hypotheses represent the therapist's 'diagnosis', which includes his/her understanding of the problem, the person, the effects the problem are having on the person's life, and appropriate management strategies. However, except for very straightforward patient problems where the clinical pattern and course of management are not in any doubt (i.e. no problem solving required), the hypotheses reached through the examination must then be tested through the management/reassessment process. As the clinician discusses here, even with a hypothesis of a dominant pathobiological central pain mechanism, physical impairments (specific or general) may still be relevant. In fact, speaking at an unpublished pain seminar in Australia, Patrick Wall discussed this very issue and shared the story of a patient whose central sensitivity and psychiatric symptoms were maintained by a specific physical impairment of his kidney. The point here is that it can be very difficult to be certain in the more complex patient presentations what is necessarily relevant and whether identified physical impairments are the result of, or the trigger to, a concomitant central sensitization. Hence, as discussed in Chapter 1, the reasoning process must continue through the ongoing management. Often it is not until physical impairments have been addressed in the management, and the pattern of response to such management is revealed, that the therapist can reach a more secure decision.

As manual therapists, teaching is a central component of our management with most patients. While some of our teaching is instrumental or procedural in the form of specific exercise instruction, much of our teaching centres around assisting patients to reflect on their own perspectives (e.g. beliefs and health attitudes); through this self-reflection and our explanations, our patients learn: that is they acquire new perspectives or understandings of their problems and their management. Similarly, through reflection, clinicians can also learn and acquire new perspectives (transformative learning, as discussed in Ch. 1). Critical self-reflection requires metacognition (higher order thinking and awareness of, for example, your own thinking, beliefs and knowledge limitations), an attribute characteristic of experts in all professions and the means by which clinicians shift their perspectives.

Reference

Butler, D.S. (2000). The Sensitive Nervous System. Adelaide, Australia: Noigroup Press.

Further reading

Gifford, L.S. (ed.) (1998). Topical Issues in Pain 1. Falmouth, MA: CNS Press.

Gifford, L.S.(ed.) (2000).Topical Issues in Pain 2. Falmouth, MA: CNS Press.

Wall, P.D. and Melzack, R. (1999) Textbook of Pain, 4th edn. Edinburgh: Churchill Livingstone.

CHAPTER 4

Chronic low back pain over 13 years

Dick Erhard and Brian Egloff

SUBJECTIVE EXAMINATION

A 30-year-old Caucasian male (David) presented to the clinic with a chief complaint of bilateral anterior groin pain, in addition to severe low back pain (LBP) and hip area pain. He indicated on a pain diagram (Fig. 4.1) that he was experiencing sharp pain in the lower portion of both buttocks and a deep ache on the anterior and posterior aspects of both thighs. He did not indicate on the pain diagram that he was experiencing groin pain, but during the interview he motioned with his hands in a manner that indicated he felt pain bilaterally in the anterior groin region. David related that the symptoms were so severe at times that they caused him to limp when walking. However, on the visual analogue scale (VAS) he rated his pain in the last 24 hours as 2/10, both at its worst and at its best (where 0 is 'no pain' and 10 is 'extremely intense' pain). He also pointed out that he felt stiff in the low back and right posterior superior iliac spine (PSIS) region in the morning, but that this resolved as he went about his morning routine. Furthermore, he related a feeling of his pelvis being 'rotated forward'. David's hand gestures when describing this pelvic rotation were consistent with a lateral shift of the lumbar spine.

Upon questioning, David explained that his symptoms began approximately 13 years ago when he sat down after a round of golf. At that time he noticed right buttock pain, and the symptoms had been episodic ever since. He reported that the current episode was the worst, although at the time of the clinical evaluation his symptoms had decreased. Four years after the onset of symptoms and following a

magnetic resonance imaging (MRI) scan, he was diagnosed by an orthopaedic surgeon as having a herniated nucleus pulposus at L4–L5. He described a series of incidents of LBP in the years between being diagnosed and the present time, associated with only minor or even no precipitating events. Each time chiropractic treatment, physical therapy, prescribed exercise or pain medication brought him some relief. David also described how treatment with methyl-prednisolone (oral steroids) brought him almost complete relief on one occasion. However, after the dose pack was completed the buttock pain returned. Most recently, David had enrolled in a yoga class. His hope was that the stretching would help to relieve his symptoms, but he felt that the stretches had actually aggravated his buttock pain and they had no effect on the LBP. He also indicated that prolonged sitting, such as at his desk at work, increased his symptoms and that movement somewhat alleviated the symptoms.

Questionnaire findings

A medical intake questionnaire revealed that David had not experienced any recent unexplained weight loss, nor any bowel irregularities or abdominal symptoms. He indicated he had experienced night pain at the onset of his symptoms, but when further questioned he related that this had not recurred in years. He also indicated on the questionnaire that he experienced weakness in his legs during walking and episodes of his legs giving way (right more so than left).

51

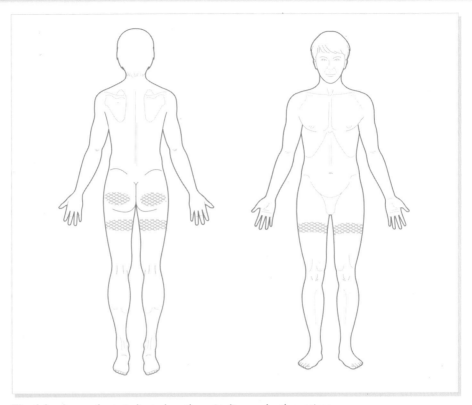

Fig. 4.1 Areas of pain indicated on the pain diagram by the patient.

When questioned further about this weakness, David added that the weakness was related to distance and that during this most recent episode he had found it necessary to rely on crutches for ambulation. At the time of his office visit, he was not using an assistive device to aid him in walking. He also indicated that there had been episodes of bladder urgency, when he had to rush to the bathroom on his crutches and quickly void to prevent urinary incontinence. Upon subsequent inquiry, he revealed he had never lost control over his bladder and had not experienced any burning sensations during urination. David denied having any paraesthesia or numbness in his extremities or groin region.

REASONING DISCUSSION AND CLINICAL REASONING COMMENTARY

1 What were your initial thoughts about the pattern of onset of the symptoms, particularly regarding their episodic nature?

Clinicians' answer

Instability is characterized by exacerbation from minimal perturbation. The fact that the patient had had numerous episodes of LBP over the years caused by insignificant or no precipitating events tended to suggest a diagnosis of instability. The onset at an early age was also consistent with this syndrome's presentation, as was the temporary help he obtained from chiropractic care. The patient's use of a supportive device (crutches) with some relief provided further support for the instability hypothesis. Finally, the patient gestured with his hands what appeared to be a lateral shift compatible with lumbar instability. Conversely, the patient did not indicate he was a 'self-manipulator', which tended to negate the hypothesis of instability, as did his gender.

2 Were you at all concerned about the episodes of bladder urgency? Did you consider investigating this problem further?

Clinicians' answer

Not really, as it was apparent these episodes were not persistent or worsening. Upon questioning the patient further, it was clear he was not describing a spastic bladder (no feelings of constant fullness or episodes of voiding abnormally small volumes of urine) nor any episodes of urinary incontinence (no dribbling as would be expected with a flaccid bladder). In addition, these episodes were not constant and ongoing, certainly not the frequent urgency one would expect from a spastic bladder. He merely had a couple of instances when he had to rush to relieve a full bladder and thus no further investigation was warranted at this stage.

Clinical reasoning commentary

The clinical diagnosis of 'instability' has been hypothesized as the cause of (or factor contributing to) the patient's symptoms, based on the recognition of typical cues associated with this clinical pattern, and probably considering the fact that this is a disorder with a relatively high prevalence. A second precautionary hypothesis related to potential mechanical causes of bladder dysfunction is given less weighting, based on an absence of typically associated cues and probably considering the fact that cauda equina syndrome is a disorder that is rarely clinically encountered. Nevertheless, it is important to note that neither hypothesis has been accepted or rejected at this early stage, which would have constituted an error in the clinicians' reasoning, with additional testing of these hypotheses to be undertaken through further questioning and standard physical examination procedures.

Analysis of the impact of pain

David filled out a Modified Oswestry Questionnaire (MOQ), a 10-category inventory of a patient's perception of the disability they have incurred as a result of their LBP (Fairbanks et al., 1980; Hudson-Cook et al., 1989). In each of the 10 categories, the patient is asked to select the statement that best applies to them from six possible responses that vary slightly in their descriptions. For example, the statements in the pain intensity category range from 'The pain comes and goes and is very mild' to 'The pain is severe and does not vary much'. In addition to questions relating to pain, the categories also include questions pertaining to functional tasks, such as sitting, standing and walking. Each category is then graded from 0 to 5 depending on which statement the

patient selects. The category scores are totalled and multiplied by two to produce a score out of 100%. Thus, the higher the percentage the more disabled the patients perceive themselves to be as a result of their back pain.

David's score was calculated to be 46%, indicating that he viewed himself as being significantly disabled when performing daily tasks. An initial MOQ score of 40–60% is one of the criteria used to assign a patient a stage I classification (Table 4.1; Delitto et al., 1995). If the initial score is extremely high (greater than 60%) and the episode is more than a few weeks old, it raises the suspicion of an affective/cognitive component to the patient's complaint. An elevated score on this questionnaire may also indicate a serious non-mechanical disease process that is not amenable to physical therapy intervention (e.g. metastatic bone disease).

Table 4.1 The Modified Oswestry Questionnaire classification system

Stage	Score	Characteristics
I	40–60%	Unable to sit for more than 30 minutes, stand for more than 15 minutes or walk for more than 400 metres without symptom aggravation
II	20–40%	Has more tolerance for sitting, standing and walking than stage I but instrumental activities of daily living, such as housecleaning or yard work, cannot be tolerated
III	<20%	Reserved for individuals whose occupation places a high demand on their lumbar spine, e.g. manual labourer or elite athlete

REASONING DISCUSSION AND CLINICAL REASONING COMMENTARY

1 At the conclusion of the interview, what were your clinical impressions? Specifically, what hypotheses were you entertaining with respect to the source(s) of (and factors contributing to) the patient's symptoms? Could you please discuss the supporting and negating evidence for each hypothesis.

■ Clinicians' answer

At this stage, the primary diagnostic hypothesis was that of lumbar instability. Supporting evidence for this hypothesis included:

- the history of multiple episodes of LBP associated with only minor or even no precipitating events
- worsening of symptoms with inactivity and relief with movement over 24 hours
- pain reduction following chiropractic treatment in the past but with diminishing returns.

The sole negating evidence was the bilateral presentation of the lower extremity symptoms.

The main competing hypothesis was a central disc herniation. This hypothesis seemed likely considering the bilateral presentation of the patient's symptoms. The reported worsening of symptoms with flexed postures (sitting) was consistent with this diagnosis. In addition, the use of crutches to assist with ambulation seemed to indicate the profound muscle weakness one might associate with a massive central disc herniation. The patient's positive response to methylprednisolone also supported this hypothesis. Initially, the report of urinary problems possibly appeared to indicate a central disc herniation, but subsequent questioning determined that the patient did not have frank bladder dysfunction. Evidence that tended to negate this hypothesis included the mechanism of injury. In a healthy individual, a disc herniation would require a large amount of force, such as compression through a flexed spine or a lifting injury. In this patient's case, a round of golf seemed to be insufficient to produce an injury of this magnitude. Furthermore, the patient did not report any kind of sensory disturbance, numbness or paraesthesia, which one might expect with a herniated disc compromising neural tissue.

2 Considering the recalcitrant nature and unusual pattern of the patient's pain, did you think at all at this time about the pain mechanisms that may have been involved?

■ Clinicians' answer

At this point, the major pathobiological pain mechanism considered was nociceptive. In keeping with an initial hypothesis of instability, mechanical nociceptive pain seemed probable. The inability to exercise the proper neuromuscular control over the available range of motion can result in the deformation of tissues, causing pain. In addition, this mechanical nociceptive pain response may lead to chronic adaptive pain and an affective component to the condition as the patient avoids activities that are known to provoke pain. The affective component to the disorder may result in fear-avoidance of activities that the patient suspects will exacerbate his pain.

3 Did you consider that psychosocial factors may have been contributing to the patient's current and/or previous episodes?

■ Clinicians' answer

No. The patient was referred to the clinic by a therapist near his home. It was this therapist's opinion that the patient's problem was not related to psychosocial issues, but that he had been misdiagnosed. In addition, the patient travelled a long distance and provided his lodging at his own expense. The patient was also self-employed, working in his family's business. He was not litigating and no avenue of secondary gain could be identified. He was well-educated and seemed content with his employment and socioeconomic status.

During the interview, his affect, mood and responses were all appropriate. His pain diagram was appropriate in that the source of pain was most likely anatomical and the diagram did not indicate an increased level of psychological distress. The area on a pain diagram that a patient marks can be related to their level of psychological distress (Margolis et al., 1986). In this patient's case, the area marked was relatively small and specific. Finally, it is not uncommon that patients with psychosocial issues have an elevated numerical pain rating. This patient's rating was only 2 on a 10 point scale.k

■ Clinical reasoning commentary

Despite the 13-year history of lumbopelvic pain and numerous health practitioners consulted, the clinicians have not erred in their reasoning by automatically assuming that psychosocial impairments would be significant factors in the maintenance of this patient's symptoms and associated activity/participation restrictions. Although, on the one hand, such impairments were obviously considered and tested for during the subjective examination, it is clear that little or no supportive evidence for a psychosocial hypothesis was thought to be present. Biased thinking, on the other hand, could have led to such an assumption being accepted (despite the evidence to the contrary) and inappropriate psychological management being implemented, possibly at the expense of appropriate physical management.

 ## PHYSICAL EXAMINATION

The physical examination began with an assessment of the patient's pelvic landmark symmetry via palpation and with the pelviometer (Piva et al., 2003), a device for measuring iliac crest level in the standing and sitting positions (Fig. 4.2). This revealed a high right iliac crest and a high right anterior superior iliac spine (ASIS) in comparison with the left side. The left PSIS and right PSIS were determined to be even. A standing flexion test was then performed, with the examiner palpating both PSIS while the patient flexed forward from an upright position. With this test, a positive result occurs when one PSIS has a greater overall excursion than its counterpart in relation to its starting position. The side that has the greater excursion is regarded as being hypomobile because the ilium and sacrum have moved as a unit (instead of moving separately as per normal). The standing flexion test was found to be positive on the right, whereas a seated flexion test was found to be positive on the left.

Active lumbar flexion, extension and both directions of side bending were non-provocative. There

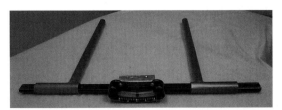

Fig. 4.2 Pelviometer for measuring iliac crest level in the standing and sitting positions.

was a slight deviation of the trunk to the left of midline with forward bending. David was able to heel and toe walk without evidence of weakness in either the dorsiflexors or the plantarflexors in both lower extremities. Muscle strength in the remaining major muscle groups of the lower limbs was tested and found to be 5/5. The knee and ankle jerks were brisk and bilaterally symmetrical. Straight leg raise (SLR) was assessed and found to be less than 70 degrees bilaterally. The end-feel suggested that the limitation was secondary to insufficient hamstring length and there was no provocation of LBP or other symptoms, as might be expected with restricted neural mobility.

The FABER test (passive flexion, abduction and external rotation of the hip joint) was performed as a quick screening test for the hips and reproduced anterior groin pain bilaterally. In addition, the lateral aspect of the knee (both left and right) failed to approximate the table when the patient was put into the FABER test position. Internal rotation of the hip joint in neutral (0 degrees hip flexion in prone lying) and also in 90 degrees hip flexion (in sitting) was then examined passively. There was significant limitation of internal rotation motion bilaterally in both of these positions. Provocation and accessory mobility testing was performed by mobilizing from the sacrum through to T11 in a posterior to anterior direction. The vertebral joints in the thoracolumbar region were found to be generally hypomobile. At this point a measurement of David's chest expansion was made.

A tape measure was circumferentially wrapped around the patient's chest at the nipple line and measurements were taken at maximal exhalation and inhalation. The chest expansion was found to be less than 1 cm. Assessment of the passive range of motion (PROM) for shoulder flexion revealed significant limitations bilaterally.

No further physical examination was carried out at this stage.

REASONING DISCUSSION AND CLINICAL REASONING COMMENTARY

1 What was your interpretation of the pelvic joint examination findings? How much importance did you place on the observational tests, particularly considering their reliability and validity? What is the mechanism by which the ASIS was high but the PSIS was even?

▮ Clinicians' answer

The interpretation of these findings was that the patient was not actually describing a lateral list, but rather a torsion of the pelvis. Normally a composite of tests is used to diagnose iliosacral or sacroiliac joint dysfunction. The tests used in this case were the comparison of various pelvic landmarks with the patient standing, and also with both the standing flexion and seated flexion tests. All of these observational pelvic tests have been shown to meet an acceptable level of reliability (NIOSH, 1988; Piva et al., 2003). The more of these tests that are positive (abnormal finding), then the more evidence there is that the patient has a pelvic obliquity (sacroiliac joint dysfunction or leg length discrepancy). Furthermore, when three out of four tests agree that there is a pelvic component to the patient's problem, the weight of the findings indicates that one can effectively and accurately intervene.

A leg length inequality will cause the appearance of a high iliac crest, ASIS and PSIS on the side ipsilateral to the long leg. A concomitant posterior rotation of the inominate (fixation at the iliosacral joint) on the same side as the long leg will cause the ipsilateral iliac crest and ASIS to appear even higher, while both PSIS may appear to be even.

2 What weighting did you give the previous diagnosis of a herniated disc? What clinical features at this stage in the examination supported and refuted this explanation?

▮ Clinicians' answer

Not much weight was given to the herniated disc diagnosis provided by the orthopaedic surgeon. A central disc herniation would be the only possible logical explanation for the bilateral symptoms. Notably, the behaviour of the symptoms was not consistent with this diagnosis. The patient complained of night pain while recumbent, a finding inconsistent with a disc herniation. Recumbency will usually provide some relief from symptoms, as the spine is unloaded. In addition, the patient's constant 2/10 pain rating suggested that the symptoms were not significantly affected by any position or movement. A patient suffering from a disc herniation will likely report radiation of symptoms with sagittal plane motion; however, this patient's symptoms were generally constant (although the symptoms were slightly worsened in a flexed or sitting posture). It is also not consistent with a disc herniation that no position was reported that afforded any significant relief. Usually a patient whose symptoms are caused by a disc herniation can find some position of comfort, or some mechanical bias to the behaviour of the symptoms. The findings of negative SLR testing and myotomal examination, in addition to pain-free and full active range of motion of the lumbar spine, also tended to refute this hypothesis.

3 Did the physical examination provide any further information to support or refute your primary diagnostic hypothesis of lumbar instability?

▮ Clinicians' answer

Some further supporting evidence for the lumbar instability hypothesis was provided by the presence of trunk deviation during forward bending.

However, several other findings tended to negate this hypothesis:

■ the lack of general muscle flexibility (limitations of SLR and FABER test motion)
■ normal lumbopelvic rhythm with forward bending
■ the lack of joint movement with posteroanterior mobility testing of vertebrae.

4 Measurement of chest expansion is not normally a routine part of a lumbar spine examination. What was the specific reason(s) that prompted you to measure chest expansion in this case?

■ Clinicians' answer

A reasonable degree of suspicion of *ankylosing spondylitis* led to the decision to measure the patient's chest expansion. It is a clinically useful test for ankylosing spondylitis because a measurement of less than 2.5 cm is 94% specific for (or likely to rule in) ankylosing spondylitis. If a patient tests positive to a test with a high specificity, it is probable he has the disease (Sackett et al., 1997). Therefore, chest expansion greater than 2.5 cm would be required for a normal test result (Rigby and Wood, 1993). The findings that raised the suspicion of ankylosing spondylitis were:

■ reported morning stiffness, alleviated by movement
■ constant 2/10 pain rating over a 24-hour period, relatively uninfluenced by movement
■ some movement was helpful, but vigorous movement (e.g. yoga) worsened the symptoms
■ bilateral hip involvement (marked decrease in bilateral hip passive range of motion, positive FABER test for decreased motion and bilateral limitation of SLR)
■ reduced vertebral mobility throughout the lumbar spine and thoracolumbar junction.

Further investigations

David was then referred for radiological investigation. The specific views requested were anteroposterior and lateral views of the lumbar spine, oblique sacroiliac joint views, and an erect anteroposterior view of the pelvis including the hip joints. This series was

5 Why did you curtail the examination at the point you did?

■ Clinicians' answer

The physical examination was ceased at this time because of an increasingly high degree of suspicion of ankylosing spondylitis. In particular, the markedly restricted chest expansion was of concern as it is a sign commonly found in patients diagnosed as having this disorder. A radiological examination was needed to help to confirm or exclude this provisional diagnosis and also to determine the extent of articular involvement (especially of the hip joints) if changes were found.

■ Clinical reasoning commentary

What led the clinicians to test specifically for ankylosing spondylitis, particularly considering that this condition is relatively uncommon and the patient had been previously examined by many other health practitioners (including medical specialists)? It would appear that the inability to 'fit' satisfactorily the various clinical findings to the more obvious mechanical diagnostic hypotheses (e.g. lumbar instability, disc herniation, pelvic joint impairment) led the clinicians to consider or 'suspect' other less frequent disorders in an attempt to explain the patient's perplexing presentation better. Although ankylosing spondylitis was not mentioned earlier in the clinical examination process as a potential mechanism/source for the symptoms, it had not been excluded either. That is, the hypothesis of ankylosing spondylitis probably rose through the ranks of hypotheses as the higher-ranked patterns/hypotheses initially generated failed to withstand testing. The clinicians have maintained an open mind and critical outlook during the examination, resisting the temptation and avoiding the reasoning error of accepting an hypothesis that may be more prevalent or favoured but which only partially explains all the clinical findings.

ordered based on a high index of suspicion of ankylosing spondylitis. Below is a synopsis of the findings detailed in the radiographic report.

Anteroposterior and lateral views of lumbar spine. Essentially a normal lumbar spine. Mild straightening of the anterior margins of the vertebral bodies is of uncertain significance. While this finding may

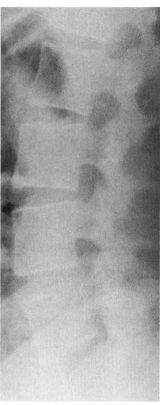

Fig. 4.3 Lateral view of the lumbar spine demonstrating mild straightening of the anterior margins of the vertebral bodies. These findings are consistent with ankylosing spondylitis.

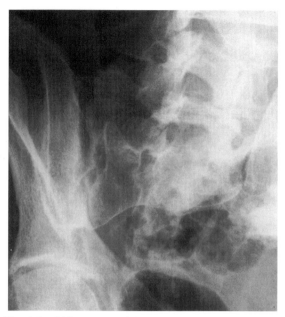

Fig. 4.4 Oblique view of the sacroiliac joint showing moderate sacroiliitis.

represent a normal variant, these changes may also be seen with early ankylosing spondylitis (Fig. 4.3).

Oblique views of sacroiliac joints. Changes are compatible with bilateral moderate sacroiliitis (Fig. 4.4).

Anteroposterior view of pelvis. Mild to moderate hip joint osteoarthritis and moderate bilateral sacroiliitis (sclerosis and joint irregularity) is evident (Fig. 4.5).

These findings led to a request for a HLA-B27 assay. The results of this test were positive for the presence of B27 antigen.

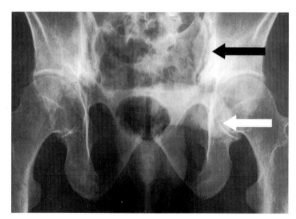

Fig. 4.5 Anteroposterior view of the pelvis showing moderate hip osteoarthritis (white arrow) and moderate sacroiliitis (black arrow).

REASONING DISCUSSION

1 Following the physical examination you were obviously suspicious of the presence of ankylosing spondylitis. Did you consider any other possible diagnoses?

■ Clinicians' answer

After the physical examination, it was almost certain the diagnosis was ankylosing spondylitis. At this point, there really was no other explanation for the patient's symptoms and patterns of movement limitation of his trunk and larger joints. The radiographs were ordered to add weight to the diagnosis and so that a referral to a rheumatologist could be made. There was no plausible competing hypothesis that could explain the results of the physical examination. Perhaps if you took a few findings from the physical examination in isolation, then you may be able to suggest some other explanations. However, if all the physical findings are considered together, along with the history and symptom behaviour, then a diagnosis of ankylosing spondylitis is strongly supported.

2 What clinical feature initially caused you to become suspicious of a systemic inflammatory disease?

 Clinicians' answer

The long history of symptoms without a precipitating event and the insidious onset of symptoms at just 17 years of age, as well as the constant nature of the symptoms, all tended to initially raise suspicions.

The patient's initial report of insidious buttock and PSIS pain also added to my suspicion, as these are common symptomatic sites for sacroiliac joint pathology. Furthermore, the patient received almost complete relief of symptoms while on oral steroids (methylprednisolone). The presence of bilateral symptoms, unprovoked by any movement and in the presence of a negative neurological examination, also increased the suspicion of a systemic cause. Additional support was provided by the bilateral loss of PROM of some large peripheral joints (hips and shoulders), the reduced mobility of vertebrae in the thoracolumbar transition region and the decreased chest expansion during inhalation.

The radiological changes added substantial support to the working hypothesis of ankylosing spondylitis. In particular, bilateral sacroiliac joint involvement (sacroiliitis) is pathognomonic for ankylosing spondylitis and is a radiological prerequisite for its diagnosis. The bilateral sclerotic changes of the hip joints in a patient of this young age also provided weight to the hypothesis, as in one-third of cases of ankylosing spondylitis there is involvement of the hip and/or shoulder joints (Koopman, 1997).

 Management

David was subsequently referred to a rheumatologist near his home. On his follow-up visit 3 weeks after commencing medical management for ankylosing spondylitis the MOQ score was 18% and his pain intensity was a constant, unvarying 1/10 on the VAS. The pain diagram remained unchanged except

that the buttock pain was no longer present. His physical examination findings were also unchanged from his initial consultation. It was decided to treat his iliosacral joint dysfunction using manipulation and a reduction of his pelvic landmarks was obtained. In other words, the pelvic obliquity was no longer present and his pelvic landmarks were now symmetrical.

REASONING DISCUSSION AND CLINICAL REASONING COMMENTARY

1 You administered a MOQ as part of your examination and following the patient's referral to a rheumatologist. What particular information were you seeking with this test and how did you use that information? Do you use it instead of asking certain questions in the subjective examination?

Clinicians' answer

The MOQ was administered in part to gather information in lieu of asking questions during the subjective examination, and in part to assess the patient's progress after being treated by the rheumatologist. A comparison of the initial and follow-up MOQ results also gave an insight into which activities were still difficult for the patient to perform and which activities were now easier. This information helped to guide the physical examination at each appointment.

2 Many practitioners would be tempted to categorize a patient with a 13-year history of LBP as beyond physical intervention and requiring psychological management. What led you to pursue a physical diagnosis despite the failure of numerous clinicians in the past?

Clinicians' answer

This patient travelled a considerable distance at his own expense and on his own initiative and presented as a straightforward patient seeking help. That is, the patient's physical limitations as found in the physical examination were consistent with his reported level of disability (as determined by the MOQ score) and with his level of distress (as indicated by his pain diagram and numerical pain score). Notably, his pain diagram, pain VAS rating and MOQ score were all reasonable. The patient's pain diagram was best described as being consistent with a nociceptive disorder, i.e. he did not complete the diagram in a non-anatomical pattern with large areas marked with multiple descriptors, as is common for the patient in psychological distress. His MOQ score was 46% and we find that most patients in psychological distress will have a score of 70% or higher. Finally, his pain VAS rating matched his demeanour and apparent level of distress. Usually patients in psychological distress will claim a pain level of 9–10/10 and yet be in no obvious cardiovascular distress, with normal heart and breathing rates evident.

In the end, this patient could be diagnosed. Perhaps it took time for his pattern of limited motion to emerge to the point where it was recognizable. It is likely, however, that in the past this patient offered clues as to his underlying condition that went unnoticed.

Clinical reasoning commentary

Two particularly important aspects of the reasoning illustrated throughout this case are the use of screening questions and the combined application of patient questioning and questionnaires to acquire information. Screening questions were used to obtain a full picture of the patient's symptoms, behaviour of symptoms, history, possible non-musculoskeletal sources and potential psychosocial factors. While patients will volunteer what they feel to be important, it is critical that manual therapists then screen further in order to gain a complete understanding of the person's pain experience. In this case, questions regarding precautions and contraindications to physical examination and physical treatment (i.e. red flags suggestive of sinister pathology) were essential. Similarly, screening for yellow, blue and black flags, as discussed in Chapter 1, are important to identify aspects in the patient's presentation that may represent obstacles to recovery, either as a manifestation of a central pain component or highlighting that the patient may be at risk of developing chronic pain.

References

Delitto, A., Erhard, R.E. and Bowling, R.W. (1995). A treatment-based approach to low back syndrome: identifying and staging patients for conservative treatment. Physical Therapy, 75, 470–489.

Fairbanks, J.C.T., Cooper, J., Davies, J.G. et al. (1980). The Oswestry low back pain disability questionnaire. Physiotherapy, 66, 271–273.

Hudson-Cook, N., Tomes-Nicholson, K. and Breen, A. (1989). A revised Oswestry disability questionnaire. In Back Pain: New Approaches to Rehabilitation and Education (M.D. Roland and J.R. Jenner, eds.)

pp. 187–204. Manchester, UK: Manchester University Press.

Koopman, W.J. (1997). Arthritis and Allied Conditions: A Textbook of Rheumatology, 13th edn, Vol. I. London: Williams &Wilkins.

Margolis, R.B., Tail, R.C. and Krause, S.J. (1986). A rating system for use with patient pain drawings. Pain, 24, 57–65.

NIOSH (1988). Low Back Atlas of Standardized Tests and Measurements. Washington, DC: US Department of Health and Human Service, Center for Disease Control, National Institute for Occupational Safety and Health.

Piva, S.R., Erhard, R.E., Childs, J.D. and Hicks, G. (2003). Reliability of measuring iliac crest height in the standing and sitting position using a new measurement device. Journal of Manipulative and Physiological Therapeutics, in press.

Rigby, A.S. and Wood, P.H.N. (1993). Observations on diagnostic criteria for ankylosing spondylitis. Clinical and Experimental Rheumatology, 11, 5–12.

Sackett, D.L., Richardson, S.W., Rosenberg, W. and Haynes, B.R. (1997). Evidence-based Medicine: How to Practice and Teach EBM. Edinburgh: Churchill Livingstone.

Unnecessary fear avoidance and physical incapacity in a 55-year-old housewife

Louis Gifford

 SUBJECTIVE EXAMINATION

Lara is a well-preserved 55-year-old woman. She is married to Raymond, who is an architect, and they have one son who is a general practitioner. They are well off and have a lovely home in a very pleasant region of rural England.

Lara has a chronic pain problem relating to her back and legs, but in particular to her feet. She has pain in both feet, but also pain and dysaesthesia in both legs, and pain in her right groin, buttock and in the middle of her back (Fig. 5.1). She also has intermittent problems

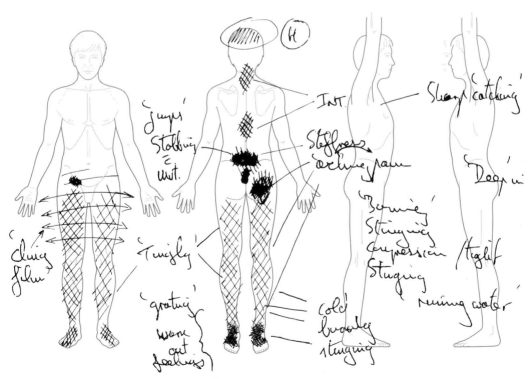

Fig. 5.1 Body chart illustrating the patient's symptoms.

in the low thoracic region and at the base of her neck, and she frequently gets headaches.

Lara came 200 miles to see me. She was recommended to me by two physiotherapists who had been working with her. She was pleasant on the phone and said that she was desperate. I interviewed, examined and began her management in two sessions spread over 2 days. The first session, which was entirely interview, took 2 hours, while the second lasted about 1.5 hours.

 ## REASONING DISCUSSION AND CLINICAL REASONING COMMENTARY

1 You decided to spend the full 2 hours of your first appointment entirely on interviewing this lady; this clearly indicates the importance you place on this initial session and on the information you will obtain. Could you briefly outline the broad aims of your initial interview and how you use this information to guide your subsequent physical examination and management.

Clinician's answer

There is no doubt that complex long-standing problems take time to understand fully. The broader more biopsychosocial approach that is taken here requires a full appreciation of patients' problems and the way in which their problems have affected them and those around them. Interview, and discussion during interview, is also a very powerful and important part of the management process. It provides the information base that dictates the best direction in which to proceed and it reassures the patient that I understand the problems that they are facing, as well as the nature of the presentation. There were several key aspects to the initial interview.

- To find out about her situation now compared with how it had been before the problem started. In particular, to find out how much she does physically in comparison to the situation previously. This gives an understanding of her disability level and some idea of shorter and longer-term goals.
- To find out what she feels is wrong, what the pain means to her, and what she feels about the future.
- I also needed to find out about her expectations of me and what she was expecting from our sessions. Much insight is gained here with discussion of previous treatments and investigations, treatment effectiveness, and how messages and information given have been interpreted.
- I needed to feel comfortable that no serious condition was present that would be more appropriately managed within or alongside some form of medical

intervention. Information here may lead to appropriate physical testing later.
- I wanted to get enough information so that together we would be able to plan a way forward.
- I needed enough information about her symptoms to be able to understand her problem in terms of pain mechanisms and all the current physical and any 'emotional/cognitive/psychological' issues relating to the problem.
- It is necessary to have a full appreciation of all psychosocial factors that may impede management.

2 With respect to your aim to ensure that no serious condition was present, were you concerned/worried at this stage that her bilateral lower limb symptoms could reflect spinal cord involvement?

Clinician's answer

Not really, although it is always a possibility and should always be entertained in every patient. Important 'special questions' and physical/neurological tests should never be left out, however confident one feels. The reason for my confidence here is threefold. First, patients with chronic pain like Lara have usually been seen by many doctors and specialists and have often been thoroughly biomedically screened already. Secondly, if there was significant spinal cord involvement, clues should be picked up during history taking. Thirdly, bilateral lower limb pain is not uncommon in many chronic pain states and may be a reflection of central processing/central mechanism factors rather than gross or frank cord pathology.

Clinical reasoning commentary

The clinician's account of the 'broader more biopsychosocial approach' he takes with this sort of complex, long-standing problem is consistent with what Mattingly (1991) has described in the clinical reasoning literature as attending to the patient's 'illness experience'. As discussed in Chapter 1, a patient's illness experience, or what is synonymously described as 'pain experience' in the pain science literature, refers to the effects patients' problems have on them, and those around them, psychosocially. Understanding the context, also called 'narrative reasoning' (Fleming and Mattingly, 2000; Jones et al., 2002), requires attempting to understand the patient as a person, including their perspective of the problem (e.g. understanding, beliefs, desires, motivations, emotions, etc.), the basis of their perspective, and how the problem is affecting their life. Understanding the person, in addition to the problem, as identified by the clinician as a key aim of his interview assessment, is increasingly being recognized as a significant variable influencing patient outcomes (Borkan et al., 1991; Feuerstein and Beattie, 1995; Lackner et al., 1996;

Main et al., 2000; Malt and Olafson, 1995; Strong, 1995; Watson, 2000).

The clinician's reference to screening for potential serious conditions (i.e. precautions and contraindications) and attempting to understand the patient's symptoms in terms of pain mechanisms (i.e. pathobiological mechanisms) reveals a structure to his knowledge and thinking consistent with the hypothesis categories discussed in Chapter 1. This is not surprising given he has personally contributed to the development of these categories (Gifford, 1997; Gifford and Butler, 1997), but it also highlights how a framework, as provided by categories of hypotheses, can assist in organizing one's knowledge and guiding examination and reasoning. The clinician's aim of gaining sufficient information 'so that together we would be able to plan a way forward' is testimonial to the 'collaborative reasoning' approach to his assessment and management.

Initial assessment interview

Lara's husband accompanied her for every session. She met me with a smile, but she moved very stiffly and sighed easily. She sat bolt upright, back in extension, knees at right angles and together, and her hands rested on her thighs in a very symmetrical and stylized way.

The history of Lara's problem can be summarized as follows.

1. About 5 years ago, she had a fairly nasty low back problem, which she was told by her physiotherapist was a disc condition. There was no history of any injuring incident and in the past she had only suffered minor, odd back pains that lasted for a few days. This episode recovered with repeated extension exercises in one week. I asked Lara if she went back to 'normal' activities after this and she replied: 'The therapist helped me understand about fluid movement inside the disc and that bending pushed the fluid backwards and made the disc bulge towards my nerves. She also taught me good posture to prevent this happening. As a result all the pain went, but in order to be careful of the fluid I stopped most of the gardening and have always been very careful with any back bending.'

2. Eight months later, Lara had a hysterectomy and colposuspension (remodelling of the vagina) operation. She had complained of some urinary leakage prior to this operation and noted that the back pain

was markedly worse following it. She regretted ever having the surgery and her husband added that he believed that her problems really stemmed from the operation. He was notably disgruntled about it. She recalled that her low back was agony at the time of the operation, but that it 'more or less' cleared up once she got moving afterwards.

3. After a further 8 months, Lara's back pain returned, again for no apparent reason. This time the pain had increased its area to include the low right buttock. The physiotherapist told her that the bulge was likely to have increased and was starting to irritate the sciatic nerve. She said that the therapist went through all the postural and movement 'dos and don'ts' and some similar previous exercises. As well as giving the exercises, the therapist treated her using 'pressures on the back' and ultrasound. She remembers often feeling very stiff getting off the couch after treatment and that the exercises often left a lingering pain further down her right leg. After 10 treatments over 6 weeks, treatment stopped. She recalled the physiotherapist saying that the disc would be healed and that further treatment was unnecessary. I asked Lara if she had felt better, to which she said. 'To be honest, I felt quite depressed; my movements were better but my pain was much the same and I had some new rather odd feelings in my right thigh and calf, which I was also starting to feel in my other leg. The overall intensity of the pain was perhaps

slightly less, but I was getting worried and it was starting to really trouble me at night.'

4. Lara was advised to see a local chiropractor by a close friend. She was diagnosed as having four major contributory problems. These were described as facial distortion ('some sort of jaw distortion'), C2 fixed in a left rotated position, unequal leg and arm lengths and what the chiropractor described as the worst sacroiliac (SI) blocking he had ever seen. I asked Lara how she had felt about that? She said, 'I remember feeling pleased to start with, that he had found something, he seemed very confident that it would all be put right very easily. Later on I started to dread going, when I think about it now I felt that he started to make me feel that the lack of progress was my fault. I also started to worry that the things he said were wrong, were impossible to overcome. By the end I got worse and stopped going.' Treatment involved a series of regular but very quick adjustments to her head and neck and some 'pressing on the roof of her mouth'. Lara was warned to stop all swimming so as not to upset her SI joint: 'He told me to stop the physiotherapy exercises and concentrate on my neck posture.'

5. A further 4 months later, Lara's doctor referred her to an orthopaedic consultant after radiographs revealed modest degenerative changes. 'He said that I had normal wear and tear on the X-rays but there was the possibility of spinal stenosis. I had a scan that revealed moderate disc bulging at L5–S1 and no significant stenosis.' What happened from there? Lara said, 'I remember feeling very empty, very tearful and almost embarrassed to start with. He made me feel as if I was making it up, I remember the comment he made, "you've got the same back as everyone else of your age on this earth", and then he said, "the best thing you can do is 100 sit ups a day and go swimming". About a week later, I started to feel very angry that I hadn't been believed, but even my husband seemed to side with his view—when he came in from work his first words were usually, "have you done your sit-ups?".'

6. Through the next few months, Lara's doctor treated her for mild depressive disorder with amitriptyline (tricyclic antidepressant). She was also given 'painkillers' (ibuprofen: non-steroidal anti-inflammatory agent) and co-proxamol (dextropropoxyphene hydrochloride plus paracetamol: compound opiate analgesic).

7. Within a couple of months, Lara started to suffer from stiffness in the back of the thighs on bending. She also had low back pain, buttock pain and lumbar stiffness. In desperation, she returned to her physiotherapist, who concentrated on the disc bulge. She had eight traction treatments, which helped to start with, but pain soon returned. In addition, she was given a corset to wear all the time. Lara could not remember any exercises being given that were not stopped because of exacerbation of the pain.

8. She returned to the chiropractor, who 'cracked' her neck and adjusted her SI joint. After four treatments and progressively worsening pain, the chiropractor referred her back to her GP, who organized an appointment with the local rheumatologist.

9. Lara saw the rheumatologist 2 months later. By now she was only walking around the house, rarely went out of doors and had stopped all social engagements. Her doctor son was keen for her to see a psychiatrist. 'I was starting to think that I had something that no one else in the world had ever experienced, and that because it was so new and nothing could be found to reasonably explain it, the only rational way for doctors to see me was in terms of some kind of madness! Even my son was seeing me as a mental case. The rheumatologist said that I was "atypical" and that I did not have any joint rheumatism. He actually took me seriously, listened and arranged for some blood tests. Once the results came through negative, he referred me to the local pain clinic. Here, I was given acupuncture and TENS (transcutaneous electrical nerve stimulation). After three treatments, I had terrible pains in the balls of my feet, which the physiotherapist said was a good thing! But the pains got worse and worse and she then referred me to hydrotherapy. She said that I had tight nerves that need moving and stretching.'

10. The hydrotherapy was the first step towards some improvement; Lara enjoyed the movement in the pool and the pain was masked by the warmth. She said she felt very safe moving in the pool and after 4–5 weeks found that she was able to do some simple back exercises lying down at home. She made further gains using the Alexander technique (Barlow, 1981).

11. She continued through early the following year 'managing' reasonably well and even getting to

about 70% of normal for several months. Lara continued with physiotherapy and the Alexander technique. Physiotherapy she described as 'lying on my tummy for 20 minutes while she loosened me, then some stretches to my legs and ultrasound on my feet. I had four major exercises. Tightening my stomach for 5 seconds ten times three times a day, then the same but also tightening my buttocks at the same time, holding this tension and arching and flattening my back 1 cm while I was sitting, and then lying on the floor and stretching my leg up the door frame. The main message was that my back was unstable and that muscle tone had to be increased to prevent it slipping out of place. I was also instructed to never bend without tightening my stomach.'

12. Five months later Lara suffered a severe setback in pain and also had treatment for depression again.

13. Lara was referred to a neurosurgeon 2 months later, who offered to do a sympathectomy. Her comment was: 'How can I go ahead with an operation when the man I saw didn't even examine me, peered at my notes, scans and X-rays, asked two questions about my cold feet and said that my only chance was to have an operation that cut nerves to improve my leg circulation?'

REASONING DISCUSSION AND CLINICAL REASONING COMMENTARY

1 What were your thoughts regarding the history of Lara's problems? Include your thoughts on the previous management.

Clinician's answer

If you really follow what happened over time, it is an unfolding story of disastrous management that sequentially reinforced the notion of structural weakness and abnormality and fear of further damage; this resulted in progressive disability with psychological distress and depressive symptoms. All practitioners have been very structurally based in their thinking and have made no attempt to understand or take on board the patient's thoughts, beliefs, attributions and feelings regarding the nature of the problem. Little has been done to allay Lara's fears and rehabilitate her back to a fuller potential with increased physical confidence. Therapists appeared satisfied that pain relief was an adequate outcome. Also, common to many similar patients, doctors dismissed the problem as trivial and inferred mental weakness on the patient's part, with the unhelpful end result being the conclusion that the patient has a psychiatric disorder. It is worth noting that the therapists/doctors who have treated Lara to date have created:

■ an obsession with upright posture: partially responsible for creating unrealistic avoidance and structural fear, or behaviour patterns caused by the fear created by therapy

■ fear avoidance beliefs and behaviour, created disability/loss of confidence; this is the result of most therapists using a 'weak/vulnerable structure' focus and not helping the patient actively and gradually to restore confidence in spinal movement and back strength alongside their treatments

■ an unnatural overfocus on the body during movements; instructions like 'never to bend without tightening the stomach' reinforces structural weakness perception, movement avoidance, and tension with movement. Normal movement should eventually be trained to be thoughtless movement but pain-focused treatment reinforces a 'back off' movement strategy

■ confusion and conflicting information: doctors and other clinicians have been adopting a blinkered view of the problem specific to their area of interest.

2 Specifically please comment on the key activity/participation restrictions and associated impairments you hypothesized would need to be addressed and the dominant pathobiological pain mechanism pattern you felt was emerging.

In the 'psychological/mental' impairments hypothesis category, it is clear that Lara is upset, unhappy, distressed, frustrated, and possibly even angry. There are also many very unhelpful beliefs and attributions about structure and cause that will need to be addressed and overcome before a gradual functional improvement approach can be started (especially those relating to bending). A thorough examination and careful explanation of pain mechanisms would be a useful start in the process. Highlighting structural integrity and soundness following examination would be important. It is likely that Lara will have altered movement patterns and significant apprehension performing many movements. A great deal of tissue testing is likely to find widespread abnormality. In particular, lumbar flexion and lumbar flexion activities may need careful addressing.

It would be unwise to try and be specific about the pain mechanism(s) in view of the chronicity of pain, the consequent neuroplastic changes in nervous system input, processing and output pathways/networks, the weak and deconditioned tissues, possible minor or moderate degeneration, lack of normal movement patterns and the psychological and social consequences of the whole episode. A single lesion approach to well-established chronic pain states like this one has to be, at best, extremely cautious. A broader biopsychosocial model that incorporates multidimensional and multi-level thinking for assessment and management is probably the most desirable option (Gifford, 2000a, 2001, 2002a; Main and Spanswick, 2000; Waddell, 1998). Importantly, this does not preclude focussing on specific physical impairments at some time in the management process.

Allocating a specific pain mechanism in this type of patient is probably detrimental in that it makes thoughts linger in a focussed way and misses a far bigger picture. A shift in focus to disability (i.e. activity and participation restriction) management is probably the singularly most important issue. Clearly though, altered, or maladaptive, central processing of sensory and motor information, central generation of pain, maintained peripheral sensitivity, peripheral nerve hypersensitivity and all output mechanisms have a role in presentations of this type. The message is that there is no specific single source targetable by passive therapy interventions. By working on the patient's thoughts and beliefs, alongside graded return of physical function and confidence, we will actually be working and manipulating neural pathways responsible for the pain and disability problem (Gifford, 2000b). A key thought is that inputs that improve things like self-efficacy, patient sense of control and understanding, levels of distress, physical function and goal achievement will have positive neuroplastic effects that will have repercussions for the health of the whole organism (see Gifford, 2002b; Lawes, 2002; Roche, 2002).

◼ Clinical reasoning commentary

A key aspect of expert reasoning we wish to draw readers' attention to here is the clear illustration of the clinician's thinking occurring on multiple levels. Recognizing apparent psychological components, activity restrictions and physical impairments within a broader picture of overlapping pain mechanisms has provided a basis on which management strategies are already being formulated. Despite the emerging pattern, the patient's problem has not been pigeon-holed into a scenario where the pain and physical impairment are seen to be completely driven by the psychosocial issues. Rather, management of specific physical impairments is hypothesized as possibly being required, and the facilitation of 'thoughtless' normal movement, consistent with motor control retraining philosophies featured in other cases in this book, is seen as important in the overall management.

Also note here, and throughout the case, the clinician uses quotations from the patient extensively. This reflects how much he listens to the patient and the importance he places on the patient's thoughts and feelings about their problems.

Lara first saw me the following month. The following summarizes the current situation and other pertinent information to her condition.

Family history

Father fine, mother diagnosed as having spinal stenosis in last 2 years (86 years old). Mother always grumbled about her back and never did any lifting. She also never did any walking or kept fit. Lara has a brother 63 years old, very inactive with a long-standing bad back.

Symptoms

Lara is constantly aware of symptoms (Fig. 5.1). These rate on the Numerical Rating Scale (NRS) as 8–9 on average; 6 at best and 10+ at worst. The main problem is with the feet and back. Symptoms are described as burning, stinging, flickers, tightness or compression feeling, and cold discomfort. Lara describes being able to hear her feet grating and has the feeling that something inside was stuck and would not move. She describes her feet as having burning pain yet feeling cold. The back produces sharp stabbing pains all the time when she moves.

Her legs feel tingly and coated in cling film from groin to lower one third of thigh. There are odd sensations in her legs: flickering, moving, wriggling, stinging nettles and running water sensations. All sensations are deep, not in the skin. There is no segmental pattern; the symptoms are deep and diffuse throughout the whole leg. The low back was a constant problem and now the right SI joint area 'jumps' and often feels weak. The pain frequently moves. She often gets pain in the coccyx region and has a sharp catching pain in the right buttock. She also has right groin pain and when groin is better, the buttock is worse. Lara does not complaint of loss of sensation.

REASONING DISCUSSION AND CLINICAL REASONING COMMENTARY

1 Lara's body chart and this list of symptoms presents a rather daunting picture. Could you highlight your thoughts at this stage? What did you consider were the key features in the body chart and was there any further support for your earlier hypothesis regarding the dominant pain mechanism?

Clinician's answer

The body chart (Fig. 5.1) clearly shows that Lara's symptoms are complex, widespread, non-segmental, and not at all typical of common acute and subacute presentations. The body chart presentation reinforces the earlier interpretations with regard to multiple mechanisms and sources (relating to input processing and output) and the importance of maladaptive neuroplastic change (central mechanisms). My main thoughts were that the only form of helpful management would be if I could successfully restructure this lady's understanding of her problem and the potential of therapy to help/not help; then I may be successful in helping her to move on.

2 Given this sort of presentation, how specific were you prepared to be regarding possible sources of her symptoms at this stage?

Clinician's answer

The key here I believe is thinking in terms of multiple tissues and at multiple levels throughout, but with the central nervous system as the main player. Being specific, with our current state of knowledge, is likely to be detrimental to a multidimensional approach and is unrealistic. The very complexity of the presentation is enough to determine that, rather than try to grapple with hypotheses about specific 'sources' of symptoms, a more productive approach would be achieved by investigating, understanding and addressing the relevant activity restrictions/disabilities/impairments. Some of the 'clues' that lead to these conclusions include the chronicity of the problem, the lack of success with interventions so far, the widespread and variable symptom distribution, and the many descriptive terms used. A final comment here is that it is probably far more productive to think in terms of sources of disability/activity restriction/impairment rather than sources of symptoms. This shifts thinking towards what can productively be improved rather than what needs to be 'fixed'.

Clinical reasoning commentary

The clinician raises an important point regarding the use of hypothesis categories. By virtue of being provided with a list of hypothesis categories to be considered when examining and managing patients, it is common for therapists to proceed and attempt to think through all hypothesis categories from the start with every patient. This is not only cognitively too demanding and hence unrealistic, as pointed out here, it also can be detrimental to understanding some patients' problems. Prematurely focussing on specific structures often occurs at the expense of gaining a broader picture of the patient and his/her problems. There are, of course, no strict guidelines that can be recommended for when specific structures should be hypothesized. Patient clues suggesting serious or sinister pathology must be recognized and immediately followed up. However, beyond that, the clinician has provided useful suggestions for when specific hypotheses regarding sources of the symptoms are less useful.

Even in nociceptively dominant problems, successful management will usually come more from treatment directed to specific function-related impairments rather than specific tissues. Therapists rarely have their hypotheses regarding sources validated and often make the reasoning error of interpreting patient improvement as substantiating the source. However, knowledge of common clinical patterns for specific structures can in many cases assist enormously the recognition of the problem, whether physiotherapy is indicated, and if so what type of management is likely to be helpful. The application of thorough assessment and balanced reasoning, wherein identified impairments are considered within the broader picture of pathobiological mechanisms, and in conjunction with known and hypothesized pathology, will enable therapists to deliver effective management while continuing to improve their understanding and expand, and eventually validate, their clinical impressions.

Behaviour of symptoms

The main ways the symptoms occur are:

- standing still causes burning/tightness in the feet, which quickly builds in intensity; it is eased by taking shoes off; 'releases immediately'
- sitting also relieves the feet symptoms quickly but it increases the back and thigh pain, making her quickly restless
- the low back and buttock symptoms increase with sitting and Lara becomes very sore or 'raw' inside; the pain, when severe is tender to touch; maximum sitting tolerance is 20–30 minutes
- never really free of symptoms: they are constant; if they do go it is only for seconds
- back pain is there all the time as a background aching but when moving gives sharp jabs all the time
- cold feet feeling improves with fast walking but walking makes pain worse afterwards
- all symptoms aggravated by movement
- shopping in local supermarket consistently aggravates the pain in the feet so avoids shopping as much as possible (tried changing shoes, adding pads in shoes and different corsets—all with modest success for a short time, but now nothing helping)
- when pain increases in feet and legs, the coldness gets worse
- the colour of the skin of her lower legs and feet change from a blotchy/purple to a deep red when going from sitting to standing
- night time results in some problems lying on back, with tail pain, and side lying is best; occasionally wakes aware of pain but always manages to get back to sleep
- poor sleeper without medication
- copes best in the morning
- evenings are horrid and ends up lying semisupine on couch
- best when half asleep
- has noticed that symptoms are worse when she is 'uptight'.

Current activity levels

Lara's current activity levels can be summarized as:

- swims once a week: manages gentle walking in the pool and about one width in total by swimming on her back
- walks 1 mile once a week if she can and walks through the pain, which spreads to toes and settles; the whole leg becomes painful when she stops and it is usually all stirred up for 3–4 days, with a level of pain that forces her to rest off her feet most of the following day
- maximum walking time is 40 minutes; prefers fast walking
- used to be very busy but describes herself now as 90% less active than prior to the problem being severe; for example, she could easily walk 5–6 miles, swim 20–30 lengths and carry all her shopping bags with no problems
- spends an average of 4–5 hours doing very little during the day, mainly shifting from sitting to lying interspersed with small household activities
- most of her life is spent inside and at home; she used to be 'out and about' all the time
- occasionally does all the housework in a morning out of frustration but pays for it for several days afterwards
- has given all hobbies up; these were gardening (regular), flower arranging, voluntary work, painting flowers and embroidery (earlier in the year she had

managed some pottering about in the garden but she had not done any flower arranging for 2 years)

- has not been on holiday since the problem started because of fear of the problem worsening and wishing she had stayed at home
- has not cooked a meal for other than her husband or been out for a meal for 2 years (previously she had been very sociable, often giving dinner parties and going out with friends).

Any form of concentration has made the problem worse and makes her very frustrated and upset. When asked why she had stopped so much, Lara said that she had a fear of doing more damage, creating more pain, and of something giving or going, with days of resting afterwards. She said she felt weak; activities made her limbs feel heavy and she got very tired very easily.

REASONING DISCUSSION AND CLINICAL REASONING COMMENTARY

1 There is a certain degree of stimulus–response predictability that is apparent in the behaviour of her symptoms. In your previous answers, you noted that you felt there was strong evidence emerging supporting a dominant processing pain mechanism in her presentation; however, elsewhere (Gifford and Butler, 1997) you have described a common feature of the nociceptive pain mechanism pattern is its stimulus–response predictability. Can you comment on what features of this lady's presentation alter the relevance of the stimulus–response predictability that is apparent in her presentation?

■ Clinician's answer

A degree of predictability in symptom response to mechanical stress is common to a great many pain states: it is just as easy to increase and decrease symptoms instantaneously using physical forces and movements in an acute injury as it is in chronic pain states. 'Processing', along with cognitive, emotional and behavioural responses, are still a feature of all pain, even presentations that are acute and deemed largely nociceptive in nature. However, in the more chronic state, inputs that produce a pain response may be coming from quite normal tissues as well as from tissues that are in various states of 'ill-health'—many of which presumably contain maladaptively sensitized and hence over-reactive nociceptors. Further, and central to chronic pain states, is the fact that the pain 'reaction' to physical inputs is often way out of proportion to what might be 'needed' by the tissues. In Lara's case, features that tend to discourage any thoughts with regard to major nociceptive mechanisms (for which the stimulus–response pattern is more in

keeping with the extent of tissue pathology) are the length of time the problem has been around, the severity and reactivity of the symptoms, and the lack of medical evidence for significant enough pathology. One would expect less reactivity perhaps from a severe rheumatoid arthritis presentation. It might be best to reason that Lara has a great deal of maladaptive nociception going on and maladaptive processing of nociceptive traffic in the central nervous system as well. Clinically this equates to too much pain and sensitivity for the state of the tissues: hurt does not mean harm.

2 Has any of this new information elicited any new thoughts/hypotheses regarding other pain mechanisms or sources?

■ Clinician's answer

Not really. There are some features that might elicit thoughts relating to circulation or even aberrant sympathetic activity: like the cold feet/legs and skin colour changes. Hence, one line of thought could be: maladaptive central processing leads to altered and inappropriate outputs, which, in turn, lead to sensory inputs and more sensations. Another side of the issue is that symptoms like alterations in temperature and blotchy skin may well represent reactions of a very unfit and deconditioned body and are hardly surprising. Also, there is the likelihood that Lara's attention system has become conditioned to focus on bodily sensations, thus changes in temperature may be going on normally but, as a result of the maladaptive bias in attention towards her soma, she has become greatly aware of them. These types of interpretation are 'better for the patient' because the message that comes across is that improved function and fitness, decreased body-related worry and attention and more physical confidence may help to overcome some of these symptoms and sensations. Allocating blame on the sympathetic nervous system or the circulation, immediately 'medicalizes' the findings and presents the patient with a problem that has no natural or guaranteed medical solution—presenting them with yet another source of worry and frustration.

3 Some features of her presentation, such as her coping best in the morning, frequent sharp jabs of pain and even her preference for walking fast, could be interpreted as support for a 'postural' or muscle control problem. Do you feel this impairment could be a component of her problem, either as a possible predisposing factor to the original onset and/or as a contributing factor to the maintenance of her symptoms? Could any 'motor control' impairment that may be present be a manifestation of her altered input–output mechanisms, that is a learned phenomenon with implications as to whether and how this should be addressed in her management?

Clinician's answer

This is a good point because it really highlights the dangers of focussing on a single 'dominant' pain mechanism. While central-processing issues are so important here, it is foolhardy to deny any input/sensory/nociceptive-related mechanisms. Tissues may be unfit, deconditioned, shortened, degenerate, prone to ischaemic effects, have scar tissues, perhaps even have a modest inflammatory component, etc. All these factors may produce a sensory barrage enough to maintain sufficient central activity to affect pain awareness.

An important point is that a 'muscle control problem' is not a direct pain mechanism, rather it is an impairment that in some circumstances may influence the sensory system. There are a great many of us with huge muscle control/weakness/imbalance problems who have no pain at all. However, in a weakened or vulnerable organism (Lara), minor impairments, like those relating to muscle control, poor muscle power or endurance properties, may be enough to play a part in maintaining hypersensitivity. It seems likely to me that the sensory nerves and pathways relevant to vulnerable tissues may somehow perceive that they have little

protection from related muscle systems and hence maintain their sensitivity to a high degree. Stronger and more efficient muscles, in parallel with increased patient 'physical confidence', may provide a sufficient environment for a sensitized tissue or sensory system to dampen down its hypersensitivity.

Dangers come when clinicians see an altered muscle control finding as key or central to this kind of problem. This is just a small hypothesis with regard to the 'bio' part of the assessment and needs to be attached very strongly to the 'psychosocial' part. I would be very wary of overfocussing on specific 'muscle control' issues in the early stages of patients like Lara.

You ask about thoughts regarding a learnt response. The answer is very much so. Pain alters movement patterns, so does fear of injury and fear of pain and loss of physical confidence. For most patients with chronic pain, these are long-standing features that result in chronically altered movement patterns, which become 'set' as new habits and for many start to feel normal. The secondary consequences to all the musculoskeletal tissues and the circuitry of movement must be vast. Thoughts like this highlight the need for reduction of fear of movement and structural weakness, and the adoption of adequate but graduated normal functional movement patterns from early on. Clearly for Lara, an essential part of her programme should involve normal movement patterns and normal recruitment. However, I would warn again about being overspecific and too focussed/complicated early in the management with a patient like Lara.

The following points are important alternative hypotheses.

■ Sharp jabs of pain can be interpreted as 'neurogenic'. For example, ectopic impulse-generating sites in sensory neurons can spontaneously discharge and, therefore, have the potential to cause a sharp jab of pain. Ectopic impulse-generating sites can also be highly mechanically sensitive; hence small movements produce massive electrical discharges and consequently sharp pain.

■ Coping best in the morning may relate to deconditioning; in the morning, the body has had some rest and may be best able to cope. Clearly muscle capacity to cope is a very likely part of this.

■ Walking fast may produce a 'gating' effect. In other words, the preoccupation with walking fast helps to inhibit sensory input relating to pain from reaching consciousness.

■ Clinical reasoning commentary

The significance of one's organization of knowledge to the clinical judgments reached is apparent throughout these answers. The knowledge of pain mechanisms and their associated clinical features, linked with the implications for management and, no doubt, prognosis, clearly underlies the clinician's views. Patient information is not interpreted in isolation but considered with respect to the broader unfolding picture that is emerging: earlier hypotheses are supported. In this way, the stimulus–response predictability common in nociceptive dominant pain states can be seen also to fit within the pattern of central sensitization described by the clinician. Specific nociceptive physical impairments are not discounted; rather the likelihood of multiple pain mechanisms is highlighted with management implications that include taking care to avoid overattention to any single physical impairment. Further, the importance of

education and explanation as an aspect of skilled clinical reasoning also stands out in the clinician's caution regarding apportioning blame to a particular structure or system with a patient where such beliefs are hypothesized to already be contributing to her problems.

The importance of re-establishing more normal movement patterns is recognized but, as with involvement of other systems, motor control is considered within the broader framework of altered central processing. Alternative interpretations for conventional clinical features of motor impairment are put forward. Clearly it is not possible to discern the precise interrelationship between the patient's altered movement patterns/muscle control and the underlying pain mechanisms within a clinical examination. However, so long as the alternatives are considered, as they are here, the manual therapist can then proceed with interventions directed at altering motor control and be guided by reassessment of the relevant outcomes.

General health and wellbeing

Her general health and wellbeing are not good:

- frequent colds and 'flu, which take much longer to shrug off than prior to problem worsening
- urinary problems still disturb her
- generally low and feels 'blue' most of the time; copes best in the mornings and is tearful on average once a week
- worries about her problem and feels very vulnerable physically
- feels her concentration and memory are not up to what they had been: 'When you do nothing you get out of practice!'.

Current pain management: treatment and medication

She uses a number of pain management methods:

- uses TENS for relief of back pain, which 'helps a little'
- hot showers and hot water bottle are 'comforting'
- takes amitryptiline 'for sleeping'; this is 'effective'
- takes co-proxamol and diclofenac (non-steroidal anti-inflammatory agent): little help but takes the edge off symptoms

- the Alexander technique audiotape has been helpful so keeps using this
- has tried visualizing pain away: not successful.

Patient understanding of problem and attributions regarding problem

Lara felt that her problem related to some weakness and instability in her back and that nerves were trapped in some way. She felt that her SI joints were still stuck and that she had pelvic torsion and leg length problems. She also thought that there was arthritis in her back, that it might be developing in her feet, and that her neck was 'weak' and vulnerable to being 'locked out'. She had no fear of sinister disease and felt that her mother was to blame for passing on her 'weaknesses'.

Coping

Generally Lara copes reasonably well, especially in the morning, but really struggles by the end of the day. Her husband and family are very supportive; however, her husband displays overly solicitous behaviour toward her, not allowing her to do much. She said that she had become far less spontaneous since the problem began: 'Normal me is in a cage; I have been so restricted physically for so long that the natural spontaneity part of me seems to have disappeared'.

Her husband added that 'she is not the same person at all; it's very sad really'.

Patient's thoughts about the future and expectations about clinician's input

Lara has come with high expectations for a cure as she has been told that I teach and write articles about 'curing' chronic pain.

Her thoughts about the future are sometimes positive; she feels it is curable and she just has to find the right therapist and therapy. Lara has been through negative phases—'I want to die'—and been through some 'bad times emotionally'.

REASONING DISCUSSION AND CLINICAL REASONING COMMENTARY

1 How has the information from the interview either supported or not supported your previous hypotheses regarding this patient's problems and the dominant pain mechanisms?

Clinician's answer

The information from these sections confirms that Lara has a number of factors contributing to her activity and participation restrictions. She is physically disabled and deconditioned; the pain mechanisms are multiple, complex and well established, and her psychological distress strongly features. It also confirms my feelings about her very passive attitude to recovery, her reliance on medical intervention, and her 'structural weakness' beliefs about the nature and cause of her pain. These findings provide much baseline information. I am starting to understand where she is now in terms of her physical and psychological health and where she would like to return, which is important with regard to short- and long-term goals, as well as providing useful starting points for discussion and action.

2 Given all the information obtained to this point, what were your thoughts regarding potential contributing factors (e.g. environmental, psychosocial, physical, biomechanical, etc.) to the development and maintenance of Lara's symptoms and activity or participation restrictions (i.e. disabilities)?

Clinician's answer

The onset of the original back episode, as in a great many patients, could not be related to any specific injuring incident. Understanding or dwelling on the original mechanism of injury may not be that helpful at this stage. It has happened; it will have had physical origins and it has now become complex and chronic. There does not appear to be anything serious biomedically at this stage, but vigilance should always be maintained. It seems that there is a family history of back pain—her mother and her brother—which should make one think in terms of 'genetic' predisposition and social learning/social modelling factors. Factors like these help us to come to terms with prognosis and help us to understand just a few possible features that contribute to the development and maintenance of a problem. It is very unhelpful to attribute blame on factors like these, for we can have little effect on familial features or the effects of the past.

As far as contributing factors in relation to maintenance of activity/participation restrictions and symptoms, a significant percentage of Lara's restrictions (i.e. disability) may be put down to the way she has been managed and the resulting beliefs and attributions she has about her problem: for instance, the images she has been given, the conflicting messages, the lack of information or interventions promoting health and function, and the lack of any convincing (to her) examination of structure. Other issues include ongoing high levels of pain that are poorly controlled, the widespread distribution of pain, ongoing and high levels of psychological distress, and a predominantly passive/avoidance coping style with low activity levels. These are all present and are known to be strong predictors of high disability and poor outcome (Watson, 2000). Her husband's understanding, beliefs and behaviours are also likely to be contributing to the maintenance of her disability/activity restrictions and participation restrictions and will need to be addressed (Newton-John, 2000).

Many of the above factors are likely to have played a major role in the maintenance of her symptoms too. Poor management leading to ongoing anxiety in relation to the problem may create a habitual focussing on pain, serving to enhance its accessibility to consciousness and further strengthen its neural representation. Deconditioning, degenerative changes or what might be termed 'physical vulnerability' must also play a part as well.

3 Given the presentation that is unfolding thus far, what are your aims for your physical examination?

Clinician's answer

Physical examination has significance for the management process, for diagnosis and for the patient. For the patient, we need to seek to reassure via a thorough examination. The patient must feel that a thorough examination has been done and that any findings have been given a reasonable explanation. It is wise always to attempt to give reassuring messages, rather than create fear. Examination is perhaps one of the most important parts of the management process; an important issue for patients like Lara is finding features that are good and highlighting them as they emerge, rather than searching out the bad and adding to the worry and confusion.

For management we need to explore the extent of physical impairment and make sense of it in relation to the type of intervention offered.

Diagnostic examination may have limited value in this type of patient with chronic pain. Clearly the clinician should always be aware of any 'red flag' features of importance. However, Lara has had plenty of medical screening tests and is, therefore, unlikely to have any serious disease process.

Examining patients like Lara, who have chronic pain and marked activity restriction, does not normally warrant any in-depth or focussed appraisal of minor impairments if a broad educational/self-management/functional recovery approach is to be adopted. Here, the early focus of examination is more on observations of function and activity restriction and perhaps some of the more blatant and relevant physical impairments, as well as patterns of illness behaviour, tension and fear in movement, and an appreciation of the extent of the problem and the degree of the deconditioned state. We basically need to know what the patient can do on their own rather than bias our investigation to more detailed findings. More specific examinations of physical impairments can sometimes be useful and relevant later in the management process. Every abnormal reaction, minor movement abnormality or loss of range is something that can be added to a list of findings that could be worked on and improved, but may not need to be. Most frequently, the restoration of confident movement patterns greatly improves or even resolves many of the physical impairments that may be noted. The primary aim is to get a disabled human being active, functional and confident again, and not to delve unnecessarily further into finding overspecific abnormalities that may be irrelevant or of little value to treatment goals—especially early on in the management process.

Clinical reasoning commentary

As discussed above, it is easy to overattend to the source of the symptoms in a classic medical diagnostic sense. While hypothesizing regarding symptom source is useful in many patient presentations, and here the clinician is increasingly more certain of a widely distributed source to much of her symptoms, identifying the contributing factors relevant to the presenting disability often will be as important, or even more important, to a successful outcome. In this case, psychosocial factors/impairments are considered the key contributing factors, although physical impairments, such as the altered motor control discussed above, may also be seen as contributing factors to the maintenance of her problems. While experience will enable therapists to recognize patterns where physical impairment is secondary to the broader psychosocial and health/fitness concerns, as is the case with this patient, prematurely discounting or not even assessing for physical impairment is as much an error as only looking for specific physical impairments without regard for the broader psychosocial and health status of the patient. That is, physical impairment can also trigger or drive psychosocial problems, and differentiation of the relevance of each is best made through thorough assessment, intervention and reassessment of both physical/functional and psychosocial outcomes.

An important aspect of skilled clinical reasoning, which is nicely highlighted here, is the clinician's incorporation of management within the actual examination. By 'finding features that are good and highlighting them as they emerge', the dynamic nature of the clinician's reasoning is evident. Clinical reasoning does not occur as a series of set steps. Rather, it is a fluid, evolving process where hypotheses are continually being reappraised.

Management is not reserved until some set point when all information has been obtained; instead it commences with the initial introductions, especially through the rapport that is established and the interest that is shown, and continues with the ongoing explanations and education that are provided.

PHYSICAL EXAMINATION

Movement analysis and testing is not a silent or totally therapist dominant affair. All the time I am asking the patient what they think about the quality, range or particular strength of a movement or test. In these types of presentation, as well as observing the poor quality of many movements, I also make a point of looking for good quality or relaxed movements and may positively reinforce what I observe, thus beginning a forward moving therapeutic process. Most examinations that these patients have had point out the abnormal findings, thus adding to their already negative state. It is useful to hear what the patient thinks in relation to your thoughts, and it is important to involve them in the process of analysis—something that has usually been denied them (Shorland, 1998).

Initial observations and functional observations

Lara sat very upright, knees together and very symmetrically poised. She looked tense and she moved very stiffly and winced going to sit and stand. She kept very still at first and talked very clearly in a slow and monotonous voice.

Before asking her to undress, I asked Lara to walk several times the length of the clinic corridor and to go up and down some steps. She walked with a relatively slow, but normal gait. Walking was recorded as 43 seconds to do four lengths of the corridor (the corridor is about 9 metres long and four lengths at a reasonably normal walking pace takes about 20 seconds). She managed the steps with great effort; she regularly winced and held herself.

She could get into the upright kneeling position with difficulty but was unwilling to go onto all fours or get down onto the floor. She could not walk on tip-toes and was very unsteady walking backwards.

Lara's husband helped her a lot in undressing. Lara avoided all bending, groaned a great deal and held her back when it hurt.

Her standing posture looked fine: leg length looked equal with no obvious major distortion or shift. There was no evidence of marked muscle wasting in any one individual group. Her balance on either leg was poor.

Physical goals

Several physical goals could be listed at this stage:

- relaxed sitting and moving, especially getting out of a chair, gait and negotiating stairs
- relaxed and faster/more normal walking pace
- improve confidence and find a 'physical pathway' or a series of graded exercises or activities to facilitate tip-toe walking, backward walking, kneeling on all fours and getting onto the floor
- independent dressing/undressing, independence from husband (he needs to be included in understanding pain and suggested process of rehabilitation)
- reducing groaning and grimacing; the aim is to enjoy movement
- improve balance.

We also need to discuss and reassure Lara concerning leg length and all the other 'structural faults' she has been told about.

Standing examination

I informed Lara: 'I want to look at some of the movements of your back and legs. I don't want you to do anything you don't feel like doing, I just want to get an idea of how good your movements are. We can discuss what you feel or anything you want to say as we go along, is that OK?'

I usually stand where the patient can see me and first perform the movements to show them what I want them to do.

Flexion

Flexion was about 10 degrees. When asked, 'What stops you going further?', Lara answered 'The pain and I know it will stir it up for hours'. We continued, doing and asking.

Extension

Extension was virtually nil: 'I hate it'.

Side flexion

Side flexion was half range and rotation was all trunk on legs with very little spinal movement.

Arm and neck movements

With Lara facing me, I asked her to copy my movements as far as she wanted to move. I did arms above head, hand behind back, and horizontal shoulder flexion, all standard neck movements, deep breath in and fully out (noted good spontaneous thoracic and lumbar extension and flexion here). Her arm and neck movements were full range, spontaneous and of good, smooth quality. When I asked Lara how her arm and neck movements felt to her, she surprisingly replied, 'extremely difficult and they feel like lead'. She then made a spontaneous comment: 'I've been examined at least 10 times in the last few years and no one has ever asked me what I think or feel with the tests. It's almost as if I have to relinquish ownership of this body thing that I live in, because nobody asks, nobody understands, because nobody has time to listen, nobody has heard anything. I think that the medical profession and all the therapists are afraid of my problem.'

Lumbar movement

Lumbar side gliding or side shifting revealed surprisingly good quality of movement.

Hip movement

Standing with one hand on the wall for balance, we did hip flexion, abduction and extension. These movements were generally half range and difficult for her to perform, with the description 'heavy' featuring strongly again. Lara was surprised at the findings and made the comment in a rather disconsolate voice: 'I'm more knackered than I thought I was'. I then commented back (it was a very opportune time to do so): 'All this is not surprising, as you haven't been at all active for a long time. I'm seeing someone in front of me who, like many others similar to you, is in quite a deconditioned state. You're weak and your body has become more sensitive, in part because it is so weak. I'll tell you more about this later, but for the time being understand that the human body has a very good capacity to get strong and healthy if its done in a careful, constructive way and in a way that you don't feel frightened.'

Tests for behavioural signs

Before moving, on I did an additional two tests: axial loading and simulated rotation. Both these tests are used to indicate what Waddell terms 'behavioural signs'. These signs and the reasoning behind them are described in detail in his book The Back Pain Revolution (Waddell, 1998). This book is strongly recommended to all manual therapists. Axial loading involves slight pressure applied to the top of the patient's head with your hands. Simulated rotation aims to rotate the patient's body without producing rotation in the lower spine. In order to do this, the examiner gently rotates the patient from the pelvis making sure the trunk does not twist. Trunk twist can be prevented by getting the patient to stand relaxed with their hands at their sides, holding the patient's wrists or hands against his or her pelvis, and passively directing rotation of the body. Both the tests were positive in that they provoked pain in the back.

The other 'Waddell signs' are:

- widespread tenderness spreading far beyond single anatomical regions and often over many segments
- distracted straight leg raise (SLR)
- regional weakness indicated by weakness over many segments and a jerky or 'giving way' response: for example, weak and jerky quadriceps testing, yet the patient can walk
- regional sensory change: losses of sensation where the boundaries are beyond the normal innervation field and dermatome distribution.

The symptoms may include:

- pain at the tip of the tailbone
- whole leg pain

- whole leg numbness
- whole leg giving way
- complete absence of any spells with very little pain in the past year
- intolerance of, or reactions to, many treatments
- emergency admission to hospital with simple backache.

Additional physical goals

Lara needs a progressive programme to restore confidence and the function of lumbar and hip movements and muscles. At some stage, a programme for the upper limbs and neck should be included.

Sitting examination

I now asked Lara to sit on a low stool. I sat in front of her, again doing the movements with her. Movements performed were head into flexion and back up, and slumping the spine. As I did the latter movement I said, 'Can you let yourself go into what I call lazy sitting, like this?' She commented back, 'I haven't done that for 2 years—I've been told to keep upright to stop the disc bulging'. Remember that her bending was 10 degrees in standing and that her husband had helped her undress—I had not seen her bend beyond this. I then hugged one knee to my chest and gently dropped my chin part way to my knee: 'What about this movement, or a part of it?' Lara tried and demonstrated quite smooth movement with spontaneous lumbar flexion using either leg. Importantly, I *did not* say something like: 'See your back is bending'. All I said was, 'That looks good, now lets try this'. I put my leg back down, placed my hands on my knees and slowly lowered my body forwards towards my knees, saying, 'See what you can do. You have your arms to stop the movement if you are not sure and you can come back up any time you like. If you don't want to do it, that's fine.' She flexed very slowly but quite well in the spine and hips, probably about half normal range.

I then looked at Lara's feet, palpated them generally and did foot movements and muscle tests while she sat with her legs dependent on the treatment couch. Her feet were cold and 'blotchy'. They were hypersensitive to palpation, particularly over the balls of her feet, but active movements were good. All muscle tests produced giving way (a notable 'Waddell sign'). Her feet looked anatomically normal, with no evidence of swelling or degenerative changes except some slight lipping of the medial joint line of the metatarsophalangeal joint of the big toe. Lara mentioned being aware of some cracking and clicking in the ankle joint. My response was, 'Is that concerning you?' She replied, 'It makes me feel that arthritis is setting in'. I responded, 'OK, that is an issue that I will put on my list of things to go into'. The point is that until a patient understands the nature of chronic pain and tissue health issues it is difficult and often unhelpful to discuss individual concerns like this. The best strategy is to listen and acknowledge all the patient's worries and concerns so that they can all be dealt with later on.

Calf and quadriceps reflexes done in this sitting position were quite normal. There was no clonus and the Babinski test was normal. Proprioceptive testing in all four limbs was normal. There was no major sensory loss to light touch, although diffuse areas of slight numbness around the foot and lower leg were revealed. The key words she used were, 'I know its not as it should be'.

Lying examination

The examination continued in a similar vein in supine lying, crook lying and side lying. Most tests were actively performed by the patient and directed or demonstrated by myself. For example, Lara performed the following active movements in lying.

- Hip flexion: patient grabs her knee and pulls it towards her. Lara was very tentative but could do it.
- Active SLR: good range to 90 degrees with the opposite leg in 'crook' position. With both legs straight she could not initiate the movement. Passive testing/assistance revealed marked pulling in the whole leg at 70 degrees (both legs). If active dorsiflexion was then added, the pulling spread into the foot quite markedly.
- Active lumbar rotation in crook lying was half range and tense.
- Active hip abduction in crook lying position demonstrated good range.
- Active pelvic rocking surprisingly showed a good range of flexion, well coordinated and with no wincing! Extension was of modest range and reasonably relaxed until pain came in.
- Leg length looked quite normal with feet together in supine and crook lying (she agreed).

I also put a long ruler across her anterior superor iliac spines to assess for any pelvic torsion. Again we both agreed that there was little difference. I even tried to get Lara to tilt the pelvis by contracting her buttock muscles on one side and then relax; always the ruler came back to level. This raised a lot of questions for her as you can imagine. Rather than dismiss the notion of pelvic torsion (which might be quite detrimental), I commented: 'I will talk about all this later and I hope you will be able to see how it fits in to a bigger picture about the modern understanding of ongoing pain. All the findings here, and the findings of those you have seen in the past, need explaining as far as possible. For now, try and think of your system as having entered into a "hypersensitivity state" with all your nerves conveying information that too easily gets processed

by your nervous system in terms of pain and danger. I will talk about it more later and I have some hand-outs so you can go over it when you are at home.'

All areas of pain were palpated to establish the extent of the sensitivity state (rather than solely using it to assess for local tissue pathology or local tissue abnormalities). For instance, in side lying it was established that very gentle palpatory tests over the back and right buttock areas were excessively sensitive, indicating marked hyperalgesia/allodynia. The reader should also be aware that widespread tenderness on palpation in atypical non-segmental patterns is one of the 'Waddell signs' (listed above). Again, an indication of a maladaptive central hypersensitivity mechanism.

REASONING DISCUSSION AND CLINICAL REASONING COMMENTARY

1 There is some concern amongst some clinicians that the 'Waddell symptoms and signs' can lead to some patients' problems unfairly and non-usefully being categorized as 'non-organic'. Can you comment on how you interpreted this lady's positive signs and the implications it held for the management plan you were formulating?

■ Clinician's answer

It should be remembered that Gordon Waddell is an orthopaedic surgeon whose primary concern when he developed these tests was to prevent any unnecessary surgery or the performance of surgery on patients who were likely to have a poor outcome. He developed the 'non-organic versus organic' symptoms and signs to help to distinguish between patients with back pain who had a specific and uncomplicated problem that was amenable to surgery and those whose pain states were far more complex and where surgery was inappropriate. Unfortunately for many patients assessed by others, the very unhelpful term 'non-organic' suggested that the patient's problem had psychogenic origins and was, therefore, to be discounted as real. What Gordon Waddell intended from the list of signs and symptoms is a great deal different from the way it has been interpreted and used. His choice of terms was very unfortunate.

Interpreted in a non-judgmental way, these signs are very useful. My preference is to use them to help in classifying the patient in terms of 'chronic

hypersensitivity syndrome': thus, offering evidence of a marked presence of a maladaptive centralized pain mechanism in the patient's problem and the likelihood of high levels of distress. I rather feel that the thinking clinician, with all the subjective information and the information gathered from the observations, should be able to see the state of affairs quite clearly without recourse to the 'Waddell symptoms and signs'. However, they are well researched and, like routinely checking reflexes, they are often well worth quickly doing. If several of the signs and symptoms are present, they are strong indicators that a multidimensional approach is vital. The fact that two of the behavioural signs are present in Lara adds supportive evidence to the emerging picture that further suggests a complex hypersensitivity syndrome, rather than a biomedically alarming presentation.

2 At this stage what were your thoughts regarding the information obtained from the physical examination?

■ Clinician's answer

Because of the chronicity and the subjective presentation findings, my thinking during the physical examination of Lara was not overdominated by thoughts relating to specific hypotheses about pathology, sources and mechanisms. However, key 'red flag' testing for neurological impairment has still been done and should never be omitted, in my opinion. My main intention was to look at function/activity restriction (and monitor the regions or 'sources' of the restrictions) and hence find out what she could and could not do, thus giving me some idea of where a process of physical recovery might begin or proceed. I guess that in a subconscious way observations of movement and willingness to move in different positions reveal features that confirm a feeling of structural confidence and that no major biomechanical or pathological issues are present. For example, I was able to observe good lumbar intervertebral movement from some starting positions in my sitting examination. What this left me with was that her back was capable of physically bending given a situation whereby fear, anxiety or the notion that the back was bending/vulnerable was eliminated or was being 'gated out' in a subconscious way. The key is that this type of situation is common, and, if anything quite normal, even in acute back injuries where patients have an understandable fear of bending. It must not be looked upon as the problem being 'non-organic'. Rather, it reveals the extent of fear of movement, but it also reveals a 'way in' to be able to restore back bending confidence for the patient.

By the end of the sitting examination, some of the important issues raised were:

- examination revealed a simple way of addressing lumbar flexion fear/movement loss
- matters relating to education about her problems, e.g. arthritis and cracking/clicking
- education about the process of physical recovery, for example, that bending of the spine is safe, normal and necessary for a healthy spine, and that it is possible to improve
- areas of hypersenstivity in the feet; a graded touch/massage programme to address this may be appropriate at some stage.

Note that findings like normal reflexes and diffuse low-grade alterations in sensitivity that are out of classic nerve root or nerve trunk patterns increases confidence in the therapist's structural and physiological interpretation. It also downgrades notions about mechanisms relating to anatomical structure, such as tissue integrity or peripheral nerve root vulnerablility.

Also note that in the lying examination a 70 degree SLR with foot dorsiflexion adding to the symptomatic response could be seen as a positive sign for neurodynamic abnormality or a peripheral neurogenic mechanism. However, I hesitate to consider this anything more than hypersensitivity relating to the neural continuum and central processing, rather than labelling it

in pathological terms, such as 'adverse neural tension' or a significant peripheral neurogenic mechanism. The symptom picture is just too long standing and too widespread to consider in an isolated way. Far better for now to label this finding as a SLR impairment that could be usefully addressed at some stage in the rehabilitation programme.

Favourable examination movements/findings

Most practitioners focus on the negative findings: the things that are wrong. While this is understandable and necessary in treatment models that chase the 'sources' of a disorder, or that seek-out the impairments to be rehabilitated, it is often worthwhile to start with summing up the positive aspects of the examination for this type of chronic problem. Most of the time these patients are presented with a rather grim scenario following standard physical examinations, so presenting some positive findings is a novel and very useful thing for many patients. The importance of using positive reinforcement has been emphasized by Shorland (1998). For Lara the positive findings were:

- walking and ascending/descending stairs
- side shifting in standing
- bringing knee up towards chin in sitting
- coming forward in sitting
- feet movements in sitting
- all knee movements in sitting
- hip flexion and active SLR in crook lying
- pelvic rocking in crook lying (i.e. arching and rounding the back)
- lumbar rotation in crook lying (i.e. taking both legs to one side then the other)
- essentially normal neurological findings, e.g. reflexes
- taking some exercise, e.g. swimming, walking.

Findings that may be focussed on for improvement

Much relates to fear of movement, fear of damage and fear of pain exacerbation, as well as lack of use and physical deconditioning:

- wincing and holding with many movements and activities
- unable to go to all fours or get down onto floor
- markedly reduced lumbar motion in standing and during functional activities, e.g. dressing
- hypersensitivity over back/buttock and feet

- heaviness/weakness in arms/neck/legs
- poor balance
- poor hip movements
- general lack of end-range capability in affected areas
- giving way with muscle testing.

Examples of some important functional findings (activity and participation restrictions):

- decreased tolerance to standing still
- decreased tolerance for sitting
- decreased walking distance
- not dressing independently
- inactive in the evenings
- sleeping problems
- limited shopping
- stopped various activities, e.g. driving, cooking, gardening, flower arranging, embroidery
- general feeling of weakness and being unfit.

Social participation restrictions include:

- entertainment and hobbies curtailed/nil
- not been on holiday
- a significant loss from what she used to do (see list above)

Mental/psychological impairment was not formally evaluated. However, it is quite clear that this lady is distressed and frustrated by her predicament and is desperate to get help in some way.

Many chronic pain management units assess levels of depression and distress as well as heightened somatic perception using questionnaires, for example the Modified Zung Depression Inventory and the Modified Somatic Perception Questionnaire (MSPQ). High scores on these measures really indicate that there may be a need for psychological input alongside the physical rehabilitation process (Waddell, 1998).

■ Clinical reasoning commentary

The continual linking the clinician makes between examination findings and implications again highlights the dynamic nature of clinical reasoning. Expert therapists do not wait until all possible examinations have been completed before forming and further testing hypotheses. Hypothesis generation and testing is an evolving process commencing from the patient interview and continuing through the physical examination and ultimately throughout the ongoing management. While expert therapists will have highly developed knowledge bases that enable them to recognize clinical patterns and management implications, they arguably only reach that level of knowledge organization through a process of reflective reasoning that allows them to integrate acquired biopsychosocial knowledge with clinical presentations learned from their practice. Even management in the form of deliberate responses to the patient and goal setting are seen to commence within the physical examination by this expert, a skill only possible when the therapist is able to think simultaneously and metacognitively on these different planes.

m | Management

■ Management stage 1

There are two initial difficulties that need to be helpfully addressed. Both relate to the patient's beliefs. First, the beliefs about the nature of the problem are very 'vulnerable/weak structure' and disease orientated. Secondly, the beliefs about treatment are orientated towards a process of finding the source or disorder and fixing or curing it. Lara seems to have high expectations that I will provide her with the cure and this is unrealistic and unhelpful.

A primary goal was to shift her understanding of the problem from a perspective where pain is seen as a reliable guide to danger (adaptive/helpful pain) to one where pain can in large part be viewed as of little value (maladaptive/unhelpful pain).

The steps that follow encourage a patient dominated role in the process of restoring physical fitness and confidence. Patients usually quickly understand the meaning of a deconditioned state and that lack of physical activity leads to loss of physical fitness and heightened sensitivity.

Education 1

The overall goal of the first 'education' input was to decrease her concern about pain meaning damage or danger, so that the process of gradual return of physical confidence might go ahead less hindered by negative and fearful thinking about structural damage and progressive disablement. This is not as easy to do as it sounds. Maladaptive pain is just as real as adaptive pain, and it can be very hard to believe that the hurt you have has little meaning or little value. Like it or not, patients are more likely to listen to and believe clinicians who in their minds have some kind of high professional status.

The second aim was to help Lara to understand that a passive treatment approach was inappropriate at this stage and that the best approach involved a great deal of input from her. Part of this involves a shift in emphasis from pain-focussed management to more function-focussed goal achievement.

Education, therefore, involved a simple brief discussion of the following.

- The nature of adaptive/acute pain and chronic/maladaptive pain: the former is useful, helpful pain as opposed to useless, unhelpful pain.
- A simple explanation was given for maladaptive and excessive sensitivity to movement, intolerance of prolonged posture, and tenderness/hypersensitivity to touch and pressures.
- The analogy was made of ongoing background pain to an annoying tune in the head all the time, i.e. the constant pain relating to abnormal nervous system 'circuitry activity' rather than a disease or abnormality in the tissue where the hurt is felt. Explaining and discussing phantom limb pain often helps here (Gifford 1998a,b).
- The gate control theory of pain is explained (i.e. that pain normally comes and goes relative to an individual's attention and the value or meaning they may put on it).

- The effect of mood on pain, activity and life in general is discussed. This helps the patient to come to terms with low mood being normal for anyone who suffers an ongoing and seemingly non-resolvable problem. It also underlines the positive message that mood state commonly improves as the patient starts to achieve progress and gradually recover better physical function.
- The effect of 'pain fear' and 'damage fear' on movements, activity and life leads on to introducing a treatment approach with a focus more on functional recovery/physical confidence rather than on getting rid of the pain or the apparent source of the pain. Patients somehow have to come to terms with the fact that pain therapies and medical interventions for chronic ongoing maladaptive pain have a very poor record of success. In contrast, approaches that focus on better physical confidence and fitness have a much better record. It is sometimes helpful to give a brief history of another patient who has been successful. Giving the patient a book like Neville Shone's Coping Successfully with Pain (1995) is often very helpful.
- The illustration from Nicholas (1996; Fig. 5.2) was used to show the patient the way in which modern pain research has begun to appreciate the complexity and difficulties that a patient with ongoing pain can have. Patients are often relieved to find that medicine is beginning to understand the impact that their ongoing pain has on their lives, and that they are not alone.

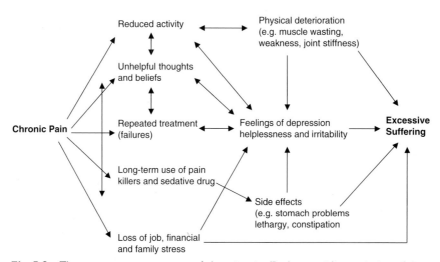

Fig. 5.2 The common consequences of chronic pain. (Redrawn with permission of the IASP, from Nicholas, M.K. (1996). Theory and practice of cognitive–behavioral programs. In Pain 1996: an updated review. Refresher course syllabus, Campbell, J.N., ed., pp. 297–303. IASP Press, Seattle, WA.)

Like many similar patients, Lara found the information very enlightening and interesting. She had many questions, and we both explored many issues that related to the hopes and fears of past management as well as issues for the future. She quickly grasped the concept of maladaptive pain and that physically getting back more relaxed and normal movements would be a good starting point for recovery. She was instantly eager to start the physical 'challenge' and we spent quite some time dealing with fear of bending/flexing the spine and the natural strength of the spine, even when degenerate.

As with so many patients in similar situations she said, 'Why hasn't anyone told me this before about pain and movements?' An answer that can helpfully be given is that, 'It is only in the last 10 to 15 years or so that science and research has started to give us a better understanding of pain, and it is only very recently that the full implications for management of pain has started to have an impact on clinical practices'. This attempts to avoid producing any unhelpful anger with previous practitioners and treatments or advice.

Pre-prepared handouts were given relating to all the above.

Starting the process

The last 45 minutes of the second consultation involved a focus on a series of simple exercises relating to the back, hip and leg, as well as two functional activities: walking and going up/down stairs. Concepts discussed included gradual mastery (graded exposure), baselines, pacing and incrementing the exercise programme.

Gradual mastery/graded exposure process

The term gradual mastery/graded exposure comes from the psychological literature dealing with phobias (Harding, 1998; Shorland, 1998). The key process is that the patient overcomes their fear (for example of a spider or of a particular movement) by gradually approaching rather than avoiding the cause of the fear. This can be a very slow process and the speed of exposure is determined by the patient rather than by therapist bullying! A successful outcome is achieved when the process is graduated (slowly more and more difficult levels are mastered), repeated regularly and prolonged. Gradually, the patient gains confidence and learns that their fears are unfounded as they achieve their goals. The key to success is starting the chosen movement or activity at a realistic and achievable baseline.

Baselines, pacing and incrementing

Most pain sufferers like Lara persist with activities until they are forced to stop by the pain. This often involves many hours, sometimes days of resting and inactivity. In order to break this overactivity–underactivity cycle, exercises and activities are paced so that this very unproductive process is overcome. A baseline is the number/repetitions/amount of time for an exercise or activity that a patient can manage to do every day regardless of the intensity of the pain. This is found by taking the average of a series of trials done over several days and then reducing the average by 20%. Incrementing or pacing from this baseline is done by increasing the number or time of each activity/exercise after a set period, for example weekly or every four days (Harding, 1997, 1998; Shorland, 1998).

The overactivity–underactivity cycle was explained and pacing of resting was discussed. Exercises were recorded for reference and handouts were given relating to exercise and functional pacing and the overactivity–underactivity cycle. The following exercises were used:

- crook-lying starting position: lumbar rotation; pelvic rocking; alternate leg flexion (possibly progress to grasping knee or if easier do in sitting as in examination)
- active SLR with non-active leg in crook position
- walking up/down stairs or step-ups (whichever preferred)
- sit to stand
- standing starting position (with support as required): hip flexion/extension, hip abduction, one leg balance, alternate calf raises
- tip-toeing practice (weight through arms as required).

Instead of walking for 2 miles intermittently and with marked exacerbation, it was decided that a short regular walk of good quality would be of greater benefit. Lara's initial task was to find a reasonable baseline starting time or distance that would not incur a massive flare up and which was manageable even on bad days.

▇ Management stage 2

Lara returned 2 weeks later. I saw her twice over 2 days, with each session being 1.5 hours.

She felt she had begun to master lumbar movements in lying (e.g. flexion using pelvic rocking and single leg flexing) and paced up her numbers from an initial baseline of 10 slow, relaxed, small-range repetitions to 15 fuller range and slightly faster repetitions. She had managed to generalize this out to modest flexing in sitting and was feeling good about it because she was needing quite a bit less help with dressing from her husband. She made a spontaneous comment: 'The most profound thing that has happened is the sense of relief. I believe what you say; it makes sense. It gives me control and it allows me to have a vision of my life with some kind of future. Whatever it is going to be it will be better than where I have been for so long—I know that.'

She had had one bout of a very bad flare up for 1 day but had managed to keep most of the programme going. For the first time, the flare up had not unduly bothered her. Her comment was, 'It taught me that my desire to progress quickly may be my worst enemy. The day before I got carried away with the exercises and paid for it. The good thing was that I recovered and haven't lost any ground.'

She found the use of regular short resting far more effective than responding with rest only when pain became severe and unmanageable.

The second half of the first session was spent going through some of the things looked at in the initial physical examination. Movements and the exercises she was doing were observed and discussed, and walking, climbing steps, balance etc. were reviewed. The focus was on patient comments about the quality and feel of each task/movement, not on pain and not on any 'therapist opinion' about the movement (unless helpful). At appropriate times, positive reinforcement was given. Difficulties were discussed and Lara was encouraged to problem solve and find out for herself rather than be told or shown alternatives by me. For example, she had found left SLR in crook lying difficult and uncomfortable to do. She had kept to a baseline of four repetitions three times per day but had not progressed it and did not like doing it much as she immediately felt sore in her leg and back. I explained that the exercise strengthens weak hip and back muscles, as well as moving and stretching leg muscles and nerves from the back. Also, that subtle adjustments of the back, the leg or the starting position were often helpful in making movement easier. I gave an example of doing the exercise in a semi-reclined position. She tried it and was not convinced. She then tried it sitting but found this even harder. After 5 minutes or so experimenting, with some ideas

thrown in from me, she came up with the notion of doing it while lying in the flexed pelvic rocking position. The result of this is that it helped her to find a way of doing the exercise much more comfortably, but it also introduced the idea of being 'allowed' to play around with or modify an exercise to make it more acceptable. For so long patients have been fearful of doing an exercise 'wrong'. In my opinion, this is very unhelpful when dealing with this type of patient and problem.

Some new exercises were added:

- sit-up in supported (pillows behind back) slouch sitting
- lumbar extension in lean forward sitting with arms supported on knees.

The first was decided on after experimenting in different starting positions to get some dynamic abdominal work going and to encourage active lumbar flexion. Lying flexion from the 'top-end' was found too difficult. Bilateral leg lifting from the crook-lying position produced sharp pain in the initiation phase of the movement, but reaching forward from a gentle slouch sitting position was enjoyable! This was because, first, she found it rewarding to try slouching after so long avoiding it and, secondly, the movement was pain-free and easy to perform. Lara could immediately see how her abdominal muscles were working quite strongly, that she was flexing her back, and that she could occasionally try a lying, or half lying, sit-up when ready to progress.

Sitting with arms supported on knees was the starting position found most useful as a progression from extension in the crook lying position. It should be remembered that Lara 'hated' extension from the standing position.

Education 2

In the second half of the session, time was taken to explain the importance of setting realistic goals in all areas of Lara's life and looking at the physical components that needed to be mastered in order to achieve these goals. The following goals were chosen and programmes worked out to help to achieve them:

- dressing independently
- getting on all fours
- swimming one length of the pool
- starting hobbies again (e.g. flower arranging).

The health requirements of tissues

Some simple information was required about the needs of musculoskeletal and neural tissue for movement and exercise to remain healthy and to improve fitness. Part of this included the notion that fitter tissues which are used in a confident way have a better chance of becoming less sensitive. Key aspects of tissue requirements include the need for regular through-range movements, comfortable stretching, progressive strengthening, endurance training, and improved coordination. A handout was given to Lara.

Understanding the multiple factors that can trigger pain

Headaches were used to illustrate the multiple triggering factors that can be involved in triggering pain. Most patients are able to come up with some of the following factors that can trigger or worsen a headache: diet, tiredness, stress and tension, a particular environment or situation, as well as more physical factors like prolonged postures or overexertion when tired or hungry. These issues are then discussed in relationship to the variability of the patient's pain and in such a way that the patient can start to understand the complexity of the problem and the difficulties in trying to relate the waxing and waning of pain to a single structure or pathology. Realising that multiple factors are often involved in precipitating flare-ups helps the patient to realise that there is more to pain and its behaviour than just physical factors.

Management stage 3

On month later Lara returned again for two more long sessions. She had achieved all the goals and was progressing the swimming and could now manage two lengths of the swimming pool without a significant flare-up. She had started some simple gardening tasks as well as getting more involved in some of her hobbies.

Movement quality and range was markedly improved. For example, she was able to get onto the floor and as a result now managed to get in and out of the bath. She was managing a few half sit-up exercises and had increased her daily walking to a comfortable 20 minutes. She had progressed to doing a full SLR from supine lying.

Time was spent discussing some new goals. These included entertaining her family to a meal and the possibility of a holiday for a few days with her husband.

Some current difficulties were discussed. In particular this included a major concern she had about the pain and the hypersensitivity: 'I am doing so much better physically, I am achieving more, I continue to improve and my confidence is gradually returning, but the pain and symptoms seem to be much the same and I am still very tender.' This prompted a review of the nature of chronic pain and hypersensitivity, but also a review of pain reduction and desensitizing strategies that may be helpful. Some of these were the use of rest and relaxation techniques, progressive desensitizing massage, heat/cold, 'nice' exercises and stretches. 'Nice' exercises are those exercises that the patient chooses which feel good and are often used to ease discomfort: they are usually a combination of relaxed through-range exercises and comfortable stretches. A simple breathing relaxation technique was taught and instruction given regarding the use and progression of massage over the tender areas. Again, information was written down and handouts given.

REASONING DISCUSSION AND CLINICAL REASONING COMMENTARY

1 The abdominal exercises you have described appear very general. Do you feel assessment of specific trunk and pelvic muscle function (i.e. awareness, recruitment, strength, endurance, etc.) is appropriate for this sort of presentation, and if so, at what stage would you assess these further?

■ Clinician's answer

This is a very personal matter, especially considering the current wave of enthusiasm for specific muscle control approaches. I would urge great caution in over-focussing on specific impairments at this stage. Muscles work in groups, and movement should normally be for the most part unconscious, thoughtless and silent; this is what needs to be rehabilitated. Recall that Lara had been given specific exercises for the trunk and pelvic region in relation to a diagnosis of 'instability' and had been told never to bend without tightening her stomach. This style of approach may enhance somatic awareness as well as increase fear that if she does not do this she is likely to cause further harm. If successful functional recovery occurs then bringing more focussed 'muscle imbalance' issues in may be worthwhile later on. It is always important for a patient to feel that they have good muscular control, especially around an area that has given a great deal of trouble for a long time. However, I do not think that it is desirable for patients to have to recruit muscles consciously before or during movements: not only is it very difficult to do for many people, it is not natural.

2 What are your thoughts regarding this patient's long-term prognosis? Please include some reference to the 'positive' and 'negative' features in her presentation that you feel assist in predicting this result.

Clinician's answer

Lara has successfully coped with a new perspective on her problem for over a year. She has made quite significant gains in function and independence and has reintroduced many of her former hobbies and interests. This was all helped by her open-mindedness, her readiness to accept new perspectives on her problem, and her eagerness to take responsibility for her own management. Her home situation and financial security were very helpful in that they allowed her to have time to devote to the programme. She got involved, she did the programme and she worked hard at it. Note her comment above that 'working with chronic pain can be very hard work'. In this respect, it is very common for patients to make changes to their lives, manage well for a while, but to then relapse into old ways and become passive and despondent about the whole situation. Lara is as vulnerable to relapse as anyone and this is a strong possibility.

Her long-term prognosis looks good. Importantly, there are two aspects to consider for the future: her disability and function and her pain and symptoms. The prognosis for function is good. Her recovery is already excellent and still improving; even if she relapses she knows the way out. Symptom prognosis is a different

matter and one that is really very difficult to predict. Everyone wants their pain to go; however, the reality of long-term well-established widespread pain with its underlying neurophysiological representations is that, like the significant memories of our lifetime, they are very hard to get rid of or forget. The reality is that the pain will probably always be there; however, many patients like Lara find that it bothers them less and it becomes easier to manage.

Clinical reasoning commentary

The application of any therapeutic intervention, be it joint mobilization, motor control retraining or explanation to alter understanding, must be based on patients' unique clinical presentations. Recipe treatments or protocols are unfortunately still common in manual therapy, although often the latest 'fad' is created by those who extrapolate from the ideas of others and not by the originators of the research on which it is based. There is clearly a continuum of impairment possible within the sensory–motor system, which, when considered along with the multitude of biopsychosocial factors that influence how that impairment will manifest in a given patient, necessitates that therapists are sufficiently open-minded and skilled in sensory–motor retraining. While a variety of techniques are used to facilitate improved motor control, it is important the underlying strategy is based on sound principles of motor control and learning theory. Again there is no recipe. Even with the growing body of research to assist us in recognizing the factors that influence motor control, application of that knowledge to our patients requires advanced assessment and teaching/training skills as well as the clinical reasoning to know which strategies are indicated and when they should be trialed. Reassessment of the effect on the different systems (e.g. psychological, cognitive/affective/behavioural, neuromusculoskeletal) should guide the progression and modification of all interventions.

Determination of prognosis may well be one of the most difficult decisions for therapists to make. However, prognosis, like the other categories of hypotheses, forms patterns. Attending to the positive and negative features from the patient's psychosocial and physical presentation is the key.

There may also be more than one prognosis, as discussed here, with different prognoses predicted for the patient's functional recovery and pain recovery. The crucial factor, as with all clinical patterns, is reflective reasoning. Not simply making a prognosis but, as time goes by, and particularly if the prognosis is not met, taking the time to reflect what may have been missed, over- or under-rated in the initial judgment, so that future predictions might be improved.

Outcome

One year after Lara first consulted me she was back to near normal levels of activity and confident that she would progress further. She moved in a relaxed way and was not frightened to bend her back. She could easily bend to touch the floor with both hands flat; she could walk happily on tip-toes and go up stairs two steps at a time. She still had low periods and occasional pain flare-ups. Her pain level overall was, in her words, 'more manageable and less intrusive'. She slept much better and managed slowly to stop all her medication. She commented: 'Working with chronic pain can be very hard work, it is a daily challenge that most often is quite conquerable, but on some days it is a long and very tough and tiring struggle'.

At the time of writing, there had been seven visits in total and she was coming to see me about once every 3–4 months. There had been no passive treatment, but there had been a great deal of skilled physical appraisal and the gradual introduction of more and more specific exercises related to more minor physical impairments. This is not always required but it had been Lara's aim to get as fit as her age and underlying condition would allow.

I picked Lara as a good example of the problems we all can have with the management of chronic pain states. She exhibits many features that can be made to fit various models and explanations, yet if her problem is really scrutinized there is a great deal that does not fit, can be viewed as odd or can be unproductively classified in some way as 'non-organic'. She had been through a large number of therapies and consultants in search of an answer to her problem with little success. She has been through periods of great hope with some of them, yet her hopes dwindled to despair as treatment after treatment failed and consultant after consultant provided inadequate or even dismissive explanations and attitudes to her and her problem.

Like many chronic pain sufferers, Lara had widespread symptoms and signs that do not fit into neat diagnostic categories or syndrome presentations. She had many maladaptive movement and behaviour patterns, and she had many unhelpful and unrealistic beliefs and attributions about the nature of her problem and the means of recovery. Her case history illustrates how an enclosed tissue-based and predominantly passive approach to treatment really did not help, and how a multidimensional and multilevel perspective and approach enabled her to recover and lead a far fuller and more confident life.

References

Barlow, W. (1981). The Alexander Principle. London: Arrow Books.

Borkan, J.M., Quirk, M. and Sullivan, M. (1991). Finding meaning after the fall: injury narratives from elderly hip fracture patients. Social Science and Medicine, 33, 947–957.

Feuerstein, M. and Beattie, P. (1995). Biobehavioural factors affecting pain and disability in low back pain: mechanisms and assessment. Physical Therapy, 75, 267–280.

Fleming, M.H. and Mattingly, C. (2000). Action and narrative: two dynamics of clinical reasoning, In Clinical Reasoning in the Health Professions, 2nd edn (J. Higgs and M.A. Jones, eds.) pp. 54– 61. Oxford: Butterworth-Heinemann.

Gifford, L.S. (1997). Pain. In Rehabilitation of Movement: Theoretical Bases of Clinical Practice (Pitt-Brooke ed.) pp. 196–232. London: Saunders.

Gifford, L.S. (1998a). Central mechanisms. In Topical Issues in Pain 1. Whiplash—Science and Management, Fear-avoidance Beliefs and Behaviour (L.S. Gifford, ed.) pp. 67–80. Falmouth, MA: CNS Press.

Gifford, L.S. (ed.) (1998b). Topical Issues in Pain 1. Whiplash—Science and Management, Fear-avoidance Beliefs and Behaviour. Falmouth, MA: CNS Press.

Gifford, L.S. (ed.) (2000a).Topical Issues in Pain 2. Biopsychosocial Assessment. Relationships and Pain. Falmouth, MA: CNS Press.

Gifford, L.S. (2000b). The patient in front of us: from genes to environment. In Topical Issues in Pain 2. Biopsychosocial Assessment. Relationships and Pain (L.S. Gifford ed.) pp. 1–11. Falmouth, MA: CNS Press.

Gifford, L.S. (2001). Perspectives on the biopsychosocial model part 1: some issues that need to be accepted?

Touch [Journal of the Organisation of Chartered Physiotherapists in Private Practice] 97, 3–9.

Gifford, L.S. (2002a). Perspectives on the biopsychosocial model part 2: the shopping basket approach. Touch [Journal of the Organisation of Chartered Physiotherapists in Private Practice] 99, 11–22.

Gifford, L.S. (2002b). An introduction to evolutionary reasoning: diet, discs and the placebo. In Topical Issues in Pain 4. Placebo and Nocebo, Pain Management, Muscles and Pain (L.S. Gifford, ed.) pp. 119–144. Falmouth, MA: CNS Press.

Gifford, L. and Butler, D. (1997). The integration of pain sciences into clinical practice. Journal of Hand Therapy, 10, 86–95.

Harding, V. (1997). Application of the cognitive-behavioural approach. In Rehabilitation of Movement: Theoretical Bases of Clinical Practice (J. Pitt-Brooke ed.) pp. 539–583. London: Saunders.

Harding, V. (1998). Cognitive-behavioural approach to fear and avoidance. In Topical Issues in Pain 1. Whiplash—Science and Management, Fear-avoidance Beliefs and Behaviour (L.S. Gifford, ed.) pp. 173–191. Falmouth, MA: CNS Press.

Jones, M.A., Edwards, I. and Gifford, L. (2002). Conceptual models for implementing biopsychosocial theory in clinical practice. Manual Therapy, 7, 2–9.

Lackner, J.M., Caarosella, A.M. and Feuerstein, M. (1996). Pain expectancies, pain and functional self-efficacy expectancies as determinants of disability in patients with chronic low back disorders. Journal of Consulting Clinical Psychology, 64, 212–220.

Lawes, N. (2002). The reality of the placebo response. In Topical Issues in Pain 3. Sympathetic Nervous System and Pain. Pain Management, Clinical Effectiveness. (L.S. Gifford, ed.) pp. 41–62. Falmouth, MA: CNS Press.

Main, C.J. and Spanswick, C.C. (2000). Pain Management: An Interdisciplinary Approach. Edinburgh: Churchill Livingstone.

Main, C.J., Spanswick, C.C. and Watson, P. (2000). The nature of disability. In Pain Management: An Interdisciplinary Approach (C.J. Main and C.C. Spanswick, eds.) pp. 89–106. Edinburgh: Churchill Livingstone.

Malt, U.F. and Olafson, O.M. (1995). Psychological appraisal and emotional response to physical injury: a clinical, phenomenological study of 109 adults. Psychiatric Medicine, 10, 117–134.

Mattingly, C. (1991). What is clinical reasoning? American Journal of Occupational Therapy, 45, 979–986.

Newton-John, T. (2000). When helping does not help: responding to pain behaviours. In Topical Issues in Pain 2. Biopsychosocial Assessment and Management. Relationships and Pain

(L.S. Gifford ed.) pp. 165–175. Falmouth, MA: CNS Press.

Nicholas, M.K. (1996). Theory and practice of cognitive-behavioural programs. In Pain 1996: An updated review. Refresher course syllabus (J.N. Campbell ed.) pp. 297–303. Seattle, WA: IASP Press.

Roche, P.A. (2002). Placebo and patient care. In Topical Issues in Pain 4. Placebo and Nocebo. Pain Management, Muscles and Pain (L.S. Gifford ed.) pp. 19–39. Falmouth, MA: CNS Press.

Shone, N. (1995). Coping Successfully with Pain. London: Sheldon Press.

Shorland, S. (1998). Management of chronic pain following whiplash injuries. In Topical Issues in Pain 1. Whiplash—Science and Management, Fear-avoidance Beliefs and Behaviour (L.S. Gifford, ed.) pp. 115–134. Falmouth, MA: CNS Press.

Strong, J. (1995). Self-efficacy and the patient with chronic pain. In Moving in on Pain (M. Shacklock, ed.) pp. 97–102. Oxford: Butterworth-Heinemann.

Waddell, G. (1998). The Back Pain Revolution. Edinburgh: Churchill Livingstone.

Watson, P. (2000). Psychosocial predictors of outcome from low back pain. In Topical Issues in Pain 2. Biopsychosocial Assessment and Management, Relationships and Pain (L.S. Gifford ed.) pp. 85–109. Falmouth, MA: CNS Press.

CHAPTER 6

A chronic case of mechanic's elbow

Toby Hall and Brian Mulligan

SUBJECTIVE EXAMINATION

Howard is a normally healthy 51-year-old male who has a sedentary lifestyle. He is right hand dominant and enjoyed the occasional game of lawn bowls prior to the onset of his elbow problem. He runs a small motor vehicle repair shop attached to a service station. He usually manages the business, but for 2 weeks he had to stand in for one of his mechanics who was away on sick leave.

The principal nature of the relief work involved fitting new exhaust systems. The majority of tasks were undertaken in a vehicle inspection pit with the car overhead. Howard noticed the sudden onset of right elbow pain at the beginning of the second week of relief work. On this particular day, he experienced extraordinary difficulty loosening a corroded nut using a socket wrench, with considerable force being required. Within an hour, he became aware of moderate lateral elbow pain with any forceful gripping activity. He persevered through the rest of the week as he was unable to restrict his activity because there was no replacement. The pain gradually increased to the point of becoming quite severe.

In the following week, he returned to his normal duties, which mainly involved supervising mechanical work and office duties. The pain continued to bother him constantly but had subsided to a moderate intensity. Being a busy person, he let the situation continue for a further 2 weeks. He then went to see his general medical practitioner, who prescribed non-steroidal anti-inflammatory drugs for 4 weeks. During this period, the pain began to change from a constant to an intermittent nature. The doctor then, over a period of 8 weeks, administered a series of three local cortisone injections in the region of the right lateral epicondyle near the common extensor origin. This had no effect in reducing the symptoms and only increased his pain for 48 hours after each injection.

Chronic stage

At this stage, Howard was having problems writing and using a computer at work. He was referred by his doctor to a rheumatologist, who ordered a bone scan. The results of the scan were normal, with an apparent coincidental finding of increased tracer uptake in the C5–C6 and T3–T4 facet joints bilaterally. The patient was then advised to see a physiotherapist for strengthening and stretching exercises.

There was no previous history of arm problems despite the fact that Howard had been a motor mechanic for 15 years of his working life. However, there was a history of recurrent neck pain for which he had never sought treatment. These episodes were caused by long periods working underneath vehicles, the last being 3 years ago.

At initial evaluation 4 months after the onset of symptoms, the patient complained of pain in the anterolateral and posterolateral aspects of the elbow (Fig. 6.1). There was no pain or other symptoms elsewhere in the left or right upper quarter.

There was no apparent stress in Howard's life and he was coping well with his problem. He had continued to work and on questioning there were no work or family issues that might have interfered with his recovery.

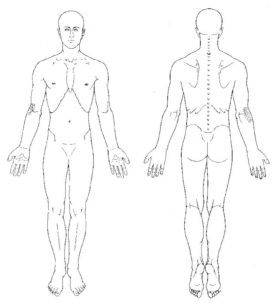

Fig. 6.1 Body chart indicating the extent of elbow pain.

 REASONING DISCUSSION AND CLINICAL REASONING COMMENTARY

1 How did you interpret the effects of the medical interventions on the patient's symptoms?

Clinicians' answer

The patient reported a gradual change in the nature of his symptoms during the 4-week period when he was taking non-steroidal anti-inflammatory medication. He felt that his symptoms changed from being constant to intermittent. This improvement may have been related to spontaneous recovery of the disorder rather than the prescribed medication, especially as he had stopped the activity that had caused the symptoms in the first place. There may have been an inflammatory element to the condition, arising from repetitive microtrauma through overuse and the sudden exertion (overload) required to loosen the corroded nut. This inflammatory component subsided with time and with the aid of the anti-inflammatory medication. The symptoms remaining after the 4-week period were probably related to mechanical dysfunction of the elbow complex. The patient reported a temporary increase in pain after local cortisone injections in the region of the lateral epicondyle, but no overall

change. Cortisone is a powerful anti-inflammatory agent: if there was any remaining inflammation some relief of symptoms would likely have resulted.

It has been demonstrated that in chronic tennis elbow (also known as lateral epicondylitis or lateral epicondylalgia) there is histological evidence of angio-fibroblastic hyperplasia (Nirschl and Petrone, 1979) and mesenchymal transformation within the common extensor tendon at its point of insertion into the lateral epicondyle (Uhthoff and Sarkar, 1980). In contrast, there is no evidence of acute or chronic inflammatory cells. Prolonged anti-inflammatory medication or cortisone injection are, therefore, unwarranted in the management of chronic tennis elbow and were (as would be expected) unsuccessful in this case.

2 What were your initial thoughts and hypotheses about the possible source(s) of the patient's elbow pain?

Clinicians' answer

In this case of localized pain in the region of the lateral epicondyle, possible structures/pain sources to be considered include local joints, musculotendinous elements and neural tissue, as well as remote structures, particularly within the lower cervical spine. Working hypotheses in order of priority were:

1. The insertion of the wrist and finger extensors at the lateral epicondyle, notably extensor carpi radialis brevis
2. The nervi nervorum supplying the radial nerve or its terminal branches (posterior interosseous nerve)
3. The lower cervical spine (C5–C7)
4. The radiohumeral and radioulnar joints.

The evidence in support of local structures includes a well-defined area of pain, without evidence of associated proximal or distal symptoms; a history of abuse of local elbow structures immediately preceding the onset of symptoms; activity involving local structures reproduced the symptoms immediately after the symptom onset; and an unvarying area of symptoms over the history of the condition. In support of contractile and associated elements as the most likely pain source is the history of excessive muscle force required to release a corroded nut. The evidence against local structures includes the failure of local cortisone injections to relieve pain, although it is highly likely that this relates to the lack of an inflammatory process rather than injecting the wrong tissue.

At this point there is little evidence to support remote structures as a source of pain, other than a tenuous link with the bone scan abnormalities at C5–C6 and T3–T4, as well as a history of stressful cervical spine postures working underneath cars. Furthermore, there is no complaint of neck symptoms to suggest somatic referred pain from cervical or thoracic structures, nor dysaesthesia or sensory loss to support cervical neural compromise.

3 What were your hypotheses regarding the pathobiological pain mechanisms involved? What evidence was there to support (and negate) your hypothesis?

Clinicians' answer

In this case, the condition is certainly chronic, being now 4 months in duration. If we assume that the original tissue damage was a tear of the musculotendinous insertion related to forcing the corroded nut, then this soft tissue damage should normally have repaired by this time. Considering the lack of evidence

of inflammatory cells in chronic tennis elbow (Nirschl and Petrone, 1979; Uhthoff and Sarkar, 1980) and the patient's poor response to powerful local anti-inflammatory agents, it would appear that inflammatory nociceptive pain is an unlikely explanation for the ongoing symptoms.

The pathobiology of tennis elbow has been proposed to involve a tear of the tendon of origin of the extensor muscles from the lateral epicondyle (Cyriax, 1936; Nirschl and Petrone, 1979). The tear occurs at the junction between muscle and bone, and healing is slow because of a lack of periosteal tissue overlying this bone area (Putnam and Cohen, 1999). It has been shown that the granulofibroblastic material laid down in the repair process contains free nerve endings (Goldie, 1964). Repetitive microtrauma from overuse or abnormal joint biomechanics may overload the repairing tissue, mechanically distort the scar tissue and thus stimulate the in situ free nerve endings sufficiently to evoke mechanical nociceptive pain. Chronicity of the problem may be related to continued use of the arm, causing repeated microtrauma to the scar tissue, which has not yet gained adequate strength to withstand normal function. In the case history, there is some evidence to support this hypothesis. The history of onset is consistent with musculotendinous overload, either by repetitive microtrauma or sudden strain. The pain has changed from a constant to intermittent nature and is related to activities (such as keyboarding and writing) that involve repetitive use of the proposed damaged musculotendinous insertion.

Alternatively, it has been suggested that ischaemia plays a part in the pain process (Putnam and Cohen, 1999). The blood supply to the muscle origin is limited and it is suspected that it would be prone to reduced flow after injury (Uhthoff and Sarkar, 1980). Ischaemia can cause nerve endings to lower their thresholds for firing (Gifford and Butler, 1997). The nerve endings may then fire more readily and with movements not normally painful. The patient's age is a significant factor in reduced vascularity of the musculotendinous insertion.

At this point in the examination, there is little evidence to support a neuropathic disorder involving abnormal nerve conduction, central nervous system changes or maladaptive behaviours. Certainly, there do not appear to be any significant psychological or social issues that could contribute to a central pain state.

■ Clinical reasoning commentary

The response to Question 1 nicely demonstrates how hypotheses relating to pathobiological mechanisms (notably tissue-healing mechanisms) have been generated early in the clinical encounter and that tentative decisions are being formed at the outset, rather than at the end, of the examination. It is also evident that the integration of propositional knowledge of pathobiological mechanisms within the broader knowledge base of the expert clinician enables the consideration of this patient's clinical presentation in the light of research-validated theory.

A number of hypotheses relating to the structural sources of the elbow pain and related pathobiological mechanisms (both tissue healing and pain) have been generated from this patient's history thus far, with ranking of these hypotheses evident. Testing of these hypotheses is apparent in that consideration has been given to the supporting features in the patient's presentation. Importantly, however, non-supporting clinical findings have also been attended to carefully, as have 'missing features' or features that would be expected with a particular clinical disorder, such as the absence of neck symptoms with the hypothesis of somatic referred pain from cervical or thoracic structures. Whereas the novice clinician often ignores features that do not fit with the favoured hypothesis, the expert clinician avoids this error and weighs both the supporting and negating evidence objectively.

These two hypothesis categories are not each considered in isolation but rather are found to be intricately intertwined, and consequently have an impact on the decision-making process proceeding in relation to the other hypothesis category. This is reflective of a richly organized knowledge base that is deep as well as broad, and is characteristic of the clinical reasoning of the expert clinician.

In addition, there is evidence of attention to the possibility of psychosocial factors (yellow, blue and black flags; see Ch. 1), which potentially could have contributed to the patient's pain state and created obstacles to his recovery.

Pain behaviour

The principal aggravating activities were writing for more than 10 minutes and use of a computer keyboard for more than 15 minutes. The pain never stopped him undertaking the activity, but at the end of a busy day involving these activities, his elbow pain would not settle until the following day. Gripping and squeezing activities (including carrying heavy objects in the right hand) were also painful. For this reason he had stopped playing social lawn bowls for the duration of his symptoms. He also described occasional pain when brushing his teeth or shaving, as he had the same difficulty holding and manipulating a toothbrush/disposable razor with the elbow flexed as he did using a writing pen in the same position.

Howard was unaware of any position or activity that would ease his pain. His sleep was only disturbed if he slept with his elbow flexed and the forearm tucked under the pillow. In the morning he generally awoke pain-free and without elbow stiffness, unless he had been sleeping with his arm in an awkward position during the night. Specific questions regarding the effect of cervical movements and sustained cervical postures provided no further information.

Specific questioning regarding general health, previous medical history and other related health issues, revealed nothing apart from dermatitis.

■ REASONING DISCUSSION

 1 Did you specifically screen for or appraise the patient's psychosocial status (including his understanding of the problem and his feelings about his management to date and the effect it is having on his life)? Did this factor have an effect on his symptoms?

■ Clinicians' answer

In response to the question of what was his main problem, the patient answered that it was pain in the region of the lateral epicondyle when writing or using the computer keyboard. The patient had never before been to a physiotherapist for treatment. His only reason for attending was because he had been asked to do so by his treating doctor. His understanding of the problem was based on what he had been told by the doctors he had consulted, in that he had tendinitis of the wrist and finger extensors.

The elbow problem certainly affected his life. He had pain through the day at work and was unable to perform his normal duties of writing and computer keyboard operation without significant exacerbation. Being in a managerial position, he felt he could not reduce his work activity by taking sick leave. In addition, his social life had been disrupted as he had been forced to stop playing recreational bowls. Even though the elbow problem was a significant intrusion in his life, Howard still felt able to cope and was not particularly

burdened by his elbow disability. He believed that auto-mechanics had to put up with some impairment during their working life as a consequence of the physical nature of their work. His previous history of neck pain bore witness to this fact.

Howard appeared quietly resigned to his lot. He felt that medical management had not really helped him and that he was probably going to have to live with a painful elbow for a considerable length of time. Because he was managing the business, he also felt frustrated that he was unable to take time off when he first hurt his elbow. He believed that the problem would have settled if he had been allowed to rest initially and that he would not have been in the present situation if his mechanic had not been off work.

PHYSICAL EXAMINATION

On physical examination, Howard had poor sitting posture, with an increased thoracic kyphosis, protracted and depressed shoulder girdle bilaterally and an increased cervical spine lordosis. In the standing position, the upper limbs were held in internal rotation at the shoulder, both elbows were maintained in slight flexion and both forearms were pronated. There was no evidence of muscle wasting, soft tissue swelling or any other sign of deformity in the elbow region.

Active movements

Right elbow and wrist mobility was full and without pain. Cervical range of motion was limited in all directions by stiffness. Rotation and side flexion was more restricted to the left than the right, and extension was

more restricted than flexion. Positioning the spine in combinations of extension with right side flexion and right rotation, in addition to flexion with left side flexion and left rotation, was pain-free, although the movements were limited in range.

Right and left shoulder mobility, specifically abduction and hand behind back, was mildly restricted by stiffness. The addition of neural tissue-sensitizing manoeuvres slightly decreased the abduction and hand-behind-back ranges of motion on both sides equally. None of these manoeuvres provoked the patient's symptoms, nor any discomfort in the lateral elbow region. However, wrist extension in combination with finger and full right elbow extension evoked the patient's elbow pain with the right shoulder in either abduction or flexion. These same movements on the left side were completely painless.

REASONING DISCUSSION AND CLINICAL REASONING COMMENTARY

1 What was your interpretation of the postural observations? Specifically, what hypotheses did you consider and how did you plan to test these?

Clinicians' answer

Abnormal posture is a frequent finding during routine clinical examination. Some studies have demon-

strated abnormal postural features related to specific pain syndromes such as cervical headache (Haughie et al., 1995; Watson and Trott, 1993), but other investigations have found no such link (Refshauge et al., 1995). This particular patient presented with a common form of spinal and upper limb postural abnormality. It has been proposed (Mack and

Burfield, 1998) that forearm muscle imbalance and abnormal radiohumeral alignment plays a significant role in the prolongation of tennis elbow. Similarly, White and Sahrmann (1994) contended that abnormal posture and related muscle function may lead to repetitive microtrauma, which may be a factor in the development and maintenance of pain syndromes. The therapist must, therefore, determine whether the patient's posture has any bearing on the development or maintenance of the presenting condition.

In this case, the postural assessment revealed no significant difference between the left and right upper limb, which may indicate that the variance in posture was not directly related to the pain disorder. However, the abnormal posture and possible related muscle dysfunction may have been a contributing factor to the problem. Lee (1986) has postulated that the type of head and neck posture seen in this patient may be a precipitating factor in the development of chronic tennis elbow, and that correction of this posture is an important aspect of treatment. The history of neck problems, abnormal bone scan findings in the lower cervical and thoracic spine, and the abnormal cervical and thoracic posture indicate the need to examine the cervical spine thoroughly. If the cervical spine was found to be a significant contributing factor to the problem, then the abnormal posture may need to be addressed. In addition, the flexed and pronated forearm posture may have been caused by muscle imbalance or joint restriction in the elbow complex, necessitating assessment of both muscle and articular function.

2 What was your interpretation of the pain provoked by wrist extension and shoulder movement?

Clinicians' answer

Clinical experience suggests that peripheral nerve trunk sensitization frequently accompanies lateral elbow pain, with this finding also reported in the literature (Yaxley and Jull, 1993). To determine the presence of nerve trunk sensitization, an assessment for active movement dysfunction is needed (Hall and Elvey, 1999). The movements of wrist extension and shoulder abduction are provocative to upper quarter neural tissue (Elvey, 1979; Kleinrensink et al., 1995; Lewis et al., 1998; Reid, 1987). Active wrist extension will also stress the origin of the wrist and finger

extensors. In contrast, shoulder flexion is usually less provocative than abduction to upper quarter neural tissue. Hence, there should be a greater pain response to wrist extension with the arm in abduction rather than flexion, if the upper quarter neural tissue is sensitized. If the source of the symptoms is the extensor muscle origin (or structures other than neural tissue), then wrist extension should be equally symptomatic in shoulder abduction and shoulder flexion, as was found in this case.

3 At this stage, were there any potential contributing factors (e.g. environmental, biomechanical) identified in either the subjective or physical examination that you considered may be relevant to the development or maintenance of his problem?

Clinicians' answer

Tennis elbow is not restricted to those that play tennis and other racquet sports (Kivi, 1982). It is common in the general non-sporting population, especially amongst those whose occupations involve repetitive or forceful forearm, wrist and hand activities (Plancher et al., 1996), particularly involving overuse of gripping and wrist extension. Following an extensive survey of 15 000 residents of Stockholm, Allander (1974) reported an annual incidence rate for lateral epicondylitis of 0.1–1% and a prevalence rate of 1–10%.

A number of factors can be identified from the subjective examination that may have contributed to either the onset or the maintenance of Howard's lateral elbow pain:

- a sedentary lifestyle, including working in an office, that suddenly changed to a physically demanding job involving repetitive and forceful wrist and arm activities, with the neck and arm in awkward positions; although he had the skills required to perform this job, he did not have the necessary musculoskeletal conditioning
- continuing to work as a mechanic for some time after the incident of loosening the corroded nut would have amplified the problem
- activities (e.g. typing and writing) after returning to normal duties may have delayed normal healing through repetitive overload stress
- age (51 years): Putnam and Cohen (1999) reported slower healing times for older patients.

In terms of the physical examination, the following factors may have contributed to the onset or maintenance of Howard's lateral elbow pain:

- overactivity of the elbow flexor and forearm pronator muscles may indicate abnormal functioning of the upper limb muscles
- active movement dysfunction of the cervical spine.

Even though the patient demonstrated full range of elbow and wrist motion, the resting posture suggests overactivity of the elbow flexor and forearm pronator muscles. This may be an indication of abnormal functioning of the upper limb muscles. A muscle imbalance may cause abnormal joint axes of rotation and repetitive microtrauma from everyday joint movement (White and Sahrmann, 1994). Mack and Burfield (1998) have proposed that imbalance between the forearm supinator and pronator muscles is a causative factor in tennis elbow.

Physical examination of the cervical spine revealed evidence of active movement dysfunction, although not symptomatic. Bone scan imaging showed increased tracer uptake in the C5–C6 facet joints bilaterally. Some authors have proposed that clinical and subclinical neuropathic disorders of the cervical spine can sometimes be a significant factor in tennis elbow (Gunn and Milbrandt, 1976; Lee, 1986).

■ Clinical reasoning commentary

Although observation is just one small part of the physical examination in this case, it is interesting to note how the findings from this common 'test' can be used to form and test hypotheses in several categories. The findings have informed decision making related to the physical impairments (e.g. joint restriction in the elbow) and sources of the elbow pain (e.g. cervical spine), factors contributing to the problem (e.g. abnormal posture), and management and treatment (e.g. postural correction), as well as directing later search strategies, such as the need to examine the cervical spine. This illustrates the ability of the expert to recognize the relevance and meaning of clinical features, and the associated implications for subsequent actions. In addition to improving the accuracy of decision making, this also enhances the efficiency of the overall clinical reasoning process. Extensive clinical experience, and reflection about such experience, is integral to developing this ability.

Muscle tests

Significant pain was reproduced on palpating the origin of the right extensor carpi radialis brevis muscle on the anteroinferior aspect of the lateral epicondyle, as well as the proximal muscle mass of the wrist and finger extensors. Gripping with mild pressure reproduced the pain with the elbow flexed or extended, but only in forearm pronation. Isometric contraction of the wrist and finger extensors also reproduced the elbow pain. Isolated isometric contraction of the middle finger extensors was notably more painful, but testing of the forearm supinators was symptom free. Stretching the wrist into flexion was provocative, particularly with the forearm pronated and the elbow fully extended. Muscle length of the forearm supinators and pronators was assessed indirectly by observing the range of active movement of forearm pronation and supination and found to be normal. Further assessment for muscle imbalance was left for a later session (if necessary) because the principal goal of the initial assessment was pain relief.

Passive movements

Mild pain was reproduced and abnormal stiffness detected on passive accessory motion testing of the right radiohumeral joint but not the humeroulnar joint, nor the joints of the left elbow complex. Pain and stiffness was more apparent with the right elbow in full extension and pronation. Neural tissue provocation tests biased to the radial and median nerve trunks did not reproduce the symptoms, and the range of movement was equal between sides. Normal responses were elicited on palpation of the nerve trunks in the upper limb. Passive physiological motion testing of the cervical and thoracic spine revealed marked restriction of movement at C5–C6, C6–C7 and from T3 to T6. Passive accessory motion testing indicated a pain and stiffness relationship at the same spinal levels. It was not possible to reproduce the arm symptoms using any provocative manoeuvres of the cervical spine.

The effect of mobilizations with movement (MWMs) (Mulligan, 1999) of the elbow was also assessed. This was considered worthwhile as they often have the effect of increasing function while at the same time reducing pain, and do not usually require a reduction in duties at home or work. MWMs are sustained mobilizations (accessory glides) of a joint simultaneously applied with the particular movement that is painful or restricted in range. In cases of soft tissue lesions (such as tennis elbow), the glide is accompanied by contraction of the muscles surrounding the joint. The most important principle to follow in using MWMs is that the pain associated with the muscle contraction or joint movement should be completely relieved by the mobilization. In some instances, pain may not be relieved at the first attempt and the therapist must adjust either the force of the glide or the plane in which it is made. Furthermore, the glide should be applied as close as possible to the joint line. If pain is not alleviated, even after adjustments are made by the therapist, then the technique is not indicated and should not be used. In cases of chronic tennis elbow, the passive accessory movement that usually relieves pain is a lateral glide of the ulna and radius on the humerus (Mulligan, 1999).

To determine whether the technique was indicated a lateral glide was trialed. The proximal aspect of the elbow was stabilized with one hand over the lateral

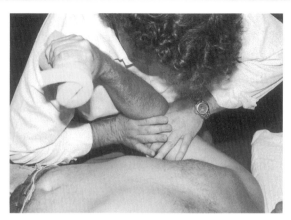

Fig. 6.2 Lateral glide of the elbow.

border of the humerus, as close as possible to the elbow joint line (Fig. 6.2). The other hand was placed just distal to the joint line on the medial border of the ulna and mobilized in a lateral direction. The glide was sustained while the patient performed an activity that normally reproduced his symptoms markedly. Gripping was chosen as it was functional and would be easy for the patient to perform at home at a later stage if necessary. It was found that the pain normally caused by gripping was not present during the application of the lateral glide.

REASONING DISCUSSION AND CLINICAL REASONING COMMENTARY

1 What was your working hypothesis at the conclusion of the physical examination? What clinical findings tended to support or discount your thinking?

Clinicians' answer

The physical examination findings correlated well with the subjective complaint and suggested a disorder characteristic of lateral epicondylitis. There was strong evidence of local structures as the source of the symptoms, namely extensor carpi radialis brevis and the radiohumeral joint. There was lesser evidence for referred pain from remote sources. It was probable that the cervical and thoracic signs were related to a coincidental degenerative disorder and there was no evidence of neural tissue involvement.

Findings in support of local structures as a source of pain include:

- symptom reproduction on active wrist extension was unchanged with either shoulder flexion or elbow flexion
- symptom reproduction on mildly forceful gripping
- symptom reproduction on isometric contraction of the wrist and finger extensors, and in particular the middle finger extensors, which are thought to indicate involvement of extensor carpi radialis brevis (Wadsworth, 1987)
- pain on stretching the finger extensors
- symptom reproduction on palpation of the lateral epicondyle at the site of the origin of the extensor carpi radialis brevis muscle (Noteboom et al., 1994)
- no pain on gripping with the MWM.

Somewhat inconsistent with this hypothesis (but not uncommon) was the finding of pain on gripping with the elbow either flexed or extended. The finding of radiohumeral joint dysfunction on passive accessory motion testing was also inconsistent with a tendinopathy as the source of pain.

Findings in support of remote structures as a source of pain include:

- cervical active and combined movement dysfunction, although not in a clinical pattern consistent with the arm symptoms
- bone scan abnormality at C5–C6, a cervical level consistent with the arm symptoms
- cervical passive physiological movement dysfunction in a region (C5–C6, C6–C7) consistent with the arm symptoms
- the pain and stiffness relationship found on passive accessory motion testing in a region (C5–C6, C6–C7) consistent with the arm symptoms.

Assessment of cervical active movements revealed limitation of movement without pain. Clinical pattern recognition for arm pain, be it a mechanical nociceptive or neuropathic disorder, is dependent in part on key active and combined movement combinations. Clinical patterns can be recognized for cervical neural tissue sensitization, cervical neural tissue axonal compromise/dysaesthesia, and cervical somatic tissue dysfunction (disc and facet joint). Combinations of the most restricted active movements did not provide evidence of a regular stretch or compressive pattern as outlined by Edwards (1992) and Oliver (1989). If right-sided cervical somatic structures were the source of the elbow symptoms, then applying increasing stress in a regular, progressive fashion either to stretch or to compress those tissues would have given a predictable pain provocative response. This was not the case. If cervical neural structures were the source

of the arm symptoms, by way of axonal compromise or dysaesthesia, then applying a combination of movements to close the right lower cervical intervertebral foramen (extension with right side flexion and right rotation) should be provocative. Again, this was not the case. Cervical active movement limitation was consistent with neural tissue sensitization (left side flexion), but further testing negated this possibility.

Tending to negate the cervical spine as a source of the pain was the inability to reproduce any arm symptoms using a range of provocative manoeuvres. There was also no evidence of a neurogenic disorder. Neural tissue provocation tests, outlined by Hall and Elvey (1999), failed to reveal any significant abnormality. A neurological examination was not undertaken as it is unlikely to be sufficiently sensitive to detect the mild signs of neural compromise that may be present in tennis elbow (Gunn and Milbrandt, 1976; Lee, 1986).

■ Clinical reasoning commentary

Thinking related to the recognition of clinical patterns is evident in this response. Pattern recognition, a hallmark of the clinical reasoning automatically used by expert clinicians, is an efficient and accurate process for handling large amounts of clinical data and making appropriate clinical decisions. Nevertheless, these patterns must still be tested to determine whether they are correct in a particular clinical case. In this case, clinical patterns were sought, but were unable to be verified, for cervical neural tissue sensitization, cervical neural tissue axonal compromise/dysaesthesia, and cervical somatic tissue impairment (disc and facet joint). Testing by way of active and combined movements, in addition to later neural mobility testing, enabled the reranking, if not almost rejection, of these hypotheses in an efficient and logical manner.

m ▎ Initial management

■ Treatment 1

The treatment chosen consisted of an MWM to the elbow using a lateral glide with gripping. A thorough explanation was given to the patient about the principles behind the technique before mobilization was commenced. It is important that the patient understands that the technique should cause no

pain at all. If pain is provoked, then the patient must inform the therapist immediately to prevent exacerbating the condition. In addition, the patient is given to understand that a positional fault of the bones in the elbow joint can cause abnormal pulling of the extensor muscles at the elbow and be a contributing factor to chronic tennis elbow. If this is the case, then correction of the positional fault by lateral gliding of the bones should allow gripping to become pain-free.

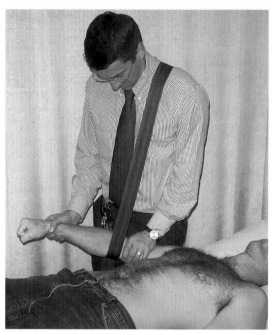

Fig. 6.3 Mobilization with movement for tennis elbow using a treatment belt.

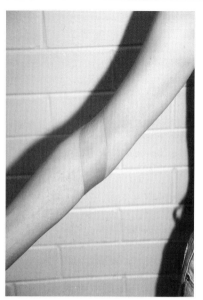

Fig. 6.4 Taping technique for tennis elbow.

A manual therapy belt was used to maintain comfortably sufficient lateral glide force to relieve pain completely while the aggravating activity of gripping was undertaken ten times in succession (Fig. 6.3).

At the end of ten repetitions, reassessment demonstrated that mild gripping was pain-free. Moderately forceful gripping and resisted finger extension were still painful. The same technique was repeated for two more sets of ten repetitions. Subsequently gripping was completely pain-free.

Strapping tape was applied to the elbow in such a fashion as to replicate the lateral glide, in an attempt to maintain the effect of the technique (Fig. 6.4). The patient was advised to wear the tape for 48 hours in order to maintain the effect of the treatment. The need to remove the tape in the event of skin irritation was stressed because of the history of dermatitis.

To determine the efficacy of the therapy, Howard was instructed to carry out his normal home and work activities, and asked to return in 2 days.

Treatment 2

On returning, the patient reported significant relief of symptoms after treatment, with less-frequent pain and the ability to type and write for longer periods without pain. The strapping tape had irritated his skin and was removed the morning after the first treatment. The skin where the tape had been applied was slightly red. No further strapping tape was used.

On reassessment, gripping was comfortable until a moderate force was applied, whereupon pain was provoked with the elbow in either full extension or 90 degrees flexion. Pain on resisted isometric wrist and finger extension, and local tenderness in the region of the attachment of extensor carpi radialis brevis, was unchanged from the previous examination. Pain was also elicited on active wrist extension with the elbow in full extension and pronation and with the arm positioned several ways, including by the side, in 90 degrees flexion and in 90 degrees abduction.

Because of the success of the initial treatment, a decision was made to incorporate a self-management programme involving the lateral glide technique. Howard was shown a simple means of replicating the technique utilizing a broad belt around the circumference of the body lateral to the humerus and just proximal to the elbow joint line (Fig. 6.5).

The patient applied the lateral glide with his left hand. He was instructed that at no time should the technique be painful. If pain occurred, then the technique was either to be adjusted until it became pain-free or abandoned. Howard was asked to demonstrate the technique and guidance was given on the appropriate method. Using this approach, Howard was able

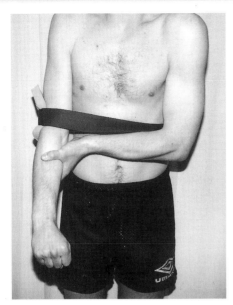

Fig. 6.5   Self-treatment for tennis elbow.

to eliminate all pain with moderate gripping force. He was advised to perform 10 repetitions of the exercise three times per day.

Therapist intervention consisted of a sustained lateral glide using a belt, while the patient performed 10 repetitions of gripping. Three sets were undertaken with the elbow in full extension and a further three with the elbow in 90 degrees flexion. On reassessment, gripping was no longer painful in extension or flexion; however resisted isometric wrist and finger extension continued to be symptomatic. Active wrist extension with the elbow in full extension and pronation and with the arm by the side, in 90 degrees flexion and in 90 degrees abduction, was less painful than at initial evaluation. Howard was advised to continue his normal daily activities and to return in 4 days.

Treatment 3

Howard reported no discomfort with writing but still complained of pain with computer keyboard and mouse activities. Shaving and teeth cleaning had not been problems. He had noticed carrying a heavy bag in his right hand had aggravated his symptoms for 1 day. Regular use of the prescribed exercise markedly relieved the symptoms the next day.

On physical examination, gripping was pain-free in full extension and 90 degrees flexion, but resisted isometric wrist and finger extension was still painful,

however not to the same degree as at the initial examination. The movement of active wrist extension with the elbow in full extension and pronation and with the arm by the side, in 90 degrees flexion and in 90 degrees abduction, was only mildly painful. Stretching the extensor muscles using full wrist flexion with an extended/pronated elbow was no longer painful. In addition, the degree of sensitivity on palpation of the common extensor origin and muscle mass was markedly reduced.

A decision was made to maintain the lateral glide but change the active component to resisted isometric wrist and finger extension, rather than gripping. The pain-free isometric contraction was sustained for 3 seconds and repeated 10 times in succession. Four further sets were included in this treatment session. The only modification to the home exercise was adding end-range wrist extension to clenching of the hand.

At the end of the treatment session, Howard had pain-free resisted isometric finger and wrist extension, as well as full pain-free grip strength. It was thought that a trial game of lawn bowls would be appropriate to determine the degree of improvement. An appointment was arranged for 1 week to review progress.

Treatment 4

Howard reported that since the previous treatment session there had been no discomfort with everyday work and home duties. He had played a full game of bowls and carried the ball in his right hand without difficulty. There had been a flare up of symptoms after working for 3 hours on his son's car. Using a screwdriver and a socket driver appeared to be the aggravating activities. This exacerbation settled after performing his home exercise the next day.

On physical examination, the only activity that reproduced pain was resisted isometric middle finger extension. There was mild tenderness on palpation of the attachment of extensor carpi radialis brevis and the associated extensor muscle mass. The movement of active wrist extension with the elbow in full extension and pronation, with the arm by the side, in 90 degrees flexion and in 90 degrees abduction, was not painful. Wrist and finger extensor muscle stretch was now pain-free. Passive accessory motion of the radiohumeral joint was still restricted by stiffness, but pain was no longer evoked.

Therapist intervention was the same as that provided at the previous session. Five sets of 10 repetitions of resisted isometric wrist and finger extension, with each contraction held for 3 seconds, completely abolished the pain with all muscle contraction tests. Howard was advised to carry on with the self-mobilization techniques on a daily basis for the next week, or longer if the elbow continued to be a problem.

In an attempt to prevent future recurrences, a tennis elbow brace (epicondylitis clasp) was provided for unaccustomed activities involving forceful gripping. The brace was recommended to reduce the stress on the common extensor origin from forceful gripping activities. It was thought that unaccustomed forceful use of the wrist and finger extensor and forearm pronator muscles could overload the common extensor origin and provoke a new episode of pain. The mechanical role of the brace was to spread the force

of gripping over the whole forearm and so reduce the overall load at the common extensor origin. It has been shown that similar clasps can significantly improve pain-free grip strength in sufferers of tennis elbow (Burton, 1985).

As this episode had been caused by overstress of the forearm musculature, Howard was also prescribed exercises for improving control of the forearm supinator and pronator muscles, as well as the wrist and finger extensor and flexor muscles. It was explained to the patient that this was to prepare the elbow joint and forearm muscles for future forceful gripping activities. Howard was also advised to resume the self-mobilization exercises in the event of recurrence and to continue with them for 1 week after the symptoms subside.

 ## REASONING DISCUSSION AND CLINICAL REASONING COMMENTARY

1 What caused to you to select the chosen MWM as your treatment?

■ Clinicians' answer

Historically, tennis elbow has been a difficult problem to treat, with a wide variety of procedures and management protocols advocated (Caldwell and Safran, 1995; Noteboom et al., 1994; Putnam and Cohen, 1999; Reid and Kushner, 1993). Generally, treatment is prolonged and long-term outcomes questionable (Mack and Burfield, 1998). When indicated, the MWM for tennis elbow described by Mulligan (1999) is a simple but extremely effective means of treating this disorder. However, an indication for use is only determined by trial application of the technique. Therefore, the reasons for selection of an elbow MWM for treatment were:

- immediate abolishment of pain during the trial
- previous experience and knowledge of efficacy of the technique
- potential for integration into a home treatment programme suitable for the patient's presentation and lifestyle.

Furthermore, the immediate and marked reduction in symptoms with the technique was helpful in gaining the patient's confidence and compliance in his rehabilitation process. This was particularly important in

this case, as the patient had been referred for strengthening and stretching exercises by his rheumatologist.

2 Could you elaborate further regarding the pathobiological mechanism for this case of tennis elbow? What did you consider caused the positional fault in the first place and what subsequently maintained it?

■ Clinicians' answer

It is probable that the patient developed lateral elbow pain as a result of unaccustomed use (as well as overuse) of the forearm pronator and the wrist and finger extensor muscles during the 2-week period he worked as a mechanic. His attempt at freeing the corroded nut also required sustained, excessive gripping, forearm pronation and wrist extension force. The patient, therefore, suffered a sudden strain, as well as repetitive microtrauma, to the musculotendinous insertion, thus causing tissue damage. The consequent scarring, possibly consisting of granulofibroblastic materials among others, subsequently became infiltrated with free nerve endings. It is known that granulofibroblastic material laid down in the repair process of tennis elbow contains free nerve endings (Goldie, 1964).

It was found that 'repositioning' the ulna and radius with respect to the humerus completely abolished the patient's pain. It was hypothesized that malpositioning of the ulna and radius was caused by the excessive forearm pronation and wrist extension force used to loosen the corroded nut. This excessive force was not matched by adequate control of the antagonist forearm muscles, particularly the supinator. This information, together with the other findings from the clinical examination, indicates that this patient's pain problem was a mechanical nociceptive disorder involving the elbow joint complex, as well as the muscles that arise from the common extensor origin at the lateral epicondyle. Abnormal positioning of the ulna and radius during activities that involved contraction of the finger and wrist extensor muscles, particularly with the forearm in pronation (typing, writing, teeth cleaning, shaving, etc.), significantly loaded the attachment of the extensor muscles and caused pain. Repeated overuse of the forearm pronator and wrist and finger extensor muscles during these activities maintained the bony positional fault at the elbow. Repeated abnormal loading of the repairing musculotendinous insertion maintained sensitization (centrally and/or peripherally) of the nociceptors and other receptors in the scar tissue, consequently maintaining the pain disorder.

The concept of abnormal bone positioning has been proposed by Mulligan (1999) as an explanation for the purported success of MWMs in the treatment of chronic tennis elbow and other disorders. Mack and Burfield (1998) similarly hypothesized that lack of eccentric control of forearm pronation leads to excessive medial and inferior displacement of the head of the radius, which subsequently increases the load on the common extensor origin at the lateral epicondyle. Eccentric control of forearm pronation, and therefore lateral elbow stability, is provided by the supinator muscle (Stroyan and Wilk, 1993) with its close attachment to the lateral epicondyle, radial collateral and annular ligaments (Mack and Burfield, 1998). The concept of abnormal humeroulnar and radiohumeral alignment in tennis elbow is supported by the results of a single case study design by Vicenzino and Wright (1995). They demonstrated that the lateral glide MWM of the elbow (Mulligan, 1999), which might potentially correct the medial radial displacement described by Mack and Burfield (1998), immediately relieved the pain experienced during gripping tasks and normal function was rapidly restored.

However, clinical experience indicates that close attention to technique with respect to the angle and plane of the glide is critical to the success of MWM. In a concave/convex joint, the plane in which the MWM

glide is directed is dependent on the orientation of the concave joint surface, often referred to as the treatment plane (Kaltenborn, 1980). Failure by the therapist to apply the glide parallel to this treatment plane will result in compression of the joint surfaces and consequently cause pain (Mulligan, 1999). In many cases, the therapist may not apply the glide precisely in the right direction initially. If the therapist is unable to relieve the symptoms with the glide, then subtle changes in the glide angle should be employed to abolish symptoms completely during the accompanying movement or muscle contraction.

Faulty joint alignment can mechanically distort scar tissue and thus stimulate the in situ free nerve endings laid down in the repair process sufficiently to evoke mechanical nociceptive pain. Correction of the joint malalignment by MWM may reduce the mechanical distortion of the scar tissue and so relieve pain.

3 Considering the proposed positional fault mechanism, what was your interpretation of the physical signs that suggested a musculotendinous pathology rather than a joint pathology?

Clinicians' answer

It is important to understand that the hypothesis of malpositioning of the ulna and radius in relation to the humerus does not preclude a problem with the musculotendinous insertion. The physical signs found are consistent with a musculotendinous pathology, as well as an elbow joint complex pathology. Malpositioning of the ulna and radius in relation to the humerus creates an increased load on the musculotendinous attachment during gripping and wrist and finger extension tasks. Nociception arises from mechanically evoked responses from receptors in the repairing scar tissue at the musculotendinous attachment, rather than from just the joint complex itself. Repositioning the ulna and radius in relation to the humerus normalizes loading on the attachment during gripping and other tasks, thereby reducing mechanical provocation of the sensitized receptors within the scar tissue.

The finding of increased stiffness to passive accessory motion testing of the radiohumeral joint was not entirely consistent with a joint instability problem. With an instability problem, one would anticipate hypermobility rather than hypomobility, unless there was associated muscle guarding.

4 How did you gain the patient's consent for the MWM intervention when he had been referred for strengthening and stretching exercises?

Clinicians' answer

The MWM is an integral part of the assessment process. The patient was informed that in the opinion of the examiner there was a positional fault of the bones that make up the elbow joint. The relief of pain on MWM testing while gripping verified this finding. The patient could see that restoring the alignment of the bones had allowed normal pain-free functioning of the wrist and forearm muscles. It was also explained that if the technique was repeated a number of times this would permit the muscles to be exercised painlessly and would hasten the recovery process. As well, it would allow the patient to perform his normal daily duties. Therefore, MWM is not inconsistent with the doctor's request for strengthening exercise. Graduated muscle activity is an integral part of the treatment procedure. The passive mobilization component of the MWM allows the exercise to be performed without pain.

5 Were you expecting the MWMs involving gripping to have a greater effect upon resisted wrist and finger extension? Why did you think that the effect was limited?

Clinicians' answer

Isometric wrist and finger extension is usually more provocative to the musculotendinous unit at the lateral epicondyle than gripping. Clinically, gripping is sometimes only mildly evocative of lateral elbow symptoms, whereas isometric wrist and finger extension is more frequently intensely evocative. However, with Howard, gripping was incorporated into the MWM because it is easier to perform both in the clinic and at home than isometric wrist and finger extension.

In many cases, using a MWM that involves gripping will subsequently relieve the pain on isometric wrist and finger extension. This was not the case with Howard, although the pain with isometric wrist and finger extension was diminished to some degree. The reason for this may be that the force required to reposition the radius with respect to the humerus for pain-free gripping was less than that required for pain-free isometric wrist and finger extension. This could be because gripping is a less-stressful activity for the musculotendinous attachment at the lateral epicondyle. Consequently it was planned to combine the MWM with isometric wrist and finger extension as a progression of treatment.

Clinical reasoning commentary

The selection of MWM for the treatment sheds light on some interesting aspects of expert clinical reasoning. This management decision was based on several reasons relating to the past, the present and the future. First, past experience with similar clinical presentations, along with knowledge of preliminary research evidence, has greatly informed the treatment decision. Recognition of this particular clinical pattern is associated with specific actions, including interventions, that have previously been found to be productive. Secondly, the present finding of immediate abolition of pain with the application of MWM is a defining result from the 'trial treatment' test. The hypothesis of local elbow musculotendinous and joint pathology receives strong support from this finding, but of greater importance is the support it provides for the application of MWM for treatment purposes, as suggested by past experience. Finally, it is anticipated that in future management the use of MWM self-treatment will be valuable, perhaps to accelerate recovery and enable patients to become more actively involved and responsible for their own care. The elimination of pain manifest with MWM is also expected to facilitate compliance with therapy as the patient is able to see immediate results. This ability to think across time—simultaneously in the past, present and future—is reflective of higher order cognitive abilities typical of the expert clinician.

Outcome

During a follow-up telephone call 1 month later, Howard said he had experienced occasional minimal discomfort but felt no need to carry on with his self-mobilization nor attend for further treatment. In the light of this outcome, no further appointments were necessary.

REASONING DISCUSSION AND CLINICAL REASONING COMMENTARY

1 Do you expect that further episodes will occur?

Clinicians' answer

If the patient carries on with his exercise programme, it is unlikely that he will have a return of his lateral elbow pain. However, it is much more likely that he will stop doing the exercise. It is also probable that he will undertake work activity in the future that involves overuse or unaccustomed use of the pronator and wrist and finger extensor muscles, and which may cause a return of his symptoms. Having had one incident of pain related to this type of activity probably predisposes him to future episodes, particularly if normal humeroulnar and radiohumeral bone alignment is not maintained. If he experiences a significant flare-up, home exercise alone may not be sufficient to relieve his pain and he would need to return for further treatment.

In the patient's favour at this point is the fact that he has been educated about his condition and now understands the importance of self-management. Howard is aware that his problem originated from unaccustomed use of the forearm muscles, leading to abnormal forces around the elbow and subsequent joint malalignment and tissue breakdown. Careful attention has also been paid to potential contributing factors such as work technique, prevention of overuse and overload, maintenance of supinator eccentric control, and the patient's active participation in his own management, all of which may help to minimize recurrence of his pain.

Clinical reasoning commentary

The prognostic hypothesis here is guarded despite the excellent outcome to manual therapy. The possibility that the patient will cease self-management and undertake ill-advised work activities is recognized. However, the broad and holistic approach to management, which includes educational and ergonomic interventions, is acknowledged as having a positive influence on the patient's prognosis. From this response, it would appear that experience-based personal knowledge has somewhat influenced this clinical reasoning decision. An understanding of the various demands and priorities in a patient's life is largely acquired from, and can only be truly appreciated from, the perspective of one's own personal experience of similar situations.

References

Allander, E. (1974). Prevalence, incidence and remission rates of some common rheumatic diseases and syndromes. Scandinavian Journal of Rheumatology, 3, 145–153.

Burton, A.K. (1985). Grip strength and forearm straps in tennis elbow. British Journal of Sports Medicine, 19, 37–38.

Caldwell, G.L. and Safran, M.R. (1995). Elbow problems in the athlete. Orthopedic Clinics of North America, 26, 465–485.

Cyriax, J. (1936). The pathology and treatment of tennis elbow. Journal of Bone and Joint Surgery, 13, 921–939.

Edwards, B.C. (1992). Manual of Combined Movements. Edinburgh: Churchill Livingstone.

Elvey, R.L. (1979). Brachial plexus tension tests and the pathoanatomical origin of arm pain. In Aspects of Manipulative Therapy (R. Idczak, ed.) pp. 105–110. Lincoln: Lincoln Institute of Health Sciences.

Gifford, L.S. and Butler, D.S. (1997). The integration of pain sciences into clinical practice. Journal of Hand Therapy, 10, 86–95.

Goldie, I. (1964). Epicondylitis lateralis humeri. Acta Chirurgica Scandinavica Supplementum, 339, 1–114.

Gunn, C.C. and Milbrandt, W.E. (1976). Tennis elbow and the cervical spine. Canadian Medical Association Journal, 114, 803–809.

Hall, T.M. and Elvey R.L. (1999). Nerve trunk pain: Physical diagnosis and treatment. Manual Therapy, 4, 63–73.

Haughie, L.J., Fiebert, I.M. and Roach, K.E. (1995). Relationship of forward head posture and cervical backward bending to neck pain. Journal of Manual and Manipulative Therapy, 3, 91–97.

Kaltenborn, F.M. (1980). Mobilisation of the Extremity Joints. Oslo: Olaf Norlis Bokhandel.

Kivi, P. (1982). The aetiology and conservative treatment of humeral epicondylitis. Scandinavian Journal of Rehabilitation Medicine, 15, 37–41.

Kleinrensink, G., Stoeckart, R., Vleeming, A. et al. (1995). Mechanical tension in the median nerve. The effects of joint positions. Clinical Biomechanics, 10, 240–244.

Lee, D.G. (1986). 'Tennis elbow': a manual therapist's perspective. Journal of Orthopedic and Sports Physical Therapy, 8, 134–142.

Lewis, J., Ramot, R and Green, A. (1998). Changes in mechanical tension in the median nerve: possible implications for the upper limb tension test. Physiotherapy, 84, 254–261.

Mack, M. and Burfield, H. (1998). A new approach in the treatment of tennis elbow. In Newsletter of the Western Australian Chapter of the Australian Physiotherapy Association Sports Physiotherapy Group, Autumn, 4.

Mulligan, B. (1999). Manual Therapy. 'NAGS', 'SNAGS', 'MWMs' etc., 4th edn. Wellington, New Zealand: Plane View Press.

Nirschl, R.P. and Petrone, F.A. (1979). Tennis elbow. Journal of Bone and Joint Surgery, 61A, 832–839.

Noteboom, T., Cruver, R., Keller, J. et al. (1994). Tennis elbow: a review. Journal of Orthopedic and Sports Physical Therapy, 19, 357–366.

Oliver, M.J. (1989). A biomechanical basis for classification of movement patterns in combined movements examination of the spine. In Proceedings of the Sixth Biennial Conference of the Manipulative Therapists Association of Australia pp. 138–145. Melbourne: Manipulative Therapists Association of Australia.

Plancher, K.D., Halbrecht, J. and Lourie, G.M. (1996). Medial and lateral epicondylitis in the athlete. Clinics in Sports Medicine, 15, 283–305.

Putnam, M.D. and Cohen, M. (1999). Painful conditions around the elbow. Orthopedic Clinics of North America, 30, 109–118.

Refshauge, K., Bolst, L. and Goodsel, M. (1995). The relationship between cervicothoracic posture and the presence of pain. Journal of Manual and Manipulative Therapy, 3, 21–24.

Reid, D.C. and Kushner, S. (1993). The elbow region. In Orthopaedic Physical Therapy (R. Donatelli and M.J. Wooden, eds.) pp. 203–232. Edinburgh: Churchill Livingstone.

Reid, S. (1987). The measurement of tension changes in the brachial plexus. In Proceedings of the Fifth Biennial Conference of the Manipulative Therapists Association of Australia (B.A. Dalziel and J.C. Snowsill, eds.) pp. 79–90. Melbourne: Manipulative Therapists Association of Australia.

Stroyan, M. and Wilk, K.E. (1993). The functional anatomy of the elbow complex. Journal of Orthopedic and Sports Physical Therapy, 17, 279–288.

Uhthoff, H.K. and Sarkar, K. (1980). Ultrastructure of the common extensor tendon in tennis elbow. Virchows Archiv A Pathological Anatomy and Histology, 386, 317–330.

Vicenzino, B. and Wright, A. (1995). Effects of a novel manipulative physiotherapy technique on tennis elbow: A single case study. Manual Therapy, 1, 30–35.

Wadsworth, T.G. (1987). Tennis elbow: conservative, surgical, and manipulative treatment. British Medical Journal, 294, 621–623.

Watson, D.H. and Trott, P.H. (1993). Cervical headache: an investigation of natural head posture and upper cervical flexor muscle performance. Cephalalgia, 13, 272–284.

White, S.G. and Sahrmann, S.A. (1994). A movement system balance approach to management of musculoskeletal pain. In Physical Therapy of the Cervical and Thoracic Spine, 2nd edn (R. Grant, ed.) pp. 339–357. Edinburgh: Churchill Livingstone.

Yaxley, G. and Jull, G. (1993). Adverse tension in the neural system: A preliminary study of tennis elbow. Australian Journal of Physiotherapy, 39, 15–22.

7

Chronic low back and coccygeal pain

Paul Hodges

SUBJECTIVE EXAMINATION

Skye is a 39-year-old female high school teacher who presented with a 6-month history of lower back and coccyx pain. She had no referral of pain laterally into her buttocks or into her legs and no anaesthesia or paraesthesia. The pain had developed gradually over a period of 2 months with no identifiable cause. There was no history of direct trauma to the coccyx (e.g. fall or childbirth) or of previous lumbar, thoracic or lower limb pain. She was generally fit and well with no neurological, respiratory, gastroenterological, gynaecological or other musculoskeletal disorders, including no change in bladder or bowel function as ascertained through general screening questions. Prior to her initial physiotherapy consultation Skye had consulted an orthopaedic surgeon, who performed a coccygectomy. This did not result in any change to her symptoms postsurgery. Functionally, Skye was able to continue to work with modification to her routine to allow frequent changes in position, but she had required several days off work because of pain. Following the surgery, a friend had recommended she start swimming three times per week. She had done this and was now relatively fit.

Skye's main complaint was an inability to sit or stand for periods greater than 30 minutes as a result of central pain in the coccyx and lower lumbar spine area. Her pain was also increased by other sustained positions, such as lumbar flexion. She generally supported herself using her arms if she had to sustain a position for any duration and often her pain would increase after returning to the neutral position. Her most comfortable position was supine lying, and as such she had no night pain or sleep disturbance. Skye was relatively pain-free in the morning, but her pain progressively increased during the day. At times, she needed to rest in supine lying in the middle of the day in order to relieve her back pain. She had difficulty in sitting through long meetings and had to change position regularly. Her work colleagues were aware of her condition and were supportive. Her main recreational activities were reading, swimming, socializing and travel. She was able to position herself comfortably to read and swimming did not provoke her symptoms. However, she found it difficult to meet people socially because this generally involved either prolonged sitting or prolonged standing, which invariably were uncomfortable. Therefore, she had limited her social interaction because of the pain. In addition, she lived alone and was now depressed about her present situation. She was also concerned that she may not be able to travel long distances again because of her inability to sit for long periods.

Skye felt angry and disappointed that the removal of her coccyx did not resolve her pain. She felt she had been let down by the orthopaedic surgeon, who had provided a simple explanation for her problem. Following the failure of the first surgery, it was recommended to her that she have a revision of the surgery and removal of further tissue. However, Skye felt that this was unlikely to help and declined to have further surgery. She had accepted that she would have pain forever and was concerned that she might 'end up in a wheelchair'. It was clear that she had no understanding of the complex nature of chronic pain or of the concept of pain referral and was not cognisant of any alternative explanation for her symptoms. Furthermore, she was unaware of what physiotherapy could offer but was willing to try anything to help reduce her pain. Her ultimate goal was to become completely pain-free and unrestricted in her recreational activities and travel.

REASONING DISCUSSION AND CLINICAL REASONING COMMENTARY

1 What were your initial thoughts at this stage? In particular, what hypotheses were you considering with respect to the source of the symptoms/impairments and the pain mechanisms involved?

Clinician's answer

My initial impression of this patient was that the coccyx was probably not the primary source of her symptoms. This was largely based on the fact that there was no provocative episode related to the onset of her symptoms and that most of the painful positions and movements would be unlikely to impact on the sacro-coccygeal area. In particular, the failure of the coccygectomy to alter the pain suggested that it was probably not the source. There were several other options that required consideration. The location of the pain was consistent with possible somatic referral from the lumbar spine or sacroiliac joints. In addition, it was anticipated that the function of the deep trunk muscles may be compromised as a result of the presence of pain. This was hypothesized because research evidence has indicated that such a change is a relatively constant finding in people with low back pain (at least of insidious onset) (Hodges and Richardson, 1996) and these changes can be induced by experimental pain (Hodges et al., 2001a). On the basis of the mechanisms that increased and decreased her symptoms (such as sustained flexion) and the insidious onset of her pain, it may be reasonable to suspect disc pathology, but this is difficult to confirm.

Because of the 6-month duration of her symptoms, Skye had moved into a chronic pain state and as such it was likely that peripheral sources of her symptoms may be reduced and central pain processes are now involved. Several factors further complicated this issue, such as her depression, catastrophizing beliefs and the reduction of her leisure activities as a result of pain. However, local processes could not be excluded, particularly if the maintenance of her pain was caused by movement dysfunction/impairment, resulting in repetitive irritation of spinal structures. Regardless, it would be important to consider changes in the central nervous system perception and interpretation of pain.

2 Did you consider that there were any significant psychosocial factors in the patient's presentation? If so, how did you plan to address these in your management?

Clinician's answer

There were several potential psychological factors that may have influenced Skye's presentation. The major factor was a feeling of loss of control and uncertainty. This was compounded by the failure of the initial surgery, which had promised a simple solution. Skye was also fearful for her future and had beliefs regarding the probable course of her symptoms (e.g. 'end up in a wheelchair'). She was also depressed that her social interaction and opportunity to travel were limited by the presence of pain. There is considerable evidence in the literature to suggest that mood and emotion have a significant effect on pain perception (Weisenberg et al., 1998; Zelman et al., 1991). Therefore, it was considered important to attempt to deal with these changes both directly and indirectly.

It was planned to use three main strategies to deal with the psychosocial issues. The first was to provide adequate education about the nature of low back pain and changes that arise when pain becomes chronic. Related discussion would also be needed to deal with expectations and misconceptions. The second was to give her back control of her situation and make her responsible for her recovery. Taking an active approach to management (predominantly involving exercise of the trunk muscles and restoration of trunk control) was considered essential for this to occur. Finally, it was planned to assist with the resolution of these factors by listening, providing support and encouragement, and answering her questions.

Clinical reasoning commentary

The responses to these two questions clearly demonstrate the breadth and depth of the clinical reasoning of the expert clinician, despite it being only early in the clinical encounter. Notably, specific and detailed hypotheses have been generated in a number of categories, including activity/participation restrictions; pathobiological mechanisms (e.g. central pain processes); the patient's perceptions of her experience (i.e. the psychosocial issues discussed); physical impairments and associated sources (e.g. lumbar disc); factors contributing to the maintenance of the problem (e.g. deep trunk muscle dysfunction/impairment); and management (e.g. exercise). This ability to consider multiple hypotheses in multiple categories simultaneously is evidence of highly developed skills in the cognitive processing of clinical data.

PHYSICAL EXAMINATION

General observations

Skye had poor posture in sitting and standing, with a general appearance of having what is commonly described clinically as 'low tone'. Her posture was slouched with a marked cervicothoracic kyphosis, rounded shoulders and upper cervical extension with a 'poked' chin. In standing she had a long shallow lumbar lordosis extending to the mid-thoracic level, an anteriorly shifted pelvis that was positioned in posterior pelvic tilt and hyperextended knees. In many positions, she relied on using her upper limbs to hold herself upright. The thoracic erector spinae were hypertrophied and there was an obvious reduction in bulk of the extensor muscles in the lumbar region. There was also hypertrophy of the hamstrings and wasting of the gluteal muscles. Activity of obliquus externus abdominis (OE) was apparent at rest in standing and sitting. This activity of OE was modulated with respiration, indicating a contribution of OE to expiration (which is normally passive and dependent on elastic recoil of the lungs and chest wall). In conjunction with Skye's kyphosis was a recessed lower rib cage (that narrowed with expiration) and a protruding lower abdomen. Relaxed breathing predominantly involved the upper chest with activity of the accessory inspiratory muscles.

REASONING DISCUSSION AND CLINICAL REASONING COMMENTARY

1 What was your interpretation of the postural and breathing pattern, and its significance to your management?

Clinician's answer

Several recent studies have highlighted the coordination between the diaphragm and deep abdominal muscles (particularly TA) for respiration and postural control (Hodges et al., 1997a; Hodges and Gandevia, 2000a). In normal relaxed standing, there should be low level tonic activity of TA (De Troyer et al., 1990; Goldman et al., 1987; Hodges et al., 1997b); however, there should be no or minimal respiratory modulation of this activity and expiration should be a passive process generated by the elastic recoil of the lungs and rib cage (De Troyer, 1996). In tasks in which respiratory demand is increased, activity of the abdominal muscles will normally occur during expiration to assist with expiratory airflow (Agostoni and Campbell, 1970). If the increased drive for respiration is involuntary (e.g. increased concentration of carbon dioxide), the respiratory modulation of abdominal muscle activity should first occur in TA, then the other abdominal muscles (De Troyer et al., 1990).

When the diaphragm contracts to produce inspiration, there should be both an anterior displacement of the abdominal wall and a bi-basal expansion of the rib cage (as a result of the vertical pull of the costal fibres of the diaphragm and the 'bucket-handle' action of the ribs (Mead, 1979)). For example, during normal relaxed respiration there should be abdominal wall displacement, bi-basal expansion of the rib cage, minimal upper chest movement and no or minimal respiratory activity of the abdominal muscles. When the demand for spinal stability is increased (for example, during repetitive limb movement) the diaphragm and TA should co-contract, with reciprocal changes in amplitude of activity to sustain intra-abdominal pressure and respiration concurrently (concentric contraction of the diaphragm and eccentric contraction of TA for inspiration and the converse for expiration) (Hodges and Gandevia, 2000a,b).

In Skye, there was unexpected activation of OE with expiration (rib cage depression and obvious muscle activity that was modulated with respiration), no tonic activity of TA (protruding lower abdomen) and a reduction in the normal pattern of diaphragmatic breathing (reduced bi-basal expansion, increased upper chest breathing). As a result, most respiration occurred in the upper chest. The reduction in bi-basal expansion is likely to be at least partly a result of the activity of OE, which limits rib cage expansion. These signs suggest that the normal coordination of respiration and postural control may have been compromised and there is excessive use of the superficial abdominal muscles. Clearly, more specific assessment of the function of TA and the other abdominal muscles is needed to confirm this observation. No study has yet confirmed a relationship between these changes in respiratory pattern and back pain, but clinically it appears to be a common finding. Furthermore, experimentally induced acute pain has been shown to produce changes in respiratory function (Tandon et al., 1997).

The mechanism for such changes is not known but it could involve both physical and psychological mechanisms. For instance, the changes may result from increased activity of OE attempting to compensate for poor TA control, or alterations in movement coordination by the central nervous system as a result of pain, which then causes increased activity of OE. Several studies have shown increased activity of specific trunk muscles following experimentally induced pain (Arendt-Nielsen et al., 1996; Hodges et al., 2001a). The changes in respiratory pattern may also occur in an attempt to limit motion of the spine (normal diaphragmatic respiration involves extension of

the lumbar spine and motion at the thoracolumbar junction and rib cage (Gurfinkel et al., 1971)). Recent data indicate that the normal postural compensation for respiration involves subtle movements of the spine and pelvis (Hodges et al., 2002a), but this compensation may be inadequate in people with low back pain (Grimstone and Hodges, unpublished data). Alternatively, psychological factors, such as those commonly associated with chronic pain, may produce changes in breathing pattern. Studies have indicated that postural activity of the trunk muscles may be affected by stress, fear and attention demand (Moseley and Hodges, 2001).

There are several postural factors that have possible implications for muscle function and movement characteristics, which need to be confirmed with further examination. First, Skye's general appearance of having 'low tone' may have several implications for the aetiology of her pain and its management. It has been reported that minor coordination deficits are common in people with chronic low back pain (Janda, 1978). The general appearance of low tone is consistent with this proposal and suggests that Skye may have had poor muscle control over an extended period. In terms of management, the likely presence of coordination deficiencies and the duration of these changes would have ramifications for the efficacy and speed of re-education of function of the trunk muscles. Secondly, Skye's standing posture and changes in muscle bulk suggest that she relies predominantly on the long thoracolumbar erector spinae and superficial abdominal muscles to move and control her spine. Although contraction of the lumbar erector spinae and superficial multifidus can produce and maintain the lumbar lordosis (Bogduk, 1997), when the thoracolumbar erector spinae muscles contract they produce thoracolumbar extension. The motion at the mid-lumbar and thoracolumbar regions may be increased, placing stress on the passive elements in the lumbar spine. This finding is consistent with the changes in respiratory pattern and requires further investigation.

Therefore, the respiratory and postural parameters of Skye's presentation provide an indication that the function of the deep trunk muscles may be compromised. Although further specific evaluation would be required to confirm these observations, they provide preliminary evidence of several factors that may need to be considered in the retraining of the deep muscle function.

■ Clinical reasoning commentary

The very detailed response regarding posture and breathing, in conjunction with the consideration of psychosocial aspects above, nicely illustrates how the three types of knowledge—propositional (e.g. studies highlighting the coordination between the diaphragm and deep abdominal muscles for respiration and postural control), professional craft (e.g. skills in postural observation) and personal—can be linked in the context of real-life patient problems, thus enhancing meaning and accessibility in the clinical setting. This linking further enriches the clinician's knowledge base through the development of a higher level of organization. As in this case, the successful understanding and management of clinical problems requires a rich organization of all three types of knowledge.

Assessment of the pelvis indicated a slightly higher iliac crest on the right side and increased anterior tilt. In addition, Skye had hyperextended knees and elbows and was generally hypermobile (she could approximate the lateral side of her thumb to her forearm and extend her fingers to become parallel with her wrist).

Movement examination

All movements of the lumbar spine were of greater than average range of motion. Pain was reproduced in the lumbar spine at the end of range of extension, lateral flexion to both sides and lateral gliding of the pelvis in either direction. Lateral glide of her pelvis to the right gave the most accurate reproduction of her lumbar spine pain. Pain remained briefly after returning to the neutral standing position. Trunk flexion in standing and on hands and knees predominantly involved movement in the regions of the thoracolumbar junction and mid-lumbar spine, with a lesser degree of movement in the low lumbar spine and hips. Minimal intervertebral movement of the lower lumbar segments was observed with trunk movement in the sagittal plane. In four-point kneeling, she was unable to control the position of the lumbar spine when moving backwards with hips towards the feet. This movement resulted in considerable flexion at the thoracolumbar junction.

Passive joint movement examination and palpation

On passive movement examination of the spine and pelvis, there was increased resistance to central posteroanterior pressures at the L4 and L5 vertebral levels. Sustained posteroanterior pressure on L4 for more than 10 seconds resulted in reproduction of the coccyx pain. Posteroanterior pressures applied to the upper lumbar levels were normal or had slightly increased mobility. Unilateral posteroanterior pressures were unremarkable. Palpation of the structures around the lumbopelvic region was undertaken to gain a general picture of the patient's presentation. Piriformis was found to be tender bilaterally, as it commonly is in people with low back pain.

Muscle function examination

The function of the deep trunk muscles was assessed following initial attempts to teach Skye to contract transversus abdominis (TA) independently from the superficial abdominal muscles, and the deep fibres of multifidus independently from the long erector spinae and superficial fibres of multifidus. Prior to performance of the test, it was necessary to educate Skye as to the anatomy and function of TA (Fig. 7.1) and the evidence which suggests that the function of the deep muscles may be impaired in patients with low back pain. She was then positioned in four-point kneeling and instructed to relax her abdomen. She had difficulty relaxing her OE completely in this position and experienced discomfort in her elbows, which were hyperextended. The elbow pain was resolved by positioning her with the weight of her upper body supported

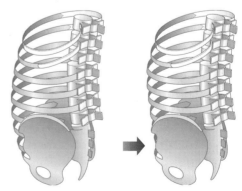

Fig. 7.1 Diagram shown to patient to demonstrate the anatomy of transversus abdominis and the performance of an independent contraction of this muscle.

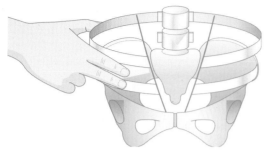

Fig. 7.2 Diagram shown to patient to demonstrate the technique for palpation of contraction of transversus abdominis and how to detect through palpation whether the contraction is correct.

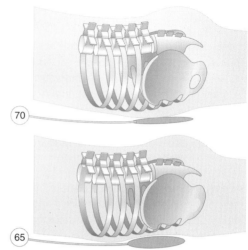

Fig. 7.3 Test for independent activation of transversus abdominis without contribution of the superficial abdominal muscles. The patient lies prone with an inflated pressure cuff placed under the abdomen. Contraction of transversus abdominis lifts the abdominal wall up off the cuff, resulting in a reduction in the cuff pressure. The normal response is a decrease in pressure of 4–6 mmHg, which can be held for 10 seconds and repeated.

on her forearms. She was instructed to breath in and out and then gently and slowly draw her lower abdominal wall up and in. Skye found this task difficult, and on observation it was apparent that most of the movement of her abdomen occurred in the upper half and her rib cage was depressed downwards and inwards. Both of these signs indicated that she had predominantly contracted her OE. Findings from palpation of the lateral abdominal wall and surface electromyography recordings from electrodes placed over the distal end of the eighth rib confirmed the presence of excessive OE activity during the performance of this task. With palpation of the abdominal wall medial and inferior to the anterior superior iliac spine (ASIS) there was no discernible contraction of TA (deep tightening) (Fig. 7.2) and only superficial contraction of obliquus internus abdominis. To assess the contraction of TA more formally, Skye was positioned in prone lying with an air-filled cuff (Stabilizer, Chattanooga, USA) placed under her abdomen (Fig. 7.3). When Skye attempted to perform the contraction in this position, she was unable to reduce the pressure but instead increased it from 70 to 72 mmHg. This pressure change was associated with the signs of superficial muscle activity outlined above.

Following education pertaining to the anatomy and function of multifidus, Skye was taught to contract the lumbar multifidus isometrically. Palpation of the back muscles and multifidus revealed rigid superficial tendons of the long erector spinae. The bulk of lumbar multifidus was generally reduced but equal between the left and right sides; it had a thickened consistency that lacked the normal elastic feel of healthy muscle tissue at the L4–L5 and L5–S1 levels. Attempts to contract the multifidus (Fig. 7.4) revealed an inability to perform this task, which she simulated by performing a posterior

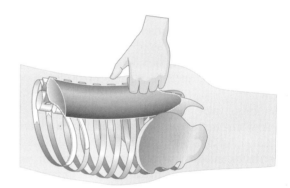

Fig. 7.4 Test for independent activation of the deep fibres of multifidus without contribution of the superficial erector spinae muscles. The therapist palpates for a gentle slow increase in deep tension in the multifidus while the patient performs an isometric contraction of the muscle.

pelvic tilt combined with contraction of the oblique abdominal muscles. The pressure in the inflated cuff under the abdomen was increased in response to the activation of the oblique abdominal muscles.

Muscle length tests

The ranges of motion found on muscle length tests for rectus femoris and iliopsoas were moderately restricted and equal between sides. Measurement of the length of the hamstring muscles was undertaken in two ways: passive straight leg raise and active extension of the knee with the hip held in 90 degrees of flexion. Both tests revealed limitation in the range of motion (approximately 45 degrees of hip flexion with straight leg raise and 40 degrees short of full knee extension with the hip held in 90 degrees of flexion) and stretch pain in the posterior thigh that was not increased by passive ankle dorsiflexion.

Examination of neurodynamics

There was no asymmetry in range of motion of straight leg raise or prone knee bend and no reproduction of lumbar or coccyx pain. The straight leg raise evoked only a stretch pain in the posterior thigh (as described above).

Adjacent joints

No pain or movement dysfunction/impairment was found in the hips or knees with active and passive movement tests. Pain provocation tests of the sacro-iliac joints and pubic symphysis were negative.

Neurological examination

Nothing abnormal was detected on examination of reflexes, muscle strength or sensation.

REASONING DISCUSSION AND CLINICAL REASONING COMMENTARY

1 What factors do you consider have contributed to the onset and perpetuation of the patient's symptoms? Can you please explain the mechanism(s) by which each factor has contributed to the pathology?

Clinician's answer

Skye has several factors in her presentation that may have contributed to the onset and continuation of her pathology. First, the changes in the activation of the deep muscles are theoretically consistent with continuing instability and irritation to the lumbar structures. It has been argued that lack of an effectively functioning deep muscle system would predispose the trunk to continued microtrauma (Gardner-Morse et al., 1995). It is not possible to determine whether the poor activity of the deep muscles was present prior to the onset of Skye's pain, but her presentation of poor coordination and poor posture suggests a long-standing history of poor movement control. It is impossible to ascertain whether the change in muscle function was responsible for the initial development of pain; however, it could be a contributing factor in the continuation of her symptoms.

There is considerable evidence that TA and multifidus are important for segmental stability of the spine. In animal models and in vitro human studies, simulation of multifidus contraction has been shown to increase stiffness of the spine and control motion, particularly around the neutral position (Kaigle et al., 1995; Wilke et al., 1995). Contraction of TA and elevation of intra-abdominal pressure have been shown to increase segmental stiffness of the spine in humans (Hodges et al., 2001b,c) and pigs (Hodges et al., 2002b). In addition, TA has been found to be active in a manner that is consistent with stabilization of the spine, but unrelated to torque production (Cresswell et al., 1994; Hodges and Richardson, 1997). Furthermore, changes in the function of these muscles have been identified in people with low back pain (i.e. delayed onset of TA activity with arm movement tasks (Hodges and Richardson, 1996) and decreased fatigue resistance of multifidus (Roy et al., 1989)). While it is difficult to obtain direct evidence to show that the change in function of these muscles leads to joint injury/microtrauma by inadequate support of the spinal structures, it is hypothesized that this may be the case.

Instability is a continuum of change in intersegmental control. At one end of the spectrum is gross instability resulting from major disruption of the passive structures (e.g. spondylolisthesis, burst fractures) (Panjabi et al., 1995). At the other end of the spectrum is poor control of intersegmental motion within the normal range of movement, and particularly around the neutral position, as a result of minor disruption of passive structures (e.g. minor tear of the annular fibres of the intervertebral disc) (Panjabi, 1992). From her presentation of pain in sustained mid-range positions and lack of frank trauma, Skye is likely to fall into the latter group. This theoretical construct has derived some direct support from biomechanical models of the spine. Several authors have argued that an operational deep muscle system is essential for maintenance of support of the spine (Cholewicki et al., 1997; Gardner-Morse et al., 1995). On this basis, it seems feasible that one factor contributing to the perpetuation of (and perhaps even causing) Skye's symptoms may be the poor control of spinal stability. Although we cannot (yet) directly measure in the clinical setting the function of TA and multifidus in stabilizing the spine, we can gain some indirect indication of function/dysfunction via the hollowing test with the pressure cuff placed under the abdomen. There is initial evidence that the ability to perform this test is related to the timing of TA in a task that challenges postural control (Hodges et al., 1996).

Second, several postural/ergonomic factors present as potential contributing factors to the onset and/or perpetuation of Skye's symptoms. For instance, her poor posture in sitting (increased lumbar flexion) and standing (thoracolumbar extension) is likely to lead to excessive strain of the intervertebral discs and other lumbar structures through increased intradiscal pressure (Nachemson and Elfstrom, 1970) and creep in viscoelastic passive tissues, resulting from sustained tension at the end of range of lumbar flexion. In addition, Skye's poor posture is associated with changes in the movement pattern of the hip-lumbopelvic region, which may lead to increased stress on lumbar spine structures. Skye has compensated for the reduced use of hip and lower lumbar movement by increasing the motion in the mid-lumbar and thoracolumbar regions. This increased movement may be responsible for increased stress on the lumbar segments and could potentially result in repeated microtrauma.

Third, there are psychological factors that may be contributing to her presentation. A major issue has been her disappointment that removal of her coccyx ('the cause of her symptoms') did not alleviate her pain. This has left her feeling helpless and frustrated, and pessimistic about her chances of recovery.

2 In a previous response, you mentioned that the chronic nature of this patient's problem suggests that central pain mechanism processes would be likely. What features in her presentation specifically supported or negated a pathological central pain mechanism?

Clinician's answer

The main features of Skye's pain that were suggestive of central sensitization were that the pain had outlasted tissue healing time, it was sometimes unpredictable, pain and relief from treatment were latent, and the pain was associated with anxiety and depression. The evidence from Skye's presentation that was inconsistent with this proposal was the strong correlation between physical signs and her pain. For instance, it was possible to reproduce her symptoms by performance of a simple physical test. Many other factors of her presentation (e.g. change in movement pattern, pain-reproducing manoeuvres) were also consistent with a peripheral source. In the case of Skye, it is critical to consider that peripheral and central changes are not exclusive and elements of both can be present. In fact the combination of peripheral sensitization and central adaptations that 'upregulate' the response of the system to pain are likely to be equally important.

3 What was your primary hypothesis at this stage regarding the source of the patient's symptoms/impairments (e.g. back and coccygeal pain with prolonged standing or sitting) and the associated pathobiological mechanism(s)? What clinical findings support and negate this hypothesis?

Clinician's answer

The primary hypothesis for the source of the symptoms was pathology at the L3–L4 lumbar motion segment resulting from a combination of poor control of spinal movement, generalized hypermobility and ergonomic or postural factors. From the evaluation, the structures involved could be either the intervertebral disc or the zygapophyseal joints. Lack of changes in sensation, muscle strength, reflexes and the absence of pain referral to the leg indicate that spinal nerve/nerve root compromise was probably not a factor. The principal location of the symptoms in the coccyx area could be explained by somatic pain referral.

Because of the absence of sensory innervation of the inner two-thirds of the intervertebral disc, pain is more likely to arise from trauma to the annular fibres and associated inflammatory processes (Bogduk, 1997). Several factors from Skye's clinical presentation were consistent with the disc hypothesis. First, reproduction of Skye's pain was achieved by central posteroanterior pressure to the L4 level. Secondly, on examination of the movement pattern, the L3–L4 level was identified as the region of transition between an area of decreased mobility (lower lumbar segments) and the mobile upper lumbar spine/thoracolumbar junction. This could result in increased stress on the passive elements at the L3–L4 level. Thirdly, the insidious onset of her pain is consistent with the commonly described clinical presentation of disc pathology. Finally, the provocative positions and movements, particularly sustained sitting and trunk flexion, are consistent with activities involving increased stress of the intervertebral disc as a result of raised pressure and loading.

The zygapophyseal joints may also be responsible for the symptoms. This hypothesis is supported by the finding that pain was reproduced by lateral flexion and extension of the spine, both of which close down the facet joints. However, several factors are inconsistent with this proposal. These include central presentation of the pain, elicitation of symptoms with trunk movement to each side and pain provocation with a central posteroanterior pressure (and not with a unilateral pressure).

It is important to acknowledge that these hypotheses are far from watertight and there is little experimental evidence to confirm the relationship between these clinical combinations and deficit in a specific structure.

5 Are there any other hypotheses you were considering as possible explanations for the patient's presentation? Why did you consider these less likely?

■ Clinician's answer

Coccyx pathology was less likely as there was no mechanical mechanism for the onset of pain (e.g. fall or childbirth). Removal of the coccyx does not necessarily exclude this possibility as there may be 'memory of pain' or central changes may have been initiated and still be present. However, the reproduction of symptoms by manual pressure to L4 is suggestive of lumbar and not coccygeal involvement. This does not completely exclude coccygeal pathology as the pressure could mechanically affect the sacrum.

The sacroiliac joint also presented as a potential source of the symptoms, through pain referral. The provocative positions of sitting and standing both place stress on the sacroiliac joint from torsional forces between the sacrum and ilia. In the first instance, this hypothesis was rejected as the pain was located centrally and was not elicited with basic pain provocation screening tests of the sacroiliac joint (for a review of these tests see Lee, 1989). However, if the symptoms failed to resolve with the initial treatment of other structures, it might then be necessary to undertake a more comprehensive examination of this region.

Of course, it is possible that the peripheral source of Skye's pain may no longer be present and the pain was now perpetuated by central changes in interpretation of normal sensory information.

■ Clinical reasoning commentary

It is clear from the responses that the clinician has not limited or reduced his thinking to just mechanical sources of nociceptive pain, although several hypotheses are obviously considered under this category in terms of the supporting and negating evidence. Due thought, however, is also given to the psychological features of the presentation (e.g. feelings of helplessness and frustration) and the potential role of central pain mechanisms in the maintenance of the patient's symptoms. Such a holistic and comprehensive approach to management facilitates both the clinician's and the patient's understanding of her clinical problem, and should enhance the chances of a successful treatment outcome. Importantly, the clinician is also metacognitively well aware of the limitations of clinical structural diagnoses. Such awareness is critical so that professional theory is not accepted as sufficient evidence in is own right. Conversely, in the absence of hard evidence, clinicians must use existing theory in attempting to understand patients and their presentations while continually remaining both critical and open minded toward alternative explanations.

_m_ Management

In collaboration with Skye, it was decided to take an active approach to management whereby minimal 'hands on' procedures would be used. However, manual techniques would be employed to provide initial pain relief so that the exercises could be performed optimally. The primary focus of treatment was to be based on Skye taking the responsibility to restore the function of her trunk muscles so as to improve her ability to stabilize and protect her spine. The evidence that training of the deep muscles of the trunk is effective in the management of certain types of low back pain was discussed, as well as the main assumptions underlying this approach to management. Time was also spent discussing the nature of chronic pain, its presentation and the problems associated with its management. The goal of the training programme for the deep trunk muscles was the restoration of the independent function of the muscles (Richardson et al., 1999). The aim of this approach is not to teach people to activate these muscles alone, but rather to activate the trunk muscles in an integrated manner to optimize the control of the spine. However, in the early stages, it is necessary to perform specific contractions of the deep muscles, so that their skilled activation can be incorporated into complex functional tasks.

Initial treatment

The initial treatment involved two applications for 30 seconds of central posteroanterior pressures to L4 at grade III-(large amplitude movement towards the end of range of movement (Maitland, 1986)). Two applications for 30 seconds of right lateral flexion PPIVMs (passive physiological intervertebral movements) to L4–L5 at grade II (large amplitude movement without moving into resistance (Maitland, 1986)) were also given. Reassessment of lateral pelvic shifting to the right after each application indicated no change or a slight increase in her symptoms, and no change in range of motion.

Attempts were made to teach Skye to perform contraction of TA independently of the other superficial abdominal muscles. The two main difficulties encountered were, first, her inability to relax OE, which made it difficult to activate TA independently, and, secondly, Skye's poor awareness of movement of the abdominal wall. Each attempt to perform the contraction was associated with strong activity in OE and minimal palpable tightening of TA. Several positions were trialed in order to achieve the greatest relaxation of the superficial muscles (particularly OE) and optimal activation of TA. It was also necessary to teach Skye to breathe without contraction of OE during expiration. Efforts in four-point kneeling, supported standing and supine lying all resulted in overactivity of the superficial

muscles. The best reduction of activity of OE was achieved in right side lying with a pillow between her knees; however, OE remained somewhat active and this activity was modulated with respiration. Verbal instructions to reduce the amount of OE activity were unsuccessful. Instruction was given in relaxed diaphragmatic breathing. With tactile feedback over her lower ribs and abdomen, she was able to inspire with basal rib cage expansion and slight abdominal wall movement, and then expire while maintaining OE relaxation. Accurate relaxation was achieved most successfully by allowing her to palpate the lateral aspect of her abdominal wall for activity of OE. After several minutes of practice, Skye was then encouraged to breath in a controlled diaphragmatic manner for several breaths, and then gently and slowly draw her lower abdomen up and in. This instruction resulted in a rapid contraction of OE. Skye was instructed to reduce her effort so as to perform a contraction that was just perceptible and to perform it slowly. This again resulted in significant contraction of OE.

Since all instructions related to the abdominal wall resulted in inappropriate contraction of OE and no palpable contraction of TA, it was decided to change the strategy and teach Skye to perform a gentle contraction of her pelvic floor muscles in an attempt to facilitate a contraction of TA. Skye was instructed to contract the pelvic floor muscles slowly and gently and to concentrate on the anterior part of the pelvic floor as if stopping the flow of urine. After several attempts Skye was able to perform the contraction. When this was done in combination with controlled breathing (prior to the contraction of the pelvic floor muscles), there was minimal activity of OE and tightening of TA was palpable inferior and medial to the ASIS. Once she had contracted TA she was unable to start breathing without increasing the activity of OE. To ensure that Skye could repeat the same procedure at home, she was shown how to palpate the lateral abdominal wall with the right hand and also taught to distinguish between contraction of TA and the oblique abdominal muscles by palpating inferior and medial to the ASIS with her left hand. After three attempts at performing the contraction of TA for 5 seconds, she was no longer able to contract TA successfully independently of the other abdominal muscles. She was instructed not to breathe for the few seconds of the contraction and that this would be incorporated later.

It was decided that Skye would have a better chance of achieving the contraction correctly at home if she was only to perform this exercise and left contraction of the lumbar multifidus to a later stage. No other treatment was implemented in the first session and she was instructed to practise the contraction of TA exactly as she had been taught three to four time per day for just three repetitions. She was advised to return for reassessment in 7 days.

Second treatment (1 week later)

Skye stated that 30 minutes after the treatment session her pain was diminished and the reduction in pain lasted for several days before returning as before with little change in intensity or duration. She had practiced the exercises daily and was happy that she had been successful.

Reassessment of active movements revealed no change in range of motion in any direction, nor in pain produced at the end of range. Pain persisted for a short period after returning to the neutral position, as had occurred during the initial consultation. Passive joint movement examination revealed resistance to central posteroanterior pressures to L5 and provocation of the coccyx pain with sustained pressure to L4.

Reassessment of her ability to isolate the contraction of TA indicated there was no improvement of her capability to reduce the pressure with the inflated pressure cuff under her abdomen in prone lying. In addition, there was no reduction in the overactivity of OE. Assessment of the lumbar multifidus indicated there was no change in her ability to perform a contraction of this muscle.

Skye stated that she had practised the exercise at home but had found it very difficult as she felt that she was doing 'nothing'. In response to this she had contracted the muscles with increased effort so that she was aware of the contraction. Although she was able to feel that this resulted in the inappropriate contraction of OE, she felt that it would be better for her because it would be making the muscles stronger. Skye was educated that the exercise was aimed at retraining the coordination of the trunk muscles and not at making the muscles stronger. She was further educated in the importance of precision in her training and that practising an exercise that was not correct would not improve the coordination of these muscles and achieve our goal of improving the stability of her spine.

Examination of the home exercise revealed that Skye had difficulty in achieving the correct contraction in side lying because of overactivity of OE. As a result, other positions were trialed. Supported supine lying was tried with the trunk elevated on pillows and the elbows supported, but Skye was still unable to relax appropriately. The best relaxation of the abdomen was achieved with Skye lying in prone supported on her elbows. The tactile contact of her ribs on the bed gave her extra feedback about the movement of her ribs and allowed her to identify whether she was using OE to move her rib cage. Unfortunately, this position made it difficult for her to palpate TA since her arms were used for support. As an alternative, a pressure cuff was placed under the abdomen to provide feedback on elevation of the lower abdomen. The exercise involved several controlled breaths followed by slow gentle contraction of her pelvic floor muscles. She was still unable to breathe while performing the contraction without increasing the activity of OE. It was reinforced to Skye that the exercise was aimed at precision and not the magnitude of the pressure change. She was also instructed to spend time in supine lying practising controlled relaxed breathing with bi-basal expansion and relaxed expiration.

Passive treatment involved application of the L4–L5 lateral flexion PPIVMs to the right at grade III and three repetitions of sustained (15 seconds) posteroanterior pressure to L4. Reassessment of lateral pelvic gliding indicated a slight increase in pain during movement to the left, but with no maintenance of pain on return to the neutral position. Muscle control was also retested after the application of the manual techniques to determine whether there was any change in task performance as a result of the intervention. If manual techniques change muscle activity or neurophysiological mechanisms, it may be possible to change control, although this has not been tested experimentally. Skye exhibited no change in performance following the manual intervention.

Skye was given advice on the use of a rolled towel for lumbar support in order to determine whether this would assist her pain control during periods of sustained sitting. She was also given general back care and lifting advice and advised to return in 1 week.

REASONING DISCUSSION AND CLINICAL REASONING COMMENTARY

1 You appear to have spent considerable time in educating the patient as part of the management of the problem. Did you specifically assess her understanding of the problem prior to providing these explanations? Could you also comment on the importance of education in your overall management.

Clinician's answer

Skye was questioned directly about her understanding of her problem and informally through conversation. From the assessment, it was clear that her understanding of the problem was limited. She had previously been informed of a simple cause-effect relationship between a single tangible pathology and her pain. Following failure of the surgery to remedy her symptoms she was not provided with any further explanation. As we were about to take on a largely self-motivated programme of exercises, it was critical for Skye to understand completely the theoretical construct upon which this approach to management was based. Education was also needed to ensure that the exercises were performed optimally. For instance, the initial exercise that Skye was to perform does not conform to the expectation that many patients share (i.e. exercise is aimed at increasing muscle strength). Therefore, it was necessary to change this perception by helping Skye to understand the reasoning behind the performance of gentle precise contractions. In addition, it was important to educate Skye about treatment efficacy (Hides et al., 1997; Jull et al., 1998; O'Sullivan et al., 1997) and realistic expectations in order to encourage motivation. Education is clearly one of the main factors when embarking on a management programme that is primarily dependent on self-management and independent exercise.

2 How did you interpret the response to the first treatment?

Clinician's answer

The conclusions drawn from the initial response were that there was a delayed (30 minute) response to the manual techniques and that the slight increase in pain resulting from the performance of these techniques was temporary. However, the improvement of her symptoms was only maintained for a limited period, suggesting that the benefit from the passive manual techniques was short term. This response did not indicate that the exercise approach was unlikely to be beneficial, as any effect from exercise would not occur until there was a change in muscle function. Because there had been no change in the deep muscle function since the first treatment, because of incorrect performance of the exercise, it was not expected that the muscular support for the spine would be improved and able to control the symptoms.

Therefore, the effect of the first treatment was consistent with the initial biomechanical hypothesis in that the selected manual techniques had resulted in improvement of symptoms, although delayed. Furthermore, the failure of the exercise to make a clinical change in symptoms was not inconsistent with the approach as Skye had not yet successfully trained the system and her exercise needed refinement. On this basis it was decided to continue with the manual techniques and to persist striving for independent activation of TA.

3 What thoughts did you have at assessing the initial treatment regarding her prognosis for mastering an automatic motor programme of improved muscle control, given the difficulties she was experiencing? Did you find it necessary to adapt or try different teaching strategies in response to the patient's ability, understanding and learning style?

Clinician's answer

Following the first experience, it became clear that it would be difficult to achieve the correct contraction of the deep muscles. Collaboratively, a decision was made to persist trying for the ideal response. However, it was important to keep in mind the need to review the situation after several treatments to determine whether Skye was progressing with this demanding cognitive approach. It was also critical that Skye did not become frustrated with the time required for her to make a change. The difficulty in achieving the correct contraction arose because, first, Skye required copious feedback and intense concentration to be successful and, secondly, she continued to believe that strength was important. Because of this, it was necessary to take things slowly and regularly reinforce the main points regarding effort and precision. It was also necessary to be more explicit about the treatment goals and management approach. As she had poor movement perception, it was essential to adapt the strategy to provide alternative sources of feedback (i.e. pressure changes using the pressure cuff under the abdomen) to enhance her awareness of the contraction. Consequently, there was no change in teaching strategy, just reinforcement of the exercise and the use of alternative strategies to provide feedback.

▮ Clinical reasoning commentary

Manual therapists must be good teachers. To promote change successfully in a patient's behaviour, and consequently in their problem, requires a collaborative approach to clinical reasoning between therapist and patient, along with explanation and reassurance. Patient learning is a crucial factor in the success of any treatment outcome, but particularly when it involves self-management. The clinician in this case has obviously learnt that, in chronic presentations such as this where the patient's own meaning perspectives, including feelings (e.g. helplessness), beliefs (e.g. muscles only require strengthening) and understandings (e.g. the coccyx is the problem), are dysfunctional/impaired, it is often fruitless, if not counterproductive, to pursue a course of treatment without addressing these issues through patient education. Manual therapists need to develop their teaching skills continually, as they would their manual skills, and to employ these skills in cultivating a collaborative approach to their patients' clinical problems.

▮ Third treatment (1 week later)

On reassessment, Skye again indicated that her pain had been improved for several days after treatment but had returned. There was little change in active movement or passive joint movement signs. However evaluation of her ability to perform an isolated contraction of TA this time indicated slight improvement. Although she was unable to reduce the pressure in the cuff placed under her abdomen, she was able to perform the contraction with less overactivity of OE. She still required encouragement to reduce the amount of effort she was using to produce the contraction and performed better without feedback from the pressure dial. In view of this, she was advised not to use the pressure biofeedback unit for training and was instructed instead to use a mirror to monitor the movement of her abdomen from the side. At this stage, she was still not able to commence breathing while holding a contraction of TA, and so she was encouraged to increase the number of repetitions to five. Passive treatment involved reapplication of the joint mobilizations used in the last treatment with increased vigour and duration, and the addition of transverse mobilizations of L4 to the left at grade III. As the use of the rolled towel had been found to be beneficial, Skye was advised to purchase a lumbar support for use in the car, during meetings and at the cinema.

Her home programme of exercises involved continuation of her TA training, with the addition of active hamstring stretches (in supine lying with her hips bent to 90 degrees). Gluteal exercises (bridging) were also superimposed on her attempted TA setting, which at this stage was still only fair. The bridging exercise was aimed at improving the activation of the gluteal muscles and was performed from crook lying using hip extension. Prior to this bridging movement, Skye was instructed to pre-contract her TA.

Postural correction exercises were also commenced at this treatment session. This involved correction of her entire spinal posture. Skye's natural attempts to sit or stand straight were associated with extension at the thoracolumbar junction rather than control of the normal spinal curves. Postural correction was commenced in sitting, where she was taught to control her lumbar lordosis actively by gently tilting her pelvis forward. To assist her to control the extension at the thoracolumbar junction, she was told to hold her thumb on her sternum and little finger in her navel, and to keep the distance between these two points stable as she moved. Cervical spine posture was corrected by telling her to imagine a string pulled up from the back of the top of her head. Skye was encouraged to adopt this posture at work each time she heard the school bell for classes to finish.

REASONING DISCUSSION AND CLINICAL REASONING COMMENTARY

1 Why do you think that the use of the pressure biofeedback unit was of no value, if not counterproductive? How does its use differ from that of the mirror?

■ Clinician's answer

Although the pressure cuff was used to provide additional feedback as to the success of the contraction, it unfortunately meant that Skye focussed on changing the pressure rather than the contraction of her abdominal muscles. The pressure in the cuff can be reduced by several mechanisms in addition to contraction of TA, such as elevation of the lower ribs and flexion at the thoracolumbar junction. When a reduction in pressure occurs without any motion of the rib cage or pelvis, it is considered to be largely a result of TA contraction (Richardson et al., 1999). However, when motion of the rib cage or pelvis is produced, other muscles are then involved (e.g. OE). Failure to instruct the patient about these other possible mechanisms for decreasing pressure (or failure to identify them) may result in practise of an inappropriate contraction. Although Skye was instructed to keep the rib cage in contact with the bed, she had found this difficult to perceive. As a result, Skye had learnt mechanisms to reduce the pressure that were not associated with TA contraction, notably flexion of the thoracolumbar junction and elevation of the rib cage by contraction of OE. Consequently, the pressure biofeedback technique had encouraged an undesirable contraction and had failed to provide improved kinesthetic awareness of the contraction. By comparison, the mirror provided more useful feedback that enabled Skye to focus on the correct performance of the contraction (i.e. lower abdominal movement) and to detect inappropriate strategies (e.g. rib cage depression, observable contraction of OE, movement predominantly of the upper abdomen, and fast or jerky contraction). Therefore, unlike the pressure cuff, observation with the mirror provided feedback of correct and incorrect performance, and so the desired movement (change in abdominal contour) could not be simulated by imprecise contraction.

2 What was your reasoning for prescribing hamstring and gluteal exercises?

■ Clinician's answer

It was considered necessary not only to train the deep muscle function but also to restore normal function of all of the muscles in the lumbopelvic region. This is critical because normal function of these muscles is essential to optimize the control of the spine, as all lumbopelvic muscles contribute to specific aspects of stability. In Skye's case, the reduction in length of the hamstring muscles acted to limit hip motion and resulted in an increased demand for motion at the lumbar spine. This would occur particularly at the level where there was a transition between the regions of high and low mobility (i.e. L3–L4). By increasing the length of the hamstring muscles, the aim was to minimize further the load/stress on the lumbar spine and increase the contribution of the hip to lumbopelvic motion. Correspondingly, it was considered desirable to restore normal gluteal activation to assist with the control of lumbopelvic motion. Although the deep muscles are able to control segmental stability, they have only a limited ability to control the overall orientation of the lumbar spine and pelvis. Therefore, the exercises for the hip muscles were not expected to have a direct effect on the control of the deep trunk muscles, but they were expected instead to reduce the reliance on lumbar motion.

3 Many therapists consider postural correction to be an almost obligatory part of the management of the patient with low back pain. What was your reasoning behind the decision to introduce these exercises for correcting Skye's posture? Is there any research evidence to support this approach?

■ Clinician's answer

Postural correction has underpinned many clinical approaches. The decision to include postural correction as a component of Skye's management was based on a number of factors. First, there are relatively consistent data to argue that the loading through the spine is more optimal in a 'neutral' position with lumbar lordosis and thoracic kyphosis (e.g. McGill and Norman, 1993). Early data also indicate that posture affects factors such as disc pressure (Nachemson and Morris,

1964). Secondly, it is suggested clinically that activity of the superficial muscles may be affected by posture (or may affect posture). For example, overactivity of OE in association with a depressed rib cage and activity of thoracic erector spinae muscles appears clinically to favour a military type posture rather than the normal neutral curves. There is evidence that these muscles are overactive in many people with low back pain (Radebold et al., 2000). Therefore, correction of posture may assist in the re-education of normal coordination of the trunk muscles.

One issue to consider is that it is not normal to adopt a neutral position and stay there. Although this may be optimal for tasks that involve sustained loading, it is abnormal to maintain a neutral spinal posture rigidly without variation. It is known that the central nervous system uses movement to assist in the absorption of forces (Hodges et al., 1999). Therefore, normal function should encourage a functional range of movement, with specific instruction for situations when ideal posture may be required, but with an understanding of allowing the spine to move.

■ Clinical reasoning commentary

Research-based evidence, whether it be empirical proof or biological bases as discussed in this response, can be used to inform the decision-making process related to the management of individual patients. What is crucial, though, is to determine clinically if the evidence is appropriate and applicable for a particular patient. As the mature organism model (discussed in Ch. 1) implies, no two people will have exactly the same presentation given their unique past experiences and current contexts. Clinical reasoning must be applied to research-based evidence to establish the similarity of the patient's presentation to that studied and to administer the intervention appropriately considering the unique features of the presentation. The effects of the research-based intervention for an individual patient should also be subject to the same clinical evaluation (or reassessment) process as an experience-based intervention.

■ Fourth treatment (2 weeks later)

On Skye's return 2 weeks later, she reported decreased pain following the previous treatment, which was maintained for a longer period (approximately 4 days), with a gradual return of her symptoms over this time. She stated that the performance of the abdominal muscle exercises gave her a subjective feeling of increased control of her spine. She could delay the onset of pain during periods of prolonged sitting and standing by performing regular TA contractions. This had been particularly beneficial during staff meetings and while attending the cinema. On physical examination, there was slight reduction of lumbar pain on lateral pelvic gliding to the right and decreased coccyx pain with sustained posteroanterior pressure to L4. Reassessment of her ability to contract TA indicated that she was still unable to reduce the pressure with the pressure cuff placed under her abdomen, but she was now able to perform the contraction easily without instruction or feedback. Palpation of multifidus during performance of the pelvic floor/TA contraction indicated a palpable bilateral contraction that was greater on the left than the right and which was able to be performed in a slow and controlled manner.

Progression involved teaching Skye to perform the contraction in the more functional position of supported standing and the incorporation of breathing with the contraction. Breathing training involved performance of a contraction of TA and then adding speech (counting) to encourage controlled airflow. It was necessary to take this intermediate step before commencing true breathing training because of her difficulty with this task. After practice holding the TA contraction with speaking, Skye was encouraged to commence bi-basal diaphragmatic breathing superimposed on the TA contraction. To assist with this integration, Skye was advised to place one hand over the lower rib cage to give feedback of basal rib cage expansion and the other hand over TA inferior to the ASIS. She was instructed to breathe with bi-basal expansion and abdominal wall movement with each breath, rather than the shallow upper chest breathing that patients often perform in conjunction with the deep abdominal muscle contraction.

In terms of progression of the exercise into functional positions, Skye could most effectively perform the contraction of TA if she stood with her feet approximately 20 cm from the wall with her pelvis resting against the wall. She was encouraged to do this exercise throughout the day between classes and to continue her training in prone lying using visual feedback from the mirror. Evaluation of the postural correction exercise indicated that she still required a great deal of concentration to achieve the desired position and was finding this difficult to accomplish at work. Passive joint movement techniques were reapplied with progression of duration of the sustained posteroanterior pressure to L4 and performance of the L4–L5 lateral flexion PPIVM at grade IV. Transverse mobilization was repeated at the same grade but in an increasing degree of lateral flexion of the trunk to the right to move further into the range of motion. In view of the improvement in her symptoms, but considering the slow rate of change in Skye's ability to perform a contraction of TA, she was given 1 month to practise the exercises independently. She was instructed to increase the number and duration of the contractions according to what she was able to manage. She was also instructed to use palpation and observation of the activity of OE as a guide to this progression.

m Further management

Over the next 6 months, Skye was seen initially monthly (for 2 months) and then every second month. The main limitation to her progress was the slow rate of change in her trunk muscle function. She required long periods between treatments in order to be able to detect a change in her ability to perform the contraction effectively.

Deep muscle control

After the first month, Skye had mastered the ability to perform a contraction of TA independently from the superficial abdominal muscles. Additional exercises were included to improve activation of the lumbar multifidus. For the first exercise, Skye palpated her multifidus in sitting and performed gentle isometric contractions in combination with TA. She required specific instruction as to the correct hand placement and feeling for the appropriate contraction. Correction of the precision of the exercise was required at several sessions before the exercise could be performed optimally. Skye was also taught to perform a co-contraction of these two muscle groups during more functional tasks such as walking. She was encouraged to palpate the muscles initially in order to determine whether they were active and then to superimpose stepping.

Incorporation of deep and superficial muscles

During this 6-month period, Skye progressed to the stage where she could perform a contraction of TA and reduce the pressure in the cuff placed under the abdomen by 4 mmHg. At this point, exercises to retrain the coordination between TA and the superficial muscles were also commenced. These exercises started with her positioned in crook lying with the inflated pressure cuff under her lumbar spine. She was instructed to let her knee gently move out to the side without changing the pressure in the cuff, in an attempt to increase further the load required for spinal stabilization while promoting dissociation with limb movement. This was gradually progressed to sliding one leg out straight and then lifting her leg. All exercises were performed without letting the pressure change during the exercise. Other exercises included single limb movements and then contralateral arm and leg movements in four-point kneeling, and arm movements while sitting on a ball. For each of these exercises, Skye was instructed to contract her deep muscles prior to the addition of the load of the arms and legs. She was also encouraged to adopt a controlled neutral spine position (using the method she had been taught previously) and to maintain this during the movements.

Exercises were progressed after she was able to perform them accurately. For most exercises, she required some form of feedback, either from a pressure cuff or mirror, to help to ensure that she kept her spine controlled. Throughout this time, Skye continued to train her TA in prone lying, gradually increasing the holding time and the number of repetitions. She also continued to train the multifidus in standing with self-palpation of the contraction. The use of passive techniques made no further change to her symptoms and were, therefore, ceased. This allowed Skye to focus on performing the active exercise regimen.

Movement pattern correction

Additional exercises were included to change her movement patterns so as to increase the movement of her hips during trunk movements without associated excessive movement at the thoracolumbar junction. This involved exercises in which she corrected the posture of her trunk (as previously instructed) and then flexed at the hips, keeping the position of the trunk stable with combined contraction of TA and multifidus.

With each treatment session, the duration of the reduction in symptoms was increased, and over the period of 6 months Skye described a gradual decrease in the overall level of her symptoms. She improved to the point where she experienced only minimal pain with prolonged periods of sitting or standing, such as traveling in a plane for greater than 3 hours. She was advised to return in 4 months for review.

Final presentation

On her final presentation, Skye was relatively pain-free. She was able to perform her work duties with minimal or no pain and was no longer limited in her ability to stand for lengthy periods. However, she continued to avoid sustained sitting and still used her lumbar support when driving long distances or during prolonged meetings. Skye commented that if she ceased the TA exercises for 3 days then her low back pain would return. It would then take 3 days of exercise for it to again subside. She had tested this on at least two occasions to convince herself that there was indeed a cause-effect relationship between exercise practice and the recurrence of pain. On examination, all active movements had full range of motion, and pain could only be reproduced slightly with overpressure of pelvic gliding to the right. Passive movement examination failed to provoke any coccygeal pain with sustained posteroanterior pressure to L4. Skye was advised to continue a daily maintenance programme each morning that involved independent contraction of TA in prone lying and multifidus in standing. She was also given a list of 10 exercises (from those she had been practising) that involved pre-contraction of TA and multifidus with the addition of slow controlled movements of the leg or arm. She was to select two exercises from this list each day and vary them between days.

REASONING DISCUSSION AND CLINICAL REASONING COMMENTARY

1 How did you see the various dissociative exercises you used contributing to the management programme? How important was the patient's cognitive awareness in facilitating these changes?

■ Clinician's answer

The dissociative exercises were added to the management programme to restore normal movement of the lumbopelvic region by reducing the excessive motion of the lumbar spine and by increasing motion of the hip. At the initial assessment, it was noted that most movement with trunk flexion occurred at the lumbar spine, with minimal contribution from the hip. The functional characteristics of several of the hip muscles (e.g. gluteus maximus and hamstrings) were consistent with this observation. Although TA and multifidus should be able to enhance spinal control throughout the range of motion, any attempt to reduce the reliance on spinal movement (as opposed to hip movement) was considered to be worthwhile. Any improvement in this regard might assist in minimizing the stress on the joint structures at the mid-lumbar level that could result from excessive movement.

Cognitive awareness is critical in facilitating changes in motor control in this approach to management. Although several other approaches to management rely on restoration of function through automatic facilitation of the correct motor pattern (for example, Janda, 1978), contemporary motor learning theory focusses strongly on cognitive correction, with accurate feedback about movement performance and outcome (Carr and Shepherd, 1987; Hodges, 2003; Magill, 2001). As the motor coordination/skill improves, the amount of attention/cognitive awareness and feedback that is required is reduced. Once the skill is mastered, then many repetitions are required in order to train the response to become automatic. There is preliminary evidence that training the trunk muscles in this manner does result in a change in automatic activation in functional tasks (Jull et al., 1998).

2 One of the problems of predominantly exercise based treatment regimens can be patient compliance. What strategies do you consider were most useful in encouraging compliance with this patient?

■ Clinician's answer

I believe that the strategy most useful for encouraging compliance with Skye was education regarding the basis for the exercise and the potential benefit of the exercise programme. If a patient can understand what the exercise aims to achieve and is provided with evidence for its efficacy, then motivation will be increased. Another factor of importance in this case was the reinforcement of the relative value of the passive and active components of the treatment. It was essential for compliance that Skye took on the onus of responsibility for her improvement. Patients need to understand that they will be responsible for a large part of the change; the passive techniques may assist with symptom reduction, but the exercise component is essential for maintenance. If a patient believes that the passive techniques will make them better regardless of what they do, then the motivation to exercise may be reduced.

3 Why does Skye appear to need regular exercise in order to control her symptoms? Is the retraining effect only temporary?

■ Clinician's answer

Clinically, it appears that many patients can cease to exercise once the control of the deep muscles has been restored. In clinical trials the benefit of exercise has been shown to be maintained for 30 months (O'Sullivan et al., 1997). However, others such as Skye appear to need continued reinforcement of the contraction. This may be because of her poor general coordination or perhaps an ongoing inhibitory process. The decision to encourage Skye to continue with regular exercise was only determined from evaluation of progress and maintenance of response, although some initial factors such as 'low tone' may have suggested the need for this approach to management. In this particular case, the likening of daily brushing of teeth to prevent tooth decay to the training of the deep muscles to prevent the recurrence of pain helped to encourage acceptance of the need for ongoing maintenance.

4 Earlier you noted that this patient had potential psychosocial problems that you felt could be contributing to her pain state, and you outlined three measures you planned to undertake to address them. Could you comment now on your reassessment of her psychosocial status and whether this was a problem?

■ Clinician's answer

In Skye's case, the reassessment of psychosocial issues was undertaken by informal questioning. It was clear from Skye's progress that she had accepted the need to be responsible for her own recovery. The clinical process required a great deal of motivation and Skye responded well to this challenge. During conversation, attempts were continually made to reinforce the non-threatening nature of pain: that the pain was no longer acting as a warning of damage to structures. Through questioning it was obvious that her attitude was changing. Her attitude to her symptoms became more positive, she catastrophized less, and she no longer expected to 'end up in a wheelchair'. While in some cases it may be necessary to undertake more formal measures (e.g. questionnaires), my belief in Skye's case was that the informal method was best as steady progress was observable; to undertake more formal examination may have unnecessarily emphasized the psychosocial issue.

■ Clinical reasoning commentary

Satisfactory patient compliance with an ongoing exercise programme is a fundamental requirement for a successful outcome in manual therapy, as is illustrated here. Poor compliance with self-management regimens leads to poor self-efficacy and eventually to poor treatment outcomes. Self-management necessitates the patient sharing responsibility for their problem, which can be a difficult step for some patients with impaired or unhelpful beliefs and understandings about their problem and its treatment, particularly if they only expect or wish to be a passive recipient of the 'healing hands' of the manual therapist. The clinical reasoning of the expert clinician in this case has again highlighted the crucial role of educating the patient, especially about the proven or likely benefits of a self-management programme, in order to foster motivation and compliance. Effective skills in communication and teaching, such as the use of a simple analogy (i.e. the preventive role of brushing one's teeth), are an important part of the armamentarium of the expert manual therapist.

It is evident in this response that just as physical impairments have been regularly reassessed (e.g. motor control), so too have psychosocial impairments (e.g. maladaptive beliefs about pain). However, the reassessment of psychosocial factors has clearly been more of an informal (albeit continual) process and has been closely intertwined with management strategies applied for the same factors. The clinician had previously identified that the patient may have had a lack of insight into the psychosocial factors influencing her problem, which could have potentially created obstacles to her improvement. Narrative reasoning and communicative management (e.g. listening, clarifying, explaining, negotiating and counselling) were, therefore, applied interactively and collaboratively to reveal and act on the patient's meaning perspectives (see Ch. 1). Change was obviously effected by this communicative approach, and validation was achieved through therapist-patient common understanding and consensus.

References

Agostoni, E. and Campbell, E.J.M. (1970). The abdominal muscles. In The Respiratory Muscles: Mechanisms and Neural Control (E.J.M. Campbell, E. Agostoni and J. Newsom-Davis, eds.) pp. 175–180. London: Lloyd-Luke.

Arendt-Nielsen, L., Graven-Nielsen, T., Svarrer, H. and Svensson, P. (1996). The influence of low back pain on muscle activity and coordination during gait: a clinical and experimental study. Pain, 64, 231–240.

Bogduk, N. (1997). Clinical Anatomy of the Lumbar Spine, 2nd edn. Edinburgh: Churchill Livingstone.

Carr, J.H. and Shepherd, R.B. (1987). A Motor Relearning Program for Stroke, 2nd edn. Aspen, CO: Aspen Publishers.

Cholewicki, J., Panjabi, M.M. and Khachatryan, A. (1997). Stabilizing function of trunk flexor-extensor muscles around a neutral spine posture. Spine, 22, 2207–2212.

Cresswell, A.G., Oddsson, L. and Thorstensson, A. (1994). The influence of sudden perturbations on trunk muscle activity and intra-abdominal pressure while standing. Experimental Brain Research, 98, 336–341.

De Troyer, A. (1996). Mechanics of the chest wall muscles. In Neural Control of Respiratory Muscles (A.D. Miller, A.L. Bianchi and B.P. Bishop, eds.) pp. 59–76. Boca Raton, FL: CRC Press.

De Troyer, A., Estenne, M., Ninane, V. et al. (1990). Transversus abdominis muscle function in humans. Journal of Applied Physiology, 68, 1010–1016.

Gardner-Morse, M., Stokes, I.A. and Laible, J.P. (1995). Role of muscles in lumbar spine stability in maximum extension efforts. Journal of Orthopedic Research, 13, 802–808.

Goldman, J.M., Lehr, R.P., Millar, A.B. and Silver, J.R. (1987). An electromyographic study of the abdominal muscles during postural and respiratory manoeuvres. Journal of Neurology, Neurosurgery and Psychiatry, 50, 866–869.

Gurfinkel, V.S., Kors, Y.M., Pal'tsev, E.I. and Feldman, A.G. (1971). The compensation of respiratory disturbances of the erect posture of man as an example of the organisation of inter-articular interaction. In Models of the Structural-Functional Organization of Certain Biological Systems (I.M. Gelfand, V.S. Gurfinkel, S.V. Fomin and M.L. Tsetlin, eds.) pp. 382–395. Cambridge, MA: MIT Press.

Hides, J.A., Richardson, C.A. and Jull, G.A. (1997). Multifidus muscle recovery is not automatic after resolution of acute, first-episode low back pain. Spine, 21, 2763–2769.

Hodges, P.W. (2003). Motor control. Physical Therapies in Sport and Physical Activity (G. Kolt and L. Snyder-Mackler, eds.) pp. 107–126. London: Harcourt.

Hodges, P.W. and Gandevia, S.C. (2000a). Changes in intra-abdominal pressure during postural and respiratory activation of the human diaphragm. Journal of Applied Physiology, 89, 967–976.

Hodges, P.W. and Gandevia, S.C. (2000b). Activation of the human diaphragm during a repetitive postural task. Journal of Physiology, 522, 165–175.

Hodges, P.W. and Richardson, C.A. (1996). Inefficient muscular stabilization of the lumbar spine associated with low back pain. A motor control evaluation of transversus abdominis. Spine, 21, 2640–2650.

Hodges, P.W. and Richardson, C.A. (1997). Feedforward contraction of transversus abdominis is not influenced by the direction of arm movement. Experimental Brain Research, 114, 362–370.

Hodges, P., Richardson, C. and Jull, G. (1996). Evaluation of the relationship between laboratory and clinical tests of transversus abdominis function. Physiotherapy Resarch International, 1, 30–40.

Hodges, P.W., Butler, J.E., McKenzie, D.K. and Gandevia, S.C. (1997a). Contraction of the human diaphragm during rapid postural adjustments. Journal of Physiology, 505, 539–548.

Hodges, P.W., Gandevia, S.C. and Richardson, C.A. (1997b). Contractions of specific abdominal muscles in postural tasks are affected by respiratory maneuvers. Journal of Applied Physiology, 83, 753–760.

Hodges, P.W., Cresswell, A.G. and Thorstensson, A. (1999). Preparatory trunk motion accompanies rapid upper limb movement. Experimental Brain Research, 124, 69–79.

Hodges, P.W., Moseley, G.L, Gabrielsson, A. and Gandevia, S.C. (2001a). Acute experimental pain changes postural recruitment of the trunk muscles in pain-free humans. In 31st Annual Meeting of the Society for Neuroscience, San Diego, CA. Abstracts 27. Washington, DC: Society for Neuroscience Abstracts.

Hodges, P.W., Eriksson, A.E.M., Shirley, D. and Gandevia, S.C. (2001b). Lumbar spine stiffness is increased by elevation of intra-abdominal pressure.

In Proceedings of the XVIII International Congress of the Society for Biomechanics, Zurich, July 2001, abstract A712.

Hodges, P.W., Cresswell, A.G., Daggfeldt, K. and Thorstensson, A. (2001c). In vivo measurement of the effect of intra-abdominal pressure on the human spine. Journal of Biomechanics, 34, 347–353.

Hodges, P.W., Gurfinkel, V.S., Brumagne, S. et al. (2002a). Coexistence of stability and mobility in postural control: evidence from postural compensation for respiration. Experimental Brain Research, 144, 293–302.

Hodges, P.W., Kaigle-Holm, A., Holm, S. et al. (2002b). In vivo evidence that postural activity of the respiratory muscles increases intervertebal stiffness of the spine: porcine studies. In 32nd Annual Meeting of the Society for Neuroscience, Orlando, FL. Washington, DC: Society for Neuroscience.Society for Neuroscience Abstracts on line.

Janda, V. (1978). Muscles, central nervous motor regulation and back problems. In The Neurobiologic Mechanisms in Manipulative Therapy (I. M. Korr, ed.) pp. 27–41, London: Plenum Press.

Jull, G.A., Scott, Q., Richardson, C. et al. (1998). New concepts for control of pain in the lumbopelvic region. In Proceedings of the Third Interdisciplinary World Congress on Low Back and Pelvic Pain (A. Vleeming, V. Mooney, H. Tilscher et al., eds.) pp. 128–131. Rotterdam: ECO.

Kaigle, A.M., Holm, S.H. and Hansson, T.H. (1995). Experimental instability in the lumbar spine. Spine, 20, 421–430.

Lee, D. (1989). The Pelvic Girdle: An Approach to the Examination of the Lumbo–Pelvic–Hip Region. Edinburgh: Churchill Livingstone.

Magill, R.A. (2001). Motor Learning: Concepts and Applications. New York: McGraw-Hill.

Maitland, G.D. (1986). Vertebral Manipulation, 5th edn. Oxford: Butterworth-Heinemann.

McGill, S.M. and Norman, R.W. (1993). Low back biomechanics in industry: the prevention of injury through safer lifting. In Current Issues in Biomechanics (M.D. Grabiner, ed.) pp. 69–120. Champaign, France: Human Kinetics.

Mead, J. (1979). Functional significance of the area of apposition of diaphragm to rib cage. American Review of Respiratory Disease, 119, 31–32.

Moseley, G.L. and Hodges, P.W. (2001). Attention demand, anxiety and acute pain cause differential effects on postural activation of the abdominal muscles in humans. In 31st Annual Meeting of the Society for Neuroscience, San Diego, CA. Abstracts 27. Washington, DC: Society for Neuroscience Abstracts.

Nachemson, A. and Elfstrom, G. (1970). Intravital dynamic pressure measurements in lumbar discs. A study of common movements, maneuvers and exercises. Scandinavian Journal of Rehabilitation Medicine 1 (Suppl.), 1–40.

Nachemson, A. and Morris, J.M. (1964). In vivo measurement of intradiscal pressure: discometry, a method for the determination of presure in the lower lumbar discs. Journal of Bone and Joint Surgery, 46A, 1077–1092.

O'Sullivan, P.B., Twomey, L.T. and Allison, G.T. (1997). Evaluation of specific stabilizing exercise in the treatment of chronic low back pain with radiologic diagnosis of spondylolysis or spondylolisthesis. Spine, 22, 2959–2967.

Panjabi, M.M. (1992). The stabilizing system of the spine. Part II. Neutral zone and instability hypothesis. Journal of Spinal Disorders, 5, 390–396.

Panjabi, M.M., Oxland, T.R., Kifune, M. et al. (1995). Validity of the three-column theory of thoracolumbar fractures. A biomechanic investigation. Spine, 20, 1122–1127.

Radebold, A., Cholewicki, J., Panjabi, M.M. and Patel, T.C. (2000). Muscle response pattern to sudden trunk loading in healthy individuals and in patients with chronic low back pain. Spine, 25, 947–954.

Richardson, C.A., Jull, G.A., Hides, J.A. and Hodges, P.W. (1999). Therapeutic Exercise for Spinal Segmental Stabilisation in Low Back Pain: Scientific Basis and Clinical Approach. Edinburgh: Churchill Livingstone.

Roy, S.H., De Luca, C.J. and Casavant, D.A. (1989). Lumbar muscle fatigue and chronic lower back pain. Spine, 14, 992–1001.

Tandon, O.P., Himani, A. and Singh, S. (1997). Pulmonary responses during cold induced acute pain. Indian Journal of Physiology and Pharmacology, 41, 16–22.

Weisenberg, M., Raz, T. and Hener, T. (1998). The influence of film-induced mood on pain perception. Pain, 76, 365–375.

Wilke, H.J., Wolf, S., Claes, L.E. et al. (1995). Stability increase of the lumbar spine with different muscle groups. A biomechanical in vitro study. Spine, 20, 192–198.

Zelman, D.C., Howland, E.W., Nichols, S.N. and Cleeland, C.S. (1991). The effects of induced mood on laboratory pain. Pain, 46, 105–111.

CHAPTER 8

Ankle sprain in a 14-year-old girl

Gary Hunt

SUBJECTIVE EXAMINATION

Tiffany is a 14-year-old female high school freshman who has been referred with a diagnosis of right lateral ankle sprain. She presents as an intelligent, energetic young lady who has been very successful in school, both scholastically and in extracurricular activities. She attended her first therapy session with her mother, who was very supportive and appropriately concerned about her daughter's lack of improvement from a sprained ankle.

Tiffany originally injured her right ankle approximately 3 to 4 weeks prior to this appointment. The injury occurred while she was participating in a practice session for her cheerleading/tumbling squad. Tiffany described the mechanism of injury as an inversion ankle sprain when she landed on another team member's foot during a lift manoeuvre. She rested for a few moments, and although the ankle was tender, she was able to continue the work-out session. Three days later she returned to the gym for a follow-up work-out and reinjured the same ankle following a jump manoeuvre. She landed on the outside aspect of her foot and described hearing a 'pop', immediately experienced severe pain and was unable to place any weight on the right foot. Her coach referred her to an athletic trainer following the second injury. The athletic trainer saw her the same day and advised that she apply ice, elevation and a compression wrap, and exercise the foot as much as possible. He also encouraged her to walk with axillary crutches while bearing as much weight as tolerable.

Following 2 days of this approach and no improvement, Tiffany was evaluated by an orthopaedic surgeon.

He ordered radiographs of the foot and ankle to rule out any fracture, dislocation or epiphyseal abnormality. Posteroanterior, lateral and ankle mortice views were taken and read as normal. She was instructed by the surgeon to use the crutches with a non-weight-bearing gait and to perform ankle dorsiflexion and plantarflexion exercises within pain tolerance. Tiffany was not improving and 2 weeks later repeat radiographs were ordered to see if any bony changes had occurred that might have suggested a healing stress fracture. This second set also read as normal. The surgeon then decided to refer Tiffany for my evaluation and management.

History

Tiffany ambulated into the clinic using axillary crutches and non-weight bearing on the right leg. She was very reluctant to place the foot on the floor. She had not been able to wear a shoe to this point because of slight ankle and foot swelling, and because of increased sensitivity, primarily over all her toes and the anterolateral aspect of the foot and ankle. Tiffany was only able to tolerate an elastic bandage and an oversized fleece stocking for ankle support and protection. She rated her pain as 0/10 at rest, but with any weight bearing or pressure the pain became very intense and throbbing just inferior to the lateral malleolus, with a tingling pain located over the anterolateral aspect of the ankle (Fig. 8.1). Upon further discussion, Tiffany stated that the foot would become a dark purple colour

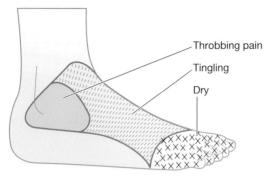

Fig. 8.1 Reported areas of symptoms.

and spotted when it was in the gravity-dependent position for even a few seconds. The throbbing and tingling in the foot and ankle also intensified when the foot was placed in the dependent position for 1–2 minutes. She also related that her toes and forefoot would begin to shake sometimes, but that it would not last

for more than a few seconds. This appeared to occur mostly when she tried to move or position her toes or ankle. She often noted that her right toes and ankle were cooler than on the opposite side.

Her physician had advised her to begin anti-inflammatory medication (naproxen 375 mg twice daily), which she took sporadically. Tiffany used the medication for the first 2 weeks after the second injury and then discontinued it, but she was unsure whether the medication had been of any benefit. She also applied extra moisturizing lotion on her forefoot daily to overcome dryness (Fig. 8.1) and maintain normal skin texture.

Tiffany said she had no previous history of ankle injuries or any history of spinal complaints. She had no present symptoms/problems elsewhere and her general health was unremarkable. Her goal is to return to her cheerleading squad as soon as possible and to participate in a cheerleading competition in 2 weeks.

 ## REASONING DISCUSSION AND CLINICAL REASONING COMMENTARY

 1 What were your thoughts regarding the mechanism of the second injury and factors contributing to the injury?

Clinician's answer

Tiffany was not exactly sure, but she thought that the ankle turned over laterally after a jump manoeuvre. By her description, I felt that she had probably sustained an inversion ankle sprain that involved all of the lateral soft tissue structures. The initial injury may have compromised her proprioceptive capabilities and/or modified her motor pattern secondary to low-grade nociceptive pain mechanisms. Furthermore, the activity of tumbling can be unpredictable concerning landings. The second injury could have occurred because the tissues were still inflamed with slight nociceptive pain present from the initial injury.

2 What were your working hypotheses at this stage about the possible sources for Tiffany's symptoms and disability? What findings so far supported and negated these hypotheses?

Clinician's answer

My working hypothesis at this time was that Tiffany had complex regional pain syndrome type II (causalgic-type pain pattern) with peroneal nerve involvement (Harden et al., 2001; Janig and Stanton-Hicks, 1996). She displayed neural impairment with vascular instability. Primary hyperalgesia from injured tissue in the ankle region, and possibly secondary hyperalgesia from adjacent uninjured tissue (Janig and Stanton-Hicks, 1996), characterized her pain. The trauma seemed to involve the peroneal nerve producing an abnormal state of afferent impulses (sympathetic fibres) leading to abnormal regulation of blood flow (changes in colour and temperature) and sweating (dryness). Distorted information processing in the spinal cord appeared to be possible as indicated by the abnormal muscle response in the toes (toes shaking). Neurogenic inflammation was also considered, as were capsular trauma and talar dome fracture. The plain radiographs eliminated any epiphyseal injury, but more sophisticated imaging would be required to rule out osteochondral injury completely. However, because of the lack of functional return and the persistence of pain, unusual for a sprained ankle which typically heals more quickly, I considered neurovascular injury the dominant diagnostic component of her clinical presentation.

3 What were your aims in taking this patient's history (subjective examination)? Did you actively search for any psychosocial implications for the management of Tiffany's problem?

Clinician's answer

My primary aim in taking the history was to help me to understand all the factors leading to her current state of disability. It helped to direct my clinical examination. Secondary aims included understanding the mechanism of injury, the state of inflammation, and the possible pathobiological mechanisms causing pain and movement impairment. I did not actively consider any psychosocial implications—she was a very outgoing and energetic individual. However, she was very goal oriented and wanted to understand why she was not getting better.

Clinical reasoning commentary

The clinician's response in regard to mechanism indicates that even at this early stage of the patient visit he was simultaneously considering hypotheses in several categories:

- physical impairments and associated structure/tissue sources (e.g. lateral soft tissue structures)
- pathobiological mechanisms, related to both tissue healing (e.g. inflammation) and pain (e.g. nociceptive)
- factors contributing to the injury (e.g. compromised proprioceptive capabilities).

Early generation of hypotheses, as in this case, largely relates to prior experience with similar clinical presentations. Expert clinicians access their well-developed knowledge base to recognize familiar initial cues, which together begin to form a clinical pattern. Previous experience with such clinical patterns or presentations will help to guide the subsequent examination and management, with newly acquired clinical data used continually to test and to refine hypotheses, thus further enriching the clinician's knowledge base.

The primary diagnostic hypothesis has obviously been further refined upon completion of the patient history. However, the clinician has recognized that the clinical findings are not entirely consistent with the typical pattern or presentation for a 'sprained ankle'. Atypical findings, notably the slow rate of recovery, have alerted him to the likelihood that he may be dealing with an unusual variation of the syndrome, providing him with a valuable opportunity to learn more about this clinical variation from his patient.

PHYSICAL EXAMINATION

Clinical inspection identified a cooler right foot and leg, which extended up to the calf. The temperature was 2.0°F (1.1°C) cooler on the right side, as measured by a biofeedback temperature thermistor (thermometer). The plantar and dorsal aspects of the lateral part of the right foot appeared dryer than those of the left foot. Although she denied any numbness in her foot, Tiffany had decreased sensation to touch in the superficial peroneal nerve distribution. She was actually surprised to discover that, in fact, she had less sensation in the nerve distribution.

The foot became mottled when placed in the gravity-dependent position, and then blanched when elevated for 20–30 seconds. No associated change in pain was noted, although she described a throbbing sensation in the foot and ankle when the foot was dangled over the edge of the examination table. Capillary filling time of the distal right great toe was prolonged compared with the left side. Posterior tibial and dorsalis pedis pulses were present and equal bilaterally. Manual muscle strength testing was deferred because of Tiffany's level of discomfort. All active movements of the toes, subtalar and ankle joints were guarded and incomplete as a result of pain. Slight quivering of the toes was at times noted during the initial examination.

Movement

Assisted active movements of the ankle were measured in prone lying with the knee extended. Dorsiflexion range of motion of the left ankle was 8 degrees, but only 2 degrees on the right side. Plantarflexion was also limited on the right side (25 degrees) compared with the left (50 degrees), as measured with a standard goniometer. Active and passive ankle plantarflexion with associated subtalar joint supination produced discomfort in the lateral anterior ankle region and Tiffany was reluctant to move in this direction. Other active foot and ankle motions were not quantified at this session because of lack of time. The end-feel of passive calcaneal inversion was soft and produced discomfort in the lateral ankle region before tension was perceived. The end-feel of calcaneal eversion was normal. Passive movement of the forefoot around the midtarsal oblique and longitudinal axes (Elftman, 1960; Manter, 1941) did not produce any notable discomfort and the end-feel was also normal. Hip and knee motion was unremarkable. No spinal examination was undertaken on the first visit as Tiffany had no history of spinal complaints.

Right straight leg raise (SLR) without prepositioning the foot or ankle produced discomfort and tingling in the right lateral ankle area at 50 degrees. Further sensitizing the peroneal nerve while performing SLR extended the discomfort and tingling into the lateral forefoot and toes. No increase in tingling occurred when the tibial nerve or the sural nerve were sensitized during the SLR test (Butler, 2000; Magee, 1997). SLR testing on the left side was accomplished to 95–100 degrees with only a stretching sensation reported in the thigh.

Remeasurement of skin temperature at the end of the physical examination demonstrated the coolness had extended up to the mid-posterior thigh. However the resting pain level had not notably changed following the examination.

REASONING DISCUSSION AND CLINICAL REASONING COMMENTARY

1 The initial part of your physical examination was largely directed at assessing vascular structures. Is this a normal feature of your routine examination for inversion injuries or were there particular cues that suggested the need for this?

■ Clinician's answer

I directed my physical examination to include an assessment of vascular structures because her symptoms and history suggested vascular involvement and I wanted to quantify the vascular responses. Coolness of the foot associated with a mottled appearance in the dependent position suggested some type of vascular involvement. Dorsalis pedis and posterior tibial pulses were normal (ruling out arterial occlusion), but capillary filling time was longer on the involved side. Dryness, coolness and the mottled appearance in the presence of normal distal pulses suggested abnormal regulation of small vessel blood flow, perhaps related to altered sympathetic nerve function (Rempel et al., 1999).

So although I routinely check vascular structures, in this case I was initially struck by the coolness, colour changes and dryness. These observations led me to perform a more thorough vascular examination (i.e. pulse check, capillary filling time and temperature measurement).

2 What was your early impression regarding the structures involved, particularly the neurovascular tissues, and the associated pathobiological mechanisms, including the stage of healing?

■ Clinician's answer

The history and clinical presentation of signs and symptoms suggested a more complicated problem than just a lateral ankle ligamentous sprain. Colour changes, cooler skin temperature and skin dryness, along with increased sensitivity to mechanical stimulation, indicated neurovascular instability.

Positive neurodynamic examination findings indicated increased irritability within neurovascular tissues, which was probably secondary to direct tensile forces at the time of injury. It appeared that the peroneal nerve (both superficial and deep peroneal sensory branches) was implicated. The vascular structures involved may have included the lateral saphenous vein and possibly the anterior lateral malleolar artery, the peroneal artery, and/or the lateral tarsal artery. The pathobiological processes in the neurovascular tissues tend to suggest the persistence of peripherally evoked neurogenic symptoms (input) and possibly centrally evoked symptoms (processing), as well as autonomic and motor (output) involvement, as evidenced by the shaking of the toes.

The ligamentous tissue should have been in stage two of healing (subacute or granulation/fibroplasia phase) and just entering stage three of the healing process (remodelling phase) because it was approximately 22 days since the second injury. Nociceptive pain should have resolved by this point in time.

■ Clinical reasoning commentary

The clinician has recognized the likely significance of those findings in the clinical examination suggestive of a neurovascular problem and which indicate that the clinical presentation is not entirely consistent with the more common syndrome of lateral ankle ligamentous sprain. Rather than ignoring symptoms and signs that are unusual, difficult to interpret or perceived as non-contributory to a favoured hypothesis, the clinician has acted upon these findings and pursued further data to enable him to test hypotheses related to trauma of neurological and vascular structures, despite the relative rarity of such injuries. A non-expert therapist may have simply focussed on the obvious injured joint structures and failed to recognize the potential significance of some key clinical features (e.g. dryness of skin), nor really considered why symptoms and signs were persisting beyond the expected timeframe for healing and nociceptive pain.

Consideration of where the patient's disorder is with respect to the normal stages of tissue healing is important in recognizing whether it is following a normal course of recovery. When this is not the case, it alerts the reflective clinician to further consideration of factors, including pain mechanisms as discussed here, which may be interfering with the healing processes.

m | Initial management

Treatment on the first day consisted of neuromobilization exercise instruction. Tiffany was advised to perform 10 repetitions of knee extension, hourly if possible, without any prepositioning of the ankle. The exercise could be carried out either in supine or sitting. She was instructed, along with her mother, to perform this exercise only to a sense of initial tension and not into pain. The aim of the exercise was to improve vascular fluid dynamics and axoplasmic flow in a non-painful manner, so as to enhance the nutrition and mobility of the neurological tissues. It was hoped this non-painful afferent input would help to start the process of normalizing the neural system.

Tiffany was also instructed to continue partial weight bearing as tolerated using the axillary crutches, but not at the expense of increasing pain. She was advised to obtain an oversized soft slipper to provide protection to the plantar foot surface. Because she felt more secure with an elastic bandage wrapped around the ankle, she was encouraged to continue with its application.

Considerable time was spent discussing with Tiffany and her mother the mechanism of injury and the tissues that could have been injured. It was explained that the presence of neurovascular instability most likely implicated neurological tissues and blood vessels, which would probably lengthen recovery time. Options for ankle supports were also discussed and it was decided that the need would be better assessed during the next couple of weeks. Tiffany and her mother were instructed on how to assess skin temperature daily, particularly following exercise, thus skin temperature acted as a 'comparable sign' for tissue stress response. They were informed that the exercise should not cause the right foot to become cooler. Timeframes for healing were also discussed, as was the probability of her competing within 2 weeks, which seemed unlikely considering her current functional status. However, follow-up assessment would be necessary to make that decision.

REASONING DISCUSSION AND CLINICAL REASONING COMMENTARY

1 You have obviously spent considerable time discussing the problem and its management with Tiffany and her mother. Why did you consider this was necessary?

■ Clinician's answer

Both Tiffany and her mother were very interested in the mechanisms of injury and healing. I felt that if they were both well informed they would be less anxious and better able to understand what needed to be accomplished to remedy the problem. In addition, our health-care system limits the number of times a patient can be seen in the clinic. This situation necessitates the patient taking responsibility for their own care, with home exercise and self-management likely to be essential components of Tiffany's rehabilitation programme.

I try to empower the patient and show them what they can do to promote the healing process. Once they understand the healing process, I then show them what they must do to accomplish their goals and improve their function. In this case, the goals of home exercise and self-management included:

- facilitating fluid dynamics to assist in resolving inflammation and to improve tissue nutrition
- remodelling connective tissue with graded progressive movements
- enhancing motor control through repetitive movement patterns.

2 What were your expectations regarding the timeframe for healing and what factors in the patient's presentation influenced your thinking? Were you at all concerned at this time about the vascular component to the problem?

■ Clinician's answer

I was hoping that in 4–6 weeks I would see functional improvement in her weight bearing and gait, taking into consideration the neural involvement. Primarily, the neurovascular dysfunction influenced my thinking. I was not absolutely sure how long it would take

to reverse this process, particularly considering the return of vascular supply to the nerve and axoplasmic flow. I expected the timeframe for connective tissue repair and remodelling to be in the order of months for full recovery.

I was not concerned that the vascular component would result in necrosis because there were palpable pedal pulses. I contacted the referring surgeon about my diagnosis, with which he concurred, and called him weekly to give him updates on Tiffany's progress.

3 Did you consider the physical (objective) examination complete at this stage or did you plan to examine the patient further at later visits? If so, what specifically were you planning to do?

■ Clinician's answer

The examination was not complete. I intended to measure calcaneal inversion and eversion and to document her weight bearing by using a bathroom scale. I also planned to evaluate her weight bearing with the podoscope when possible and to look at the thoracic spine for possible dysfunction that might influence sympathetic function. Inability to weight bear was a significant impairment preventing normal ambulation. It was considered her weight-bearing pattern on the podoscope and the magnitude of force on the scale could be used for reassessment. This was not possible on the first visit because of time constraints.

■ Clinical reasoning commentary

With the expert clinician, clinical reasoning does not occur in isolation. While it is heavily dependent on factors or attributes internal to the therapist (e.g. clinical experience, communication skills), it is also somewhat influenced by factors external to the therapist, including the attributes of the patient and the environment. Such factors are evident in this case, notably the willingness of Tiffany (and her mother) to participate in her management, the limitation on the number of treatments imposed by the health-care system, and the inevitable time restrictions of clinical work. It is apparent that the expert clinician's reasoning is

carried out in a collaborative framework with relevant parties: the patient, her mother, the referring surgeon, as well as the funding body and the workplace (see discussion of collaborative reasoning in Ch. 1).

Reassessment and further treatment

At the second visit (5 days later), Tiffany stated that she had been faithful in carrying out her neuromobilization exercises and was able to perform them without any notable increase in pain. She also reported that she had only experienced one temporary episode of numbness in the ankle, which had extended up the posterior thigh.

On examination, the right calf was 3.0°F (1.6°C) cooler than the left, but the posterior thighs were equal in temperature. Tiffany was still using axillary crutches with a non-weight-bearing gait on the right side. Active and passive motion of the toes and ankle were unchanged from the initial visit. During this session, calcaneal inversion and eversion were 35 degrees and 15 degrees bilaterally, respectively. Attempts to activate the toes using a toe-curling exercise with a towel were unsuccessful as a result of discomfort and lack of toe control. However, the colour of the foot in the dependent position was improved.

Tiffany had no complaints of thoracic spine pain, but thoracic spine mobility was assessed because of the possibility of associated sympathetic nervous system influence (Blumberg et al., 1997; Butler and Slater, 1994; Cleland et al., 2002). Active thoracic

spine rotation to the right was found to be limited and slightly uncomfortable at end-range compared with left rotation.

The second treatment session involved neuromobilization exercises for the sciatic and peroneal nerves, and this was accomplished without any adverse tissue temperature response (Fig. 8.2). Tiffany was also instructed in how to perform toe curls using a towel and ankle motion (plantarflexion and dorsiflexion) using a tilt board while sitting, without increasing any of the symptoms. She was issued with an elastic stocking to replace the elastic bandage and told to remove it if her symptoms increased.

Thoracic spine mobilization was instituted with the aim of positively influencing the sympathetic nervous system to facilitate neurovascular stability. The first exercise required the patient to be positioned in hook lying with her lower thoracic spine over a crosswise-positioned foam roll, while her hands were clasped behind her neck. She was instructed to take a deep breath while in a curled position and then to exhale as she lowered her upper thoracic spine to the table. She was cautioned not to move into significant pain nor to allow the lumbar spine to extend during this movement. This exercise was repeated three times at each thoracic spine level up to T6. Tiffany noted that right thoracic rotation movement was easier afterwards and less uncomfortable. Tiffany and

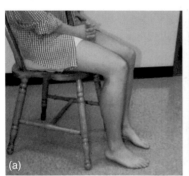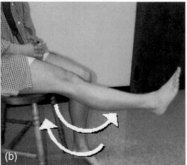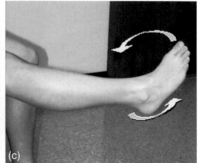

Fig. 8.2 Neurodynamic mobilization for the sciatic and peroneal nerves: (a) starting position; (b) sciatic mobilization only; (c) peroneal mobilization added.

her mother were then instructed in the use of an airbag for spinal mobilization to be performed in the supine lying position. The second exercise involved the use a foam roll against a wall for thoracic soft tissue mobilization. The patient leans on the roll against the wall in a standing position and flexes and extends the knees to move the roll over the soft tissues of the spine. Tiffany was able to perform this exercise without difficulty while only partial weight bearing on the right leg. She tolerated thoracic spine self-mobilization without incident.

A follow-up telephone conversation 2 days later with Tiffany's mother indicated that the new exercises were going well and the elastic stocking seemed more comfortable and effective than the elastic bandage. Tiffany was still unable to perform the towel toe curl exercises because of lack of motor control. The temperature pattern of the right leg was improving and it was actually feeling warmer. The colour of the foot was improving as well. The mother was advised to continue the plan of care and a reassessment would be performed at the next visit.

 ## REASONING DISCUSSION AND CLINICAL REASONING COMMENTARY

1 Why did you suspect there could be involvement of the sympathetic nervous system in an apparent inversion injury? Could you please further elaborate regarding your rationale for the thoracic spine mobilization exercises?

thoracic spine rotation to the right side. If we could improve the fluid dynamics of the vascular supply and the axoplasmic flow in the area, then this might have a positive impact on the nutrition of the sympathetic fibres.

Clinician's answer

I would not routinely suspect sympathetic nerve involvement but her symptom presentation suggested that I consider that possibility. The colour, temperature and sweating changes indicated potential involvement of sympathetic fibres. This was rather a 'shot in the dark' but the rationale relates to thoracic spine impairment influencing the sympathetic chains within that anatomical region (Blumberg et al., 1997; Butler and Slater, 1994; Cleland et al., 2002). I was trying to see if there was an association between thoracic spinal mobility and her symptom complex. My hypothesis was that maybe joint and connective tissue restriction in the thoracic spine might have had a contributing influence on sympathetic dysfunction. This was supported by the finding of decreased

Clinical reasoning commentary

The 'shot in the dark'—that is, treating the thoracic spine to help to alleviate the foot and ankle symptoms—is an example of lateral thinking on the part of the clinician. Although arguably an unlikely association, despite the pathoanatomical rationale given, it is largely through such lateral thinking processes that the professional craft knowledge of manual therapy has developed. Neural mobilization (Butler, 2000), repeated movements (McKenzie, 1981), mobilizations with movement (Mulligan, 1999) and many other interventions have resulted from a clinician daring to think 'outside of the box' and reflecting about what they had found. Both the individual manual therapist and the community of manual therapists grow from such insights.

Outcome

Third visit (1 week later)

Tiffany reported less colour change with the dependent foot position and that the foot was warmer. She was

able to wear a sandal for the first time but still needed to use crutches, although she could move around with some weight through the foot. She also related that her toes seemed to have increased sensitivity and that her thoracic rotation had improved and was more comfortable.

Physical examination revealed ankle motion was improving both in quality and quantity, especially right ankle plantarflexion (35 degrees). The temperature of the right calf was now only 1.0°F (0.6°C) cooler than the left. Capillary filling time in the right great toe was equal to the left. Tiffany was also able to flex her toes and perform toe curling with a towel and pick-up packing popcorn with her toes. Thoracic spine right rotation was now equal to left rotation without any discomfort.

The newfound ability to bear weight enabled the objective assessment of weight bearing using a bathroom scale. Right foot pressure applied to a bathroom scale while sitting measured 12 pounds (5.5 kg) compared with 45 pounds (20.5 kg) on the left. Tiffany was even able to ride a stationary bicycle for 15 minutes without pain.

Tiffany recognized and accepted that participation in the upcoming cheerleading competition was not going to be possible. She was instructed to continue her home exercise programme as previously outlined and to utilize a stationary bicycle, progressing up to 20–30 minutes of cycling daily.

Fourth visit (1 week later)

Tiffany reported that she was continuing to improve and was pleased with her progress. She was able to place more weight through the right leg during walking; the colour of the foot was still improving and it was becoming less hypersensitive. The mother had noted normal temperatures in the calf and ankle.

On examination, the temperature patterns were now normal. The right SLR had improved to 70 degrees before tightness was perceived and the neurodynamic test for the peroneal nerve was less provocative. Active right ankle dorsiflexion was now 10 degrees and plantarflexion was 40 degrees. The bathroom

scale press test in sitting measured 18 pounds (8.2 kg) on the right side. Tiffany's weight-bearing ability was further evaluated using a podoscope (a plexiglass standing box that allows the opportunity to observe an individual's weight-bearing pattern). She demonstrated decreased pressure in both the heel and forefoot (Fig. 8.3).

Tibia vara in simulated single limb stance measured 10 degrees bilaterally. This compared favourably with the calcaneal eversion of 15 degrees measured during the second visit. In other words, she did not have a varus calcaneus that would predispose her to ankle sprains. Ligament testing of the right anterior talofibular ligament revealed slight laxity compared with the left ankle.

A leg-hindfoot orthosis was fabricated to provide stabilization and proprioceptive input to the ankle region (Fig. 8.4). Tiffany was able to stand more

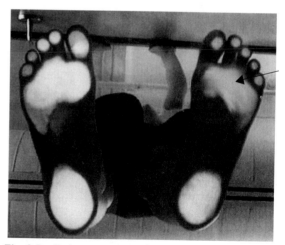
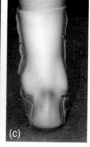

Fig. 8.3 Podoscope image demonstrating decreased right heel and right forefoot pressure (arrow).

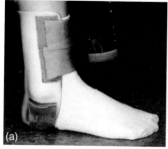
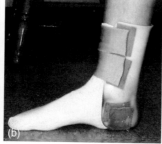

Fig. 8.4 Leg-hindfoot orthosis: (a) lateral view; (b) medial view; (c) posterior view.

comfortably with the orthosis and was able to apply 50 pounds (22.7 kg) of force in a standing position without notable pain production. At this point she was advised to increase her weight-bearing activity.

Additional instruction included various SLR exercises (no weight and 10 repetitions per position), resisted ankle plantarflexion and thoracic rotation using resistive elastic exercise bands (repeated to fatigue), and the use of a bathroom scale for visual feedback on progressive weight bearing in sitting and standing positions. Tiffany was also instructed to wear the leg-hindfoot orthosis throughout the day and to watch for any signs of skin irritation. She was encouraged to increase her ambulation and decrease her reliance on the crutches.

Fifth visit (1 week later)

Tiffany reported significant functional improvement with ambulation. She was able to ambulate with one crutch for long distances and even take a few steps without any ambulatory device for shorter distances, all without an increase in pain.

The temperature patterns were normal and shifting her weight to the right leg in standing registered 70 pounds (31.8 kg) on the bathroom scale. Right SLR was almost equal to the left, and right ankle motion had improved to 12 degrees for dorsiflexion and 47 degrees for plantarflexion without any pain. Tiffany was now able for the first time to stand on her right leg (single leg balance) for approximately 5 seconds while wearing the orthosis, with only one finger assisting her balance. The podoscope examination indicated improved heel and forefoot pressure, but still lacked good pressure under the first metatarsophalangeal joint and toes.

The addition of the orthosis fabricated during the previous visit seemed to have significantly improved Tiffany's weight-bearing status. She was encouraged to continue her home exercise programme and to concentrate on balancing activities and a normal heel-toe gait pattern using one crutch.

Sixth visit (one week later)

Tiffany was now approximately 9 weeks post-injury and was able to wear a regular shoe for the first time, although she continued to wear the leg-hindfoot orthosis. She felt that the orthosis allowed her to ambulate more effectively and with minimal discomfort. She also related that the bicycle exercise seemed to be very beneficial and that pain was no longer a significant issue, including during plantarflexion and supination of her foot. Her gait was now accomplished without crutches and with only a slight limp. For long distances, however, she still preferred to use one crutch.

On examination, the limp appeared to be related to prolonged heel contact during the terminal stance phase on the right leg. The bathroom scale test in standing produced 90 pounds (40.9 kg) without pain on the right side. The podoscope examination revealed improved pressure under the toes, but she still lacked appropriate pressure under the first metatarsophalangeal joint. No swelling was noted in the foot and ankle and the skin appeared healthy without evidence of dryness. Slight discomfort and weakness was noted with resisted peroneus longus muscle testing. Other muscles tested around the ankle were normal, except for right gastrocnemius/soleus, which was slightly weak compared with the left. Right SLR reached 80 degrees before tightness and slight tingling was produced.

Tiffany was instructed to continue her home exercise programme and progressively increase stress to the tissues, always being guided by pain.

Final visit (three weeks later)

Tiffany had been re-evaluated by the referring physician since the previous visit. He was pleased with her progress and decided to discharge her from his care. Tiffany noted that pain was no longer an issue. She experienced only occasional arch fatigue and cramping with prolonged weight bearing. It was reported the temperature, skin texture and skin colour were normal, and she no longer needed the crutch.

Physically she demonstrated improved active control of her toe and ankle muscles. Neurodynamic testing of the right peroneal nerve was improved to 85 degrees before the onset of tightness and slight tingling. Temperature patterns continued to be normal. Tiffany was able to ambulate without the leg-hindfoot orthosis, but she still felt more confident while wearing it. Her gait demonstrated good functional velocity and the late heel-off in terminal stance phase previously noted was improving. Single leg balance was accomplished for about 5 seconds without a finger assisting her balance. She still had difficulty performing a heel rise on the right leg because of weakness and possibly lack of confidence. The podoscope examination revealed symmetry between the feet (Fig. 8.5).

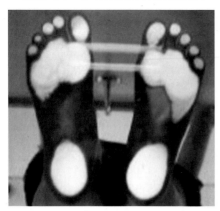

Fig. 8.5 Podoscope image demonstrating symmetrical heel and forefoot pressure.

Tiffany and her mother felt confident that she could continue on the home exercise programme with occasional telephone updates on her progress. Tiffany was advised to concentrate on balance (proprioception) and neuromobilization exercises. She was also instructed in retro-walking and eccentric loading exercises for the ankle plantarflexors to facilitate strengthening of the non-contractile tissue components as well as the contractile elements of the muscles. It was emphasized that pain should guide her exercise and activity. She was also encouraged to continue monitoring temperature as an indicator of tissue stress.

Approximately 6 months after the injury, Tiffany participated in a cheerleading squad competition without pain, using the leg-hindfoot orthosis, and winning the state championship for her school's division. At 13 months after the injury, she considered herself to be 90% normal and at 22 months after injury she considered herself to be 98% normal, with the only complaint being slight numbness over the dorsolateral aspect of the foot. She continues to wear a soft ankle support during participation in cheerleading activities.

 REASONING DISCUSSION AND CLINICAL REASONING COMMENTARY

1 What is your long-term prognosis for Tiffany?

■ **Clinician's answer**

Tiffany has a good long-term prognosis. Despite having significantly injured multiple tissues, she is now fully functional, with only slight persisting numbness over the superficial peroneal nerve distribution in the foot. However, her cheerleading activities, which include tumbling, could possibly open her up to reinjury in the future. The ankle support she uses probably assists by providing additional proprioceptive input and giving her confidence during cheerleading activities.

■ **Clinical reasoning commentary**

This case, like the others, highlights the specialized knowledge manual therapists require to practise at the highest level. However, as discussed in Chapter 1, it is not how much an individual knows that is important, but rather how that knowledge is organized. Expert clinicians possess a rich store of clinical patterns derived from a combination of propositional (research-based) and non-propositional (professional craft and personal) knowledge. Usually, examination and management of ankle sprains is straightforward given that most will resolve through normal healing processes, with advice and minimal intervention typically being all that is required. Nevertheless, as this case illustrates, problems can present in multiple ways ranging from simple to complex, as in all areas of the body. Hence, there are no recipes for examination or management that will apply across the full spectrum of possible presentations.

Recognition and management of more complex ankle sprains, as in this case, requires advanced knowledge of somatic, neural and vascular anatomy, pathobiological pain and tissue mechanisms, specialized examination procedures (e.g. thermistor assessment, neurodynamic assessment biased to specific peripheral nerves, ankle and foot biomechanics assessment) and specialized management procedures (e.g. orthotics). This advanced knowledge is not retained in abstract academic constructs. Instead expert clinicians possess highly developed knowledge bases where these different areas of knowledge are interlinked through clinical patterns. It is our belief that the hypothesis categories discussed in Chapter 1 are a useful strategy for facilitating this linking of knowledge across different areas in a clinically meaningful way. This level of knowledge organization cannot be achieved from books or journals alone. Experts acquire their clinically relevant knowledge organization through their never-ending reflection and integration of the available research and experience-based evidence.

References

Blumberg, H., Hoffman, U., Mohadjer, M. and Scheremet, R. (1997). Sympathetic nervous system and pain: a clinical re-appraisal. Behavioral and Brain Sciences, 20, 426–434.

Butler, D.S. (2000). The Sensitive Nervous System. Adelaide, Australia: Noigroup Press.

Butler, D.S. and Slater, H. (1994). Neural injury in the thoracic spine: a conceptual basis for manual therapy. In Physical Therapy of the Cervical and Thoracic Spines, 2nd edn (R. Grant, ed.) pp. 313–338. Edinburgh: Churchill Livingstone.

Cleland, J., Durall, C. and Scott, S.A. (2002). Effects of slump long sitting on peripheral sudomotor and vasomotor function: a pilot study. Journal of Manual and Manipulative Therapy, 10, 67–75.

Elftman, H. (1960). The transverse tarsal joint and its control. Clinical Orthopedics and Related Research, 16, 41–46.

Harden, R.N., Baron, R. and Janig, W. (2001). Complex Regional Pain Syndrome. Seattle, WA: IASP Press.

Janig, W. and Stanton-Hicks, M. (1996). Reflex Sympathetic Dystrophy: A Reappraisal. Seattle, WA: IASP Press.

Magee, D.J. (1997). Orthopedic Physical Assessment, 3rd edn. London: Saunders.

Manter, J.T. (1941). Movements of the subtalar joint and transverse tarsal joints. Anatomical Record, 80, 397–410.

McKenzie, R. (1981). The Lumbar Spine. Mechanical Diagnosis and Therapy. Lower Hutt, New Zealand: Spinal Publications.

Mulligan, B. (1999). Manual Therapy. 'NAGS', 'SNAGS', 'MWMs', etc., 4th edn. Wellington, New Zealand: Plane View Press.

Rempel, D., Dahlin, L. and Lundborg, G. (1999). Pathophysiology of nerve compression syndromes: response of peripheral nerves to loading. Journal of Bone and Joint Surgery, 81A, 1600–1610.

Headache in a mature athlete

Gwendolen Jull

 SUBJECTIVE EXAMINATION

Shirley was referred by a sports physician who she had consulted regarding her asthma. She was also suffering from almost daily frontal headaches. She has been having regular physiotherapy on and off for the past year in conjunction with massage but had achieved no permanent relief. She had a motor vehicle accident (MVA) 35 years ago at which time she fractured her thoracic spine. Although Shirley had some cervical stiffness, radiographs had shown only mild exit canal narrowing with no deterioration in the past 5 years. The sports physician believed that the stiffness was contributing to her headaches.

Shirley is a 54-year-old female who owns and works in her own retail business. She is also an athlete who trains and competes in canoeing and has been successful at International Masters Games level. She had been training and competing in canoeing for 15 years but in the last 2 years she has suffered from asthma and has had to ease off her training. The asthma is now under control and she is starting to train again more seriously. This is more for her recreational pursuits and desire for fitness rather than to compete at international level as her work commitments and other newly acquired responsibilities preclude her from dedicating the required time for this level of competition.

Shirley reported that she had been suffering from headaches for a long time and they certainly may have started before her MVA 35 years earlier. However, since the accident, she has always had troubles with her neck in some form, including wry neck

episodes and neck stiffness, as well as headaches. She reported that often she can limit her wry neck episodes by concentrating on relaxation, but if the episode does not ease quickly, she consults a physiotherapist and attains relief. She also injured her vocal chords in the car accident, resulting in a hoarseness in her speech. Her new responsibilities include quite a deal of public speaking and for the past 6 months she has been consulting a speech pathologist to assist with these problems.

Currently Shirley suffers from almost daily headaches of variable intensity. Some are severe and she is unable to function while they are in the intense phase, which can last for several hours. These severe headaches are not frequent and Shirley could not give any particular pattern that related to their occurrence. The moderately intense headaches are the more frequent ones. They last for variable times from a few hours to the whole day depending on how well she can intervene with either medication or attempts at relaxation or neck exercise. Shirley felt that she suffered only one form of headache and that all headaches were the same, except for the intensity.

The headaches are right sided, unilateral and in the frontal, retro-orbital area. The neck pain is less specific and is more a feeling of general neck pain and stiffness. There was no pain or discomfort reported in the rest of the face, upper limbs, thoracic or low back area. The headaches, whether moderate or severe, are consistently on the right side and do not change sides within or between headache episodes.

With the intense headaches, Shirley reported that she was often nauseous and occasionally vomited but had no other associated symptoms when headaches were either intense or moderate. She has never suffered a prodroma in association with any headache.

The time of onset of headache was variable. Shirley reported that she could wake with headache or they could come on during the day. The headaches would start in the frontal region. They never started as neck pain, but a stiff, sore neck always accompanied her headaches.

Shirley could not identify any particular provocative factors for her headaches or factors that may precipitate them. She could not predict the onset of the severe headaches. Normally Shirley slept on her side and used one normal sized pillow and one soft pillow. She considered that she was comfortable in bed and on the whole slept well even though she could wake with a headache. Her work involved a variety of activities and a variety of tasks and she had not noticed that any particular task either specifically aggravated her neck or was likely to produce a headache. She was usually quite physically active during the day.

Shirley reported that she tries to control and relieve the headaches with simple analgesics or aspirin and neck exercises (stretching) with variable success.

There was a family history of headache in that her mother had suffered from migraine.

She has not attended for physiotherapy over the last 6 months but in the preceding 12 months she had been receiving physiotherapy for her headaches. The physiotherapy, which consisted of manual therapy and muscle stretching exercises, gave some temporary relief but overall it had not had any permanent effect on her headache condition. What she had noticed in the last 6 months was that her headaches were a little less frequent and this she attributed to returning to paddling, as well as the postural advice and neck relaxation strategies taught to her by the speech pathologist in her speech rehabilitation. Headaches were still suffered on at least 3 or 4 days per week. It would be unusual for her to go for more than 2 days without a headache of some sort.

Shirley related that what she wanted was some exercises or strategies that she could use to alleviate or at least help her to control her headaches.

REASONING DISCUSSION AND CLINICAL REASONING COMMENTARY

1 At the conclusion of the subjective examination, what was your primary hypothesis regarding the source of the headaches? Could you please discuss the findings that you thought supported this hypothesis? What were the features that you considered tended to negate this hypothesis?

■ Clinician's answer

There were certain features that were consistent with a cervical spine cause or contribution to the headache syndrome, while others were not suggestive of a cervical musculoskeletal cause of headache, based on a combination of knowledge of the available research-based evidence of headache presentations and classifications and my own personal clinical experience.

The factors supportive of a cervical cause or component to her headache were:

■ an initial history of trauma involving an MVA, which the patient associated with a 35-year history of neck problems

■ the temporal pattern of the headaches, namely daily, with variable duration and intensity

■ easing of headache with relaxation of her neck and exercises

■ sidelocking of headaches to the right side (migraine not infrequently changes sides)

■ reduced frequency of headache with increased physical exercise in the past 6 months.

The factors that tended to negate a cervical cause or component to her headache were:

■ the headache onset was in the frontal region rather than associated with neck pain or stiffness (it is common for migraines to start in the head with later spread to the neck, with the opposite applying for cervical headache)

■ some headaches were of such severity to prohibit normal function (this is more common with migraine)

■ provocative factors, especially mechanical factors involving her neck, could not be identified

■ a family history of migraine

■ previous physiotherapy to her neck appeared to assist the neck pain but not her headaches to any great extent.

2 Considering the chronicity of the problem, did you at this stage consider the pain mechanism(s) that may have been mediating the patient's symptoms?

■ **Clinician's answer**

At this stage, with the amount of information obtained about the patient and her condition, hypothesizing about pain mechanisms was not a priority. It was considered that more informed consideration could be given to the proposed pain mechanisms once knowledge of the presence or not of symptomatic physical impairments had been gained from the physical examination. The chronicity of the headache was not a concern at this time. Many cervical and frequent common migraine headaches have lengthy histories. The length of history of cervical headache does not preclude a peripheral nociceptive source amenable to manual and other therapies and has not necessarily been an important factor in influencing treatment outcome in my past experience. The major aim at this time was to try to sort out if the patient suffered from a cervical headache, a migraine or a mixed headache form.

3 From the history, were there any factors that you thought may have contributed to the onset or maintenance of the headache problem? In particular, were there any psychosocial or stress factors?

■ **Clinician's answer**

There were no indicators at this time, or indeed later, that there were any psychosocial or adverse stress factors involved in the pathogenesis of this patient's headaches. From the history of neck pain dating back to the MVA, there was every likelihood based on available evidence that there would be degenerative changes in the upper cervical joints. The presence of joint pain and dysfunction would probably also be accompanied by muscle dysfunction. Previous treatment had not specifically addressed any neuromuscular dysfunction and the presence of this dysfunction could be a major contributing factor.

■ **Clinical reasoning commentary**

The answer regarding initial hypotheses demonstrates that the clinician is actively attempting to match findings from the subjective examination to elicited clinical patterns relating to her primary diagnostic hypothesis of cervical headache. This is typical of the pattern recognition process commonly used by experts. In particular, her knowledge of the pattern of presentation of cervical headache, partly based on skilled, reflective clinical reasoning and partly research based, enables her to recognize the significance of clinical findings matching (or supporting) elements of the clinical pattern she holds in her memory. Importantly, the clinician has also recognized findings that are inconsistent with (or which negate) the cervical spine hypothesis and has kept her mind open to the possibility of a migraine headache or a mixture of the two. That is, she has not ignored the clinical findings that do not fit with the primary cervical headache hypothesis and has thus avoided committing a common reasoning error of being biased toward the favoured hypothesis, particularly if it is one usually amenable to manual therapy.

It is worth noting that some potential pathobiological mechanisms underlying (and other factors contributing to) any cervical component to the headache have been hypothesized, as evidenced by consideration of degenerative joint processes and neuromuscular impairment. It is implied that further information obtained in the physical examination will be used to test these hypotheses, as well as the source of the headaches.

In addition, the clinician has made the judgment that there are no significant psychosocial or stress factors in the patient's presentation.

 PHYSICAL EXAMINATION

Posture

The basic shape of the postural curves was unremarkable, with good head, neck, and thoracic alignment. Sitting posture approached an upright neutral position. The shoulder girdles were slightly elevated, downwardly rotated and protracted. The pectoral muscles were slightly hypertrophied and appeared tight. The bulk of the levator scapulae was evident. The scalenes also appeared to be overactive, with fullness in the supraclavicular fossae.

Active movements

The patient was currently experiencing no pain. Cervical spine movements were as follows:

- flexion: full range of motion (ROM), no pain reported
- extension: slightly restricted but with no pain, and some hypomobility in the cervicothoracic region; the pattern of return to neutral from extension revealed a lack of control of upper cervical initiation of the movement
- rotation left and right: 75% ROM with a general feeling of stiffness, but no pain
- lateral flexion left and right: 50% ROM with scalene tightness restricting movement, but no reported pain
- upper cervical flexion: full ROM, no pain
- upper cervical extension: full ROM, no pain
- C1–C2 rotation left and right: some general restriction, but no reported pain.

Thoracic spine movements were unremarkable and pain-free. Shoulder movements were full range and pain-free, with the pattern of control of the shoulder girdle revealing no obvious deficiency.

Neural system

The Brachial Plexus Provocation Test (BPPT; Elvey, 1998) performed on the left and right sides demonstrated no muscle resistance to gentle scapular depression. The completion of the tests was unremarkable and produced no pain other than a cubital fossa stretch. Upper cervical flexion was not restricted, and the quality of the passive upper cervical flexion movement was unchanged when the left or right upper limb was prepositioned in the BPPT position and when the left or right leg was prepositioned in a straight leg raise position.

Manual examination

Anterior palpation

A poor ability to relax was noted. Anterior palpation of the discs was unremarkable. There was some

heightened activity palpable in the soft tissues: in the anterior and middle scalene and sternocleidomastoid muscles bilaterally. Both first ribs were slightly elevated and hypomobile. Some slight tissue thickness was detected around the C2–C3 and C3–C4 zygapophyseal joints on the right side.

Passive physiological intervertebral movements

There was a slight restriction in lateral flexion and rotation bilaterally, most notable at C2–C3 and C3–C4. Some slight restriction in rotation was also detected at C1–C2 bilaterally.

Anteroposterior glides

A slight to moderate movement restriction was found on anteroposterior gliding of the C2–C3 and C3–C4 zygapophyseal joints on the right side, and to a lesser degree on the left side.

Posterior palpation

Time needed to be taken to achieve adequate relaxation of the neck. There was thickening of the right C2–C3 and C3–C4 zygapophyseal joints.

Posteroanterior glides

Local pain of moderate intensity and muscle reactivity was provoked over the right C2–C3 and C3–C4 zygapophyseal joints, which were also moderately restricted to movement. These findings were evident to a lesser extent on the left side. The cervicothoracic junction was moderately hypomobile. Thoracic examination was unremarkable.

Tests of neuromuscular control

The pattern of activation and holding capacity of the scapular synergists is tested by active repositioning of the scapulae onto the chest wall in the prone lying position (scapular retraction, depression and upward rotation), with no arm loading. Shirley's performance was fair, with some unwanted contribution from latissimus dorsi, rhomboids, and levator scapulae muscles. There were signs of fatigue after five repetitions. The performance on the right side was slightly inferior to that on the left side.

The pattern of activation of the neck flexors and holding capacity of the deep neck flexors is tested with the patient in supine lying, with the head and neck in a neutral position. Slow and controlled upper cervical flexion is performed to target incremental pressure levels, with the pressure sensor inserted behind the neck and preinflated to 20 mmHg. Shirley's performance was poor. There was excessive recruitment of the superficial neck flexors, as well as visible recruitment of the platysma muscle. She could not control a steady pressure reading beyond 22 mmHg, and even at this level she showed evidence of fatigue after three repetitions.

Reassessment

During posteroanterior gliding of the right C2–C3 and C3–C4 zygapophyseal joints, the provoked pain and muscle reaction had decreased to a minor level, and the joint motion restriction had slightly reduced. There was no change in the ROM of active cervical lateral flexion.

Provisional diagnosis

Shirley was likely to have a mixed headache form, with a combination of migraine and a cervical component. Conversely, the musculoskeletal dysfunction may have been underlying the complaint of neck stiffness and neck discomfort but not the headache. Physical examination suggested right C2–C3 and C3–C4 zygapophyseal joint arthropathy (segmental degenerative condition) and poor neuromotor control, especially involving neck flexor synergy.

REASONING DISCUSSION AND CLINICAL REASONING COMMENTARY

1 Prior to examining the mobility of the neural system, were there any possible indications suggesting that this may have been a potential factor contributing to the symptoms? If not, what was your reasoning for undertaking this testing?

Clinician's answer

There were no particular indicators that mechanosensitivity of the neural system was contributing to the headache syndrome. The neural system was being screened for any involvement to allow it to be removed from further consideration. It is also my practice to attempt to exclude any limitation of upper cervical flexion caused by mechanosensitivity of neural structures, because if this is present it can influence the craniocervical flexion muscle test, giving false-positive findings. Conducting these muscle tests without due consideration of any neural tissue sensitivity (if present) can result in an unnecessary aggravation of headache.

2 What led you to reassess joint signs (posteroanterior glides) following the

neuromuscular examination and what is your interpretation of the reassessment findings?

Clinician's answer

Testing the cervical flexors and scapular retractors and depressors has the side benefit of inducing reciprocal relaxation of the cervical extensor muscles, including the deep cervical extensors such as the segmental multifidus. This allows the symptomatic joint to be repalpated with posteroanterior glides, temporarily devoid of protective muscle guarding. Pain provoked and perceived motion are again evaluated and compared with the original assessment. The result gives some approximate indication as to how much of the originally provoked joint pain and restriction of motion is caused by reactive muscle spasm and how much is from articular changes. This can help to guide treatment and often gives a direction for the balance between the components of manual therapy and therapeutic exercise.

The therapeutic exercise is aimed towards improving neuromotor control, thus relieving the joint of provocative strains. When joint changes are not present or not marked, the amount of manual therapy required is often less or has more of a neurophysiological rationale than a mechanical one. In the case of this patient, the re-evaluation indicated that articular changes were present, as the motion restriction was perceived to reduce only slightly. However, as pain and provoked muscle reactivity had decreased substantially, this gave a good prognostic indication that decreasing adverse muscle forces could relieve the joint pain. This gave a rational basis for, and indicated the potential value of, therapeutic exercise to retrain good neuromuscular control.

3 In view of the patient's history of asthma, did you consider assessing the breathing pattern?

Clinician's answer

This was discussed with the patient. The patient was well aware of her breathing patterns and control of air intake and exhalation. The speech pathologist and the patient were working on this aspect to improve her voice control, and the patient was already employing basal expansion breathing exercises as part of this management, as well as relaxation and postural control strategies. An emphasis was placed in the treatment on relaxation of the scalene muscles, especially in the re-education of the neck flexors in the craniocervical flexion action.

4 Your provisional diagnosis appears to suggest two alternative explanations for the patient's headache symptoms. What further information would you require from the physical examination in order to be more confident in attributing at least some of the headaches to musculoskeletal dysfunction?

Clinician's answer

I would have been a little more confident if the manual examination had reproduced the headache, although this in itself is not totally conclusive. I was prepared to give a trial of treatment to help to clarify the situation and to come to a more conclusive diagnosis. I was aware that previous treatment had assisted the neck pain but seemed not to make a substantial impact on the headache symptoms.

Clinical reasoning commentary

The response regarding mechanosensitivity of the neural system indicated that the BPPT was undertaken for three separate reasons:

- as a scanning strategy to rule out an unlikely source (neural structures) for the headaches
- to enhance the validity of a subsequent important clinical test used to evaluate the possible contribution of neuromuscular impairment in the precipitation and maintenance of any cervical component to the headache
- as a precautionary procedure to eliminate the possibility of aggravating sensitized neural tissues during the craniocervical flexion muscle test and worsening the patient's headaches.

Thinking simultaneously on several levels, such as indicated in this response, is typical of expert clinicians. The clinician is enhancing her efficiency and accuracy by maximizing the value (or 'payout') gained from this test procedure.

The decision to reassess joint signs (posteroanterior glides) illustrates how the information obtained from one test can be of use in refining hypotheses in several categories, and thus again demonstrates efficiency in thinking consistent with a maximizing principle. In this case, reassessment of posteroanterior accessory movement following the cervical and scapular muscle testing provided information of value in the following hypothesis categories: source (cervical joint hypothesis), contributing factors (neuromuscular impairment hypothesis), pathobiological mechanisms (mechanical versus neurophysiological joint component), management (balance between joint versus muscular intervention or manual therapy versus exercise therapy) and prognosis. In order to derive the maximal value from one test response the clinician must undertake reflective thinking both during and following each clinical encounter, so as to broaden and deepen the repertoire of maximizing principles.

The clinician's thoughts on a trial of treatment reinforce the notion that the treatment itself is often needed to establish the diagnosis/hypothesis more confidently when this hypothesis (source and/or contributing factors) is still provisional or tentative. Consequently, the treatment and the subsequent reassessment of the patient's signs and symptoms are integral elements in testing the hypothesis as part of the hypothetico-deductive reasoning process.

Treatment plan

Poor muscle function is likely to have had a predominant role in aggravating the C2–C3 and C3–C4 zygapophyseal joints. This is supported by the clinical finding that the reciprocal inhibition of the extensor muscles afforded by the tests of muscle function led to a reduction in provoked pain during the application of posteroanterior gliding. This indicates the need for an emphasis in treatment on neuromuscular re-education and manual therapy to the symptomatic joints. The cervicothoracic region may also need to be mobilized as a potential contributor to the problem.

Explanation of treatment

I explained to Shirley that my initial thoughts were that she was possibly suffering from either a mixed headache form, with a mixture of migraine and neck headache, or that she was experiencing frequent common migraine and had a separate and unrelated problem in her neck. Treatment was capable of influencing headaches arising from the neck but was unlikely to have any marked effect on a genuine migraine component to her headache. In light of the poor response to previous physical treatment in relation to any real affect on her headaches, a trial of treatment was suggested with critical appraisal of the results. The poorest result would be that her complaints of neck stiffness could be lessened but there would be no change in her headache pattern, with the best result being elimination of her headaches. The patient agreed to this approach, involving a realistic appraisal of treatment effects.

Explanation was given as to the importance of correct muscle control and function for the protection of joints. The rationale provided was that if the joints regained good muscle support, this would relieve joint strain and pain; hopefully this would, in turn, alleviate the headaches. As Shirley was a sportsperson and used to high-load exercise, time was taken to explain that the form of exercise that she would be taught was different from exercises undertaken for strength, endurance or fitness. The approach emphasized precision and control, and an analogy of skill training was given. The different functional roles of various muscles was explained, with an emphasis on the postural and deep supporting role of muscles that the exercises would target.

Exercises

Upper cervical flexion

To control unwanted activity in the superficial neck flexors, the patient was taught the rest position of the mandible and retaught the pattern of slow and controlled upper cervical flexion while in supine lying. The emphasis was on control and precision, and the 22 mmHg mark was targeted on the pressure sensor (attempts at any higher levels resulted in recruitment of excessive superficial muscle activity). Shirley was taught to palpate the anterior neck region and to perform the movement without feeling tension developing in the superficial muscles. She was to practise the movement and hold the position for 10 seconds.

Scapula 'setting' exercise

The scapula 'setting' exercise was retaught to the patient in prone lying with correction of the action and with emphasis on precision and control. The focus was on gently positioning the scapula back and down onto the chest wall and holding the position. The previous unwanted use of latissimus dorsi was corrected and the activity of the lower trapezius was inspected and palpated. Shirley was taught the exercise on the right and left sides separately.

Postural exercise

The use of these muscles was incorporated in a postural exercise in sitting. First, the assumption of neutral upright posture was taught with correction from the pelvis to achieve a neutral upright pelvic position with a normal lumbar lordosis. Shirley was then taught to lift her scapula gently to position it back and down onto the chest wall, right and then left, and to hold the position. A submaximal effort was encouraged.

On reassessment, pain and muscle reaction provoked had decreased to minimal levels during posteroanterior gliding of the right C2–C3 and C3–C4 joints. Joint motion restriction was still present but reduced. Active cervical lateral flexion was unchanged.

Home programme

Shirley was given written instructions for a home programme for the three retraining tasks: upper cervical flexion, the scapular exercise in prone lying, and the postural exercise. The upper cervical flexion and scapular exercises were to be performed twice per day. The aim was to achieve 10 repetitions of each exercise, holding for 10 seconds. The importance of precision was emphasized and it was explained that at the point of fatigue, or when she considered that she could not accurately control the exercise, she was to stop rather than reinforce an incorrect pattern.

The postural exercise was to be practiced repeatedly during the day and cues to remind her to perform the action were discussed. These included every time she answered the telephone and any time she walked up stairs (both common activities in her daily routine at work).

REASONING DISCUSSION AND CLINICAL REASONING COMMENTARY

1 Your initial management involved a detailed explanation of likely diagnoses, recommended treatment and rationale, and required patient contribution. Could you please elaborate as to why you considered this important?

Clinician's answer

Informing the patient is an important aspect of any management programme. The patient presented with an expectation from her referring doctor that treatment of her neck would alleviate her headache. I was unsure after the initial examination how much of the headache syndrome was cervical in origin. It was undesirable for the patient to have unrealistic expectations of treatment and I also needed a realistic and critical evaluation of treatment effects to assist in differential diagnosis. I also required of her a more critical appraisal of the nature of her headaches and aggravating factors to help in differential diagnosis. In my experience from seeing patients with headache who have previously received physiotherapy or chiropractic management without any relief, one of the primary reasons for the lack of success is that the headache is not originating from cervical spine dysfunction.

Patient compliance in the therapeutic exercise (and any other treatment) is obviously critical to its potential success. A full explanation as to how the exercise will assist their condition, and the pain-relieving benefits of re-educating muscle control, will also assist with compliance. Shirley was a sportsperson and more used to high-load exercise. The therapeutic exercise was directed toward muscle control and enhancing the active muscle support of the joints. It is skill learning and emphasizes low-load exercises with precision and control. As this was different to her concept of exercising for strength, careful explanation was considered important for compliance.

Clinical reasoning commentary

The importance of collaborative clinical reasoning is emphasized by this discourse. Not only is effective communication needed to ensure that the active interventions are performed appropriately (exercise compliance), but the role of the patient in accurately reporting the behaviour of her headaches following treatment and at other times is seen to be crucial in determining the relative contribution of the cervical spine. Therefore, the patient is somewhat responsible for both the management of her problem and its diagnosis. Consequently, it is important that the patient does not have inappropriate or unrealistic expectations of the clinician and of her own role in the rehabilitation process, and education is the tool required to overcome such problems.

Further treatment

Further treatment occurred over seven sessions. Each session involved a re-evaluation of Shirley, further treatment and a reassessment of her progress.

Treatment 2 (1 week later)
Re-evaluation

Shirley reported that she had had headaches on the 2 days following treatment, but for the last 5 days she had been without headache. This was a break from her normal pattern, which she found pleasing. The neck aching and stiffness had not perceptibly changed.

On physical examination, lateral flexion to the left and right was still restricted to approximately 50% range with scalene tightness evident. Posteroanterior gliding of the right C2–C3 and C3–C4 joints provoked less pain and muscle reaction than at the original assessment, although hypomobility was still present in the joints. During the upper cervical flexion task, Shirley could target and hold at the level of 22 mmHg, but activity of the superficial flexor muscles could be observed with attempts at any higher levels. Correction was needed with speed of performance. Scapular setting in prone lying was performed without sufficient precision and used latissimus dorsi.

Treatment

The pattern of interaction of the deep and superficial flexor muscles was again retrained. Electromyography (EMG) biofeedback was used for this, in addition to pressure biofeedback (Fig. 9.1). The EMG was placed on the sternocleidomastoid and anterior scalene muscles, and Shirley's task was to progressively target 2 mmHg increments in pressure while preventing audible feedback from the EMG biofeedback machine, which would indicate increasing superficial muscle activity. A level of 24 mmHg was achieved.

The scapular setting action in prone lying was retaught and practised. Both the correct and incorrect actions were used to help Shirley to identify the correct action. The sitting postural exercise was checked (the action was too strong) and corrected.

In addition, treatment involved mobilization of the right and left C2–C3 and C3–C4 joints, using a combination of anteroposterior glides and segmental lateral flexion mobilization. The cervicothoracic spine and first rib were also mobilized.

Reassessment

Lateral flexion demonstrated better quality movement, although the range was unchanged. Postero-anterior glides applied to the right C2–C3 and C3–C4 joints provoked little pain despite the presence of slight to moderate hypomobility. Some tissue relaxation was perceived on palpation of the scalene muscles and first rib area. Shirley was loaned a

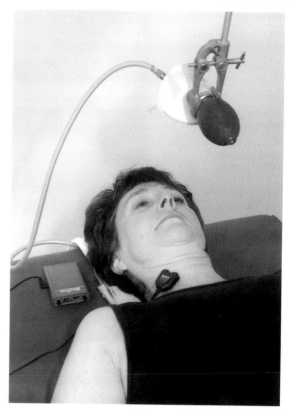

Fig. 9.1 The craniocervical flexion action (the anatomical action of the deep neck flexor muscles) performed in supine lying. The pressure cuff monitors the slight flattening of the neck that occurs with the action. The patient is instructed to perform the upper cervical flexion action to produce and hold incremental increases in pressure. The presence of inappropriate superficial flexor muscle activity is monitored using electromyography.

pressure biofeedback for home use. The home programme was reinforced, with targets of 22 and 24 mmHg set.

▇ Treatment 3 (1 week later)

Re-evaluation

Shirley reported that she was controlling the neck pain with the exercises, although she still had occasional neck pain. Notably, she had had no headaches in the past week.

Physical examination revealed that both left and right lateral flexion were still restricted to approximately half range, but showed better quality of movement.

Posteroanterior gliding of the right C2–C3 and C3–C4 joints provoked slight pain and muscle reaction, with reduced hypomobility. During the upper cervical flexion task, Shirley could target and hold at the level of 24 mmHg, with a good quality of performance evident. Scapular setting in prone lying was performed well and she could achieve 10 repetitions on each side holding for 10 seconds.

Treatment

In retraining the upper cervical flexion action, use was again made of EMG and pressure biofeedback, with the target of 26 mmHg being achieved. A new kinaesthetic task was introduced, involving randomly targeting pressures between 22 and 26 mmHg with precision.

Scapular setting retraining progressed to a position involving prone lying while supported on the elbows. Emphasis was placed on setting the scapulae and activating the serratus anterior by drawing the chest wall up to the scapulae and holding the position. Two further tasks were introduced in this position: first, patterning of the neck flexor synergy through retraining the correct pattern of upper cervical and cervical flexion/extension and, secondly, performing cervical rotation and lateral flexion ROM exercises while maintaining a neutral head/neck alignment (Fig. 9.2).

The C2–C3 and C3–C4 segments were again mobilized using anteroposterior glides and lateral flexion, but with more emphasis on the right-sided joints. The cervicothoracic region was also mobilized.

Reassessment

Lateral flexion quality of movement improved, with slightly better ROM. No pain was provoked on posteroanterior gliding of the right C2–C3 and C3–C4 joints, although there was some residual hypomobility.

The home programme was changed to incorporate the progressions to the exercises.

▮ Treatment 4 (2 weeks later)

Re-evaluation

Shirley reported that she had experienced two headaches in the past fortnight but was able to control them using the exercises. For one episode she had required analgesic tablets. Her neck became a little

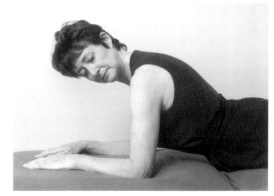

Fig. 9.2 Cervical range of movement exercises into rotation maintaining the prone lying on elbows position with scapula control.

tight after paddling, but she was able to ease it with the exercises.

Lateral flexion both directions was now approximately 75% range, with an increasing lateral curve evident. Posteroanterior gliding of the right C2–C3 and C3–C4 joints provoked very little discomfort, although slight hypomobility persisted. During the upper cervical flexion task, Shirley could target and hold at the level of 28 mmHg with a good quality of performance. Similarly, scapular setting in prone lying (supported on the elbows) was performed well.

Treatment

Upper cervical flexion action retraining again made use of EMG and pressure biofeedback to target 28 mmHg. The kinaesthetic task to test the accuracy of targeting pressures between 22 and 28 mmHg was performed with the eyes open and closed.

Scapular setting retraining was reviewed, with instructions given to continue at the same levels, both in the prone lying and prone lying on elbows positions.

Mobilization of the C2–C3 and C3–C4 segments was repeated, moving gently but more firmly to the end of available range. The cervicothoracic region was again mobilized, with notable improvement in tissue quality and movement of the first rib area.

The home programme was changed to incorporate these progressions to the exercises. In addition, Shirley was to start using the pressure biofeedback as a checking device, rather than as a training device, in preparation for removing the aid.

Reassessment

No reassessment was performed.

■ Treatment 5 (4 weeks later)

Re-evaluation

Shirley reported that her neck had been good and she had had no headaches. She had been doing exercises and they were now part of her routine. She was also working quite hard with her paddling training.

Lateral flexion movement both ways was unchanged. Posteroanterior gliding of the right C2–C3 and C3–C4 joints was now pain-free, although slight hypomobility persisted. With the upper cervical flexion task, Shirley could target and hold (for 10 seconds) at the level of 28 mmHg, with a good quality of performance over the 10 repetitions. The exercises performed in prone lying supported on the elbows were also performed well.

Treatment

All retraining of muscle performance was performed without the assistance of the biofeedback devices. Mobilization of the C2–C3 and C3–C4 segments was repeated addressing the hypomobility and prepositioning the joints into lateral flexion. Mobilization of the cervicothoracic region was also repeated.

No formal reassessment was undertaken. The home programme was adapted to emphasize self-monitoring strategies.

The plan was for one more treatment to assess the performance of the exercises, and then undertake a review.

■ Treatment 6 (3 weeks later)

Re-evaluation

Shirley reported that her neck had been good, and she had experienced one mild headache, which she could control with the exercises. However, 2 days earlier she had awoken with a severe headache and vomiting. She had tried to relieve it with exercise but was unable to do so, and so took some medication before it eventually settled. She reported that she still felt a little tight in her neck but the experience had made her realise that she was probably suffering from two different forms of headaches.

Active lateral flexion was again unchanged, but there was now slight discomfort on posteroanterior gliding of the right C2–C3 and C3–C4 joints, along with the persistent minor hypomobility. In fact, the whole neck region was a little less relaxed. The upper cervical flexion task demonstrated a good quality of performance (could target and hold at the level of 28 mmHg), as did the exercises in prone lying supported on the elbows.

Treatment

All the retraining exercises for muscle performance were checked and the performance was good. Mobilization of the C2–C3 and C3–C4 segments was repeated, addressing the hypomobility and slight discomfort.

A maintenance home programme was established. Formal exercises were to be performed once per day and postural exercises had been routinely incorporated in daily activity. The review was planned in 6 weeks.

Review (6 weeks later)

Shirley telephoned to say she had to go interstate on business and was unable to attend for the review. She reported she had been feeling good and was performing the exercises.

A letter was written to the referring doctor.

■ Treatment 7 (4 months later)

Shirley reported that she had been very well for about 3 months and so she then started easing off the exercises. Over the last 2 to 3 weeks the headaches had started to return. She had stepped up her exercises and they were helping again, but she felt that they were not as effective as before and she wished to have them checked again.

Re-evaluation

There was still some general reduction in ROM of rotation and lateral flexion active movements, but the movement range had been retained. The right-sided C3–C4 joint was slightly painful to posteroanterior glides but C2–C3 was asymptomatic. The joints had not regressed to any significant extent, with only slight residual hypomobility persisting. The holding ability during the upper cervical flexion task had decreased slightly at the target level of 24–26 mmHg. She was also performing the exercise with too much speed. The scapular setting in prone lying exercise was still performed well.

Treatment

All exercises in the training regimen were reviewed and corrected. Shirley elected to acquire her own pressure biofeedback device for home use as it gave her feedback on performance and an incentive check. Mobilization of the C2–C3 and particularly the C3–C4 segments was performed, and the cervicothoracic region was checked. Self-maintenance was restressed and Shirley reported she now had a good understanding of the effect of the self-maintenance exercises.

Treatment 8 (2 weeks later)

Re-evaluation

Shirley reported only having had one headache in the last fortnight. She was paddling regularly with no ill effects. She had been doing the exercises routinely and felt she again had them under control.

The right C2–C3 and C3–C4 joints were asymptomatic but with residual slight hypomobility. The sternocleidomastoid and scalene muscles were quite relaxed. She had regained her holding ability during the upper cervical flexion task and could target and hold 28 mmHg. The scapular girdle exercises were being performed well.

The self-care programme was fully reviewed and rewritten for the patient.

Shirley was formally discharged from treatment but informed she could call for a review if she felt it was necessary.

REASONING DISCUSSION AND CLINICAL REASONING COMMENTARY

1 The improvement of neuromuscular control of key muscle groups appears to be a primary goal of your management. What were the reasons that led you to this treatment decision?
For example, did you recognize a familiar pattern of presentation that you knew often responded favourably to this intervention? Or did you base your decision on research evidence?

■ Clinician's answer

Joint pain and dysfunction will always be accompanied by muscle dysfunction, whether it is a spinal or extremity joint problem. The assessment of Shirley's muscle system revealed very poor muscle control. The nature and extent of this impairment directed the nature and prescription of the exercise programme. There was also knowledge gained from previous treatment that manual therapy alone, while giving relief, did not address the neck dysfunction in the long term.

Research into cervical headache has identified this pattern of muscle dysfunction and evidence is emerging of the efficacy of re-education of the muscle dysfunction in the management of cervical headache. Therefore, this approach was also based on research

evidence (Beeton and Jull, 1994; Jull et al., 1999; Jull et al., 2002).

2 At the early stages in the patient's management, did you formulate a prognosis? What factors did you weigh in coming to this decision?

■ Clinician's answer

At the early stage, I was not prepared to offer a prognosis. There was some improvement in joint signs and muscle function, but not enough to relate this conclusively to the improvement in the headaches. Headaches, as with many other pains, can improve by virtue of the fact that the sufferer has sought and been offered an intervention. Any prognosis in this case would be more valid at a later stage when it could be assessed whether progress was maintained over time and if symptomatic improvement was in line with improvement in physical signs of cervical joint and muscle dysfunction.

3 Is there a reason why you decided not to reassess after treatment 4 and also after some later treatments?

Clinician's answer

Reassessment of segmental joint hypomobility, as one of the main outcomes of manual treatment, was being incorporated in the treatment. There was no expectation at this stage that lateral flexion would change dramatically and it was not a primary outcome.

The muscle system was evaluated by the performance of the exercise as it was being taught. Its immediate effect on joints was evaluated as manual therapy followed the exercise. There was no perceived need to have any other reassessment at this stage.

Clinical reasoning commentary

The clinician's thoughts suggest that the treatment decision to implement specific neuromuscular exercises was influenced by knowledge gained from both past clinical experience (recognition of the clinical presentation/pattern together with associated usual responses to treatments) and from research evidence as to the clinical efficacy of this intervention. However, it is also clear that there were individual clinical findings from the examination of this patient that indicated the appropriateness of the treatment in this particular case. That is, the clinician did not adopt a 'recipe-like approach' but instead adapted a particular treatment approach to an individual patient presentation.

The importance of reassessment in the testing and reformulating of hypotheses is evident in the responses to the questions. Although at times no formal reassessment has been undertaken, the clinician is constantly interpreting the stream of information that becomes available during the application of treatment. This information largely guides decisions related to hypotheses in the categories of treatment (including the need for progression or change) and prognosis, as well as the source(s) (such as cervical joints) and factors contributing (for example, neuromuscular impairment) to the headache.

Outcome

Shirley presented with acute hip pain 9 months later, following a canoeing trip. She reported that she was doing well with her headaches and had probably only experienced one or two severe migraine headaches in the time since her last visit. Very occasionally, she had a milder 'neck headache' but could relieve it with the exercises. She was conscientious about the exercises and there were not many days that she failed to do them.

Examination and treatment were directed to her hip problem and, at the end of this session, her neck exercises were reviewed.

 ## REASONING DISCUSSION AND CLINICAL REASONING COMMENTARY

1 Was there any feature about this case that at any time in the course of the management was not entirely consistent with your expectations?

Clinician's answer

There were really no unexpected features of this case. It is not uncommon for a patient to present with a headache syndrome that is not clear cut and easily classifiable. In such cases, it is necessary to have firm evidence of the presence of a pattern of impairment in the cervical articular and muscular systems in order to justify offering treatment directed at the neck dysfunction. The presence of some neck aching or tenderness on palpation is insufficient alone to justify therapy, as these are symptoms common to many headache forms. For Shirley, there was clear evidence of cervical articular and muscle system impairment, which justified a trial of treatment. There can be quite marked overlap between the symptoms of frequent common migraine without aura and cervical headache. As in this case, when a neck condition is present it is often not possible to predict the contribution of the cervical dysfunction to the headache from an initial assessment. Therefore, a trial of treatment is necessary as part of the diagnostic process. Although I was unable to predict the outcome of treatment from the first assessment, the outcome was not unexpected but just the same very pleasing.

■ Clinical reasoning commentary

These thoughts reveal that the clinical pattern for cervical headache recognized by the clinician was not just limited to diagnostic cues (significant clinical findings) and underlying theoretical pathobiological mechanisms. The fact that the clinician was not surprised at any stage of the management process suggests that the clinical pattern was also associated with knowledge as to the best options for treatment and the likely responses to these interventions (prognosis). This indicates a highly developed knowledge base pertaining to headache presentations and an active effort on the part of the clinician to cultivate this knowledge through clinical reflection and by the relating of clinical experience to research evidence.

■ References

Beeton, K. and Jull, G. (1994). The effectiveness of manipulative physiotherapy in the management of cervicogenic headache: a single case study. Physiotherapy, 80, 417–423.

Elvey, R. (1998). Commentary: treatment of arm pain associated with abnormal brachial plexus tension. Australian Journal of Physiotherapy, Monograph 3, 13–17.

Jull, G.A., Barrett, C., Magee, R. and Ho, P. (1999). Towards clinical characterisation of muscle dysfunction in cervical headache. Cephalalgia, 19, 179–185.

Jull, G., Trott, P., Potter, H. et al. (2002). A randomized controlled trial of exercise and manipulative therapy for cervicogenic headache. Spine, 27, 1835–1843.

Thoracic pain limiting a patient's secretarial work and sport

Diane Lee

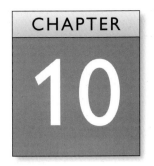

left sides pain

SUBJECTIVE EXAMINATION

Ms Thomas (Julie) presented with pain in three thoracic locations that had commenced after a motor vehicle accident. Eighteen months previously, she was on her way home from work when the vehicle she was riding in (front seat passenger) was broadsided by another, which ran a stop sign. The point of impact was just behind the passenger's door. Julie was wearing a three-point seat belt that activated such that the force of the impact drove her thorax into right rotation and flexion. She remembers feeling an immediate sharp pain on the left side of her mid-back (pain one).

This pain was localized lateral to the spine and medial to the vertebral border of the left scapula. She was able to get out of her vehicle, even though it was substantially damaged by the impact, and immediately noticed that certain movements, including breathing, aggravated her pain.

Later that evening, Julie's pain began to spread as a deep ache and reached the left lateral aspect of the thorax.

Each full breath was accompanied by a sharp shooting pain that ran from T6 beneath the left sixth rib to the rib angle (pain two). Julie was sent for X-ray scanning by her attending physician and no osseous abnormalities were found. She was advised that this was a 'soft tissue injury' and that she would heal in time. Over the next few months the intensity of both pain one and pain two softened somewhat but never disappeared.

After 6 weeks, Julie returned to her physician with reports of ongoing pain that continued to limit her activities. Prior to this accident, she was an avid snow skier and a sailor but she had not been able to return to any level of activity that involved pushing or pulling with her arms. Anti-inflammatory medication was prescribed and she was referred for physiotherapy. Julie received ultrasound, heat and massage, from which she felt only temporary relief. When any exercises were prescribed, she found both the local mid-thoracic pain and the lateral costal pain were aggravated. Julie continued to work as a legal secretary throughout this experience, although she required the use of analgesic medication to complete her day. The anti-inflammatory medication began to aggravate her stomach after 3 weeks and so she discontinued them. A mild sense of indigestion persisted even after the cessation of medication (pain three).

With respect to her feelings regarding the effect this problem was having on her life and its management to date, Julie conveyed her distress about the non-resolution of her symptoms and the limitations they had imposed on her lifestyle. She expressed some concerns regarding ever being able to return to the level of sports she had previously enjoyed; however, she did not appear to be pain focussed or exaggerate her complaints, and her concerns seemed to be very appropriate and realistic. Both her home and work environments were good with family, co-workers and her employer all being supportive.

Symptom behaviour

When first seen, Julie's pain was persisting in its original location (pains one, two and three). Most movements and/or sustained postures, particularly left rotation combined with extension of the thorax, aggravated the mid-thoracic and left lateral costal pains. Cervical movements on their own were not a problem. Julie felt that she had never been able to take a deep breath since the time of the impact. She was able to type for 10 minutes and to sit unsupported for 30 minutes. She frequently changed positions for relief. She woke often during the night and her most comfortable place/position to sleep was semireclined in a chair.

Screening with respect to possible precautions and contraindications to physiotherapy examination and treatment (e.g. general health, present and past medications, spinal cord, unexplained weight loss, cardiac/visceral dysfunction, special investigations, etc.) were all negative.

REASONING DISCUSSION AND CLINICAL REASONING COMMENTARY

1 What were your thoughts at this stage?

Clinician's answer

Possibly a mechanical dysfunction (joint shift or fixation) had occurred during the impact and had not been corrected nor spontaneously recovered. When an articular block is present, exercise tends to increase the local pain. When the problem is mechanical, anti-inflammatory medication has little long-term effect since inflammation is not the primary source of nociception. Analgesic modalities do not affect the biomechanics of a blocked joint; therefore, any pain relief would only be temporary.

2 Within the hypothesis category 'activity and participation capabilities/restrictions', the patient clearly has a number of general functional limitations including difficulty breathing, typing/prolonged sitting, and any activity requiring pushing or pulling. In addition to these, were there any psychosocial (e.g. cognitive or affective) problems apparent in her presentation? Could you briefly explain whether these were an issue in this patient's presentation and if so how they influenced your examination and management.

Clinician's answer

I did not feel that Julie presented with a cognitive or affective problem. While she did convey a degree of distress and concern regarding her continued symptoms and inability to return to the activities she enjoys, this did not appear to be creating any dysfunctional health beliefs or behaviours and I did not feel these emotions were going to interfere with her commitment to recovery. I always include psychosocial considerations in the management of my patients since we treat human beings not just their body parts. I try to create a positive environment with realistic expectations (for both myself and the patient) so that treatment can be optimized.

3 At this stage of your examination what were your thoughts regarding pathobiological pain mechanisms, specifically did you feel one mechanism was dominant? What clues in the subjective examination have led you to this impression?

Clinician's answer

The information supported my original impression that a joint fixation was present. Her symptoms were aggravated by certain postures, thus implying a peripheral nociception and not a centrally mediated situation. The inability to lie down is common when a joint fixation exists in the thoracic spine.

4 With respect to the hypothesis category of 'precautions and contraindications to examination and management', could you outline the key features at this point that guided your plans regarding extent of examination and choice of treatment. Specifically were there any precautions or contraindications?

Clinician's answer

There were no contraindications that I identified from the subjective examination. Precautions are important and whenever there is a latent nature to the symptoms or a sense of neural involvement (lateral referral of pain as well as potential neural mediated visceral symptoms) the examination of the motions that stress the neural system should be approached with care. In other words, no forceful movements are used and symptom responses are monitored with more time given for onset.

5 What were the range of hypotheses you were considering here for possible sources to each of the this lady's symptoms? Can you briefly indicate of these what you considered most likely and why?

Clinician's answer

At this point, I felt the symptoms were coming from local tissues in the thorax rather than being referred from the cervical spine since it was movements from the thorax and not the cervical spine that were aggravating. In addition, the quality of pain (sharp and fairly localized within the thorax and consistently aggravated by certain movements) was suggestive of a local source and not a referred one. I believe consistency, reproducibility and focussed location are qualities of a local source as opposed to a referred source of pain.

A key point in the subjective examination that caused me to focus on her thorax was her breathing complaints. This is common when the biomechanics of the ribs are affected and rarely seen when thoracic pain is referred from the cervical spine. While it is not possible to specify precisely which tissues are involved based on information from the subjective examination alone, my experience with similar presentations suggests pain one was likely to be from a left zygapophyseal joint or costotransverse joint in the mid-thoracic region (T3–T8). Pain two could also be from these local somatic structures or quite possibly a neurogenic pain from an intercostal nerve on the left in the mid-thoracic region, an impression supported by the shooting nature of that pain. Pain three, the mild indigestion, was likely a direct result of anti-inflammatory intolerance but could also have been a referred symptom mediated by the sympathetic nervous system in the mid-thoracic spine.

Clinical reasoning commentary

Even in the opening moments of the patient encounter, it is clear that the clinician is already beginning to formulate her thoughts on a broad range of hypotheses, with consideration given to the patient's activity/participation restrictions (i.e. physical limitations in breathing and activities involving pushing and pulling, as well as inability to resume skiing or sailing, with no psychosocial impairment apparent at this stage), dominant pain mechanisms (i.e. nociceptive), source of the pain (i.e. local thoracic tissues), contributing factors (e.g. motor vehicle accident, exercises) and prognosis (i.e. not impeded by patient's cognitive or affective status).

Not all joint restrictions or fixations will be painful or stay painful. The neurological explanation for why some do and others do not must relate back to the extent of fixation that exists and the contribution of the other contributing physical, environmental, processing and output mechanisms, which combine to form each patient's unique presentation. This underscores the importance of a holistic reasoning approach that is diagnostic in both a pathobiological and a narrative (i.e. seeking to understand how the problem has impacted on the patient's life) sense. The clinician's consideration of psychosocial factors in her assessment of patients' problems highlights her attention to this key area of reasoning and to her patients' unique pain experiences.

For Julie, the clinician has highlighted a key feature supporting a nociceptive dominant pain mechanism, that is the clear stimulus–response relationship between the patient's posture and her symptoms, a relationship also seen with the other aggravating activities. Long-term problems such as this often have or develop abnormal central nervous system processing. However, when the supporting evidence of a nociceptive pain mechanism pattern is combined with the negating evidence of an apparent healthy psychosocial presentation, the nociceptive dominant pain mechanism hypothesis is logical given the information available at this stage. This is a nice clear example of experts' abilities to access quite specific patterns of clinical presentation, which is built up from years of reflective clinical experience (i.e. pattern recognition). It also illustrates the expert's ability to think on multiple levels; in this case, considering multiple hypotheses simultaneously and then refining them in light of further information (i.e. hypothetico-deductive reasoning). As with all hypotheses though, and pointed out by the clinician here, this represents only an initial impression and will have to be considered further in light of the physical presentation that emerges. Similarly, the response to the ongoing management will further support or negate this hypothesis and, in turn, contribute to the evolving understanding of the problem and recognition of management required.

PHYSICAL EXAMINATION

Posture

On examination of the spinal curves, hypertonicity of the erector spinae muscle was noted bilaterally in the mid-thoracic region. This increased activity was not segmental and tended to hold the mid-thorax extended relative to the cervicothoracic (C7–T3 region) and thoracolumbar regions (T11–L1) of the spine. Julie's breathing pattern was shallow and apical.

Functional movement and positional tests

When Julie was examined, all movements of the mid-thorax were limited and a 'kink' in the spinal curve was apparent at the sixth thoracic ring (T5–T6 and left and right sixth ribs). This kink was most apparent in both right and left rotation. On positional testing, T5 was right rotated relative to T6. The left sixth rib was posterolateral relative to the seventh and the right sixth rib was anteromedial relative to the seventh. These findings did not change when positional analysis was done in flexion, neutral or extension of the mid-thorax.

Passive physiological mobility tests (osteokinematic function)

All motions (flexion, extension, left rotation, right rotation, left side flexion and right side flexion) were limited with an end-feel of reactive muscle spasm. The passive mobility at T5–T6 was restricted in all directions (flexion, extension, left rotation, right rotation, left lateral bending and right lateral bending) when compared with the levels above and below.

Passive accessory mobility tests (arthrokinematic function)

Both the left and right zygapophyseal joints (T5–T6) were able to glide superiorly and inferiorly, although more force was required to achieve full motion.

Both the left and right costotransverse joints (sixth rib and T6) were able to glide superiorly and inferiorly, although again more force was required to achieve full motion.

Horizontal translation (T5 and left and right sixth ribs relative to T6) was markedly blocked for right lateral translation of T5 and the sixth ribs relative to T6, with a hard end-feel to this motion (Fig. 10.1). Left lateral translation was limited compared with the segment above and below, with a softer end-feel than that of right lateral translation (Fig. 10.2).

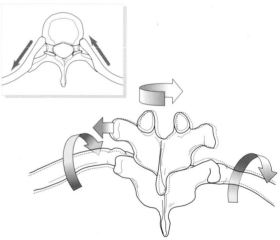

Fig. 10.1 The biomechanics proposed to occur in the mid-thorax during right rotation of the trunk. (Reproduced by kind permission of Delta Orthopaedic Physiotherapy Clinic, from Lee 1994b.)

Passive stability tests of arthrokinetic function

On the first examination, all tests were normal for segmental articular stability at T5–T6, between T6 and sixth ribs and between the sixth ribs and sternum (Fig. 10.3). These tests included:

■ vertical (compression, traction)

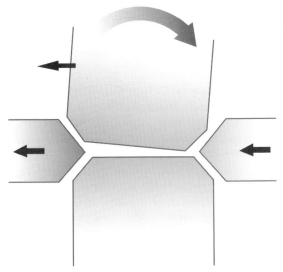

Fig. 10.2 At the limit of left lateral translation, the superior vertebra side flexes to the right along the plane of the pseudo 'U' joint formed by the intervertebral disc and the superior costovertebral joints. (Reproduced by kind permission of Delta Orthopaedic Physiotherapy Clinic, from Lee 1994b.)

- anteroposterior, posteroanterior translation T5–T6
- transverse rotation left and right T5–T6
- anterior translation T6/sixth ribs left and right
- anteroposterior costochondral joints, sternochondral joints
- horizontal translation left and right T5 and sixth ribs/T6.

Muscle function tests

Given the marked articular findings, a complete muscle balance analysis for spinal stabilization and scapular control was not done on the first examination.

Neural function tests

Conduction and mobility were assessed.

Conduction. All tests for upper motor neuron conduction through the spinal cord were negative (Plantar response test, clonus). The skin beneath the left sixth rib was hypersensitive to light touch and pinprick laterally to the mid-axillary line. There was no evidence of decreased motor innervation of the left sixth intercostal muscle.

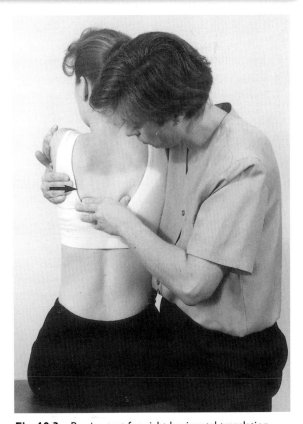

Fig. 10.3 Passive test for right horizontal translation stability of T5 and the left and right sixth ribs relative to T6. The patient sits, arms crossed to opposite shoulders, and the therapist stands beside the patient. With the right hand/arm, the therapist palpates the thorax such that the fifth finger of the right hand lies along the left sixth rib. The transverse processes of T6 are fixed with the left hand. A pure right horizontal translation force is applied to the thorax through the left sixth rib. This will translate the sixth ribs and T5 to the right relative to T6. Note the quantity of motion and in particular the end feel of motion. (Reproduced by kind permission of Delta Orthopaedic Physiotherapy Clinic, from Lee 1994b.)

Mobility. The full slump position aggravated the left lateral costal pain and this pain could be sensitized (brought on and relieved) by varying the position of Julie's head/neck when she was in full mid-thoracic flexion. If right rotation was added to the full slump position, she began to feel very unwell (slightly nauseated) and a sympathetic response could be precipitated if this position was sustained.

REASONING DISCUSSION AND CLINICAL REASONING COMMENTARY

1 Please discuss your use of functional movement and position tests, in particular your interpretation of a 'fixation'.

Clinician's answer

Functional movements tests evaluate the quality of movement, segmentally and collectively, during active range of motion. The movements tested include cardinal plane motion (pure sagittal, coronal and transverse planes) or combined movements. Positional tests are passive tests that involve observation (looking) and palpation (feeling) of bones. We look for *marked* differences in the resting position of one bone relative to a cardinal body plane as well as relative to one another. These tests help to detect joint fixations.

With fixations we are talking about a joint that is held beyond its physiological motion barrier and yet within its anatomical motion barrier (it is not dislocated). What holds it there? The joint becomes excessively compressed by muscle forces, which during the injury contract to prevent dislocation. Sometimes, like in the knee, an intra-articular structure (meniscus) can maintain the joint fixation. More often, the position is held by compression from the muscles that cross the joint. When a joint is fixated, the resting position of the bones does not change when it is examined in flexion, neutral or hyperextension. By comparison, positional changes that are the result of muscle imbalance frequently change from the extended to flexion position, thus the need to test in all three positions.

2 Please explain your analysis of the physical findings and how they relate to your choice of treatment.

Clinician's answer

In order to explain the abnormal biomechanics that have occurred here and, therefore, the clinical reasoning behind the treatment chosen, it is necessary to understand what occurs normally in rotation of the mid-thorax. During right rotation of the mid-thorax (T3–T8), the following biomechanics are thought to occur (Lee, 1993; 1994a,b). The superior vertebra rotates to the right and translates to the left (see Fig. 10.1). Right rotation of the superior vertebral body 'pulls' the superior aspect of the head of the left rib forward at the costovertebral joint, inducing anterior rotation of the neck of the left rib (superior glide at the left costotransverse joint), and 'pushes' the superior aspect of the head of the right rib backward, inducing posterior rotation of the neck of the right rib (inferior glide at the right costotransverse joint). The left lateral translation of the superior vertebral body 'pushes' the left rib posterolaterally along the line of the neck of the rib and causes a posterolateral translation of the rib at the left costotransverse joint. Simultaneously, the left lateral translation 'pulls' the right rib anteromedially along the line of the neck of the rib and causes an anteromedial translation of the rib at the right costotransverse joint. An anteromedial/posterolateral slide of the ribs relative to the transverse processes to which they attach is thought to occur during axial rotation. When the limit of this horizontal translation is reached, both the costovertebral and the costotransverse ligaments are tensed. Stability of the ribs both anteriorly and posteriorly is required for the following motion to occur. Further right rotation of the superior vertebra occurs as the superior vertebral body tilts to the right (glides superiorly along the left superior costovertebral joint and inferiorly along the right superior costovertebral joint). This tilt causes right side flexion of the superior vertebra at the limit of right rotation of the mid-thoracic segment (see Fig. 10.2).

In Julie's case, the sixth thoracic ring (T5–T6, the left and right sixth ribs and all of their related joints) was not able to translate laterally to the right. This dysfunction involved all four bones of the sixth thoracic ring and was not just the consequence of a restriction of one zygapophyseal joint nor one costotransverse joint. The passive accessory mobility tests revealed full motion at the zygapophyseal joints as well as the costotransverse joints, although a greater passive force was required to produce the motion. This resistance to movement (as opposed to lack of movement) produced a kink in the mid-thoracic spinal curve during all of the functional movement tests as well as in the passive physiological mobility tests of the sixth ring. The marked block (high resistance) to right lateral translation of the sixth ring prevented the anteromedial translation of the left sixth rib, relative to the left transverse process of T6, and the posterolateral translation of the right sixth rib, relative to the right transverse process of T6, necessary for left rotation of T5–T6 and the sixth ribs.

During forced or sudden uncontrolled rotation of the mid-thorax, a segmental thoracic ring can become 'stuck' or held at the limit of motion. It is currently thought that excessive compression of the articular surfaces occurs at the moment of injury, and this compression maintains the altered resting position. This compression is the result of the central nervous system's response to the sudden afferent input it is receiving from the deforming articular structures. The central nervous system increases the segmental muscle activity to prevent further deformation of the articular structures (Lee and Vleeming, 1998). This efferent motor response is sustained by the distorted afferent input from the displaced articular structures. When the neural tissue becomes sensitized by the excessive central afferent bombardment, further lengthening of the system can provoke symptoms. This could, in part, explain the positive slump test as well as the aggravation of symptoms with right rotation. A spontaneous efferent discharge through the sympathetic system could be responsible for the visceral symptom of nausea.

Treatment, therefore, requires the normalization of the afferent input to the central nervous system such that the efferent output to the segmental muscles (and viscera) is reduced, the articular compression is relieved and the amplitude of the joint's neutral zone (detected through passive accessory mobility testing of horizontal translation) is restored. In a biomechanical approach to treatment, this can be achieved through specific manual therapy followed by motor control re-education.

3 With the poor reliability of manual techniques to judge positional alignment and mobility, and the normal variation across the population, how do you weight the significance of your manual examination findings in reaching a diagnosis and selecting a treatment?

Clinician's answer

I firmly believe (but unfortunately cannot prove) that when we test the inter-tester reliability of a manual technique we often start by asking the wrong question. If the question is inappropriate, then the answer is not useful. For example, If we ask, 'How much is this joint moving?', we have to apply a standard of what we think is normal. In other words, is this joint moving more, less or the same as we think it should. As you mentioned, there is a wide variation of movement possibilities across the population and, therefore, an accurate answer to this question is impossible because 'normal' is a moving standard. What are we really comparing the motion with? Even if we ask the question, 'Do I feel the same amount of movement as the next tester?', I must apply a scale of motion (i.e. normal, stiff, hypermobile) to categorize what I am feeling. Where does the standard come from? Someone who writes a book saying each segment should have so many degrees of motion? Where does this information come from and, given the wide variation of 'normal', how can one number be adequate? When we interpret what we are feeling in terms of amount of movement, there will be less consistency between testers. Instead, we need to evaluate motion within the same individual by comparing motion to levels above and below and on the left and right sides. Instead of emphasizing the quantity of motion (i.e. stiff or loose), which we know is highly variable and unreliable, we should be examining quality of motion. This resistance to motion, or lack thereof, is an examination of the size and shape of the neutral zone of motion (from zero to R1 or first resistance), which every joint has. This is a dynamic feature of a joint's internal and external environment and is under articular, myofascial and neural influence.

Researching quality of motion, and not quantity, may provide us with better reliability between testers. When you watch an experienced clinician work and ask them what they are feeling, they often say, 'This joint doesn't feel right, it's gummy, or it gives way too easily'. The inexperienced clinician will try to interpret what they feel into a quantity of motion, 'I think this joint is stiff or hypermobile'. They have yet to develop an inventory of 'common feelings'. I suppose this is what you call pattern recognition of sensory input. This, for me, is the development of skilled manual technique.

So to answer the second part of your question, I weigh the significance of my manual examination findings (of resistance not quantity of motion) highly when reaching a biomechanical diagnosis. I do not reach a diagnosis based on the findings of one test but rather on the results of the entire examination process. I look for resistance to motion or giving way to implied forces and put less emphasis on the amount of movement I am feeling.

Clinical reasoning commentary

As discussed in Chapter 1, physiotherapy knowledge comprises biomedical research-validated propositional knowledge/constructs, empirically acquired non-propositional knowledge/clinical inferences and personal knowledge. It is important to relate, where possible, our examination and treatment interventions to the available biomedical knowledge, such as the anatomical and biomechanical rationale outlined here by the clinician. However, as the clinician discusses, some of our judgments, such as motion of a joint, cannot be accurately quantified in a clinical setting. Instead, those clinicians that carefully attend to sensory cues such as quality of movement and reflectively relate those patterns of sensory input to other features in the patient's presentation are able to learn from their clinical experiences. The clincian's comments regarding the limitations of movement testing, and subsequent approach of basing her physical diagnosis on the results of the entire examination rather than any single test, illustrates a key tenet of reasoning, that is looking for consistency/support for hypotheses across a number of findings. Even when some findings are weighed more heavily than others, this style of reasoning minimizes the common error of overfocussing on your favourite hypothesis and not excluding competing hypotheses. Similarly, given that our knowledge of pain and physical impairment is still far from complete, as acknowledged by the clinician in her previous comments regarding the lack of tissue specificity with physiotherapy procedures, it is critical to monitor the effect of all interventions through re-assessment of local tissue, functional and psychosocial/quality of life effects. This aspect of clinical reasoning theory in practice is evident in the clinician's comments regarding re-assessment of horizontal translation following treatment, whereby her hypothesis regarding pain mechanisms, sources and management strategy are further tested. This critical level of reflective reasoning enables therapists to challenge their theories or presuppositions continually and adjust their reasoning appropriately.

m Management

First treatment

In simple language that Julie could understand, the first treatment involved explaining what had happened to her thorax. The symptoms were co-related to her pathobiomechanics and in this manner patient/therapist rapport and confidence was developed. After 18 months, the motor pattern that sustained the pathomechanics was well established and treatment may well have provoked her symptoms initially. There must be a good understanding between patient and therapist if pain provocation occurs and trust is to be maintained.

A Grade 5 technique (manipulative thrust) was used to reduce the articular compression. The specific technique when the sixth thoracic ring is held in right rotation (left lateral translation) is described below.

The patient is in left side lying, the head supported on a pillow and the arms crossed to the opposite shoulders. With the left hand, the right seventh rib is palpated posteriorly with the thumb and the left seventh rib is palpated posteriorly with the index or long finger. T6 is fixed by compressing the two seventh ribs towards the mid-line. Care must be taken to avoid fixation of the sixth ribs, which must be free to glide relative to the transverse processes of T6. The other hand/arm lies across the patient's crossed arms to control the thorax. Segmental localization is achieved by flexing and extending the joint until a neutral position of the zygapophyseal joints is achieved. This localization is maintained as the patient is rolled supine only until contact is made between the table and the dorsal hand.

From this position, T5 and the left and right sixth ribs are translated laterally to the right through the thorax to the motion barrier. Strong longitudinal distraction is applied through the thorax prior to the application of a high-velocity, low-amplitude thrust. The thrust is in a lateral direction in the transverse plane (Fig. 10.4). The goal of the technique is to translate T5 laterally and the left and right sixth ribs relative to T6.

After the sixth segmental ring was decompressed, the functional movement, positional, mobility and stability tests were repeated. No kink in the spinal curve was noted on functional movement testing. The

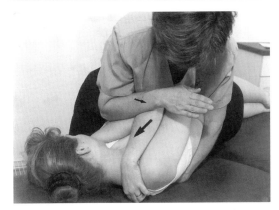

Fig. 10.4   Grade V manipulation technique used to reduce a fixated left lateral shift of T5 and the sixth ribs relative to T6. Strong axial distraction must be maintained throughout the technique. (Reproduced by kind permission of Delta Orthopaedic Physiotherapy Clinic, from Lee 1994b.)

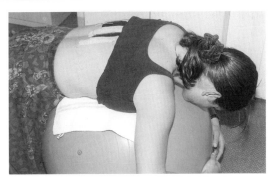

Fig 10.5   Isolation of the segmental spinal stabilizers can be facilitated using neuromuscular stimulation. (Reproduced by kind permission of Delta Orthopaedic Physiotherapy Clinic, from Lee 1994b.)

positional tests revealed symmetry between T5 and T6 as well as the left and right sixth ribs in flexion, neutral and extension of the mid-thoracic spine. The passive physiological and passive accessory mobility tests revealed less resistance to motion at the zygapophyseal joints between T5–T6 and the costo-transverse joints of the left and right sixth ribs.

An underlying instability of left lateral translation (horizontal) and right rotation was detected. A sense of giving way was felt during left lateral translation as opposed to a larger amplitude of motion. In addition, atrophy of the segmental stabilizing muscles (rotatores and deep multifidus) was noted.

The full slump position remained provocative, although the position had to be held longer for the symptoms to be aggravated.

The thorax was taped to remind Julie to avoid rotation in either direction (X tape across the T5–T6 region). She was reminded that she may experience some increase in both her local and referred pain but that this would settle over the next 2–3 days and a sense of improved mobility should follow.

Subsequent treatments

The first group of muscles that must be addressed in stabilization therapy of the thoracic spine are the transversospinal (multifidus) and erector spinae groups. Hides et al. (1994, 1996) have found that the deep fibres of multifidus atrophy quickly following an acute low back injury, and that recovery is not spontaneous without specific exercise instruction. Clinically, the same appears to be true in the thorax. The principles used in the thorax are identical to those advocated by the research team from the University of Queensland in Brisbane (Richardson et al., 1999).

Essentially, the patient is taught specifically to recruit the segmental muscles isometrically and then concentrically while prone over a gym ball (Fig. 10.5). Electrical stimulation can be a useful adjunct at this time. In side lying, specific segmental rotation can be resisted by the therapist both concentrically and eccentrically to facilitate the return of multifidus function. The programme is progressed by increasing the load the thorax must control. Initially, scapular motion is introduced, in particular lower trapezius work. The patient must control the neutral position of the mid-thorax throughout the scapular depression. The goal is to teach the patient to isolate scapular motion from spinal motion so that the scapula does not produce spinal motion during activities involving the arm. Once control is gained over the scapula, exercises involving the entire upper extremity may be added (Fig. 10.6). By increasing the lever arm and then the load, the mid-thorax is further challenged. Gymnastic ball, proprioceptive, balance and resistive work can be integrated into the programme as needed. The velocity of the exercises can be increased according to the patient's work and recreation demands. Initially, the load should be applied bilaterally and then progressed to unilateral work. At the completion of the programme, the patient should be able to isolate specific spinal extension without scapular motion and control both bilateral and

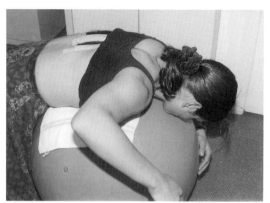

Fig. 10.6 The exercise programme progresses from central spinal stabilization to increased loading with scapular control and finally upper extremity control.

unilateral arm motion throughout mid-range. They are advised to avoid any activity that places the mid-thorax at the limit of rotation in the direction of their instability.

This was the programme of instruction given to Julie. Subsequent to the manipulation, she reported increased local mid-thoracic pain, a decrease in the lateral costal pain and no aggravation of her visceral symptoms. She felt that she could take a much deeper breath immediately after the manipulation. She used caution with all loading through her thorax and was

very fearful of any rotation for the next 3 days. She felt a sense of weakness in her chest accompanied by a deep ache when unsupported in sitting. She was able to learn specifically to recruit the deep segmental stabilizers at T5–T6 very quickly and progressed to scapular work within 1 week. If she increased the lever arm or the load too quickly, the multifidus could be felt to 'shut down' or turn off, and she had difficulty sensing when this was happening. This is a difficult area of the spine for patients to palpate themselves; however it is critical not to overload the spine beyond it's ability to achieve motor control. Julie was keen to return to her sporting activities, all of which required upper extremity pushing and pulling. Our most difficult task was pacing the exercise programme without provoking frustration. Throughout this programme, the segmental ring remained 'unstable' to static or passive testing in right rotation and left lateral translation. Over a 3-month period, she was able to learn to control her spinal position and gradually increase the loading through her upper extremities. Unilateral loading through one arm (left or right), which involved thoracic rotation, remained provocative for her. She was able to return to a high level of skiing and as long as she used both arms bilaterally was able to manage the sail on her boat. Unilateral pushing or pulling activities with her right arm remains provocative.

REASONING DISCUSSION AND CLINICAL REASONING COMMENTARY

1 At your first treatment session, you seemed to place a lot of emphasis on explaining the problem to the patient. Can you comment on the role you see of teaching and explanation in your patient management?

Clinician's answer

I have found that the more the patient understands regarding their condition, the more focussed and committed they become in the recovery process. Learning requires concentration and focus; in other words, a patient must be aware of the processes that are occurring in their bodies in order to effect a change. This is true whether we are explaining symptom behaviour

(pain) or principles of stabilization therapy. When exercises are done with awareness of what is, or should, be happening, learning is facilitated. The non-thoughtful approach to exercise (move 2 kg 10 times in this manner, three times per day regardless of how you feel or how you achieve the task) can be dangerous or, at minimum, may merely reinforce the poor motor programme that is maintaining the dysfunction. So, right from the beginning, education is a critical part of the rehabilitation process.

2 Having detected the underlying instability, please elaborate on your rationale for your further management with this patient.

Clinician's answer

Physiotherapy cannot restore articular integrity (form closure); therefore, the emphasis of treatment must be on the restoration of motor control (force closure) (Vleeming et al., 1990a,b). The goal is to control the excessive neutral zone of lateral translation and rotation during functional activities and to avoid the end-ranges of rotation, thus limiting the chances of further articular compression. This is accomplished through specific exercises augmented with muscle stimulation.

3 Seeing how the onset of this lady's symptoms was trauma, do you feel there were any contributing factors (physical, environmental/ ergonomic, psychosocial, etc.) that were partly responsible for prolonging her symptoms and disability?

Clinician's answer

This was a straightforward situation where the trauma most likely resulted in a joint fixation that did not resolve spontaneously, as some will, resulting in continued symptoms and disability. While you would expect a musculoskeletal soft tissue injury to complete its healing much sooner than the 18 months this lady's symptoms have persisted, it has been my experience that such problems can frequently be maintained this long when a joint fixation is present.

When recovery does not occur when expected, patients begin to fear that they will never get completely better. This fear can lead to psychological states that can amplify the symptom experience. Chronic pain from a body part can result in dissociation in the body–mind connection. Even after the biomechanics are restored, the body–mind connection must be addressed; this is not necessarily automatic. Exercises for range of motion, or what has been called 'motor programming' or 'sequencing of movement patterns', should be taught, emphasizing the 'awareness' component of the exercise to re-establish appropriate neural connections.

Clinical reasoning commentary

The importance the clinician places on the patient's understanding and learning is consistent with the significance of patient cognition in the mature organism model highlighted in Chapter 1. Patients' understandings and feelings are now recognized as significant aspects of their pain experience, contributing to their unique presentation and potential for recovery. Evaluating patients' understandings as potential contributing factors to their health and also as a necessary prerequisite to guide the explanation and education that will be required to effect a change in their health attitudes and behaviours is an important focus that must be incorporated in therapists' reasoning. That is, improving patients' health requires much more than physical diagnostic reasoning; therapists must also be able to recognize the other psychosocial and environmental determinants of health and use their skills as teachers to effect the necessary changes. This dimension of our reasoning is promoted when clinicians adopt a broader model of health and disability, as encouraged in the mature organism model, and practise the shared decision-making strategy depicted in the collaborative reasoning model.

The clinician's answer to reasoning question 3 nicely highlights how impairment in the mind–body connection can manifest not only as an unhelpful perception, contributing to or driving a patient's pain, but also as faulty motor programmes, as reflected in a patient's learned postural and movement patterns. Again teaching as a focus of reasoning becomes important. Education to alter a patient's awareness is central to this clinician's approach in promoting improved motor programmes and is consistent with modern theories of learning.

Outcome

Julie sustained an injury that caused a static instability of her mid-thorax. The passive structures that restrain right rotation and left lateral translation had become stretched and she required an optimal force closure mechanism to remain functional. The T5–T6 segmental ring is vulnerable should she sustain another right rotational injury. In the meantime, she has received the education she needs to maintain her dynamic stability and if she continues to take care of this segment and control the degree of loading through this part of her spine, she should be able to control her symptoms.

References

Hides, J.A., Stokes, M.J., Saide, M., Jull, G.A., Cooper, D.H. (1994). Evidence of lumbar multifidus muscles wasting ipsilateral to symptoms in patients with acute/subacute low back pain. Spine, 19, 165–177.

Hides, J.A., Richardson, C.A., Jull, G.A. (1996). Multifidus recovery is not automatic following resolution of acute first episode low back pain. Spine, 21, 2763–2769.

Lee, D.G. (1993). Biomechanics of the thorax: a clinical model of in vivo function. Journal of Manual and Manipulative Therapy, 1, 13–21.

Lee, D.G. (1994a). Biomechanics of the thorax. In Physical Therapy of the Cervical and Thoracic Spine, 2nd edn (R. Grant, ed.) pp. 47–64. New York: Churchill Livingstone.

Lee, D.G. (1994b). Manual Therapy for the Thorax—a Biomechanical Approach. Delta BC: Delta Orthopaedic Physiotherapy Clinic.

Lee, D.G. and Vleeming, A. (1998). Impaired load transfer through the pelvic girdle: a new model of altered neutral zone function. In Proceedings from the Third Interdisciplinary World Congress on Low Back and Pelvic Pain, November 1998, Vienna, Austria.

Richardson, C., Jull, G., Hodges, P. and Hides, J. (1999). Therapeutic exercise for spinal segmental stabilization in low back pain. Edinburgh: Churchill Livingstone.

Vleeming, A., Stoeckart, R., Volkers, A.C.W. and Snijders, C.J. (1990a). Relation between form and function in the sacroiliac joint. 1: Clinical anatomical aspects. Spine, 15, 130–132.

Vleeming, A., Volkers, A.C.W., Snijders. C.J. and Stoeckart, R. (1990b). Relation between form and function in the sacroiliac joint. 2: Biomechanical aspects. Spine, 15, 133–136.

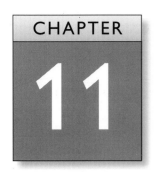

CHAPTER 11

Bilateral shoulder pain in a 16-year-old long-distance swimmer

Mary Magarey

 SUBJECTIVE EXAMINATION

Sally is a 16-year-old school girl undertaking her final year of schooling at an exclusive coeducational private school. She is from a family of three children and one adopted daughter. Her father is a doctor and her mother a teacher at the same school attended by Sally. She is a high achiever academically and appears a well-adjusted, if quiet, girl. She is also a high-level distance swimmer, with freestyle and butterfly her main events. At 14 years of age, she was a national level swimmer but had not been able to achieve this standard for the last 2 years because of difficulties with shoulder pain. She came to me on the recommendation from the physiotherapist mother of one of her swimming contemporaries.

History

Sally's presenting problem was one of bilateral shoulder pain, as indicated on the body chart (Fig. 11.1), worse on the left, though the side dominance varied from time to time for no apparent reason. She had the pain in both shoulders whenever she swam and developed an ache in the same areas after swimming. This ache lasted for 2 to 3 hours after swimming and her shoulders generally felt 'sore' at all times when she was in peak swim training. Her worst pain was with butterfly, on both recovery and mid pull-through aspects of the stroke. She also had similar pain with freestyle, particularly at the catch and mid pull-through, though the level of pain was lower. The pain was present as soon as she started swimming, was not

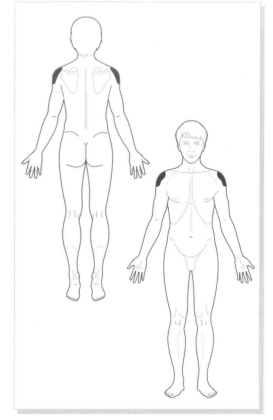

Fig. 11.1 Body chart demonstrating Sally's presenting pain picture. The pain was intermittent with swimming with the ache in the same area after swimming. There was no pain in the cervical or thoracic areas, arms or hands. There were no pins and needles in the hands or feet.

sufficient to prevent her from swimming, but inhibited full training and progressively worsened through a training session. She had no specific pain or difficulties with other activities but did not play other sports that would put the same load or challenge on her shoulders. At the time I first saw her it was the end of the summer swimming season, during which she had been swimming for eight 2 hour sessions every week with a predominance of training in freestyle. She had just started a 1 month lay-off from training before beginning a slightly lighter load through the winter.

Sleeping was no problem, even lying on her side, and she had no morning stiffness. She took no anti-inflammatory or pain medication. Sally was in good general health and appeared to have no other identifiable problems. Investigations included plain radiographs, diagnostic ultrasound and computed tomography (CT) arthrography; none of which demonstrated any abnormality.

Several years earlier, when Sally was training for the national swimming championships, she lifted a heavy suitcase and felt something 'pull' in her right shoulder with immediate pain in the anterior subacromial/superior capsular area. This pain was not severe but did not go away, disrupting her swimming

training. Her left shoulder pain, in the same area as the right, began some time later with no apparent specific precipitating incident. Since then, both had followed the pattern described above.

We discussed swimming technique, with Sally's mother indicating that Sally was a 'shoulder swimmer', getting little effect in her stroke from her kick. I explained how improving body roll and kick power could decrease the load on her shoulders and, therefore, might reduce the pain associated with her swimming, even though the kick is not as significant a component of distance swimming as it is of sprints (Maglischo, 1993). We discussed the possibility of working on these aspects of her stroke with her coach, in addition to whatever specific problems were identified in her shoulders.

Her mother, who did most of the talking at most visits, told a saga of attendance at multiple health professionals in an attempt to find a diagnosis for and resolution of Sally's shoulder pain. Of particular interest to me was the information that she had attended five different physiotherapists, none of whom, in Sally's or her mother's opinion, appeared to have given satisfactory treatment. I found this information quite daunting! The sequence of investigations and management is given in Table 11.1.

Table 11.1   Previous professional consultations before presentation

Physiotherapist 1	Treatment provided was ultrasound and interferential, with no benefit
Orthopaedic surgeon	Ordered plain radiograph, ultrasonography and computed tomographic arthrography, all of which were negative. He injected what appeared to have been her subacromial space, with no relief of symptoms, even temporarily. He was not prepared to offer arthroscopic investigation because of her age and lack of findings on the diagnostic imaging
Physiotherapist 2	This physiotherapist worked in a sports specific physiotherapy clinic and had many years of experience with national level sports teams. Treatment provided included further electrotherapy and some basic rotator cuff exercises, again with no benefit
Sports physician	He indicated that she had sloppy shoulders and that she needed an exercise programme directed at her shoulders. He referred her to physiotherapist 3
Physiotherapist 3	This physiotherapist had considerable experience in treatment of postoperative shoulders and worked in a sports-specific clinic. She was also experienced with national level sports teams. Treatment provided was shoulder and scapular stabilizing exercises (as far as could be ascertained from the description). Sally worked at the exercises but became disillusioned when the physiotherapist would not allow her to get back in the water to swim. It appeared that Sally probably did not give this programme a fair trial before looking elsewhere for assistance. Her mother's comment was 'It is hard to fit all that exercising in and swim and do homework'.
Physiotherapist 4	This physiotherapist was a national level swim coach who had practised more as a swim coach than a physiotherapist, but who had specialist knowledge of swimming requirements and a depth of understanding of the psychological issues related to working with swimmers.

Table 11.1 Previous professional consultations before presentation

	In particular, he understood how important it is for swimmers to be able to stay in the water during any rehabilitation. Treatment provided included further exercises and stretching with an emphasis on medial rotation of the shoulder. My understanding was that neither Sally nor her mother got on with this physiotherapist and the decision to cease treatment was based more on this than any failure of the treatment regimen.
Chiropractor	No specific details of the chiropractic treatment were elicited, except that the chiropractor told Sally to 'swim through it'.
Physiotherapist 5	This physiotherapist was also a sports-oriented physiotherapist with extensive national and international team experience. The comment from Sally's mother was that this was 'going down the same old path' and they did not persist with her.
General practitioner	This general practitioner had an interest in natural medicine and gave Sally eight injections of glucose over a period of some months. This treatment appeared to help Sally more than any other, although Sally's mother was unable to explain to me the theoretical basis of pain relief related to glucose injections. The benefit of these injections lasted approximately 12 months, but she had not returned for further therapy when the shoulder pain returned.

REASONING DISCUSSION AND CLINICAL REASONING COMMENTARY

1 Based on the initial information regarding the patient's personal profile, her presenting symptoms, general health and investigations as well as the history of onset for the symptoms in both shoulders, what were your hypotheses at that stage regarding dominant pain mechanisms, possible sources and contributing factors for the symptoms and activity/participation restrictions she was experiencing in her two shoulders?

▮ Clinician's answer

Dominant pain mechanisms

The dominant pain mechanism I considered with this girl was an input nociceptive mechanism. My reasoning for that related to the very mechanical nature of her symptoms with the on/off features related to her swimming and the localized site of symptoms. However, there were elements of her presentation that made me also consider other mechanisms. For example, while the history of onset of the right shoulder pain sounds mechanical and, therefore, supports a nociceptive disorder, the onset of similar pain in the left shoulder without a provoking incident could indicate the presence of some central sensitization of her symptoms. There were also a number of features that could have supported this hypothesis.

The bilaterality of her pain, while common with a sport that involves bilateral load on the shoulders, could also be a reflection of a neural processing impairment, while the anxiety created in an elite athlete by impairment that prevents participation in the chosen sport could contribute to the presence of an affective component to her problem.

The apparent dominance of her mother in the interview situation also raised questions about Sally's ability to make decisions for herself or speak her own mind, with the inherent potential of not taking responsibility for her symptoms and their management. I also wondered whether her mother's level of involvement in telling the story indicated that she was the driving force behind Sally's continued pursuit of a swimming career, rather than Sally herself. This thought may seem a bit harsh, but this is a common scenario in individual sports such as swimming and athletics. If this were the case, it would be likely to have a significant influence on Sally's motivation for compliance with any management strategy suggested.

Sally's family situation seemed financially secure, settled and happy, but the older adopted sister was a high-level sprinter, so there was the possibility of Sally feeling that she needed to achieve to keep up with this older family member, again with potential influence on the outcome of any management.

Sally was also in her last year at school, a high academic achiever who indicated that she was keen to try to study medicine on leaving school. This goal would obviously create significant pressure to achieve academically, possibly altering the perspective with which swimming was seen from that of earlier years.

These features raised the question about whether Sally was using her shoulder pain as an excuse to back away from swimming without seeming to be giving up or failing to achieve in the same way as the older sister.

However, a typical feature of high-level junior swimmers is hypermobility of the glenohumeral joints coupled with altered muscle balance and control around the shoulder girdle in particular (Pink et al., 1993; Scovazzo et al., 1991). The history of a traction injury to the right shoulder as the original provoking incident seemed to fit a nociceptive presentation, with the likelihood that the other shoulder became painful as a result of Sally adapting her swim technique to try to avoid pain in the right shoulder. With the likely underlying hypermobility in both shoulders and the high load generated by swimming, particularly butterfly in which symmetry of stroke is essential, such a scenario seemed reasonable. With the advent of pain, muscle function around the shoulder girdle, and in particular in the rotator cuff, is likely to have been affected, such that an imbalance already present from the involvement in swimming would be accentuated. Therefore, while the potential for central sensitization and an affective component to be features of the presentation was definitely there, my favoured hypothesis at this stage was one related to altered motor output, with her pain perpetuated by excessive load on structures not adequately stabilized to cope with it. Poor muscle control and dynamic support of her shoulders and shoulder girdles seemed most likely to be a dominant feature of her presentation.

Sources of pain

My main hypothesis about the source of Sally's shoulder pain was the capsule of the glenohumeral joint, with the possibility of involvement of the superior labral structures adjacent to the biceps anchor and of the biceps tendon itself. I also considered the rotator cuff as a possible contributing source of her symptoms. The bilaterality of symptoms meant that I had to consider the cervical and thoracic spine as a potential source, with somatic referral to the shoulders.

However, with an understanding of the load placed on both shoulders with swimming, particularly with butterfly, I considered it more likely that her problem related to similar mechanisms in both shoulders rather than somatic referral from a spinal source.

Contributing factors

As indicated above, I considered it highly likely that Sally had a strong contributing component of poor dynamic control of her shoulders. The particular features of her story that support this hypothesis are the history of the pain associated specifically with a sport that involves large repetition of the same action undertaken almost daily, with little chance, therefore, for recovery, added to little involvement in alternative physical activity and coupled with the stress of final year schooling.

Knowledge of the loads required of the joints and muscles in swimming also led to support of this hypothesis and recognition of what is, in fact, a very common clinical pattern in high-level swimmers. Therefore, the reasoning supporting my hypotheses was based in part on Sally's particular presentation but also on my underlying recognition of the particular clinical pattern.

2 What were your thoughts after obtaining the history of previous management? Specifically what hypothesis categories were most informed by this additional information and in what way?

Clinician's answer

I had a number of thoughts about the history of previous management. Initially, I was disappointed to hear what appeared to be tale of mismanagement of an elite athlete, even by health practitioners attuned to the needs of such patients. It also reinforced for me the importance of understanding a patient's sport and the particular needs of athletes within that sport, and relating management to those needs as much as is reasonable. Even if it is not possible to relate management to the specific requirements of a particular sport, at least demonstrating an understanding of the needs of the athlete and providing reasons for a particular management goes a long way to addressing the cognitive/affective components of a problem. In establishing this history in such detail, I was also trying to find out whether the approach to treatment that I anticipated would be effective had been tried in the past, because if it had the chance of success from my management was lower.

3 Did you judge the mother's apparent dominance of the interview to be simply typical of a parent or could this and their apparent understanding and beliefs about what was required to rehabilitate Sally's shoulders be seen as potential contributing factors to her lack of success to date and something that would have to be addressed?

■ Clinician's answer

This question is somewhat difficult to answer, as the parent who is supportive and tuned into the needs of an adolescent athlete showing considerable potential will tend to do anything to help them to succeed. Such people, as athletes themselves often do, tend to want a quick answer to a problem and will 'shop around' in the hope of finding one. Therefore, Sally's mother could be viewed in this light and, at the time, this was my main interpretation of her motives. However, so-called 'pushy' parents are commonly seen associated with individual sports such as swimming and this image did come to mind somewhat, particularly listening to her description of the list of attempts to find an answer to Sally's problems. My hypotheses, outlined in the answer to Question 1 about Sally's mother's influence on prognosis in particular, continued through this part of the interview. The comment about difficulty fitting in the exercise with studying and swimming did make me question their commitment to success of a management programme.

I did find it interesting that this family had abandoned traditional pathways in their attempts to solve Sally's problems, with their use of a chiropractor, although this sounded like it was short lived, and the apparent success of glucose injections despite their inability to explain the hypothesized mechanisms by which glucose injections would help painful shoulders in an adolescent swimmer. Clearly, the injections had been beneficial, but what surprised me was that neither mother nor daughter had any idea of the proposed mechanism of their effect. The fact that use of the chiropractor and a somewhat alternative method of management of musculoskeletal disorders were sought late in the piece suggests a failure of the more

traditional approaches to satisfy this family's needs, even though that was the background from which they came.

These considerations highlighted to me how important it was to provide a rational explanation for my suggestions for management if I was to have any success in convincing them of its potential value.

■ Clinical reasoning commentary

In discussing hypotheses at presentation regarding dominant pain mechanisms, possible sources and contributing factors for the symptoms and activity/participation restrictions, the clinician illustrates her thinking on multiple levels. While her thinking has occurred now in hindsight in response to the specific question asked, expert clinicians are also able to think in this manner as they work through an examination. The clinician's answers here also reflect a hypothesis-oriented ability to recognize a broad range of diagnostic issues, including pain mechanisms, sources and physical contributing factors, in addition to psychosocial features in the patient's presentation, including her relationship with her mother. The hypotheses considered are not closed at this early stage; rather they are clearly informed by considerable experience with shoulder problems and provide an initial picture against which subsequent information will be considered.

Understanding a patient's problem requires understanding the patient. The clinician's thinking goes well beyond analysis of shoulder impairment, with serious consideration also given to this patient's personal context, including the specific needs of her sport and the relationship she has with her mother. While the likely need for active management has been hypothesized, the importance of teaching (e.g. explanation) in this patient's management is also emphasized, that is not simply teaching to do (i.e. instrumental learning) but teaching to promote altered understanding and feelings (i.e. transformative learning). This level of teaching must be based on assessment of the patient's (and in this case the mother's) understanding and feelings, including the basis of those thoughts and emotions (i.e. previous advice, past medical experiences, personal goals and pressures). Expert clinicians must be expert teachers.

PHYSICAL EXAMINATION

For the physical examination, Sally undressed to her swimsuit. Observation demonstrated the broad shoulder, narrow hip posture typical of an elite swimmer, with very horizontal shoulder girdle, widely placed scapulae and slightly medially rotated shoulders. There was no apparent asymmetry in her shoulder girdle posture or muscle development. Her upper quarter muscle development was not outstanding. Spinal posture revealed a slightly exaggerated thoracic kyphosis and lumbar lordosis, also typical of swimmers, and the tone in her abdominal muscles, gluteal muscles and legs appeared good.

Active shoulder movements

Glenohumeral joint flexion and abduction. The glenohumeral joints were hypermobile and there was excessive scapular rotation. There was no pain at end-range nor with overpressure.

Glenohumeral joint medial rotation, measured in abduction and full flexion. There was normal range in both shoulders in both positions, with some slight discomfort on overpressure to medial rotation in full flexion. This position was tested as it is a movement emphasized by swimming coaches as important for obtaining maximum power during the catch phase of the freestyle or butterfly stroke.

Glenohumeral joint lateral rotation measured in abduction and full flexion. There was a slightly increased range compared with what might be expected as normal, with a 'loose' end-feel. No symptoms.

Hand behind back. In this posture, there was normal mobility of both shoulders, combined with excessive winging of the medial border of the scapulae. Stabilization of the scapulae did restrict glenohumeral joint range; however, it could still be considered within normal limits.

Horizontal flexion and extension. Generally hypermobile, with no reproduction of symptoms. With all active physiological movements, excessive movement of the scapulae was evident, with poor stabilization of the medial border so that arm movement was accompanied by scapular medial border winging.

Further tests

Isometric rotator cuff tests. There was no pain but the impression of poor power, particularly in lateral rotation. Specific tests for long head of biceps in different positions were negative.

Active movements of the cervical and thoracic spine. This was generally mobile to hypermobile with no pain locally or in the shoulders.

Neural provocation tests of the upper limbs. No abnormalities were detected in the upper limb tension tests 1, 2B or 3 (Butler, 2000). Test 2A was not carried out as I considered that any abnormality in the median nerve component of the neural structures would have been detected with test 1 and any abnormality related to scapular depression and protraction would have been obvious with test 2B.

Glenohumeral joint stability tests. The mobility rating scale used to evaluate shoulder translation tests is similar to that used for measurement of mobility with a Lachman's test for the anterior cruciate ligament. (Normal mobility is rated as zero, with three measures of increased laxity: +, slightly increased translation; ++, moderately increased translation; and +++, markedly increased translation, to subluxation. This rating scale is used by local orthopaedic surgeons and physiotherapists but has not been validated.) Using this rating scale, the anterior drawer was hypermobile (+) with right greater than left. Posterior drawer was hypermobile (++) with left greater than right. The inferior and anteroinferior glide was slightly hypermobile on both sides. No apprehension or pain with any stability test. All tests had a slightly loose end-feel

Passive physiological and accessory movements of the glenohumeral joint. All movements were hypermobile with a loose end-feel. Quadrant position, on the low side of the quadrant, reproduced Sally's pain on both shoulders. Differential testing in that position demonstrated increased pain with subacromial distraction, decreased pain on subacromial compression and a slight increase on glenohumeral compression, indicating a probable capsular source to her pain with a possible slight contribution from something

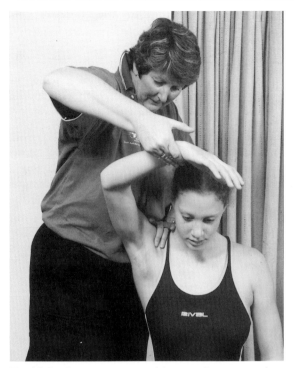

Fig. 11.2 Dynamic rotary stability test demonstrated in the catch position of the freestyle stroke, the position in which Sally's symptoms were most evident (Magarey and Jones, 2003a).

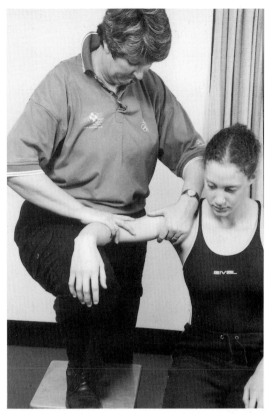

Fig. 11.3 Rotator cuff dynamic relocation test (Magarey and Jones, 2003b).

intra-articular (Magarey and Jones, 1991; Maitland, 1991).

Passive movements of the scapulothoracic joint. All movements were hypermobile with a loose end-feel, with a particularly mobile scapular abduction and lateral tilt (winging).

Passive movements of the acromioclavicular and sternoclavicular joints. All hypermobile, particularly posteroanterior glide on both acromioclavicular joints and posteroanterior glide on the left sternoclavicular joint.

Palpation. No specific areas of tenderness or altered tissue texture could be found. In particular, long head of biceps, supraspinatus insertion, the subacromial and subcoracoid spaces and the posterior joint lines were clear.

Dynamic rotary stability test. This test is shown in Figure 11.2 (Jones and Magarey, 2001; Magarey and Jones, 2003a,b). No shifting of the humeral head could be detected during testing in any position, but there was poor quality of contraction of both medial and lateral rotators, particularly in positions above

90 degrees of flexion, abduction or scaption, with quite marked weakness in these positions.

Rotator cuff dynamic relocation (concavity compression) test. This test is shown in Figure 11.3 (Jones and Magarey, 2001; Magarey and Jones, 2003a,b). With the arm in the plane of the scapula and approximately 60 degrees of abduction, Sally's ability to generate a stabilizing co-contraction of the rotator cuff was very poor. With considerable facilitation, she was eventually able to achieve it, but with poor-quality contraction.

Side-lying scapular proprioceptive neuromuscular facilitation (PNF) diagonals. Awareness of the position of the scapula and difficulty in movement of the scapula in the four diagonals, even following facilitation, was tested (Magarey and Jones, 2003a) (Fig. 11.4). Sally's ability to maintain any of the four corner positions (up and forwards, down and back, up and back, down and forwards) against any resistance was poor, particularly down and back, which is predominantly lower trapezius

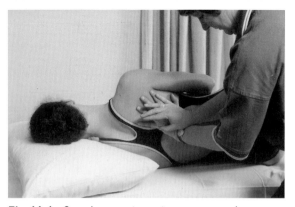

Fig. 11.4 Scapular proprioceptive neuromuscular facilitation pattern of 'down and back'—the direction in which Sally's awareness and control was found to be particularly poor.

contraction. In the up and forwards movement, she had a tendency to go into forward movement of the shoulder girdle rather than upwards, with this forwards movement representing a protraction and anterior tilt of the scapula with a lack of the elevation component. While this movement was not ideal, it was not as significant as the lack of down and back movement.

I chose to omit examination of accessory movements of the cervical or thoracic spine on Day 1 because I wanted time to assess dynamic stabilization of the glenohumeral joint and the scapula on the chest wall.

REASONING DISCUSSION AND CLINICAL REASONING COMMENTARY

1 Please highlight how the information from the physical examination did or did not support your previous hypotheses regarding dominant pain mechanisms, source of the symptoms and contributing factors?

Clinician's answer

Pain mechanisms

My physical findings supported my primary hypothesis of an input nociceptive problem coupled with an impaired output motor mechanism. The support for this hypothesis was partly the lack of findings that would support any other mechanisms. Sally demonstrated none of the physical features that tend to be identified with centralization: for example, hyperalgesia, inconsistencies in response to physical testing, and spontaneous pain. Also, she showed no features that readily supported the possible affective component that had been hypothesized during the subjective examination, with Sally cooperating fully and openly with all aspects of the physical examination. Her responses to physical tests were consistent and she did not display an obvious fear-avoidance or inappropriateness in her responses. The mechanical nature of any symptoms found and the poor muscle control of her glenohumeral joint and scapulothoracic articulation also supported my primary hypothesis.

Sources of symptoms and contributing factors

The only physical test that reproduced Sally's pain was the glenohumeral quadrant test (Maitland, 1991). The quadrant is not a test that identifies specific structures at fault, but it does appear to be a sensitive clinical test for detecting abnormalities around the shoulder complex. The details of how to undertake this testing can be found in Maitland (1991). Further discrimination of source can be made with the differential testing described above. Differential testing involves altering the stress on structures within the subacromial space, the glenohumeral joint capsular structures, intra-articular structures and the acromioclavicular joint. The responses to such testing with Sally indicated positive responses for a glenohumeral capsular source to her symptoms, with her pain exacerbated by increasing the stretch on the capsule with the shoulder in the provocative quadrant position (subacromial distraction) and decreased when the stretch was reduced (subacromial compression). Extrapolation from anatomical and biomechanical analysis related to restraints to movement would indicate the rotator interval/coracohumeral ligament region as the structures most likely to be responsible for this pain. There was also weak support from differential testing for an intra-articular component to the pain (there was some slight increase in her symptoms with the addition of glenohumeral compression to the quadrant position), in this case, probably superior labral in origin.

Therefore, my hypothesis related to the glenohumeral joint as the primary source of symptoms, with the superior capsular and labral structures associated with the biceps anchor as the most likely source, was supported by the physical findings. The hypermobility of the whole shoulder girdle also supported my hypothesis. The fact that the findings related to pain provocation were minimal also supported my hypothesis that there was little or no intrinsic pathology, with the pain primarily related to irritation of these structures as a result of poor muscle control of the hypermobility.

Lack of findings related to the neural provocation tests and normal active mobility of the cervical and thoracic spine negated these structures as sources, although I recognized that this could not be completely eliminated from my thinking as the examination of the spine was not complete.

The hypothesis related to contributing factors of poor muscle control was strongly supported by the physical findings of lack of dynamic control of the glenohumeral joint and scapulothoracic articulation during dynamic and functional testing.

■ Clinical reasoning commentary

The hypothesis testing for physical impairments and associated sources that was initiated in the subjective examination is continued through the physical examination. Importantly, the clinician does not simply follow a predetermined series of shoulder assessments; rather tests chosen are directly related to earlier hypotheses generated and the patient's particular presentation. The depth of the clinician's physical examination is apparent in her assessment of muscle function, which incorporated important aspects such as patient awareness and timing of activation, assessed through a combination of functionally relevant procedures.

Also apparent in the clinician's reasoning is her open mindedness with regard to the hypotheses considered. A common error in clinical reasoning is bias, and the greatest hindrance to pattern recognition is the difficulty clinicians have in truly considering and disproving competing hypotheses (see Ch. 26). Here the clinician entertains a number of different hypotheses, noting those that are supported and those that are not supported by the physical examination.

m | Management

■ Treatment 1

It seemed to me at this stage that any success with Sally would rely as much as anything on gaining the confidence of both Sally and her mother. Therefore, I explained what I considered to be Sally's problem, indicating that she had hypermobile shoulders and scapulae with inadequate muscular control for the demands she placed on them. The majority of her pain was likely to be related to generalized low-grade capsular inflammation from the continual irritation caused by stress created by the high levels of swimming. I brought the skeleton into the cubicle and showed them where these structures were, the reason why the rotator cuff is well positioned to function as the primary glenohumeral joint stabilizer and what was happening with Sally's scapulae when she loaded her shoulders. I talked to them about core stability and the findings of research undertaken by David et al. (2000) and Carr et al. (1998), demonstrating consistent firing of the rotator cuff and biceps group prior to activation

of the deltopectoral muscles during isokinetic rotation at the glenohumeral joint, and the significance of these research findings, particularly for swimmers. I indicated to Sally and her mother what I felt was the most appropriate course of treatment I could offer. I realised that as this was not substantially different from what had been offered by other health professionals in whom they did not have confidence, it was important that this approach was 'sold' very strongly to convince them that it was not simply 'more of the same'. It was also important that any rehabilitation programme be adapted to a regimen of swim training, as this was obviously important to both Sally and my credibility. I pointed out that the next 4 weeks when she was out of the water would be an ideal time to work hard on improving her muscle function. Once swimming recommenced, a reduction in swim training coupled with time spent on her rehabilitation programme through the winter would be advantageous, hopefully putting her in an optimal position to return to full training without pain in the spring. I emphasized that the primary responsibility for the programme would rest with Sally herself and that, therefore, Sally had to want to do the programme for it to be successful. I gave them the opportunity to decide whether they wanted to try the programme.

Once they indicated that they did want to try, I spent some time teaching Sally rotator cuff activation with the dynamic relocation manoeuvre, so that before she left she was able to produce a relatively isolated rotator cuff co-contraction of both shoulders in this position and hold it while lifting and lowering her hand with her arm in a supported position. I also taught her simple scapular awareness strategies, with particular emphasis on scapular depression and retraction, as this movement was the one identified as least effective. Since Sally was only able to maintain the contraction without loading, these movements were undertaken without additional load. She was encouraged to do these exercises at least once a day in a set exercise time and to work on increasing awareness of shoulder and scapular stabilization with movement during the day. The aim of this was to facilitate activation of correct timing of contraction in these stabilizers.

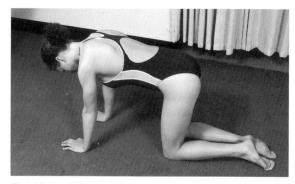

Fig. 11.5 Sally's scapular control in four-point kneeling on first assessment.

when tested in supine. She was only able to maintain the contraction and lift and lower one leg from crook lying. She was also able to maintain a TA contraction during bridging with segmental lifting and lowering; these two exercises were also added to the programme, together with an explanation of how they should help her shoulder problem.

Treatment 2

The next treatment took place 1 week later. At this time, Sally had been pain-free (she was not swimming) and both her rotator cuff and scapular retraction contractions were improved. The pain on the low side of the quadrant position was also less. She was able to maintain the rotator cuff contraction while lifting her forearm off the support. Awareness of scapular position during PNF patterns was a little improved. Importantly, in review of the rationale for this approach to management, both Sally and her mother appeared to have a good understanding of what would be required and why.

Assessment of scapular control in four-point kneeling was undertaken, demonstrating good ability to isolate scapular protraction (Fig. 11.5) but poor endurance when loaded by lifting one arm, demonstrated by winging of the medial border of the scapula. Assessment of isometric lower and middle trapezius function revealed considerable weakness of lower trapezius, such that she could only maintain a stable scapula in depression with the arm supported in approximately 120 degrees glenohumeral abduction and elbow flexion. In this position, rotator cuff co-contraction and humeral lateral rotation could be achieved. This exercise was added to her programme. Transversus abdominis (TA) function was also poor

Treatment 3

By the third visit, Sally had minimal pain on the low side of the quadrant. She was able to maintain a rotator cuff dynamic relocation contraction during isolated glenohumeral joint rotations against light theraband resistance in approximately 100 degrees of flexion, while simultaneously maintaining a stable scapula. Her ability to stabilize her scapula in four-point kneeling was also improved, so that maintaining this position during PNF pattern movements against theraband resistance with the opposite arm were included in her programme. Isolated lower trapezius exercises were replaced with functional PNF scapular diagonals also against theraband, while maintaining the humeral head dynamic relocation. Abdominal function had improved considerably, indicating that her poor control on first testing was likely to be a result of poor motor awareness/programming rather than true weakness.

At this point, TA control during rotary leg movements in supine was assessed, as was gluteal function on a stable TA contraction in prone. Appropriate levels of exercise for both these functions were added to the programme. I also described how to make an exercise bar to facilitate abdominal function with an exercise colloquially known as 'twisties', as described by Peter Blanch, physiotherapist to the Australian Swim team at the Australian Institute of Sport (Fig. 11.6).

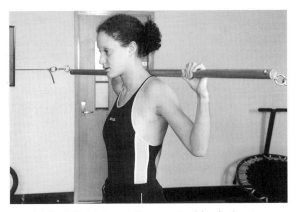

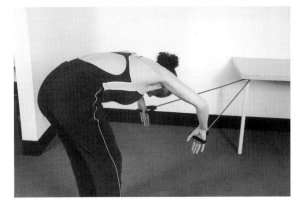

Fig. 11.6 The 'abdominal/twisties bar' for facilitating external oblique contraction and body roll in swimmers with shoulder pain. The twisties bar consists of a broom handle of approximately 180 cm length, with bolts and rings at each end, each facing in opposite directions. Theratubing of appropriate strength is then attached to the bolts and connected to similar bolts on the wall, so that one is pulling at right angles to the body position behind the patient and the other in the same direction from in front of the patient, thus providing a rotary resistance. The patient can then line their trunk up so that the resistance work is performed from neutral towards inner range or from outer range towards mid-range. For swimmers, the particular benefit of this exercise is that they can learn to initiate the rotation from the pelvis and then integrate the trunk movement, thus mimicking the action required at the catch phase of the swim stroke. More challenging rotational load can be provided specifically for swimmers with the bar overhead. Movement is still initiated from the pelvis, but the longer lever provided by having the bar overhead provides more challenge to the abdominals in a position similar to that required at the catch phase, albeit with both arms overhead not one.

Fig. 11.7 Warm-up exercise with theraband in a simulated catch position for the butterfly stroke, in which Sally worked on setting the scapulae in a neutral stable position, relocating the head of humerus in the glenoid and maintaining control of both while pulling against the theratubing into the downsweep part of the stroke.

Treatment 4

Following this visit a 3-week break in treatment was provided, during which time Sally began swimming training again. At the next visit, she indicated that she had less time for the exercises and that she still had some pain during swimming, but it seemed to be less. She was only swimming three mornings a week at this stage. Her quadrant assessment indicated a slight increase in pain with the same degree of resistance applied to the movement. Assessment of abdominal and gluteal function demonstrated marked improvement, while improvement in scapular and rotator cuff function was less apparent. As a result of the return to the water, I spent some time teaching

Sally three specific pretraining exercises: one aimed at facilitating rotator cuff co-contraction during swimming, the second at facilitating the combination of rotator cuff co-contraction and scapular control (Fig. 11.7) and the third at encouraging Sally to lead her body roll from the hips by using her oblique abdominal muscles, facilitating a stretch-shortening contraction in these muscles and thus reducing the load on her shoulders. I checked the remainder of the exercise programme and modified it appropriately. We decided to review the situation in 2 weeks to evaluate the effect of these specific pretraining exercises on her return to swimming.

At this point, I decided that I should try to make the programme more interesting for a 16-year-old girl. I decided to try to incorporate some Swiss ball work and spent some time working out ways in which I could adapt her exercises to be done on the ball. My main aims at this stage were to improve her abdominal and pelvic/hip strength and control as quickly as possible to try to reduce the load through her shoulders, while continuing to work on her shoulder and scapular stability, which I anticipated would take longer to improve, particularly since she was swimming. Therefore, her abdominal and pelvic work could be quickly progressed onto the ball and the upper quarter exercises made more challenging by doing them on the unstable surface provided by the ball. The intention was to do this at the next visit.

Treatment 5

At this next visit, Sally indicated that she had done the pretraining exercises fairly conscientiously, though usually before she left home to go to the pool rather than at the pool itself, as much so that she did not stand out from the crowd as difficulty completing them poolside. While this was not ideal, the time difference was relatively small and I decided that the facilitation would probably still be valuable. The programme certainly seemed to have been effective, as Sally reported reduced pain with swimming and more awareness of her scapular position and a sense of control in her shoulders. She was also more aware of her body roll, though could not see that it made much difference to the load through her shoulders. She was not swimming competitively at this stage, so any effect on her swim times by her concentration on these strategies could not yet be determined.

REASONING DISCUSSION AND CLINICAL REASONING COMMENTARY

1 From your comments earlier about the importance of gaining the confidence of Sally and her mother and the time you gave to explaining and educating them on both the problem and its management, you clearly place a lot of emphasis on education. Could you comment on your reasoning behind this?

Clinician's answer

My decision to spend a considerable amount of time on explanation and education was based on the principle that patient management should be a shared responsibility and that it will be more successful if the patient has been an active contributor to the development of the management plan. This conviction is supported by the observation that many patients with chronic problems tell stories of management imposed on them or management that they do not fully understand, so that they feel they lose control of the situation. Empowerment seems to be an important component to any successful management strategy. With Sally's particular situation, I hypothesized that a lack of empowerment appeared to be one factor that was common to most of the strategies attempted. It seemed that nobody had ever explained to Sally or her mother what the likely mechanism of symptom production was and, therefore, why any particular approach to management should be undertaken. If the therapists had, in fact, explained these points, neither Sally nor her mother appeared to have grasped the concept.

I recognized that I had an initial advantage with Sally and her mother as I had been recommended to them as a 'shoulder expert', so that they had come with a positive perception of my ability—whether well founded or not!

This perception had the potential to provide a degree of positive outcome on the basis of placebo. I feel it is important to build on such advantages, so that the time spent on explanation of the problem was intended to reinforce the 'shoulder (and swimming) expert' perception. This also allowed me to present a potential programme to them that was not unlike what they had been exposed to before without eliciting an immediate 'more of the same' reaction, thus enhancing compliance.

Patient understanding of the problem is also important for self-management. If Sally could understand that swimming while she had poor control of her scapular and glenohumeral hypermobility was likely to exacerbate her symptoms, she was more likely to agree to a modified training programme than if I had simply told her she must stay out of the water. Similarly, such understanding meant that she was highly motivated to improve her muscle control so that she could return to swimming as soon as possible. Sally was far less likely to do something silly that would exacerbate the problem if she understood the reasons why she should behave as suggested.

Part of the proposed programme included increasing Sally's awareness of body roll and kick, with the need to improve her strength and awareness of abdominal and pelvic muscle function; this was intended to reduce the load on her shoulders. Without an adequate understanding of her problem and the mechanics of swimming, it is unlikely that Sally would have seen the point of a programme aimed at abdominal and gluteal strengthening and would not have complied with it.

A further point that was important to make to Sally and her mother was that a programme such as that suggested had the potential to slow Sally's race times, at least in the short term, while she was learning the stabilization strategies in the water. As with any new technique, its mastery takes some time and performance is usually reduced during the mastery phase. Sally had to be prepared to accept this and work through it. However, this was not an issue for Sally, as her times for the season just completed had been slow anyway as a result of the shoulder pain. The potential for improvement was sufficient to make her prepared to try the programme. We also had the advantage that she had come to see me in the quieter season, so that a short-term reduction in times was not as disastrous as it might have been at the beginning of a new season.

▮ Clinical reasoning commentary

Explanation/teaching, patient understanding (cognitive and motor), empowerment, shared decision making and self-management are all evident through the clinician's management described and discussed above. These dimensions of management

fit well with the attributes of expert manual therapists described by Jensen et al. (1999). Reassessment, a form of hypothesis testing and medium for reflection, also features strongly in the clinician's management. Importantly, the reassessments here include patient understanding as well as physical joint and muscle control impairments/dysfunctions. Manual therapists often place a great deal of emphasis on education and explanation, yet their reassessments may only focus on physical signs. In Chapter 1, teaching was presented as a focus of clinical reasoning. If patient (and supporters) understanding is judged to be a potential problem, as in this case, then reassessment of explanations provided is essential to ensure learning has occurred. If their understanding was still judged to be faulty, further exploration for the basis of their views (an important step for some patients to revise their understanding/beliefs) and/or altered strategies of explanation may be required.

m ▌ Further management

Reassessment of all dynamic features indicated continued improvement, with the least improvement in the rotator cuff function—predictable as these are the muscles most inhibited by the shoulder pain. We transferred abdominal and lower limb work onto the Swiss ball as planned, with Sally doing a series of exercises aimed at improving her abdominal control and strength available for kicking. One involved maintaining control of her trunk and pelvic position while balancing on her thoracic spine on the ball. In this position she did alternate hip flexion, followed by knee extension, trying to replicate the muscle activity and movement required in the upbeat of her kick (Fig. 11.8a). A second exercise undertaken in prone involved Sally balancing through her hands, maintaining a stable glenohumeral joint and scapula, with the ball under her abdomen. From this position, with her toes assisting the balance, Sally maintained a TA contraction while alternately lifting one leg from the hips, ensuring that she used predominantly gluteals to perform this action (Fig. 11.8b). As her balance improved with both these exercises, Sally increased the rate of the 'kick', thus substantially increasing the load required of her trunk stabilizers. This series of exercises was fun and challenging to do and it seemed like Sally would be

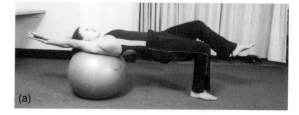
(a)

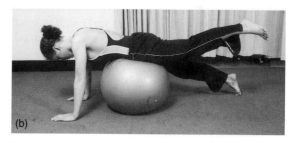
(b)

Fig. 11.8 Facilitated kicking function on a Swiss ball while maintaining abdominal control. (a) In supine over the ball, Sally was required to maintain her balance through one leg and her trunk, ensuring appropriate abdominal and gluteal activation while going through the kicking motion with the other leg, trying to replicate the upbeat action of the kick. (b) In prone over the ball, Sally was required to maintain an appropriate abdominal contraction and balance, assisted by her weight on one toe, while she worked on the kicking action with the other leg, ensuring that she emphasized a relatively straight leg and gluteal function in performing this action.

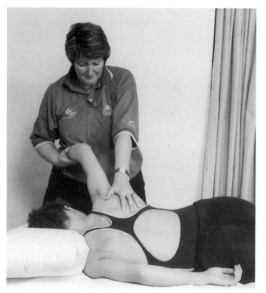

Fig. 11.9 Side-lying facilitation of dynamic control of scapular and glenohumeral positions at the catch phase of the swim stroke. Sally is using the therapist's body to simulate the water in the catch position, while the therapist applies tactile stimulation to encourage, first, scapular setting in a neutral position and then, rotator cuff relocation prior to Sally pulling the arm down through the downsweep action of the swim stroke; this is similar to her warm-up pool-side exercise.

enthusiastic to continue them at home. This she was to do in addition to the twisties exercises and the rotator cuff and scapular stabilizing work.

In addition, I spent some time working with Sally in side lying, using tactile facilitation and manual resistance to improve her rotator cuff and scapular stabilization further, initially at the catch phase (Fig. 11.9) and later at the final stroke of the pull-through phase of her freestyle stroke. This manoeuvre was similar to the pretraining facilitation exercise but was enhanced by the manual contact. During these exercises she was encouraged to maintain the TA contraction.

I asked Sally and her mother whether they were happy with the progress to date and whether they had any particular questions; they seemed enthusiastic about how things were going. We discussed maintaining a realistic schedule for Sally within the context of her schoolwork and swimming requirements. It was decided that Sally should do one exercise session per day working specifically on the tasks set. In addition, she would work on a repetition/awareness programme during the day to facilitate correct motor programming of scapular and glenohumeral stabilization and would

continue to do her facilitation exercises prior to training. Sally's mother indicated that her coach was happy with this arrangement. I asked about attending a training session and talking to the coach, but we quickly realised that this was not a practical option at the time as training was at 5 a.m.

Treatment 6

The next visit took place 2 weeks later. Sally appeared a little despondent, indicating that improvement seemed to have plateaued, with some return of her shoulder pain during swimming. She had increased the distance travelled during each session and her swim training to 5 days a week. Sally certainly could see some improvement in her shoulder control and awareness while swimming, and her use of body roll and kick, but was disappointed because of the return of shoulder pain. Her quadrant position, which had been painful early on, was certainly more painful than the last time it was assessed, with a slightly spongy end-feel. There also appeared to be some subtle swelling in the subacromial/superior capsular region of her shoulder. Isometric resisted rotations in 90 degrees of flexion now reproduced the same pain as provoked with the quadrant position.

Clearly the additional swimming was aggravating the shoulder problem and Sally's rotator cuff and scapular control was not yet sufficient to cope with the extra load. I pointed this out to her and asked how much of a problem it would be to return to the regimen of 3 days swimming. She was reluctant to do this as winter pennant championships were only 3 weeks away and she was keen to compete well in these. I indicated that I felt that this would slow down her progress and that, if the championships were important, she would have to accept the slower rate of progress and do more to reduce inflammation in her shoulders following each swim session. I suggested gentle through-range movement with rotator cuff control while in the warmth of a shower immediately after training, followed by ice massage to the sub-acromial space/rotator interval area, with a further brief but deliberate rotator cuff facilitation session after the ice. I also suggested that she increase her rotator cuff stabilizing work during her exercise sessions, aiming to increase the rate of improvement in this function.

In addition, treatment that day included gentle mobilization (Grade IV---) (Magarey, 1986; Maitland, 1991) of her glenohumeral joint into the quadrant position, with Grade IV-- subacromial distraction performed short of pain, followed by Grade III-- mobilization in the same direction. Pain on testing of the quadrant and on isometric rotator cuff testing was reduced following the mobilization and Sally was able to generate a dynamic relocation contraction more strongly in the 90 degree flexion position. More side-lying facilitation work on rotator cuff and scapular stabilizing was then added, as at the last treatment.

Sally's mother phoned a week later to say that the shoulder pain during swimming was less and that the pain she did have was reduced considerably following the post-training regimen. Sally felt more confident that she would be able to control the pain better and, therefore, the concern expressed at the last visit was alleviated somewhat. I suggested to Sally's mother that they continue to work on the same regimen, with appropriate progressions until after the winter pennant competition unless they had further difficulties. I also suggested that Sally take her theratubing to the pool and do her rotator cuff/scapular facilitation exercise immediately prior to entering the water and again three times during the training session, to try to maintain the pre-activation throughout the training session.

Treatment 7

Three weeks later following the championships, at which Sally's times were improved, both Sally and her mother seemed much more reassured and enthusiastic about her progress. I pointed out to them that Sally was not ideally built for the load she wanted to put on herself and that she was likely to have to put up with some shoulder pain if she wanted to continue to train hard and aspire to great achievements in swimming. However, she had shown herself that she could minimize this with appropriate work on general strength and technique and facilitation of her rotator cuff/scapular stabilizers. Also, when the pain was present she could reduce it with the pretraining and post-training regimen we had instituted. This empowerment and control over the pain seemed to have made a profound difference to Sally, who was much happier and outgoing at this visit than at any other time. She seemed no longer scared of her shoulder pain and no longer saw it as the end of her swimming career.

When I asked what effect intermittent exercising through the training session had had on her pain both during and after training, Sally indicated that she had initially been reluctant to do it as it would make her

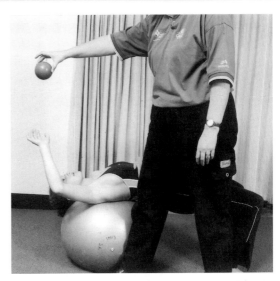

Fig. 11.10 Mini-plyometric throwing exercise with a weighted ball in a simulated catch position while balancing on the Swiss ball.

different from the rest of the squad. However, she found that the regimen reduced the amount of pain during the session and also seemed to improve her stroke and so was happy to continue with it.

Her quadrant position was less painful, the subacromial area less swollen, and her rotator cuff and scapular stabilizing contractions had improved—more than I might have anticipated based on the rate of progress to date. Treatment consisted of more rotator cuff and scapular stabilizing work in different positions and showing Sally how she could work on this with some 'mini-plyometric' drills to make her exercise sessions more interesting. This was achieved by maintaining the stabilizing contractions while throwing a tennis ball a short distance to a wall, catching it on return and throwing it again as quickly as possible. This was done with Sally's arm in a position of approximately 120 degrees of flexion in the plane of the scapula. She was able to achieve this quite readily, even as the speed of throw and catch was increased. I showed her how to progress this exercise while still maintaining the control. Later, Sally progressed to use of a small weighted ball, either in the same way or in conjunction with trunk stabilization on the Swiss ball (Fig. 11.10). She also began some plyometric wall push-ups with her arms in different positions of flexion, maintaining rotator cuff control while working the scapular muscles (Kibler, 1998; Wilk and Arrigo, 1993; Wilk et al., 1993; Wilk and Voight, 1994).

REASONING DISCUSSION AND CLINICAL REASONING COMMENTARY

1 Could you comment on the role of palliative treatment, such as the mobilizations you added, in the broader management of a predominantly muscle control problem?

Clinician's answer

Initially, Sally's presentation indicated very little pain with any active or passive movement, but an excessive range of movement and poor muscle control. At that time, emphasis on addressing this contributing factor was clearly the highest priority. My hypothesis at the time was that there was little intrinsic tissue damage and what was present related more to continual irritation than true pathology. However, at the point where palliative mobilization was added to the treatment, there was evidence of more obvious provocation of symptoms and some physical changes around the shoulder. Continued work with the muscle control approach and a reduction in swimming would have allowed this aggravation to settle in time. However, it was important to Sally at that time to keep swimming and not reduce the intensity of her training. Short-term benefit could be gained from palliative treatment aimed at reducing the inflammation in her subacromial/superior capsular area, thereby reducing her pain, so that she could continue swimming. While this treatment was recognized as having no long-term effect on her problem, it did provide the necessary immediate pain relief and also allowed Sally to see that she should be able to control her pain herself with similar measures if she found that the long training aggravated her symptoms.

This episode also gave me the opportunity to provide Sally with further insight into the requirements of elite sports performance. If swimming continued to cause pain in her shoulders, she would be able to understand why and be able to come to terms with it and not necessarily assume that the therapy provided was of no value. A common feature of high-level athletic performance is that athletes live and perform with some level of pain. To an athlete, the value of the athletic performance is greater than the pain and the potential damage inflicted. When a young athlete attends for treatment of a painful problem for the first time, it is the therapist's responsibility to explain the mechanisms for production

of the pain and strategies that can be employed, both by the therapist and the athlete, to reduce or eliminate the pain. The therapist should also point out that high-performance athletic endeavour often places forces on structures that are beyond our ability to control completely. This is particularly the case if the athlete's biomechanical make-up is not ideal for the particular sport, as was the case with Sally with her hypermobile shoulders. While a programme designed to improve muscle performance and control around her shoulders should reduce her pain and, therefore, improve her swimming, it was important that she understood that the repetitive load with swimming might have been more than her biomechanical make-up could cope with in the long term. The muscles simply may not have been able to work sufficiently to stabilize her shoulders fully. Providing her with immediate palliative strategies to reduce symptoms that were provoked gave her more confidence to work with some discomfort, rather than to let the discomfort overpower her.

2 What was your clinical and physiological rationale for incorporating plyometric exercises into her programme when swimming does not require the quick eccentric–concentric change over that occurs with throwing?

Clinician's answer

There is a small plyometric component to swimming that is being increasingly recognized by swimming coaches and related health practitioners. Immediately following hand entry, the arm reaches as far forward as possible, placing a stretch on the oblique abdominals, the scapular retractors and glenohumeral medial rotators. This stretch provides some storing of elastic energy in the series elastic components of the relevant muscles (Wilk and Arrigo, 1993; Wilk et al., 1993; Wilk and Voight, 1994), thereby enhancing the concentric contraction required at catch. Recent advances in technique emphasize initiating the catch from the pelvis, similar to the initiation of the forward movement of a throw, to generate more power through the powerful trunk rotators rather than relying only on the smaller, less-efficient shoulder girdle and glenohumeral muscles. The side-lying PNF procedures described above placed Sally's trunk and shoulder girdle in a similar position to that at the catch point in the swim cycle, thereby attempting to replicate the muscle load, enhance the control required in this position and create a small stretch-shortening component. However, manual handling and dry land exercise cannot fully replicate the muscle requirements in the water, and training of the muscles in a stretch-shortening cycle in positions similar to those required in the catch phase was included to replicate (as closely as was possible on dry land) the action that was required of these muscles at catch. Use of a throw-catch routine also encouraged a quicker changeover from eccentric to concentric contraction than is normally possible in the water.

Physiological evidence (Komi, 1986) also indicates that eccentric muscle work is more energy efficient than concentric, so that greater force can be created for the same amount of work. Therefore, if a patient has poor endurance, working eccentrically should allow tolerance of longer workouts with the potential for faster improvement (Bennett and Marcus, 1994). In addition, gains from eccentric strength training are greater than those from equivalent concentric training, with reduction of oxygen consumption during eccentric activity indicating improved neural coordination (Friden et al., 1983). Therefore, the inclusion of eccentric work in Sally's programme was justified.

3 Given Sally's overall presentation, including her unique 'pain experience' and response to your management thus far, what were your thoughts regarding prognosis. In answering this could you highlight those features of her presentation that you felt supported a positive prognosis and those supporting a negative prognosis?

■ Clinician's answer

My thoughts regarding prognosis at this point were very positive in the short term—more so than I had expected when we started out. Sally had been very compliant with her programme; her understanding of the problem and the requirements to address it were sound. She had demonstrated herself to be far more assertive and enthusiastic about her swimming than first appeared, and the response to the management programme had been very good so far. Sally appeared to have little intrinsic pathology in her shoulders; her basic swimming technique was sound, as evidenced by her success prior to the development of the shoulder problem, and her motivation to succeed was very high. She also had a very supportive and stable family and all the privileges that go with an affluent lifestyle: opportunities to train and compete at whatever level her talent took her to, the safety and security of good friends, and the life experiences provided by an exclusive private school. The questions raised earlier about a 'pushy' mother were not supported during the management period; her mother was shown to be compassionate and concerned but not overbearing. Her domination of the early sessions was more related to Sally's teenage shyness and, therefore, unwillingness to speak for herself than anything else. As Sally became more confident with me and happy with the progress, her own personality came to the fore and her mother's dominance receded. There had been no support for the hypotheses related to possible central mechanisms considered initially and little to support the affective obstacles identified as possible.

However, there were some features that did not support such a positive prognosis, particularly if a long-term view was taken. The main one was Sally's intrinsic hypermobility. Such hypermobility meant that her shoulders would always be disadvantaged when she swam compared with a swimmer of similar ability with less-mobile shoulders. She was unlikely to be able to generate the same levels of power through her shoulders as the less-mobile swimmer, thus reducing her chance of achieving the fast times necessary to compete at the top level. If Sally wanted to achieve close to those times she would be required to continue with a maintenance programme of scapular and glenohumeral stabilizing training throughout her swimming career. Even with the discipline required to maintain the training necessary to compete at elite level, continued compliance with the stabilizing programme may not be as good, with the potential for exacerbation of her symptoms.

There is a high incidence of shoulder problems in elite swimmers resulting from the highly repetitive nature of the sport and the long distances swum in training by these athletes. Hypermobile shoulders, subjected to a highly repetitive load, are likely to develop intrinsic wear and tear pathology over time, even if their muscle control is maintained at an optimal level. Superior labral damage, from the repetitive shearing at the catch phase, and anterior labral damage, from compression during the pull through phase of the stroke, are likely to be coupled with general capsular irritation. The muscle control required in a hypermobile shoulder is greater than that in a shoulder with less mobility. Again, over time, this may lead to wear and tear pathology within the rotator cuff, with associated degenerative changes. The anatomical placement of these muscles also makes them vulnerable to outside influences in the presence of poor control. With fatigue of the rotator cuff and hypermobility of the shoulder, the likelihood of developing subacromial or subcoracoid impingement is high as a result of loss of centring of the humeral head, with rotator cuff tearing associated with friction trauma from the impingement. Therefore, the long-term prognosis for Sally, if she continues to swim, is not as positive as the shorter-term prognosis.

■ Clinical reasoning commentary

The clinician's answer on the role of palliative treatment in management highlights a difficult decision manual therapists regularly face, that is, should treatment be directed at a hypothesized source of the symptoms or at a potential contributing factor. Even when it is clear that both are necessary, a decision is still required as to which to treat first. There is no simple rule to follow. In the end, as evidenced by the clinician's reasoning here, the decision must be based on the weighting of the patient's clinical presentation (strength of evidence behind each pain mechanism, source and contributing factor considered) and the associated contextual issues (psychosocial status, beliefs/expectations, personal goals, etc.). It is common for some manual therapists to take an either/or approach, whereby once a dynamic approach is recognized as important, passive movement treatment is no longer even considered. Passive mobilization can be an effective adjunct to treat pain and also can improve muscle function/motor control through the relief of the inhibitory effect of pain on muscle function. In this case, while recognizing that passive treatment would not have a long-term effect on Sally's problem, the clinician judiciously used passive mobilization as a means to provide immediate pain relief and to identify measures the patient could use herself in her own future self-management.

The clinician's prognostic reasoning is both broad and realistic in its considerations. The exercise of identifying positive and negative prognostic indicators can be very useful to facilitate therapists' critical reflections. The patient's immediate pain and functional status and the broader contextual factors must all be taken into account. When predictions are not realised, a retrospective critique of what was judged positive and negative, as well as other previously less-considered factors, can assist therapists to recognize where they may have overemphasized, underemphasized or perhaps completely dismissed as not relevant different aspects of the patient's presentation and pain experience.

Outcome

Sally continued with this programme for several weeks, and she now understood how to progress it appropriately. She continued to get some shoulder pain with swimming, particularly when she increased distance or number of sessions, but over the remainder of the winter she found an optimal training regimen (including sessions of specific exercises) that allowed her swimming to continue to improve without significant exacerbation of the shoulder pain. She certainly found that she needed to keep up the exercise sessions and the facilitation exercises during training or she quickly developed pain again. Sally also found that her awareness of pre-activation and her functional rotator cuff strength reduced quickly if she did not do the specific exercises aimed at its facilitation. She was happy to continue with this regimen for an extended period, with the arrangement that she would phone for a further appointment if she wanted some more ideas for exercise progression, if she felt she needed manual facilitation to improve her shoulder function, or if she had any questions. I emphasized that I considered she would need to continue specific facilitation activities as long as she continued swimming, and the commitment to these would need to be proportional to the amount of swim training, as she had already shown that the improvements gained were not maintained without continued work. I encouraged her to continue with the trunk stabilization and to work hard on kicking strength and technique with her coach to lighten the load through her shoulders as much as was possible.

Sally was typical of many young athletes needing to come to the realisation that top-level competition tends to come with a price: the pain associated with training and competition. She continued to suffer from some shoulder pain with her swimming, but she had found ways in which she could control that pain and she was able to understand the mechanics of its production and perpetuation. Consequently, she was able to cope with her problem and continue to train and compete at the top level.

References

Bennett, J.G. and Marcus N.A. (1994). The decelerator mechanism: eccentric muscular contraction applications at the shoulder. In The Athlete's Shoulder (J.R. Andrews and K.E. Wilk, eds.) pp. 567–575. New York: Churchill Livingstone.

Butler, D.S. (2000). The Sensitive Nervous System. Adelaide, Australia: Noigroup Press.

Carr, A., David, G., Magarey, M. and Jones, M. (1998). Rotator cuff muscle performances during glenohumeral joint rotations: an isokinetic and electromyographic study of freestyle swimmers. In Proceedings of the Australian Conference of Science and Medicine in Sport, Adelaide, p. 84.

David, G., Magarey, M., Jones, M., Türker, K. et al. (2000). Electromyographic activity of rotator cuff and delto-pectoral muscles during isokinetic gleno-humeral joint rotations. Journal of Clinical Biomechanics, 15, 95–102.

Friden, J., Seger, J., Sjostrom, M. and Ekbolm, B. (1983). Adaptive response in human skeletal muscle subjected to prolonged eccentric training. International Journal of Sports Medicine, 4, 177–183.

Jensen, G.M., Gwyer, J., Hack, L.M. and Shepard, K.F. (1999). Expertise in Physical Therapy Practice. Oxford: Butterworth-Heinemann.

Jones, M. and Magarey, M. (2001). Clinical reasoning in the use of manual therapy techniques for the shoulder girdle, In Evaluation and Rehabilitation of the Shoulder: An Impairment Based Approach (B. Tovin and B. Greenfield, eds.) pp. 317–346. Lansdale, PA: F.A. Davis.

Kibler, B. (1998). Shoulder rehabilitation: principles and practice. Medicine and Science in Sports and Exercise, Supplement S40–S50 (online at http://www.wwilkins.com/MSSE)

Komi, P.V. (1986). The stretch-shortening cycle and human power output. In Human Muscle Power (N.L. Jones, N. McCartney and A.J. McComas, eds.) pp. 27–39. Champaign, France: Human Kinetics.

Magarey, M.E. (1986). The First Treatment Session. In Modern Manual Therapy of the Vertebral Column (G.P. Grieve, ed.) pp. 661–672. Edinburgh: Churchill Livingstone.

Magarey, M.E. and Jones, M.A. (1991). Clinical examination and management for minor instability of the shoulder complex. Australian Journal of Physiotherapy, 38, 260–280.

Magarey, M.E. and Jones, M.A. (2003a). Clinical evaluation, diagnosis and management of the shoulder complex. 2: Dynamic evaluation and early management of altered motor control around the shoulder complex. Manual Therapy, in press.

Magarey, M.E. and Jones, M.A (2003b). Specific evaluation of the function of force couples relevant for stabilisation of glenohumeral joint. Manual Therapy, in press.

Maglischo, E.W. (1993). Swimming Even Faster. Mountain View, CA: Mayfield Publishing.

Maitland, G.D. (1991). Peripheral Manipulation, London: Butterworth-Heinemann.

Pink, M., Jobe, F.W., Perry, J., Browne, A., Scovazzo, M.L. and Kerrigan J. (1993). The painful shoulder during the butterfly stroke. An electromyographic and cinematographic analysis of twelve muscles. Clinical Orthopedics and Related Research, 288, 60–72.

Scovazzo, M.L., Browne, A., Pink, M., Jobe, F.W. and Kerrigan, J. (1991). The painful shoulder during freestyle swimming. An electromyographic, cinematographic analysis of twelve muscles. American Journal of Sports Medicine, 19, 577–582.

Wilk, K.E. and Arrigo, C. (1993). Current concepts in the rehabilitation of the athletic shoulder. Journal of Orthopedic and Sports Physical Therapy, 18, 365–378.

Wilk, K.E. and Voight, M.L. (1994). Plyometrics for the shoulder complex. In The Athlete's Shoulder (J.R. Andrews and K.E. Wilk, eds.) pp. 543–566. New York: Churchill Livingstone.

Wilk, K.E., Voight, M.L., Keirns, M.A., Gambetta, V., Andrews, J.R. and Dillman, C.J. (1993). Stretch-shortening drills for the upper extremities: theory and practical application. Journal of Orthopedic and Sports Physical Therapy, 17, 225–239.

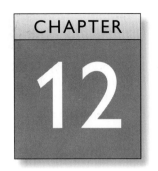

CHAPTER 12

Medial collateral ligament repair in a professional ice hockey player

David Magee

SUBJECTIVE EXAMINATION

Tom is a professional hockey player who was injured during the first period of a game. At the time, he was body checked by an opposing player and at the same moment his foot caught in a rut in the ice while he was weight bearing on the limb. With the body check, a valgus stress was applied to the leg and the athlete fell to the ice. During the contact, Tom experienced pain and when he got up and tried to skate he noted that the knee did not feel right, and so he skated off the ice. The trainer questioned Tom on the bench and then took him to the dressing room where the team doctor, an orthopaedic surgeon, saw him. This game was the fourth game of this season. Tom had missed all of the pre-season training camp and the beginning of the season because of prolonged contract negotiations. So, in addition to the mechanism of injury, conditioning and timing may have been factors that contributed to the injury.

On initial assessment, the orthopaedic surgeon determined that there was a valgus laxity in the knee, without the 'abrupt stop' end-feel one would normally expect to find with an intact ligament. There appeared to be some positive anterior drawer motion indicating injury to both the medial collateral ligament (MCL) and the anterior cruciate ligament (ACL). All other tests were negative, although muscle spasm was beginning to manifest itself, with the range of motion being limited. Strength was slightly less on the injured side as a result of reflex inhibition caused by pain. Tom was immediately given anti-inflammatory medication (diclofenac; Voltarin Rapide) and started on a programme of ice, compression, and elevation to prevent

swelling and to give the injury a chance to 'settle down'. A primary concern at this time was the instability of the knee, as well as the possibility that the injury might be season ending. During the surgeon's assessment, both the team trainer and team physical therapist were present and the findings stated were based on the examination of the surgeon. It was felt that for the team trainer or physical therapist to repeat the tests would be counterproductive because of Tom's apprehension, the starting presence of muscle spasm, which may have affected the accuracy of some tests, and the desire to ensure the vascular clotting mechanism would be interfered with minimally. Because the mechanism of injury was seen by the medical personnel at the time of injury and because the injury was replayed several times on video playback, it was felt there was no need to clear other joints or to do neurological testing. It was a consensus opinion that the MCL had suffered a third degree sprain and the ACL had probably suffered a first degree sprain. As muscle spasm had begun to set in a definitive diagnosis was impossible and so treatment to minimize swelling and pain was immediately instituted.

At the time of the incident, Tom was very apprehensive about the extent of the injury and what effect it would have in the short term, in addition to his long-term prospects as a hockey player. Although he had an understanding of the injury, he was also agitated at being injured so soon after returning to the team to play. He partly felt he was 'letting the team down'. It also bothered him that he should be injured when he was in 'the best shape he had ever been' after spending a great deal of time working on his fitness over the summer. Because of the apprehension on Tom's part, the medical team decided that treatment would be very conservative.

After the application of ice, compression and elevation, Tom was placed in an immobilization brace with crutches to protect the knee and was given analgesics for pain control. In this case, the knee immobilizer brace consisted of an open foam sleeve, which was closed with six velcro straps (three above knee, three below knee) and medial and lateral articulated bar supports. The brace was removed for rehabilitation.

The next day Tom was seen by the athletic trainer, who continued the ice, compression and elevation treatment, and in addition, instituted quadriceps setting (isometric quadriceps in extension) and co-contraction of quadriceps and hamstring exercises to maintain muscle activity. Tom was able to do the exercises with no apparent difficulty. This same treatment was continued for 2 days. Two days after Tom was injured, he underwent a magnetic resonance imaging scan, which indicated that the ACL was intact and that the MCL had suffered a third degree strain or rupture, thus confirming the clinical diagnosis. Over the next two days until surgery, Tom received ice, compression, elevation, and range of motion exercises to the knee to control the swelling and to keep the pain at a minimum. The knee was taken out of the brace while the athlete performed the exercises. Crutches with partial weight bearing were still used by Tom.

Surgery

Five days after the injury occurred, Tom underwent arthroscopic surgery to the right knee to repair the MCL and to reattach the meniscotibial fibres. The previous history indicated that Tom had injured the same knee while playing in college. It was recorded in his preseason assessment by the professional hockey team 6 years earlier that he had a grade II Lachman's test (an anterior

translation of 10–16 mm) and a grade I medial opening (a valgus gapping on the medial side of 5 mm on testing in extension) (Kennedy, 1979; Muller, 1983). He also had a knee that hyperextended. As Tom did not complain of any problems, no special programme for the knee was instituted in the intervening years.

At surgery, the patellofemoral articulation was found to be normal and the medial and lateral femoral gutters were devoid of loose bodies. The suprapatellar pouch was normal and only mildly hyperaemic. The lateral femoral condyle and lateral tibial condyle were normal, as were the medial femoral condyle and medial tibial condyle. On first viewing, the medial meniscus looked normal throughout its length; although it appeared firmly attached around the periphery, there was a small amount of fraying at its posterior attachment. There was no tearing within the intersubstance of the medial meniscus, but there was some disruption of the meniscotibial fibres in its undersurface, giving a small amount of increased mobility to the meniscus when probed. The surgeon decided that this small loose part of the meniscus could be 'caught' or anchored in the suture used to repair the MCL. The intercondylar notch showed a cruciate ligament with all fibres intact, but the fibres themselves demonstrated a small amount of looseness when probed, as if there had been a previous second-degree tear of the intersubstance tissue. There was a small amount of fresh bleeding around the femoral attachment of the fibres of the ACL. The surgeon felt that the new injury to the ACL was probably insignificant and it was deemed unnecessary to tighten the structure. Having inspected the knee joint, the surgeon removed the arthroscope and made a small medial incision. On viewing the MCL, the surgeon noted a complete tear, which was then repaired through the same incision. Finally, the incision was sutured and a pressure dressing applied. The surgeon's postoperative plan was for a very controlled rehabilitation programme avoiding valgus stress to the knee.

REASONING DISCUSSION AND CLINICAL REASONING COMMENTARY

1 What was your interpretation of the findings at surgery and the subsequent surgical repair with respect to your plans for management, precautions required and the patient's prognosis for recovery?

■ Clinician's answer

Based on clinical findings, the magnetic resonance and surgical findings, a decision was made to begin strengthening and range of motion exercises using pain as a guideline as soon as the athlete was able. The surgeon's philosophy was that there was no need to restrict exercises to certain ranges of motion as long as the exercises were done carefully and with control, although no attempt was made to initiate any valgus stress motion at this stage. The surgeon's thinking was that, if he had done a proper repair, controlled range of motion exercises within the pain-free range would not have an adverse effect on the repair. In addition, cryotherapy was used to control swelling and pain. The prognosis for recovery was excellent because the surgery was successful and there were no complications, the patient was very fit and motivated, and the rehabilitation programme was initiated before surgery and continued with only one day off for surgery.

Clinical reasoning commentary

The clinician's reference to the surgeon's philosophy and thinking regarding postoperative management highlights the collaborative decision making essential in a multidisciplinary team approach. Although not always thought of as such, prognoses, like diagnoses, represent clinical patterns. Consideration of prognosis, along with positive and negative features of the presentation that may influence the prognosis (relating to both the person and the problem), will assist clinicians to improve their prognostic decision making. Importantly, when a prognostic hypothesis does not eventuate, the clinician should then take time to reflect on why, including consideration of aspects of the patient's presentation that perhaps were under- or overweighted at the initial assessment.

m | Initial management

Stage 1

Because of the nature of the injury and the anticipated long rehabilitation programme, it was team practice that the team physical therapist become the dominant caregiver, providing regular reports (at least two or three times a week) to the team trainer, who is the coordinator of medical services, and the team physician, an orthopaedic surgeon who performed the surgery.

When Tom was seen by the sports physical therapist following surgery, a regimen of ice, compression, elevation, and quadriceps setting and co-contraction isometric exercises was instituted immediately. On the second day, a range of motion exercises were added within the pain-free range to try to restore range of motion. Analgesic medication was used as well to control pain. Although this pain was real to Tom, it must be remembered that his pain tolerance was judged to be low. Depending on the state of the knee, anti-inflammatory medications were used from time to time by the sports physical therapist in consultation with the orthopaedic surgeon. If there was evidence of overuse in the knee (swelling or pain), the anti-inflammatory drugs were used to control symptoms and treatment was modified.

When first seen by the sports physical therapist, Tom presented with the knee held in slight flexion in an 'off-the-shelf' knee brace. Although the therapist had been involved in the initial assessment, a postsurgical assessment of the knee was required. History indicated the knee was painful following the surgery. Observation showed the knee to be held in approximately 15 degrees of flexion, with a 15 cm wide elastic/ace/tensor bandage applied. On removing the elastic bandage, the wound area was clean and showed no indication of infection. On palpation, the knee was cool, although slightly warmer than the uninjured knee, especially adjacent to the surgical scar. Active movement testing demonstrated that the range was restricted to 10–45 degrees by pain and a soft tissue capsular end-feel, with obvious muscle weakness, notably of the vastus medialis. This was confirmed on resisted isometric testing, with a graded strength of 3/5 for the quadriceps in the range of motion available. The hamstrings demonstrated a strength of 4+/5 in the range of motion available. Passive movement indicated a soft capsular end-feel into both flexion and extension. As Tom had just had his surgery the previous day, no ligamentous testing was performed. Sensory testing was negative except for a 5 cm area distal to the medial surgical scar, which was numb. Interstitial swelling in the knee was evident, but swelling in the joint was minimal. Mobility of the patella was found to be slightly restricted medially and laterally because of interstitial swelling, but patellar tracking appeared normal.

Stage 2

Early in the treatment programme, Tom showed that he was anxious to improve and demonstrated a certain amount of frustration at the slow (in his estimation, not the therapist's) rate of improvement. The therapist treating Tom found that he continually had to advise him that he was progressing at a rate that would be considered quicker than normal, but that tissue recovery would take time progressing from the inflammatory phase to the fibroplasia phase, and finally to the maturation phase. While Tom seemed to understand what the therapist was saying, it did not make it any easier for him to accept that he had been injured. Part of the reason for this is that he was late in returning to the team because he was a 'hold out' caused by salary negotiations with the team and had not attended the training camp at all. In fact, he did not return to the team until well after the first month of league play. He felt he was in the best shape he had ever been in prior to the start of the season; to have this injury occur during only his fourth game after returning presented a quite significant psychological block for the player. The other factor was Tom's relatively low pain tolerance, which led him to believe he was not improving quickly enough.

REASONING DISCUSSION AND CLINICAL REASONING COMMENTARY

1 You have described a psychological block. How did this manifest? What were the key features that emerged in either the subjective examination or in later discussions through the treatment that enabled you to recognize this pattern?

Clinician's answer

The psychological block was indicated by Tom's anxiety at not getting better or not improving as fast as he thought he should. This frustration was continually demonstrated by Tom in his questioning of his progress and his injury, such as why he was not getting better faster and why the pain was not going away, and the depression he demonstrated when things did not go the way he wanted. Tom would demonstrate this depression by his demeanour (slouching, swearing to himself, grabbing and squeezing things).

2 The indications of a psychological block were identified at only 3 days after surgery. At this stage, what were your thoughts on the significance of the psychological aspect of his presentation for your management?

Clinician's answer

While it is common for an individual to be concerned about his/her injury, Tom spent an inordinate amount of time discussing his injury, its progress and his resulting frustration at not being back with the team.

Given the injury, Tom continued to work out to maintain his general fitness. Part of this was probably a way of channelling his frustration at his (in his view) slow progress, but this activity was to later lead to problems of general fatigue and concern about the effect of fatigue on the healing process of his injury. Because he was one of the top athletes on the team, his inability to contribute to the team probably also led to frustration and the feeling he was letting the team down. In addition, Tom may have had a feeling of guilt because he was late joining the team as a result of the contract hold out. Tom's low pain tolerance was also a complicating factor. Throughout the treatment, Tom was continually assured that he was progressing very well and that any setbacks he experienced were part of the healing process and, in part, a result of the aggressive treatment. The clinician had to monitor progress very carefully and watch that Tom was not being pushed 'too hard'. Later in the treatment programme (when he began skating), Tom was given an opportunity to accompany the team on one of the road trips, which helped his psyche a great deal. The psychological overlay may also have affected his pain tolerance. However, even before and since the injury, Tom showed similar low pain tolerance with other injuries. While one might think it would be worthwhile to 'send him fishing' or some similar relaxing activity, such an action would be even harder on the athlete because he would feel he was not doing everything he should to get better. During the season, these athletes only get about 1 day per month in which they are not involved in hockey-related activities.

■ Clinical reasoning commentary

The key issue here, as discussed in Chapter 1, is that patients' psychological status, including their understanding of their problems and management and how they are coping with the effects their problems are having on their lives, can have significant influence on their pain perception, the responsibility they take in the management process and ultimately their outcomes. Like physical clinical syndromes, patients' psychosocial status will present in patterns. However, as with patterns of physical impairment, care is needed not to overly 'box' a patient's psychological status. Rather, cues of psychosocial problems should be attended to, and even screened for, with the view of identifying where the patient's psychosocial status may be interfering with or counterproductive to their recovery. By giving this dimension of a patient's presentation the same consideration that is normally paid to physical impairment, therapists can develop greater skills in assessing for and recognizing patterns of psychosocial presentations that are productive versus counterproductive. As is the case with this patient, management can then be varied accordingly and prognosis viewed with appropriate consideration to these issues.

In an attempt to alleviate Tom's frustration, he was put on a fitness programme for his upper body and uninjured leg 3 days after surgery. This action was taken to get Tom's mind off his injury and to maintain his cardiovascular fitness. The fitness programme was developed by the team fitness consultant with input from the team physical therapist. Seven days post-surgery, Tom began to use the bicycle ergometer with no resistance in an attempt to restore more of the flexion range of motion. Initially, Tom was given electrical muscle stimulation to the quadriceps because he was having trouble 'turning on' the quadriceps to extend the knee. Once a good contraction of the quadriceps was achieved (two treatments), the electrical stimulation was discontinued. An interesting finding with this patient was that he demonstrated only minimal swelling (swelling only slightly evident with the swipe test) after the surgery and throughout the full rehabilitation programme. The main guide used by the physical therapist in determining how far Tom could exercise was the pain level. Because Tom's pain tolerance was low, however, he was encouraged to do controlled activities even if they were uncomfortable. Provided the pain or discomfort ended relatively quickly after stopping the activity, it was felt the injury was not being overstressed. Swelling played a very insignificant role, and even when pushed, the restricting factor was pain not swelling. During this time and subsequent weeks, Tom wore an off-the-shelf fibreglass knee brace prescribed by the surgeon to protect his knee medially and laterally, while allowing flexion and extension within the available range of motion.

Nine days after the injury, Tom experienced a sudden extension force on his knee when he slipped on ice walking outside while wearing the brace (it was winter in Canada). While the increased pain caused Tom some concern, the resulting irritation settled down within 1 day and he was able to continue with his normal treatment and fitness regimens. Ten days after the operation, the surgeon removed the sutures. Tom still demonstrated a lack of 10 degree extension because of capsular stiffness. In the early stages of treatment, it is common practice with this medical team to work within the range available but not to push through pain into full extension. If full extension had been available, naturally Tom would have been worked into that range. Flexion had improved to about 120 degrees. Quadriceps strength had increased to 4/5 within the existing range, while hamstring strength within the available range was normal. Passive movement testing at this stage indicated a capsular end-feel. However, because the tissue was in the early fibroplasia phase of healing, it was felt that increases in range of motion would be attempted primarily by active range of motion exercises, with some gentle passive range of motion elastic stretching to provide only a small amount of healing stress to the tissues.

■ Stage 3

In order to retrain the proprioceptive feedback system affected by the surgery, proprioceptive and control exercises were begun. Exercises included weight shifting, balance exercises (one legged) in combination with body blade (Fig. 12.1), balance board exercises (Fig. 12.2), use of a balance machine, as well as more vigorous closed kinetic chain quadriceps and hamstring exercises (Figs 12.3 and 12.4), including single

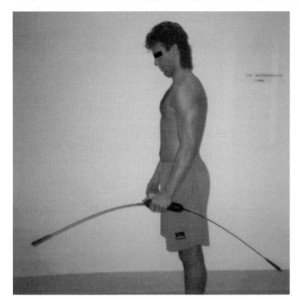

Fig. 12.1 Example of oscillating body blade used for proprioceptive training.

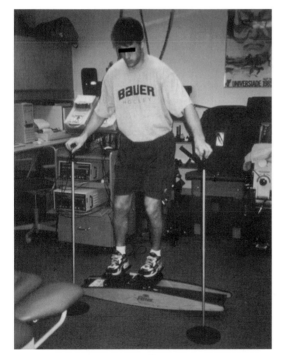

Fig. 12.2 Athlete on 'Profitter'® (dynamic balance apparatus, reproduced with permission of Fitter International Inc).

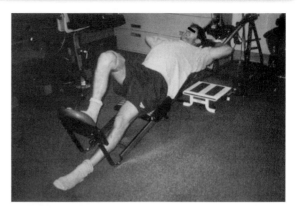

Fig. 12.3 Athlete on incline plane using body weight as resistance. Note the unstable base.

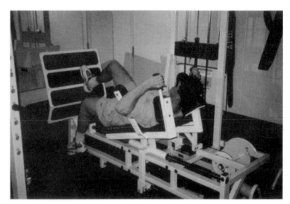

Fig. 12.4 Athlete doing single leg press. Note knee flexion does not go past 90 degrees.

leg wall slides and tubing into extension while weight bearing. When doing the exercises, the therapist watched to ensure that correct, controlled motion occurred. Often, because of injury, proprioceptive feedback and the ability to control motion is lost to some degree. Consequently, only motions that Tom could do correctly in the available range were allowed. These exercises provided a small healing stress to the injured tissues, as well as range of motion and strengthening effects. The progression of exercises was based on the ability of Tom to control the exercise he was asked to do and on the pain response. Very specific instructions were given to Tom and if he deviated he was stopped to prevent incorrect movement patterning from developing. When Tom demonstrated an ability to do an activity, the repetition, weight used or time were increased. At the same time, Tom's work on the bicycle ergometer increased from 5 minutes with no resistance to 20 minutes with resistance now being implemented. The seat height was modified as he went through the exercise regimen, with the height lowered every 5 minutes until knee flexion became uncomfortable.

One of the problems that had to be dealt with early in the rehabilitation process was the noticeable quadriceps lag that developed before full extension was achieved. Diligent work by Tom, however, led to full

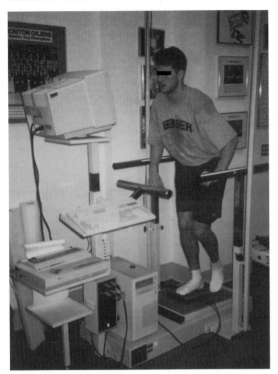

Fig. 12.5 Athlete on balance machine. Base may be static or dynamic. Athlete is concentrating on keeping his centre of gravity by viewing the computer screen and either statically or dynamically maintaining the 'ball' image centred.

active extension within about 10 days of accomplishing full passive extension range of motion. This lag was of initial concern because, as long as it was present, it indicated that he did not have control in part of his extension range, making him potentially vulnerable to injury or re-injury. The exercises included quadriceps setting exercises, wall slides, 90 degree squats and extension against tubing resistance. With full extension and the ability to do closed kinetic chain activities with no difficulty and no adverse effect, more vigorous open kinetic chain activities were instituted beyond the quadriceps setting and leg straightening exercises. Tom began jogging very slowly forwards and backwards,

as well as ascending/descending stairs at speeds (slow) at which he felt comfortable and the therapist felt he could control. In addition, on the balance machine, target training was instituted with the targets designed to increase the valgus stress to the MCL (Fig. 12.5). By concentrating on keeping the 'dot' on target, Tom was working on maintaining control while stressing the MCL and facilitating the mechanoreceptors in the joint and muscles.

Stage 4

About 3 weeks following the surgery, ultrasound was instituted to facilitate further the healing and fibroplasia phase of the tissue. It was felt by the physical therapist that, given the normal continuum of soft tissue healing (clotting phase, inflammatory phase, fibroplasia phase and maturation phase), Tom was now well into the fibroplasia phase of healing and at this stage ultrasound would be effective in helping stimulating collagen formation. The end-feel at this point was still tissue stretch, but the pain Tom was feeling on passive stretch was decreasing. It was also found during application of the ultrasound to the medial side of the knee, which was the area of original numbness, that this area had become extremely hypersensitive to the movement of the sound head. This appeared to represent a true decrease in pain threshold rather than just a low pain tolerance. By continued use of the ultrasound over the area and by giving instructions to Tom to rub the area gently with a skin cream to help to desensitize the tissues, the hypersensitivity decreased over a period of time although the numb area remained. Tom continued to work out to maintain his physical fitness. In fact, it was felt by the physical therapist that he was working out too hard, spending 6–8 hours a day working on his physical fitness. Because he was becoming exhausted from working the other parts of his body so hard to maintain and improve his fitness level, it was hypothesized that this may have been impeding the healing process.

  REASONING DISCUSSION AND CLINICAL REASONING COMMENTARY

1 What is the pathophysiological basis for general fatigue to interfere with the healing process?

Clinician's answer

General fatigue can be the result of several factors. Fatigue may be central or peripheral, both of which may directly or indirectly affect the healing process. Metabolic fatigue is primarily peripheral, leading to reduced ATP, lower blood glucose levels, muscle glycogen depletion, dehydration, and loss of electrolytes. Neuromuscular fatigue, which may occur peripherally or centrally, can result in substances competing for receptor sites, with cholinesterase increases and acetylcholine decreases leading to impaired neuromuscular transmission and/or propagation of a muscle action potential, as well as reduced motor unit recruitment and a psychological overlay, especially if the fatigue is chronic. Electrophysiological fatigue leads to decreased membrane potentials. All of the types of fatigue affect the force-generating capacity of the muscle as well as affecting the 'building blocks' of repair through stress on the endocrine system, which will, in turn, slow the rehabilitation progression.

2 Do you feel this patient's psyche, which you have already highlighted as a problem, could also be contributing to his fatigue and healing capacity?

Clinician's answer

Tom's psyche may have compounded the fatigue and overtraining problems. Often, especially in the early stages, Tom reported difficulty with sleeping and tiredness, not because of the injury, but because of having 'nothing to do' during the day and evening, although he spent an inordinate amount of time 'working out'.

Clinical reasoning commentary

The biomedical knowledge evident in this answer, along with the clinical implication noted in the clinician's last statement, highlights the combination of biomedical and clinical knowledge that contribute to expert therapists' organization of professional knowledge. The clinician's hypothesized involvement of the endocrine system illustrates a broad perspective beyond the obvious local tissue injury/repair and supports the value of including pathobiological hypotheses in one's clinical reasoning. Such considerations should encourage therapists to be alert to the links between the various input, processing and output mechanisms that are known to exist. For example, similar to the fatigue, this patient's observed frustration may also have been contributing to stress-related endocrine effects such as altered sleeping and compromised healing. Skilled clinical reasoning requires a highly developed and contextually relevant organization of knowledge. Contemporary manual therapy requires that this knowledge base includes understanding of the inter-relationships between the different body systems (e.g. psychological status, sensory-motor, endocrine and immune systems), screening questions for symptoms of impairment in the different systems, and how best to modify management, including appropriate referral when impairment is suspected. While it is not possible for the manual therapist also to be a psychologist, endocrinologist and immunologist, we are often the first person with which the patient shares such symptoms, and as such it is critical that manual therapists at least have the knowledge and awareness to seek further consultation.

Stage 5

By 3 weeks, Tom was doing one-legged wall slides as well as balancing exercises, lunge exercises, and several different quadriceps exercises. Ball bouncing exercises were instituted to improve further flexion range of motion, proprioception and ballistically controlled motion. As well, resistance was continually added to the bicycle ergometer exercise. The amount of resistance set on the bicycle ergometer was determined by the desired stress to be placed on the knee, and not by a desired cardiovascular training effect. The desired level of stress was determined subjectively by

Tom's reaction to the new load. Tom was continually monitored during the exercise, with the therapist noting any change in symptoms while riding the bike, after treatment, and before beginning treatment the next day. Tom was made to understand the difference between stress pain, which disappeared when activity stopped, and pain that lingered after the activity stopped, indicating too much stress was applied to the knee. By 4 weeks, Tom had progressed on the bicycle ergometer to approximately 100 watts resistance and the seat had been lowered close to normal functional levels.

As well as doing exercises with the therapist offering resistance or using tubing, the use of exercise machines was also instituted (leg press, hamstrings machine, abduction/adduction machine with resistance above knee). Repetitions and weight were set depending on Tom's ability to do the required repetitions without adverse symptoms. Alternate days were used for strength (high load, low repetitions) and endurance (low load, high repetitions) training. Tubing was also progressively used with more and more functional activities, such as resistance in proprioceptive neuromuscular facilitation (PNF) patterns and oblique movement, as well as resistance in skating type motions. Resistance was initially applied above the knee, but as the healing process progressed the resistance was applied to the tibia to increase the healing stress to the tissues that had been repaired. With these functional activities, Tom's ability to control the movement was the deciding factor concerning repetitions and load. As soon as Tom demonstrated loss of control (altered movement patterns, altered muscle contraction patterns anywhere in the kinetic chain but especially at the knee or more proximally in the lumbopelvic-hip stabilizers), the exercise was stopped.

REASONING DISCUSSION AND CLINICAL REASONING COMMENTARY

1 With pain assessment forming a significant component to the progression of rehabilitation for this patient, can you comment on the difficulties that can arise when the athlete does not accurately report the onset or severity of pain? Were there any patient-induced rehabilitation problems with this patient, such as inaccurate pain reporting or taking of analgesics, that resulted in his programme being advanced too quickly?

Clinician's answer

Because of Tom's low pain tolerance, the pain 'scale' had to be adjusted downward. Also, an understanding of the difference between the pain of injury and pain of activity had to be determined and the difference had to be understood by Tom. In this case, Tom truly felt the pain but with his tolerance so low

(relative to what would normally be expected), care had to be taken when considering the number of repetitions and progression in the rehabilitation programme so that the 'progression envelope' was not pushed too far. Continual closely supervised monitoring enabled the clinician to keep within an acceptable envelope of progression.

Clinical reasoning commentary

The clinician's recognition that pain is a different and unique experience for each patient and should be accepted as such is evident here. He does not 'judge' the patient or discount his pain experience as non-genuine. Rather, the 'progression envelope' is adjusted for this particular patient while taking care not to reinforce the unhelpful belief that pain necessarily equals harm, a yellow flag that can predispose to chronic pain.

 ## Further management

Stage 6

Five weeks after the surgery, it was decided by the physical therapist that as much range of motion as could be accomplished by doing active exercises had been accomplished, and therefore plastic stretching (therapeutic creep) of the tissues was instituted. The end-feel was still a tissue stretch (capsular), but the

limiting factor to range was now felt to be the tight capsule rather than muscle weakness. The therapist felt the tissue healing was sufficiently progressed that plastic stretching to increase the range of motion was the best route to follow without disrupting the healing tissue. In order to do this, the knee was placed so the foot rested on a padded bar with the knee itself not supported. A 6 lb (2.7 kg) weight was applied to the knee along with hydrocollator packs and a 15 minute stretch was instituted (Fig. 12.6). To accomplish

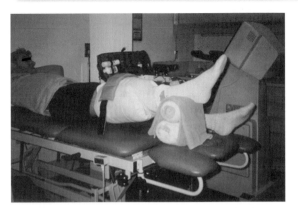

Fig. 12.6 Plastic stretching (therapeutic creep) of posterior knee structures. Note hotpacks around knee and weight applied on top.

therapeutic creep of collagen tissue, a slow progressive stretch should be instituted lasting 15–30 minutes for maximum effect (Kottke et al., 1966; Sapega et al., 1981). Stretching for less than 5 minutes is unlikely to have much permanent effect on the collagen tissue. Fifteen minutes was chosen because of Tom's discomfort level after 5 minutes. Maximum load when doing plastic stretching should be 8–10 lb (3.6–4.5 kg) (Kottke et al., 1966; Sapega et al., 1981). By heating the tissues, therapeutic creep is more easily achieved. Tom was able to tolerate this very well for the first 5 minutes and then felt the stretching become more and more uncomfortable for the remaining 10 minutes. Within five treatments, significant improvement in range of motion was noted, with full extension range of motion and a normal tissue stretch end-feel accomplished within 2 weeks. At the same time, flexion range of motion had virtually returned to normal through the exercise programme without plastic stretching.

Stage 7

By 6 weeks, Tom began doing Cybex isokinetic exercises at slow speed settings of 30, 60, 90 and 120 degrees per second maximum (three sets of 10 depending on fatigue and symptoms). At this time, Tom would have some good days and some bad days depending on how hard he pushed both his exercise for his knee and his cardiovascular fitness. A 'bad day' experience for Tom was the knee not feeling as good as the previous day, with some aching combined with a negative psychological overlay and difficulty sleeping. Tom's frustration with his progress, which in reality was excellent, was almost palpable. It was eventually hypothesized that his cardiovascular fitness programme was creating major fatigue problems for Tom. This was later shown to be true as Tom made even better progress with his knee rehabilitation when he cut back his fitness programme. There was also a certain psychological overlay on how well the athlete felt he was improving, how quickly he would get back and what effect the injury would have on his performance. This particular athlete was the top athlete and one of the leaders on the hockey team; therefore, considerable pressure was being put on him (both by himself and the team) to return to play and also to perform at a very high level when he returned. At this stage, the fitness programme (controlled by the team fitness consultant at another location) was fully integrated into the knee rehabilitation programme, with the physical therapist having final say as to what Tom would be allowed to do in both the fitness and the rehabilitation programmes. Tom had the seat at a normal level while using the bicycle ergometer and was cycling for 30 minutes. The intensity (load) placed on the bicycle ergometer was now determined by the desired cardiovascular effect rather than the stress on the knee.

Tom began by working at 70% of his maximum heart rate for this effect and worked up to 85%. Other exercises continued including quadriceps exercises, using the balance machine, balancing exercises, and more functional exercises such as slow jogging forward and backward, carioca exercises (running sideways with cross-over steps), pylon running (slow) forwards and backwards (running around pylons so person turns right and left), figure-8 running (slow), and ascending/descending stairs. During this period, Tom was fitted with a custom functional brace, which he began wearing during his exercise programme in order to become used to it, as he would be wearing this brace when he returned to competition. As the leg dimensions are usually altered following injury, it is common practice for the medical team to fit the athlete with an 'off-the-shelf' brace initially to protect the knee because it is less expensive. Once the leg dimensions are close to normal (compared with the uninjured leg), a custom brace is fitted for the athlete to return to competition. Commonly this brace is then worn at least until the end of the season. The custom brace was a brace designed by a local orthotist to provide medial and lateral protection to the knee.

Stage 8

By the seventh week, in addition to the above programme, Tom began skipping and doing high-speed Cybex isokinetic exercises (speeds: 120, 180, 240 degrees per second; 1 minute exercise, 1 minute rest, three repetitions at each speed) for endurance. Also, based on Tom's ability to control his knee motion both in closed and open kinetic chain activities, more difficult kinetic chain activities were instituted, such as one-legged hop exercises forwards, backwards, to the side, and around a cross (+). At the end of 7 weeks, in addition to the above programme that continued, Tom had demonstrated adequate strength, control, endurance and agility improvements to begin skating. His initial skating episode was 15 minutes of easy skating with no equipment except skates, elbow pads, helmet, gloves, and stick. As Tom improved, the time, speed and difficulty of the skating exercises were increased. Initially Tom did not have a puck to handle or shoot, but a puck was included as he progressed to make the activity more complex. Because Tom was a highly skilled hockey player, it was necessary that the physical therapist be present for all the initial skating sessions as Tom had a very strong tendency to want to do too much at each session. Consequently, his activity had to be very carefully controlled. Skating drills at the early stage included skating hard between the blue lines (straight ahead) and coasting around the ends (curves), figure-8 skating, crossing the 'T' at centre ice (skating forwards, backwards and sideways within the centre ice circle), as well as just skating with the puck doing various skating drills (Fig. 12.7). In addition, Tom continued with his skipping (forward and backward), riding the bike for 30 minutes, climbing stairs, and working on the exercise machines.

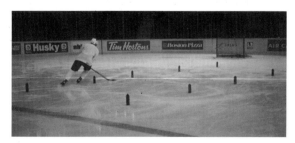

Fig. 12.7   Player doing pylon skating as part of his functional retraining.

Stage 9

By the eighth week, skating was more rigorous and Tom was using the exercise machines at higher levels and higher weights. Tom's skill level of skating even at this stage was better than many professional hockey players and he had to be controlled to ensure he did not overstress the knee. Skipping and hopping were continued as was stair work. Because of the control, strength and endurance demonstrated by Tom during skating and during his exercises, plyometrics were instituted to improve further the reactive ability of the lower limb neuromuscular system. Activities included jumping on and off a bench and jumping over a bench.

By the end of 8 weeks, Tom was skating up to 45 minutes and the bicycle programme varied from one day to the next: one day being an endurance (aerobic) programme and the next day being a sprint (anaerobic) programme. This enabled training of the two primary energy systems (80% anaerobic and 20% aerobic) used in ice hockey, as well as improving the aerobic system to facilitate recovery following exercise. Throughout the programme, Tom received treatment 6 days per week on a one to one basis with the physical therapist. This high level of treatment visits is common for professional athletes where funding is not an issue but where getting a highly trained and paid athlete back to playing his sport is of prime importance.

Stage 10

By the end of 10 weeks, Tom was cleared to skate with the team in practice. This is classed as a controlled skating with controlled activity as the athlete goes through specific passing and skating drills along with the rest of the team, but there is no body contact. If the athlete is allowed to return to practise with the team, he is expected to do everything other team members do, except for body contact. Initially, the athlete is not allowed to scrimmage (play a controlled 'game' with other players) until the medical team is sure the athlete has no problem with team drills. If he has no problems with the drills, as was the case with Tom, he is allowed to scrimmage. If he has no problems with scrimmaging and tests (Cybex tests, functional tests, physical examination) show no problems, the athlete is allowed to return to competition if he feels he is ready. By the twelfth week, Tom returned to play.

REASONING DISCUSSION AND CLINICAL REASONING COMMENTARY

1 Can you comment on why you think the flexion improved with active exercise while the extension required passive stretching?

■ Clinician's answer

Why flexion required no plastic stretching while extension did is difficult to ascertain. It may have been because the hamstrings demonstrated greater strength following surgery, being able progressively to 'stretch' or stress the anterior capsule more markedly. Alternatively, flexion may not have stressed the MCL as much (in flexion, the anterior fibres of the ligament are primarily stressed), allowing the athlete to work on flexion to a greater degree with less discomfort.

2 What guided your decision to adjust the principal aim of the bicycle ergometer exercise from one based on the local stress placed on the knee to one of cardiovascular fitness?

■ Clinician's answer

Once the point was reached when Tom's knee was able to stand the stresses of normal closed kinetic chain activity, and because no symptoms resulted from these stresses, it was felt that he could do normal cardiovascular training using both legs. Up to this point, Tom was using an upper body ergometer for his cardiovascular fitness.

3 There seems to be a number of health professionals involved in this athlete's rehabilitation. Could you comment on what was required of the therapist in his interprofessional communication with the other health professionals, the coach, manager, team owner, etc.? How does this impact on the decisions made by the therapist and how can risk of conflicting information be minimized when so many people are involved? There is clearly pressure to get the player back to his sport as soon as possible. Can you also comment on how certain strategies, such as the surgeon taking the responsibility of liaising with management or other professionals, may be used to lessen such pressures on the therapist and the athlete?

■ Clinician's answer

It is common practice with the team involved that the physical therapist is the primary care giver and determines the course of treatment, in conjunction with the physician and team athletic trainer, in situations when physical therapy is required after surgery. Initially, there was a breakdown in communication with the fitness person because this was the first year such a person was available to the team. The surgeon was readily available if the physical therapist had any questions, since the surgeon, physical therapist and fitness person attended all home hockey games (average of one to two per week). This allowed the situation to be continually reviewed and discussed with the athletic trainer, coach and general manager (if necessary). Tom was seen by all people involved. Although there was pressure to return Tom to playing as soon as possible because of the player's value to the team, there was never so much pressure that he was forced to return too early. With this team, the health of the athlete is of primary importance.

4 What was your clinical reasoning and scientific rationale for implementing plyometric exercises at the eighth week (stage 9)?

■ Clinician's answer

As plyometrics is a high-stress activity that requires good control, it was not instituted until Tom could demonstrate satisfactory control in functional activities. The purpose of the plyometric exercises was to enhance the neuromuscular system by improving its reactive ability through combining speed of movement (doing the bounce in the jump quickly) and strength (lifting his body weight). The activity involves eccentric landing, activating the stretch reflex, and concentric push off. This action of landing on the toes and pushing off quickly is used when skating and helps to improve reaction time, which is important in a fast moving sport such as hockey.

4 Would you describe what precautions were observed during the rehabilitation for this patient?

Clinician's answer

Tom's treatment was designed to 'push the envelope' of healing and, provided no adverse signs and symptoms appeared, he was continually pushed. Red flags, which led the physical therapist to modify or 'back off' on treatment, included increased pain, persistent stiffness and strength plateauing. Other factors that could have been included but were not factors here include swelling in the joint or tissues, continued muscle burning, onset of crepitus and fasciculations or cramps in muscle.

Clinical reasoning commentary

In response to question 3, the clinician has provided a nice example of collaborative reasoning in action. Collaborative reasoning, as portrayed in Chapter 1, is the shared decision making between patient, health-care providers (in this case the physical therapist, orthopaedic surgeon and the athletic trainer) and relevant others contributing to management decisions or being affected by such decisions (in this case the coach and general manager). In other patients, significant stakeholders may include family, employers and funding bodies. The benefits of shared decision making are increasingly being recognized across the health professions (Ersser and Atkins, 2000) and developing expertise in manual therapy requires that practitioners acquire these skills.

The strategic introduction of plyometric exercises highlights the specificity of training required when working with high-level athletes such as this patient. Even when postoperative protocols exist (i.e. the surgeon's and rehabilitation team's approach to rehabilitating this type of repair), this case nicely highlights how individual patient treatment selection and progression decisions are based on that patient's particular presentation and his response to treatments, as determined by the ongoing reassessment of specific physical impairments and functional indicators. Physiotherapy expertise in this setting requires special surgery- and sport-specific knowledge in order to implement and progress the optimum rehabilitation strategies for maximum speed of recovery without compromising the healing tissues or incurring a risk of recurrence.

Outcome

At 1 month following Tom's return to play (16 weeks), he still had not reached his full potential following the injury. This was evident to both the coaches and the medical team. Tom was not performing at the level that he was at before the injury. Although he could skate as fast, he was tentative in his play making and showed hesitation when there was the potential of body contact. Tom stated that he felt the knee was fine although he still had some 'twinges' in the knee when playing. As a precaution against swelling or pain, Tom received ice to the knee for 15 minutes after every practice, game or workout. From the beginning, he was told by the physical therapist and the orthopaedic surgeon that it would be a long-term process and that the healing would probably take at least a year to be completed, but Tom felt he could overcome these things and compete with no difficulty. It must be remembered that the majority of athletes are young, very healthy and very good at their sport, with high expectations especially in professional sport. To receive a major injury often makes them face their own mortality, and many people have difficulty dealing with this along with their injury. Tom found that although he was able to skate and play he was not able to bring his level of play up to that he had previously achieved, although there was improvement. Psychologically this was very hard for Tom, but the therapist continued to work with him to try to ensure that he would return to his full level of ability. At 24 weeks, Tom had almost returned to his full potential. However, a sport psychologist was also enlisted to help him to deal with his apprehension and frustration.

REASONING DISCUSSION AND CLINICAL REASONING COMMENTARY

1 In hindsight and with the presence of the early indicators of psychological factors, do you think that the sports psychologist should have been consulted sooner in this particular case?

Clinician's answer

On reflection, it probably would have been of benefit to consult a sports psychologist earlier in the rehabilitation programme. One thing this case has illustrated to me, now that I watch more closely for these adverse psychological reactions, is how fragile is the psyche of many athletes, which in many ways is surprising given the high demands and sometimes viciousness of contact/collision sports. Athletes, probably more than most patients, require a great deal of positive reinforcement on how they are progressing. The fear of losing their livelihood (and sometimes high salaries) is very real to them.

Clinical reasoning commentary

The key word from a reasoning perspective in this answer is 'reflection'. It is often incorrectly assumed that experts have such good knowledge and vast experience that they do not make 'mistakes'. Every expert represented in this book would certainly discount this assumption. Experts do make mistakes, but because they tend to possess superior metacognitive skills, including continual reflection, they learn from their patient experiences, continually building and refining their knowledge and skills for use with future patients. Experts have superior knowledge, not superior memory. They have superior knowledge because their reasoning is open-minded, critical and reflective.

References

Ersser, S.J. and Atkins, S. (2000). Clinical reasoning and patient-centred care. In Clinical Reasoning in the Health Professions (J. Higgs and M. Jones, eds.) pp. 68–77. Oxford: Butterworth-Heinemann.

Kennedy, J.C. (1979). The Injured Adolescent Knee. Baltimore, MD: Williams & Wilkins.

Kottke, F.J., Pauley, D.L. and Ptak, R.A. (1966). The rationale for prolonged stretching for correction of shortening of connective tissue. Archives of Physical Medicine and Rehabilitation, 47, 345–352.

Muller, W. (1983). The Knee: Form, Function and Ligament Reconstruction. Berlin: Springer-Verlag.

Sapega, A.A., Quedenfeld, T.C., Moyer, R.A. and Butler, R.A. (1981). Biophysical factors in range of motion exercise. Physical Sports Medicine 9, 57–65.

Further reading

Ellenbecker, T.S. (2000). Knee Ligament Rehabilitation. Edinburgh: Churchill-Livingstone.

Griffin, L.Y. (1995). Rehabilitation of the Injured Knee. London: Mosby.

Hughston, J.C. (1993). Knee Ligaments: Injury and Repair. London: Mosby.

Scott, W.N. (1991). Ligament and Extensor Mechanism Injuries of the Knee. London: Mosby.`

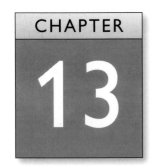

CHAPTER 13

Patellofemoral pain in a professional tennis player

Jenny McConnell

SUBJECTIVE EXAMINATION

A 27-year-old professional tennis player presented with a 6-month history of gradually worsening left knee pain. The player complained of anteroinferior pain, as well as lateral knee pain. The lateral knee pain, which only became a complaint 6 weeks ago when the player changed orthotics, was extremely severe, particularly when the knee was flexed in both the stance and swing phases of gait. The pain was so severe that he was forced to pull out of a tournament. It was less intense at the time of presentation, but he had not been stressing the knee at all as for the past month he had been non-weight bearing on crutches.

This was because the magnetic resonance imaging (MRI) scan showed a bone bruise on the lateral side of the trochlear notch. The enforced rest on crutches had resulted in marked atrophy of the quadriceps muscle but had not changed his inferior patellar symptoms to any great degree, although the lateral symptoms had subsided. He was now very depressed as his tennis ranking was sliding and his knee was not improving. He was unsure of his future and was contemplating retiring from tennis on medical grounds, but this was not his preferred option.

REASONING DISCUSSION AND CLINICAL REASONING COMMENTARY

1 From the information elicited at this early stage, were you at all able to recognize a clinical pattern in his initial presentation? What were your principal hypotheses for the two pains, and were there any other potential sources that you considered and planned to test through further examination?

Clinician's answer

From the initial part of the history, it was clear that the athlete had two different types of knee pain, which could possibly be related. The more recent lateral pain

was suggestive of an iliotibial band (ITB) friction syndrome, because the player was complaining of the lateral knee pain during flexion, even unweighted flexion, of the knee. In the flexed position of the knee, the ITB is under tension, and if tight it will rub over the lateral femoral condyle, causing a tendonosis of the ITB or an inflammation of the intervening bursa (Brukner and Khan, 1993). Additionally, the change in orthotics may have been sufficient to alter the balance of the structures in the lower extremity and place more stress on the ITB. If the orthotic is made from a rigid or semi-rigid material, then shock attenuation at the foot may be poor, particularly if the patient has a stiff rearfoot (Grelsamer and McConnell, 1998). This decrease in shock absorption places increased stress on the distal end of the ITB, as the internal rotatory force of the tibia, which should occur with knee flexion, is blocked by the distal external rotatory force created by the orthotic. The long-standing inferior pain could be caused by a patellofemoral problem or patellar tendonosis. More information from the history about the behaviour of the pain is required before a provisional diagnosis can be formulated.

The MRI had ruled out a stress fracture. Whether there was underlying chondromalacia and whether it was contributing to the patient's symptoms could not be definitely determined at this stage. The state of the articular cartilage can only be assessed with a T_2-weighted image on MRI, so it is possible the patient had some chondral degeneration, which is common in tennis players. However, recent evidence has suggested that articular cartilage degeneration is usually asymptomatic (Dye et al., 1998). Nonetheless, symptoms a clinician would need to be aware of to determine the presence of articular cartilage degeneration include swelling and locking, as well as pain.

Therefore, chondromalacia is a less likely diagnosis in this case.

■ Clinical reasoning commentary

The early formulation of hypotheses relating to the source of the pains (e.g. patellar tendonosis) and potential contributing factors (e.g. change in orthotics) is evident in this response. In particular, the identification of initial cues (the location of the lateral pain in an elite athlete and its behaviour) appears to have triggered the recognition of a familiar clinical pattern, i.e. ITB friction syndrome. Diagnostic accuracy in pattern recognition is largely dependent on previous clinical experience with similar presentations and is, therefore, not usually an important feature of the clinical reasoning of novice practitioners but is heavily relied upon by experts, such as in this case. It is important to highlight that the clinician has also drawn on information from knowledge gained indirectly from the literature and that this has been effectively integrated with knowledge directly gained from her own personal clinical experiences.

The inferior knee pain did not keep the patient awake at night, but it did cause him considerable discomfort when he was standing and going up and down stairs. The knee did not lock, click or give way, but it had been swollen. The swelling was mostly infrapatellar, but he did occasionally notice minor joint effusion after playing. When the player was first aware of his knee symptoms 6 months ago, he had been playing on grass and was running back from the net to reach a high backhand smash. He won the point, but as he made contact with the ball he felt a pinching sensation distally in his knee. That evening the knee was slightly puffy, so he iced it and sought some treatment. The treatment consisted of electrotherapy (ultrasound and interferential current), as well as quadriceps muscle stretching and strengthening. The quadriceps strengthening involved straight leg raises and isokinetic leg extension. The knee initially was only intermittently painful, but after 3 weeks of treatment it had worsened from being painful only when the player was returning low volleys, to being painful during all aspects of play.

Additionally, the patient reported that non-steroidal anti-inflammatory medication (the only medication he was taking) did not have any effect on the symptoms. He had never taken steroids, nor experienced any symptoms in the hips, feet, lumbar spine or any other joint. This was his first episode of left knee pain. He had experienced medial pain in the right knee 5 years ago, which improved with the fitting of flexible orthotics in his shoes. The orthotics were prescribed for his forefoot valgus deformity, which caused excessive pronation at midstance. He used flexible orthotics until recently, when a computer-generated pair was made. It was after this that the left lateral knee pain developed.

His general health was good with no recent weight loss, and the only surgery he had undergone was an appendectomy 3 years ago. The plain radiograph of the knee was unremarkable, but the MRI showed a bone bruise on the trochlear notch. It was this finding that prompted the orthopaedic surgeon to put the patient on crutches. However, as the patient was not improving and becoming increasingly anxious with each day away from training, the surgeon referred the patient to me.

REASONING DISCUSSION AND CLINICAL REASONING COMMENTARY

1 What was your interpretation of the worsening of the athlete's knee problem? Did the additional information regarding the mechanism of symptom onset enable you to narrow your hypotheses further regarding the source of the inferior knee pain?

Clinician's answer

At this stage, it became clear that rapid extension of the knee (retrieving the high backhand smash) produced the initial pain and that the treatment may have been instrumental in worsening the symptoms. Therefore, the most likely diagnosis for the tennis player's inferior patellar pain was an irritated fat pad, because it was triggered initially by a rapid extension manoeuvre, manifested returning from flexion (returning a low volley) and was also exacerbated by treatment. It is unlikely that the electrotherapy part of the treatment was the culprit, but it was possible that the quadriceps work, particularly the strengthening exercises, may have contributed to the increase in symptoms. The strengthening exercises emphasized extension of the knee, which can cause an increase in symptoms when the fat pad is inflamed. Once the fat pad is inflamed, forced extension of the knee, which causes a posterior tilting of the inferior pole of the patella as a result of the attachment of the patellar tendon on the tibia, may further irritate the fat pad. The fat pad has been found to be the most pain-sensitive structure in the knee (Dye et al., 1998).

At this stage, the differential diagnosis of patellar tendonosis could be largely discounted for three reasons.

1. There had been no reported increase in eccentric loading of the quadriceps during training or match play. Tendonosis is usually provoked by an increase in eccentric loading of the quadriceps muscle.
2. The particular quadriceps exercises given should not have markedly worsened the symptoms as there is less tension in the tendon during knee extension and straight leg raise than during eccentric activities.
3. The MRI did not demonstrate any degenerative change in the patellar tendon, which usually occurs when tendonosis is present.

2 What weighting did you place on the MRI finding of a bone bruise?

Clinician's answer

The bone bruise may have been incidental to the patient's symptoms in so far as the patient was complaining primarily of inferior patellar not retropatellar pain, which was the location of the bone bruise. In addition, being on crutches (rest) for a month had not changed the patient's inferior patellar symptoms at all, which would have been anticipated if the symptoms were arising from the bone bruise.

3 How did the working hypotheses you entertained influence your planning of the physical examination?

Clinician's answer

At the completion of the history, the provisional diagnosis for the patient's lateral knee pain was ITB friction syndrome and the provisional diagnosis for the inferior knee pain was an irritated infrapatellar fat pad. Both conditions are usually the consequence of poor patellofemoral biomechanics, such as a tight ITB, poor pelvic control and excessive foot pronation. The aim of the physical examination was to test further possible sources of the symptoms and to determine which of the biomechanical variables were contributing to the patient's symptoms, so that treatment could be directed accordingly.

There were several examination procedures of particular importance with respect to testing the working hypotheses:

- the Thomas test, which assesses the tightness of the tensor fasciae latae (TFL), as well as the rectus femoris and psoas muscles
- Ober's test, performed in side lying, usually elicits pain when the knee is flexed and extended from 0 to 30 degrees if the ITB is tight; this is because it flicks over the lateral femoral epicondyle causing inflammation and pain
- when the condition is acute, the lateral femoral epicondyle is often quite tender on palpation and the fat pad is frequently enlarged and when palpated feels quite 'boggy' compared with the other side, with the patella buried in the fat pad such that the inferior pole is difficult to palpate

inferior patellar pain is often exacerbated by an active quadriceps contraction in full extension, as well as during passive extension performed by the therapist.

Clinical reasoning commentary

Following the early generation of diagnostic hypotheses based on recognition of initial cues from familiar clinical patterns, the information obtained from subsequent enquiry strategies (e.g. the worsening of the problem) is used to test the competing hypotheses. The picture that unfolds is one in which there is growing evidence that supports one hypothesis (irritated fat pad) and other clinical data that tend to negate the alternative hypothesis (patellar tendonosis), often an absence of an expected finding. A plausible pathomechanical hypothesis consistent with the clinical presentation and with scientific understanding of knee pathology lends further weight to the favoured diagnostic hypothesis.

The assessment of the MRI finding of a bone bruise demonstrates testing of a diagnostic hypothesis (bone bruise as both source of the symptoms and associated pathobiological mechanism) with other findings from the history (location of pain and response to rest), which are found not to support the hypothesis. Consequently, the hypothesis has been rejected and the main supporting clinical evidence (MRI scan) reinterpreted as an incidental finding.

PHYSICAL EXAMINATION

Observation

Examination of the patient in standing revealed an internally rotated femur, tibial varum, an enlarged fat pad on the left side, stiff rearfoot and compensatory midfoot pronation. The rearfoot was deemed to be stiff because the talus was quite prominent on the medial side when the patient was viewed from the front but the calcaneum was straight when viewed from behind. If the talus was prominent on the medial side in standing, the calcaneum should be everted if the rearfoot had adequate mobility. The left quadriceps muscle, although smaller than the other side, was well defined. The ITB appeared taut on both sides. The gluteus maximus muscle was well developed, but the gluteus medius muscle was suboptimal in bulk bilaterally.

The patient was examined dynamically to evaluate the effect of muscle action on the static mechanics, as well as to reproduce symptoms. The least stressful activity of walking, which did not reproduce any symptoms, was examined first. There was minimal knee flexion evident at heel strike on the left side during walking. The patient also demonstrated increased trunk side flexion on the left side during the stance phase of gait, often suggestive of weakness of the gluteus medius and perhaps more proximal weakness of the trunk. In this case, it was probably poor gluteal control contributing to the problem rather than proximal trunk weakness, as the patient was regularly doing Pilates exercise classes as well as abdominal strengthening activities in the gym. The inferior patellar pain was reproduced at 60 degrees of knee flexion when descending stairs, during which the trunk lateral flexion was even more pronounced.

Passive examination procedures

In supine lying, the inferior pain was slightly elicited on passive extension overpressure of the knee. All other passive movement tests were clear, including flexion overpressure (straight and with an abduction and adduction bias), McMurray's test for the meniscus, and Lachman and pivot shift tests for the anterior cruciate ligament.

Muscle length tests

The TFL muscles were found to be bilaterally tight during the Thomas test. The iliopsoas, rectus femoris and TFL muscles may all be tested using the Thomas test (Hoppenfeld, 1976; Kendall and McCreary, 1983). To perform the Thomas test, the patient stands with his ischia touching the end of the plinth. One leg is pulled up to the chest to flatten the lumbar lordosis, and then the patient lies down on the plinth keeping the flexed leg close to the chest. The other leg should be resting such that the hip is in the neutral position (i.e. on the plinth, at the same width as the pelvis) and the knee should be flexed to 90 degrees. If the hip is in the neutral position but the knee cannot be flexed, then rectus femoris is tight. If the hip is flexed but lying in the plane of the body, the iliopsoas muscle is tight. If the hip remains flexed and abducted, then TFL is tight.

Lack of flexibility of TFL can be further confirmed in side lying by Ober's test (Brukner and Khan, 1993; McConnell, 1996). The Thomas test needs to be performed on both legs so a comparison between legs can be made. The other muscles acting around the knee were more than adequately flexible. In fact, the hamstring muscles were almost too flexible, with a straight leg raise of 100 degrees bilaterally.

Patellar position

Although determining the position of the patella relative to the femur has been found to be somewhat unreliable when performed as an isolated procedure (like most manual palpation tests), it still remains an important part of the examination process and can be used to help to guide treatment choice (McKenzie and Taylor, 1997; Potter and Rothstein, 1985; Watson et al., 1999). The left patella was laterally tilted and displaced, with the inferior pole tilted posteriorly into the fat pad. This was determined by examining the patellar position relative to the trochlea. An optimal patellar position is one where the patella is parallel to the femur in the frontal and sagittal planes, and the patella is situated midway between the two condyles when the knee is flexed to 20 degrees (Grelsamer and McConnell, 1998; McConnell, 1996). The distance from the middle of the patella to the medial femoral epicondyle was greater than the distance from the middle of the patella to the lateral femoral epicondyle, indicating a laterally displaced patella. The posterior edge of the lateral border of the patella was difficult to palpate, with the medial border sitting further from the femur, thus indicating a laterally tilted patella. There was also a posterior displacement of the inferior pole of the patella.

Flexibility of lateral structures

The side-lying position was used to assess the flexibility of the lateral structures, notably the lateral retinaculum (superficial and deep fibres) and the ITB. To test the superficial retinacula structures, the knee was flexed to 20 degrees, from where the patella was moved passively in a medial direction. The lateral femoral condyle was not readily exposed, indicating the superficial retinacula fibres were tight. The deep fibres were tested with the patient in the same position. The slack of the glide was taken up in a medial direction and then an anteroposterior pressure was applied to the medial border of the patella. The lateral border did not move freely away from the femur, which indicated that the deep fibres were also tight. Tightness of the ITB was further confirmed by Ober's test (McConnell, 1996). In this test, the underneath hip and knee are flexed to stabilize the pelvis, while the knee of the upper leg is flexed to 90 degrees and the hip is abducted, externally rotated and slightly extended. The thigh remained abducted when the leg was released, indicating tightness of the band (McConnell, 1996).

Other examination procedures

Testing of hip extension and external rotation range of motion in prone lying revealed tightness of the anterior hip structures. The patient was examined in a figure of four position, with the underneath foot at the level of the tibial tubercle. The distance of the left anterior superior iliac spine to the plinth was 10 cm, whereas the right was only 6 cm from the plinth. Additionally, the stiffness of the subtalar joint was confirmed in this position. The lumbar spine was not palpated at this time because there was nothing in the history to indicate lumbar involvement.

REASONING DISCUSSION AND CLINICAL REASONING COMMENTARY

 1 How did the initial observation of the patient fit in with your working hypotheses?

Clinician's answer

Patellofemoral dysfunction may arise from abnormal gait patterns, primarily caused by poor dynamic lower limb mechanics. Internal rotation of the femur is usually associated with a tight ITB and poor functioning of the posterior fibres of the gluteus medius muscle. Tightness in the ITB results in overactivity in the TFL and diminished activity in vastus medialis obliquus (VMO) and the gluteus medius posterior fibres. The faulty alignment pattern remains because the muscles in a shortened position (usually two joint muscles) are readily recruited and are strong, whereas muscles in an elongated position (usually postural muscles) are difficult to recruit and are weak (Sahrmann, 2002). A patient with a shortened ITB often demonstrates excessive medial rotation of the hip during the stance phase of gait, which means that the pelvis on the opposite side drops, giving a Trendelenburg-like appearance (Sahrmann, 2002). This hip movement will increase the dynamic quadriceps (Q) angle (D'Amico and Rubin, 1986) and hence increase the potential for patellofemoral pain.

Initial shock absorption should occur with knee flexion of 10–15 degrees, because the foot is supinated when the heel first strikes the ground. This knee flexion, which is accompanied by internal femoral rotation, should immediately be followed by rapid pronation of the foot. Reduced knee flexion on heel strike means that the ground reaction force is not minimized at the knee, so greater load will need to be taken through the foot (Powers et al., 1997). If the foot is also stiff, as in this case, then the shock absorption must occur at the pelvis, with increased anteroposterior tilt or rotation movement or lateral flexion movement. The normal pelvic range of motion during gait is 4 degrees of lateral flexion, 7 degrees of anteroposterior tilt, and 10 degrees of rotation (Perry, 1992). Reduced knee flexion on heel strike may also result in poor inner-range eccentric control of the quadriceps muscle.

As this patient presented with internally rotated femurs, tibial varum, a high-arched foot and 'locked back knees', then his shock absorption was diminished at the subtalar joint and the knee; consequently, he had to absorb more shock at the pelvis. This caused an increase in the lateral tilt and rotation of the pelvis as his hip external rotator and abductor muscles were inadequate for controlling his pelvis. The locking back of his knee further aggravated his fat pad problem.

2 Could you please describe your principal diagnostic hypotheses at the end of the examination (with supporting and negating evidence), including any significant biomechanical or other factors contributing to the problem?

Clinician's answer

The principal diagnostic hypotheses were:

- fat·pad irritation causing the inferior pain; supportive findings included:
  — the enlarged fat pad
  — the posterior tilt of the inferior pole

— the lack of knee flexion at heel strike, causing the patella to further irritate the inflamed fat pad
— tight ITB, which the patient rests on when standing on one leg with a fully extended knee, further irritating the fat pad
— tightness of the anterior hip structures, which decreases hip extension and external rotation, thereby decreasing gluteus medius posterior fibre control and increasing TFL tightness
— increased stiffness of the subtalar joint, thus transferring the shock absorption further up the kinetic chain to the pelvis; if the subtalar joint does not take some of the load, the load is then transferred from the foot through the knee, which also does not absorb the stress, up to the pelvis, causing a 'jarring' at the knee that loads the inflamed fat pad
— lack of pelvic control, increasing the internal rotation of the lower extremity and increasing the dynamic Q angle.
- ITB friction syndrome causing the lateral pain; supportive findings included:
  — tight ITB, so it 'rubs' on the femoral epicondyle
  — laterally tilted and displaced patella, which indicates tightness of the ITB because most of the lateral retinaculum arises from the ITB
  — new rigid orthotics, which further minimized the shock absorption through the foot, providing to the knee an externally rotating distal force on an internally rotating proximal force
  — increased stiffness of the subtalar joint
  — poor pelvic control.

These last three findings are important because load is transferred through the lower extremity to the pelvis if shock absorption is reduced through the foot; as a result, there will be increased dynamic pelvic movement. The lower leg needs to rotate internally on heel strike; however, a rigid rearfoot and an unforgiving high corrective orthotic will create an external rotatory moment, so the ITB attempts to absorb the force from these two opposing moments. If the pelvis exhibits an increase in lateral tilt, then the TFL tightens, decreasing its flexibility. This can affect the distal course of the structure, that is the distal end of the ITB, predisposing the patient to ITB syndrome.

3 Bearing in mind your response to the previous question, what then were your specific goals for treatment, both short and long term?

Clinician's answer

The specific short-term goals were to:

- minimize the fat pad irritation by unloading the painful structures
- improve the mobility of the anterior hip structures to increase hip extension and external rotation; this will decrease ITB tightness
- improve gluteal and eccentric inner range quadriceps muscle control.

The specific long-term goals were to:

- improve the endurance capacity of the VMO and the gluteus medius muscles
- increase the subtalar joint mobility
- return the patient to competitive tennis
- teach the patient how to recognize symptoms and provide him with strategies to self-manage his condition to prevent recurrences.

Clinical reasoning commentary

The process of generating and prioritizing a hypothesis, in whatever category it may fit, requires the ability to recognize salient clinical findings, retain those findings in short-term memory, and synthesize the patient data to determine the dominant hypothesis. As discussed in Chapter 1, a number of clinical features will provide supporting and negating evidence, and it is rare that a single feature will completely confirm or completely negate a particular hypothesis. In this response, the clinician has highlighted how all the patient information must be weighed, with the strength of the supporting data versus the strength of the negating data determining the dominant hypothesis.

m Initial management

First treatment

Initial treatment involved loosening of the tight deep lateral retinacula structures by soft tissue massage, while the patella was being medially tilted. The patient was given a stretching exercise in prone lying for the tight anterior structures (adductors, TFL, psoas, anterior capsule, iliofemoral ligament), which he was instructed to do twice a day for five repetitions.

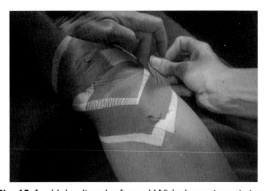

Fig. 13.1 Unloading the fat pad. With the patient sitting on the edge of the chair, the unload tape is started at the tibial tubercle and lifted out to the joint line. The soft tissue is lifted up to the patella. (From McConnell, 2002.)

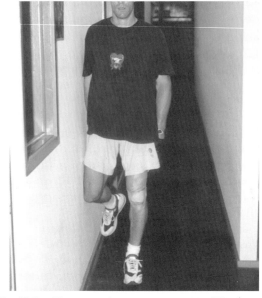

Fig. 13.2 Gluteus medius posterior training. The patient stands side-on to a wall, with the leg closest to the wall flexed at the knee so the foot is off the ground (the hip is in line with the standing hip). All of the patient's weight should be back through the heel of the standing leg, which is slightly flexed. The patient externally rotates the standing leg without turning the foot, the pelvis or the shoulders. (From McConnell, 2002.)

With the patient in supine lying, tape was applied to the patella. The first piece commenced at the superior margin in the middle of the patella to tilt the inferior pole and the lateral border of the patella anteriorly. The second piece was also anchored superiorly at the lateral border of the patella in order to correct the glide. This was followed by a 'V' taping from the tibial tubercle to the medial and lateral joint lines to unload the fat pad (Fig. 13.1), as well as another strip of tape from the lateral femoral condyle diagonally across the ITB to decrease the tension on the band. After the tape was applied the patient was retested on the stairs and did not experience any symptoms.

Training the posterior fibres of the gluteus medius muscle in weight bearing was also an immediate priority for treatment, both to decrease TFL tightness and to improve pelvic stability. The patient stood on the left leg against the wall. The hip of the right leg was in line with the left hip, but the knee was flexed

and resting against the wall. The patient was instructed to rotate the standing leg externally without moving the hip or the foot and to hold the position for 15 seconds (Fig. 13.2).

Once this exercise was sufficiently familiar to the patient that he could repeat it regularly at home, dual channel biofeedback training was commenced with the electrodes on the VMO and vastus lateralis (VL) muscles. Emphasis was on the timing and intensity of the VMO contraction. Initially when the patient performed small-range squats, the VMO activation was delayed and the VL contraction was greater in magnitude, ensuring the knees were not locking back (being forced into end-range extension). The patient was also shown how to tape his knee while sitting on the edge of a chair with the leg extended but relaxed. In addition, he was shown how to massage and stretch the deep lateral retinacula structures in sitting.

REASONING DISCUSSION AND CLINICAL REASONING COMMENTARY

1 What clinical findings led you to suspect that the VMO required retraining? In addition to your own clinical experience, what evidence supports this approach?

Clinician's answer

The left VMO activity was measured relative to the VL activity, and this was compared with the ratio on the asymptomatic side. The VMO muscle was not activating early enough during small knee bends and was exhibiting less activity than the VL. However, the signal was not normalized. The issue of VMO and VL timing is still controversial. Voight and Weider (1991) found that the reflex response time of the VMO was earlier than that of the VL in an asymptomatic group, but in a symptomatic patellofemoral group there was a reversal of the pattern. These findings were confirmed by Witvrouw et al. (1996), but curiously these investigators found that there was a shorter reflex response time in a symptomatic patellofemoral group relative to a control group. Further support is provided by the work of Koh et al. (1991), who examined isokinetic knee extension at 250 degrees/s^{-1} (following hamstring muscle preactivation) and found that the VMO

activated 5.6 milliseconds earlier than the VL. Even though this finding was statistically significant, the authors questioned the functional relevance.

The above results are at odds, however, with the findings of other investigators (Gilleard et al., 1998; Karst and Willett, 1995; Powers et al., 1997), who reported that the VMO did not fire earlier than the VL in asymptomatic volunteers and that the VMO activation was not delayed in symptomatic individuals. It is of interest to note, therefore, that Cowan et al. (2001) found that, even though the majority of patellofemoral sufferers had a delayed onset of VMO relative to VL on a stair-stepping task (67% concentrically, 79% eccentrically), there were still some whose VMO activation preceded their VL activation. Additionally, these investigators found that some of the control subjects (no history of patellofemoral pain) exhibited a delayed onset of VMO relative to VL (46% concentrically, 52% eccentrically) on the stair-stepping task. This study by Cowan et al. may clarify some of the discrepancies evident in the literature with regard to timing, in which some researchers have found a delayed onset of VMO relative to VL but others have not. The stratification of the groups only occurs when there are sufficient subject numbers to tease out the differences. The findings of some of the earlier studies may not have reached statistical significance because there were too few subjects.

Although the early literature suggests there is a difference in the ratio of the VMO and VL activity, with the VL activity being greater than that of the VMO (Mariani and Caruso, 1979), more recent literature has not supported this contention. This may be because the earlier studies did not normalize the electromyographic (EMG) data. Normalization involves obtaining a ratio of the recorded muscle activity and muscle activity from the maximal voluntary contraction (MVC), which then permits the comparison of the ratio of one muscle relative to its MVC with another muscle relative to its MVC. For example, if the recorded VMO activity is $50\,\mu V$ and the MVC is $200\,\mu V$ and the measured VL activity is $100\,\mu V$ and the MVC is $400\,\mu V$, then the ratio VMO:VL is 1:1. There has been some discussion that normalization is affected by the presence of pain, which will mask differences because there could be error in the MVC and this may appear in the error of the recorded EMG (Yang and Winter, 1983). There has also been some debate about the reliability of the maximal contraction, casting doubt on the normalization process. Howard and Enoka (1991) found that there was considerable variation in the MVC of the VL EMG, even though the force exerted by the leg remained constant. Interestingly, Yang and Winter (1983) found that the averaged rectified EMG had a coefficient of variation (standard deviation/mean) of 9.1% within 1 day and of 16.4% between days.

A recent randomized, double-blind, placebo-controlled trial of an intervention programme, similar to that received by the tennis player, showed that the treatment group demonstrated significantly greater improvements in pain and functional activities than the placebo group (Crossley et al., 2002). There were 36 patients in each group and all patients received 1 hour of treatment per week for 6 weeks. The treatment group received patellar taping, figure of four stretches, hamstring stretches, gluteal training and specific VMO training with a dual channel biofeedback device. The placebo group received placebo taping, which was applied at 90 degrees of knee flexion in the line of the femur, detuned ultrasound and massage around the patella with medicated gel. The symptoms in both groups decreased, but the treatment group had a far greater improvement (visual analogue scale, $p = 0.001$; functional assessment scale, $p = 0.0001$). Another interesting finding was that the VMO was firing earlier than the VL in the treatment group (both concentrically and eccentrically) after 6 weeks, whereas the timing of the VMO in the placebo group was unchanged after this time (i.e. it remained delayed compared with the VL).

■ Clinical reasoning commentary

The use of both research- and experience-based evidence is apparent in this answer. Expert clinicians, such as this clinician, routinely consider the two types of evidence in their decision making, even though the evidence may not always be in complete harmony. However, it is an error of clinical reasoning to take any single research finding in isolation, as it is for a single clinical finding. When research findings are at odds with skilled reflective clinical experience, the practice strategies in question should not simply be discarded. Rather, further critical reflection on the clinical use of those strategies must be undertaken, along with further research, possibly with greater attention to various subgroups, which may respond differently. Here, the clinician's critical awareness of the quality of the research evidence and her willingness to retain an open mind on this whole issue (which is as yet still clearly unresolved) is a hallmark of clinical expertise.

m Subsequent management

The patient returned after a week and was considerably improved; he was not experiencing any pain on stairs and was anxious to start playing tennis again. His VMO activity relative to his VL activity had somewhat improved, but it was still delayed in onset and was of lesser magnitude as measured on the biofeedback machine. An inhibitory VL taping was firmly applied to the thigh to enhance VMO activity (Fig. 13.3). This immediately decreased the VL activity, resulting in VMO becoming more active. After 20 repetitions of the small squats, the patient began to feel fatigue in the VMO region.

At subsequent visits, further fine tuning of the quadriceps contraction occurred, with the patient

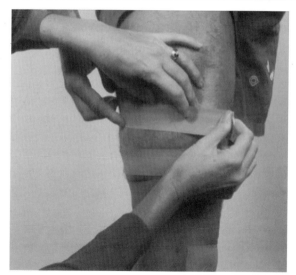

Fig. 13.3 Inhibiting the vastus lateralis. This involves applying three pieces of firm tape from mid-thigh anteriorly, passing laterally to mid-thigh posteriorly. The soft tissue is firmly compressed over the vastus lateralis and the iliotibial band. (From McConnell, 2002.)

practising sideways movements, and simulated forehand, backhand and service manoeuvres. The subtalar joint was mobilized in side lying, with the foot in neutral (plantargrade), the tibia and talus stabilized, and

the calcaneum being moved laterally. This position was adopted to simulate the moment immediately after heel strike when the subtalar joint should be pronating.

After six visits (over a period of 2 months) the VMO was activating earlier than the VL and was several times greater in magnitude. The gluteal exercise had been progressed to 30 seconds, with the patient practising in front of a mirror standing on the left leg and rapidly moving the right leg back and forth, while keeping a stable pelvis. He was also maintaining a steady pelvis while lowering his right leg down off a small step and returning back up to the step. He repeated this exercise slowly 20 times without pausing in order to increase the endurance of the VMO and gluteal musculature.

After 3 months the patient was back playing tournament tennis. His knee was still taped for playing, but not for daily activities. At this stage, the activity of the VMO relative to the VL was four times greater, as measured on a dual channel biofeedback device. The patient was not experiencing any pain on repeated one-leg squatting activities but was fearful about pain returning when he went back to tennis. The patient perspired greatly when playing so the tape had to be reapplied during his matches. It took a further 3 months before the patient felt sufficiently confident to play without taping.

REASONING DISCUSSION AND CLINICAL REASONING COMMENTARY

1 There appears to be some psychosocial issues with this athlete's presentation. Could you elaborate on any of these you considered to be clinically significant? What strategies (if any) did you employ to manage this aspect of the problem?

Clinician's answer

The player was very concerned and anxious about his ranking and his fitness, which he felt was deteriorating by the second. It was imperative that I worked in closely with the player's fitness coach, who was writing programmes to maintain cardiovascular fitness and upper body strength during his rehabilitation. Together, we devised a rehabilitation plan for the

player in which he could see the short-term and long-term goals and how we were going to measure them (principally measuring pain and EMG activity).

Initially the player was doing quite a bit of water running, which not only increased his heart rate but also helped to maintain his running form. Other cardiovascular work included cycling on a stationary bike (which became part of his programme) as soon as he had no pain doing that activity. The coach and I also examined some of the player's techniques from old video footage. We were particularly interested in the open stance forehand and discussed strategies with the player to minimize pivoting excessively around the knee and use more trunk rotation. These technique adjustments were worked on during the rehabilitation of the knee.

At the end of the second month, the player commenced interval training: short sprints followed by longer slower runs. Slowly, plyometric training was introduced into the training programme as the core stability improved, particularly gluteal work.

Clinical reasoning commentary

Manual therapists are often criticised for relying on a tissue-focussed and reductionist approach to chronic musculoskeletal problems and for inadvertently encouraging patient passivity and dependence on the therapist. They are also often guilty of working in isolation and failing to seek appropriate input in the management process from other relevant professionals. In this case, the importance that the expert clinician places on a holistic and team approach to the patient's problem is well illustrated. Consideration is given to the patient's psychosocial issues, maintaining his general fitness and upper body muscle strength, and involvement of the coaching staff, such as in addressing his playing technique. The patient is also very much involved in his rehabilitation programme and has been empowered with the means and responsibility to make a significant contribution to his own recovery. Such a comprehensive approach to recalcitrant clinical problems is critical to a successful outcome and only serves to enhance the standing of manual therapists in the eyes of their colleagues and patients.

Outcome

When the tour came back to Australia, the patient returned for review. He was still doing his maintenance exercises consisting of the standing gluteal exercise, small-range squats, and the figure of four stretch in prone lying. His VMO activity was still four times that of the VL and he had been symptom-free for 12 months.

References

Brukner, P. and Khan, K. (1993). Clinical Sports Medicine. New York: McGraw-Hill.

Cowan, S.M., Bennell, K.L., Hodges, P.W. et al. (2001). Delayed onset of electromyographic activity of vastus medialis obliquus relative to vastus lateralis in subjects with patellofemoral pain syndrome. Archives of Physical Medicine and Rehabilitation, 82, 183–189.

Crossley, K.M., Bennell, K.L., Green, S. et al. (2002). Physical therapy for patellofemoral pain: a randomized, double-blind, placebo-controlled trial. American Journal of Sports Medicine, 30, 857–865.

D'Amico, J.C. and Rubin, M. (1986). The influence of foot orthoses on the quadriceps angle. Journal of the American Podiatry Association, 76, 337–339.

Dye, S., Vaupel, G., Dye, C. et al. (1998). Conscious neurosensory mapping of the internal structures of the human knee without intra-articular anaesthesia. American Journal of Sports Medicine, 26, 773–777.

Gilleard, W., McConnell, J. and Parsons, D. (1998). The effect of patellar taping on the onset of vastus medialis obliquus and vastus lateralis muscle activity in persons with patellofemoral pain. Physical Therapy, 78, 25–32.

Grelsamer, R. and McConnell, J. (1998). The Patella. A Team Approach. Aspen, CO: Aspen Publishers.

Hoppenfeld, S. (1976). Physical Examination of the Spine and Extremities. New York: Appleton-Century-Crofts.

Howard, J. and Enoka, R. (1991). Maximum bilateral contractions are modified by neurally mediated interlimb effects. Journal of Applied Physiology, 70, 306–316.

Karst, G. and Willett, G. (1995). Onset timing of electromyographic activity in the vastus medialis oblique and vastus lateralis muscles in subjects with and without patellofemoral pain syndrome. Physical Therapy, 75, 813–822.

Kendall, F. and McCreary, L. (1983). Muscle Testing and Function. London: Williams &Wilkins.

Koh, T., Grabiner, M. and DeSwart, R. (1991). In vivo tracking of the human patella. Journal of Biomechanics, 25, 637–643.

Mariani, P. and Caruso, I. (1979). An electromyographic investigation of subluxation of the patella. Journal of Bone and Joint Surgery, 61, 169–171.

McConnell, J. (1996). Patellofemoral pain and soft tissue injuries. In Athletic Injuries and Rehabilitation (J.E. Zachazewski, D.J. Magee and W.S. Quillen, eds.) pp. 693–728. London: Saunders.

McConnell, J. (2002). The physical therapist's approach to patellofemoral disorders. Clinics in Sports Medicine, 21, 363–387.

McKenzie, A.M. and Taylor, N.F. (1997). Can physiotherapists locate lumbar spinal levels by palpation? Physiotherapy, 83, 235–239.

Perry, J. (1992). Gait Analysis. New York: Slack Corporation.

Potter, N. and Rothstein, J. (1985). Intertester reliability of selected clinical tests of the sacroiliac joint. Physical Therapy, 65, 1671–1675.

Powers, C., Landel, R., Sosnick, T. et al. (1997). The effects of patellar taping on stride characteristics and joint motion in subjects with patellofemoral pain. Journal of Orthopedic and Sports Physical Therapy, 26, 286–291.

Sahrmann, S. (2002). Diagnosis and Treatment of Movement Impairment Systems. London: Mosby.

Voight, M. and Weider, D. (1991). Comparative reflex response times of the vastus medialis and the vastus lateralis in normal subjects and subjects with extensor mechanism dysfunction. American Journal of Sports Medicine, 10, 131–137.

Watson, C., Propps, M., Galt, W. et al. (1999). Reliability of measurements obtained using McConnell's classification of patellar orientation in symptomatic and asymptomatic subjects. Journal of Orthopedic and Sports Physical Therapy, 29, 378–385.

Witvrouw, E., Sneyers, C., Lysens, R. et al. (1996). Comparative reflex response times of vastus medialis obliquus and vastus lateralis in normal subjects and subjects with patellofemoral pain syndrome. Journal of Orthopedic and Sports Physical Therapy, 24, 160–166.

Yang, J. and Winter, D. (1983). Electromyography reliability in maximal contractions and submaximal isometric contractions. Archives of Physical Medicine and Rehabilitation, 64, 417–420.

CHAPTER

14

Self-management guided by directional preference and centralization in a patient with low back and leg pain

Robin McKenzie and Helen Clare

SUBJECTIVE EXAMINATION

Jamie is a 32-year-old carpenter who for the past 2 years has been self-employed building houses, requiring only occasional assistance. He complained of back and right leg pain radiating below the knee (Fig. 14.1) and had experienced a similar problem on two previous occasions, the most recent being 2 years ago. Jamie was advised 3 years ago that he had a degenerated disc at L4–L5. He refused surgery and went to a chiropractor with a successful outcome.

The symptoms had been present for 5 weeks and had commenced on the right side of his back. The leg pain had appeared more recently. The patient believed the leg pain was getting worse with the passage of time.

Jamie stated that the pain in the centre and right-side of his lower back was constant. He complained that the pain radiated into the right buttock and thigh on performing certain movements, but these pains ceased when he returned to a more upright position. His pain was worse with prolonged bending and sitting. When driving his truck, the pain extended into the lower leg and his foot tingled and at times becomes 'dead'. His back and leg pain also increased if he stood erect for prolonged periods. He had particular difficulty getting out of bed in the morning because of increased back and buttock pain. Coughing and sneezing produced or increased pain in the right buttock.

The patient noted the back pain was partially relieved, and the buttock and leg pain abolished, when he lay face down. His leg pain decreased when he walked short distances but increased if walking was prolonged. He could then obtain relief temporarily if

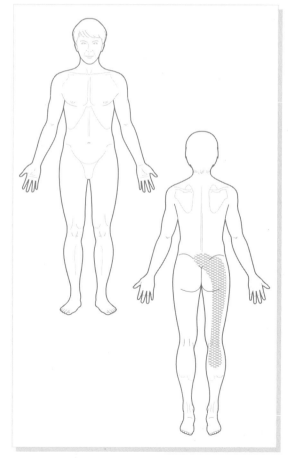

Fig. 14.1 Area of patient's pain.

he bent slightly forward. All symptoms were also relieved if he lay in bed face up with his knees bent. However, the symptoms never completely ceased in the back or upper thigh.

The patient's general health was good, there was no weight loss, and until recently he refused medication.

He was now taking two Digesic (dextropropoxyphene 30 mg + paracetamol 325 mg) tablets three times per day for pain relief. Radiographs showed slight narrowing at L4–L5.

REASONING DISCUSSION AND CLINICAL REASONING COMMENTARY

1 At this stage what were your initial thoughts? Which hypotheses (if any) were you considering with respect to the source of the patient's symptoms?

Clinicians' answer

It was noted that the patient's age placed him in an age group with a high incidence of low back pain and that in his job he must flex and lift frequently. The patient's description of increasing peripheralization (McKenzie, 1981) of pain and paraesthesia typically occurs in the presence of intervertebral disc pathology or prolapse. The peripheralizing of back and leg symptoms over time also suggested the problem was progressive and his condition was worsening. As this disorder has marked consequences if neglected, it would be unwise to ignore the significance of progressively increasing radiating symptoms in the search for more obscure causes for his problem.

It was likely that the back and leg symptoms were related, but back and leg pain are not always connected. Supportive evidence was needed, which could be obtained by increasing and decreasing the lumbar lordosis (flexing and extending the lumbar spine in sitting) to test the effect of spinal loading on the leg symptoms.

2 At the conclusion of the history, did the behaviour of the symptoms with movement tend to support or discount your hypothesis? Were there any factors (e.g. environmental, psychosocial, biomechanical) that you considered had contributed to the onset or deterioration of his disorder?

Clinicians' answer

Pain can arise from either chemical or mechanical causes (Wyke, 1980). Pain of chemical origin will usually be felt constantly as long as the concentration of chemicals is sufficient to activate pain receptors. Pain can also be experienced constantly when mechanically dislocated tissue (such as discal tissue) is displaced and deforms adjacent normal soft tissues. The concentration of chemicals in an inflammatory condition does not generally reduce with change of position or unloading or exercise. Therefore, if the symptoms are intermittent or influenced by position, they are unlikely to be inflammatory in origin. Similarly, repeated movement or prolonged loading will either have no effect or will increase rather than decrease the symptoms. However, if the symptoms result from internal derangement of a lumbar disc, repeated movements in one direction may increase displacement and cause an increase in pain, while movement in the opposite direction may decrease displacement and cause a decrease in pain.

In this case, the pain was constant and so it could have been chemical in origin or have arisen from constant mechanical deformation, such as might occur with an internal disc derangement. The behaviour, however, suggested the pain was not primarily chemical in nature. It is improbable that pain related to inflammation would appear and disappear on change of position. The behaviour did tend to support the hypothesis that the symptoms were likely to have arisen from increasing and decreasing mechanical disc deformation. The constant back pain was, therefore, most probably caused by an·internal disc derangement, which could increase or decrease, thus provoking intermittent pain in the leg according to the patient's position or movement.

The reduction in leg pain on walking a short distance may have been a consequence of the lumbar spine extension effect of walking. However, walking longer distances may have caused prolonged compression loading of a posterior disc bulge, leading to peripheralization. Perhaps the relief noted while bending (i.e. in slight spinal flexion) was a result of reduced compression of the posterior displacement. Unloaded flexion decompresses the disc but is unlikely to reduce or alter the location of displaced tissue.

The reported difficulty getting out of bed in the morning was also consistent with a mechanical disc problem. Compressive forces on a nocturnally imbibed disc would, under these circumstances, increase back pain and the patient is at increased risk of aggravation of symptoms in the first few hours of the day. Interestingly, it has been reported that recurrence of low back pain is most likely in the first few hours of the day (McKenzie, 1981; Snook et al., 1998). Differentiation between chemical and mechanical causes should be aided by the use of repeated movements during the physical examination. If pain location changes or its intensity reduces with repeated movement testing, then the pain cannot be chemical in nature.

Sitting in a truck elicited tingling and numbness in Jamie's right foot. Sitting in this position flattens or flexes the lumbar spine. The intermittent neurological symptoms confirmed intermittent mechanical compression or irritation of the spinal nerve root was occurring, probably as a result of lumbar flexion. The fact that the tingling and numbness was not constant also suggested that the condition may have been rapidly reversible. If root compression spontaneously ceases, it is usually possible to identify the position that causes the decompression. In this case, he described centralization occurring in unloaded extension of the spine (e.g. lying prone). This suggested a good outcome would likely be achievable with the use of extension principles of treatment.

The only obvious factor that may have contributed to the problem, and which may have predisposed the patient to recurrence, was environmental, that is his work. This involved frequent and sustained spinal flexion. Despite the risks, the patient was reluctant to cease work.

Clinical reasoning commentary

Pattern recognition is typical of the clinical reasoning process of expert clinicians, as is evidenced in this response. Early in the clinical session, cues are recognized (e.g. area of the symptoms, age of the patient) that relate to a familiar clinical pattern or syndrome (e.g. peripheralization of pain possibly as a result of intervertebral disc prolapse). Significant previous clinical experience with similar clinical presentations is integral to this process. However, it is still necessary that the diagnostic hypothesis be tested by further examination (e.g. increasing and decreasing the lumbar lordosis to determine the effect of lumbar posture on the symptoms) before it can be fully accepted and the problem well understood.

Hypotheses are not limited to just the structural source of a patient's complaint (e.g. lumbar disc). As illustrated in the clinicians' second answer, they may also fall into other categories including activity/participation restrictions (e.g. walking long distances), pathobiological mechanisms (e.g. chemical), factors contributing to the problem (e.g. work environment), management and treatment (e.g. 'extension principles of treatment'), and prognosis (e.g. 'good outcome would likely be achievable'). These hypotheses together guide the ongoing examination by a reasoning process in which they are eventually either refined or rejected on the basis of the clinical findings obtained.

 ## PHYSICAL EXAMINATION

On examination, Jamie sat slouched with a rounded back (i.e. in lumbar flexion). Correction of his sitting posture increased his leg pain. He stood with a flattened lumbar spine and leant to the left. Attempting to stand fully erect was impossible and increased both back and leg pain.

Flexion in standing did not increase his back pain, but after 10 repetitions he complained of increasing right lower leg pain and slight ill-defined numbness in the foot. Extension in standing increased his back and leg pain and repetition worsened his symptoms overall.

Loaded correction of the left lateral shift (Fig. 14.2) increased his right back pain but abolished the pain in his right lower leg and decreased the pain in the buttock and thigh (i.e. it centralized the pain). Repeated loaded correction of the lateral shift reduced and then abolished all symptoms below the buttock. The

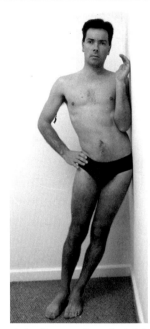

Fig 14.2   Loaded self-correction of a left lateral shift.

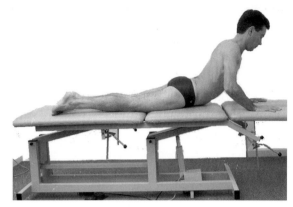

Fig. 14.3   Extension in lying with the pelvis displaced to the left.

symptoms centralized as a result of lateral shift correction but did not remain better.

A further series of corrections of the lateral shift again resulted in a reduction of intensity and centralization of pain. This, also, was of a temporary nature. Complete reduction of the disc derangement was not achievable in the loaded position, probably because of the difficulty of achieving an adequate extension force in the standing position.

After placing the patient in prone lying and moving the pelvis away from the side of pain and fixing him in this position (lumbar spine right lateral flexion in this case), the patient repeated extension in lying

(Fig. 14.3). There was a steady reduction in the leg pain as symptoms centralized. Simultaneously with centralization, Jamie's range of extension steadily improved until it appeared a full and almost painless range was achieved.

The patient was instructed to retain a lumbar lordosis when he arose from the treatment table and to maintain it when standing. On standing erect, Jamie reported minor levels of central and right low back pain only. He was asked to remain very erect and walk about for a few minutes. After 10 minutes walking, he reported that his symptoms had remained centralized and he was not aware of any leg pain or other untoward sensations.

No further examination was conducted. A neurological examination was not performed as the symptoms in the leg were intermittent. There is no evidence that muscle length or muscle control relates to intervertebral disc pathology so tests for these were not performed.

REASONING DISCUSSION AND CLINICAL REASONING COMMENTARY

1 Earlier in the examination, it was found that extension and repeated extension peripheralized and worsened the patient's symptoms overall. What, therefore, prompted you to add repeated extension to the shift correction? Did any other findings from the physical examination influence your decision making?

■ **Clinicians' answer**

McKenzie reported in 1979 and 1981 that extension performed in the presence of a lateral shift could worsen symptoms of disc prolapse and that correcting the shift is the first step in the reduction of a derangement, prior to complete reduction using extension.

Although attempting to force extension in standing in the presence of a lateral shift usually results in an unacceptable level of pain, this problem can be overcome by placing the patient in the unloaded prone lying position. Conceptually, this procedure applies a compressive force to the right posterolateral aspect of the intervertebral disc. This, will in turn, theoretically cause a posterolateral displacement of the disc nucleus to move to a more central location. Any obstruction to extension should be reduced by this process and the patient's range of extension concomitantly improved.

In this case, it was found that the patient stood off-centre with a left lateral shift away from the side of pain (i.e. a contralateral shift). Lumbar spine extension was limited to 25% of anticipated normal range and lateral flexion to the right was impossible past the midline. It was likely that right posterolateral disc fissuring with nuclear displacement was responsible for this pattern of movement limitation and forced the patient to adopt an antalgic posture. However, loaded extension was causing peripheralization of pain and was, therefore, contraindicated until reassessment indicated otherwise. Although the symptoms were centralized for only a short period with lateral shift correction, the response identified the direction of movement that had the potential to centralize and suggested that shift correction was the first motion to apply as part of the therapeutic procedure. Therefore, unloaded shift correction combined with extension was most likely to achieve reduction in these circumstances.

Other findings of note included the flexed posture (reversed lumbar spine lordosis), which probably explained why prolonged sitting increased his back and leg pain and produced numbness in his foot. Peripheralization was likely occurring as a result of prolonged flexion, which increased spinal nerve root compression. One flexion movement was not sufficient to cause root compression, but repeated loaded flexion also caused peripheralization and progressive root compression. Therefore, loaded flexion was now contraindicated until later assessment demonstrated otherwise.

2 Did you expect that the improvement from the extension exercise obtained in the unloaded position would be maintained in loaded postures, particularly considering the patient's pain was worse in sitting and standing? If so, why?

Clinicians' answer

Provided that the patient maintained lumbar spine extension on moving from the unloaded position to the loaded posture, it was expected that any benefit obtained in prone lying would remain stable on standing. This would not have happened if the patient had been permitted to flex. By maintaining extension, further posterior displacement of the disc nucleus was prevented (Donelson et al., 1991). As the pain remained centralized following ambulation, the reduction of the displacement was likely to be stable.

Clinical reasoning commentary

Although the clinicians have presented their thinking within a conceptual framework about a specific structure (i.e. the intervertebral disc), these answers indicate that their clinical reasoning is not limited to just a consideration of the structural source of the patient's symptoms. Indeed, it is apparent that this framework has enabled them to process the information from the movement examination in many ways and explore hypotheses in several other categories, such as management (e.g. 'as part of the therapeutic procedure'), contraindications to treatment (e.g. 'loaded flexion was now contraindicated'), and prognosis (e.g. 'reduction ... was likely to be stable').

Importantly, relevant physical impairments were identified through a systematic assessment of postural (shift or list) correction, active movements and repeated movements in both standing and prone lying (as indicated in the history by the reported relief found when lying face down). Similarly, attention to consistency in symptom responses (e.g. centralization versus peripheralization) provided evidence for a viable treatment strategy to be tested.

m Initial management

Jamie was advised not to remain at work. He agreed to this as he had no financial concerns and was impressed with his new-found ability to manage his own pain. Instruction was given to carry out the procedure that centralized his symptoms (i.e. extension in lying with his pelvis moved away from the side of pain), 10 repetitions every 2 hours at home and to avoid totally flexed postures or movements. He was also instructed to maintain his lumbar lordosis when sitting and was provided with and instructed in the use of a lumbar roll for all sitting occasions.

The patient was advised to continue with the prescribed routine for several days until he had little or no pain. It would then be necessary to re-evaluate him to ensure that his function was full. It was explained to Jamie that when he had the ability to flex fully without pain, he could be reassured the present episode was over. However, as his occupation required frequent bending and lifting, he would need to perform extension movements regularly during the course of the day to prevent any recurrence.

REASONING DISCUSSION AND CLINICAL REASONING COMMENTARY

1 At this stage did you have in mind any other treatment options?

Clinicians' answer

No, because with such a clear-cut positive response to loading with the extension inlying exercise (i.e. the centralization of symptoms, indicating a good prognosis), it would be premature to consider other treatment options at this point. Furthermore, the use of repeated movements plainly demonstrated the optimal direction in which to apply loading (directional preference) and the best procedure to achieve a reduction in the mechanical deformation of pain-sensitive structures. This treatment is also consistent with the literature, which suggests that activity, especially self-applied activity, is beneficial for recovery from back pain (ACC and NHC, 1997; AHCPR, 1994; CSAG, 1994; DIHTA, 1999).

2 What specific outcome measure(s) did you consider was most important in determining if progress was satisfactory and why?

Clinicians' answer

The main specific outcome measures used were pain drawings by the patient and pain and range of motion responses demonstrated during lumbar spine movement. The pain drawing is particularly important as it indicates the extent of the pain experienced. Harms-Ringdahl (1986), Kellgren (1977) and Kuslich et al. (1991) have all described that increasing stimulus increases pain intensity and the radiation of pain, with the radiation usually traveling distally; on reduction of stimulus, the pain reduces in intensity and becomes localized to the point of origin.

In the present case, both subjective (pain drawing) and objective (lumbar spine movement) improvement needed to be demonstrated for progress to be deemed satisfactory. This would indicate that the mechanical forces being applied (extension in lying with the pelvis displaced to the left) were successfully reducing posterior displacement of the nucleus of the disc, a response known as the 'extension sign' (Kopp et al., 1986). The extension sign is described by Kopp et al. as the ability to recover full extension range.

Clinical reasoning commentary

The recent shift toward evidence-based practice may, at first glance, appear to be at odds with the need for skilled clinical reasoning. However, the two are not mutually exclusive. The expert clinician recognizes that evidence-based treatment guidelines are a convenient form of propositional knowledge that may help inform their clinical decision making, for example the clinical guidelines cited in response to Question 1 supporting the use of self-applied activity. It should be considered, as the mature organism model suggests (see Ch. 1), that no two patients will present exactly the same, and managing patients' problems requires understanding their unique pain experiences. Therefore, treatment also needs to be based on the patient's individual responses to examination and progressed according to measurable outcomes. Consequently, interpretation of these examination findings and outcomes, and hence the ongoing selection of treatment for a given individual, still requires practitioner skills in clinical reasoning.

m Continued management

Session 2 (1 day later)

Jamie reported a moderate reduction in the severity of his pain the next day. On questioning regarding the location of the pain, he reported that the pain was no longer radiating into the leg and was more localized to the right lower lumbar region. He also reported experiencing an ache and stiffness across his lumbar spine, which he was able to relieve by doing the prescribed exercises (i.e. extension in lying with his pelvis displaced to the left). He could now complete daily activities with considerably less discomfort, and he was sleeping better. He had been compliant with the instructions given and had performed the exercises 2 hourly, avoided flexing and used the lumbar roll when sitting.

On examination, there was no evidence of a lateral shift. Although the lumbar spine remained flattened, there was a 50% increase in the range of lumbar spine extension. Lateral flexion to the right remained limited by 25%. The patient was asked to demonstrate how he had been performing the extension in lying exercise. His technique was correct. He reported right lumbar spine pain at rest, which shifted to the centre of his back and was then abolished after 10 repetitions of extension in lying with his pelvis displaced to the left. The pain remained abolished when the patient returned to the standing position and walked about for a few minutes.

Jamie was advised to continue performing the exercise on a 2 hourly basis, and to continue sitting for short periods only, utilizing the lumbar support, and to avoid flexion movements.

Session 3 (2 days after initial assessment)

The patient reported experiencing no thigh or buttock pain but continued to experience an ache across the lumbar spine and a sensation of stiffness. He stated that he no longer felt the need to take medication for the pain and there was less discomfort sitting and standing. The exercises were becoming easier to perform and he had been able to carry them out regularly.

On examination, there was no evidence of a lateral shift and the lumbar spine now exhibited a lordosis in standing. The range of both extension and right

lateral flexion were significantly improved. Ten repetitions of flexion in standing did not produce back or leg symptoms.

Jamie's exercise was again reviewed. Extension in lying produced a 'strain-like' discomfort across the lumbar spine and this was not influenced by positioning the pelvis to the left. As he no longer reported unilateral symptoms and because displacing the pelvis to the left no longer altered the symptom response, instructions were given to discontinue shifting the pelvis while performing the exercise. The extension in lying exercise was further modified by asking the patient to breathe out at the limit of the movement. The aim of this request was to achieve a slightly greater range of extension by providing a form of 'self-overpressure' to the movement.

Session 4 (1 week after initial assessment)

Jamie reported feeling significantly improved. He had been able to move more freely, stay upright for longer periods and sit for a considerably longer time. When questioned regarding the effect of coughing and sneezing, he reported that he no longer experienced any pain. Occasionally he was reminded of the central back pain when he attempted to perform an activity in flexion, otherwise he was experiencing minimal or no pain.

On examination, there was no lateral shift present. In standing, the only lumbar spine movement that reproduced pain and remained limited was flexion. This movement reproduced back pain at the mid-thigh position. However, when flexion was performed repeatedly the pain did not worsen. Flexion in lying also reproduced central back pain at the end of the available range, but the pain did not increase, spread or remain after the movement ceased.

The patient was informed that the next progression of treatment was to restore his flexion mobility. This needed to be introduced carefully so as not to cause an exacerbation of the original symptoms. His home exercises were now to include extension in lying (10 repetitions), flexion in lying (10 repetitions), followed again with extension in lying (10 repetitions). This sequence was to be performed 2 hourly if possible. The patient was given warnings to monitor the location and frequency of the pain and to discontinue the flexion exercise if it was causing an aggravation of the symptoms. Extension in standing was to be used as a preventative stretch after any flexion activity and after prolonged sitting. Maintenance of a lumbar lordosis when sitting was to be continued.

At this point Jamie was advised he could resume work on reduced hours doing selected duties, but with no lifting or carrying permitted.

Session 5 (2 weeks after initial assessment)

The patient reported he had returned to work without any effect on the symptoms. He had been symptom-free except for when he sat incorrectly or had to stay in a semi-flexed position to perform a task at work. The sensation he then experienced was a stiffness across the back, which made it slightly difficult to straighten. This feeling dissipated rapidly when he performed extension stretches in standing. In addition, there was no longer any discomfort experienced with the flexion in lying exercise and he felt that his flexion range of motion in standing was back to normal for him.

Examination did not reveal the presence of a lateral shift or flexion deformity. There was a good range of spinal mobility evident, with no reproduction of symptoms. The performance of 30 repeated flexion movements in standing did not reproduce any symptoms or subsequently cause any difficulty with extension. Flexion and extension in lying were both full range and pain-free. The patient demonstrated that he was able to correct his standing and sitting postures and maintain these positions for a lengthy period.

A prophylactic self-management programme was discussed with Jamie, consisting of:

- regular performance of extension in standing after sitting, sustained flexion, and before and after lifting
- continued use of a lumbar support when sitting
- continued performance of a set of 10 extension in lying exercises morning and night
- at the first sign of recurrence, repeat the sequence of exercises that led to recovery.

At this point Jamie was discharged.

REASONING DISCUSSION AND CLINICAL REASONING COMMENTARY

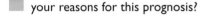 **What was your prognosis for this patient and your reasons for this prognosis?**

Clinicians' answer

The prognosis for this patient was excellent because of the rapid centralization of symptoms that had been achieved after a 5-week history of deterioration and his willingness to engage actively in his own self-management. Several studies have shown that movements or positions that centralize symptoms in patients with low back and leg pain can be used to identify those patients with a good prognosis for a successful outcome and may be therapeutically beneficial (Delitto et al., 1993; Donelson et al., 1990; Erhard et al., 1994; Long, 1995; Karas et al., 1997; Sufka et al., 1998; Werneke et al., 1999; Williams et al., 1991). Conversely, patients whose symptoms fail to centralize or whose symptoms peripheralize

with repetitive motion are likely to have a less-favourable prognosis and are less likely to respond to mechanical interventions.

Clinical reasoning commentary

As discussed in Chapter 1, self-management is a goal more readily achieved when patients receive appropriate explanation and education regarding their disabilities or activity/participation restrictions and associated impairments. When self-management is successfully initiated, patients take greater responsibility for their immediate and ongoing health care, leading to, as identified here, a better prognosis. Self-management has clearly featured strongly throughout this case, both with respect to the primary treatment and prevention of recurrence.

References

ACC and NHC (Accident Rehabilitation and Compensation Insurance Corporation of New Zealand and the National Health Committee) (1997). New Zealand Acute Low Back Pain Guide. Wellington, New Zealand: Accident Rehabilitation and Compensation Insurance Corporation of New Zealand and the National Health Committee.

AHCPR (Agency for Health Care Policy and Research) (1994). Acute Low Back Pain in Adults. Washington, DC: US Department of Health and Human Services, Agency for Health Care Policy and Research.

CSAG (Clinical Standards Advisory Group) (1994). Report on Low Back Pain. London: HMSO for Clinical Standards Advisory Group.

Delitto, A., Cibulka, M., Erhard, R. et al. (1993). Evidence for use of an extension-mobilization category in acute low back pain syndrome. Physical Therapy, 73, 216–222.

DIHTA (Danish Institute for Health Technology Assessment) (1999). Low Back Pain. Frequency, Management and Prevention from an HTA Perspective. Copenhagen, Denmark: Danish Institute for Health Technology Assessment.

Donelson, R., Silva, G. and Murphy, K. (1990). Centralization phenomenon: its usefulness in evaluating and treating referred pain. Spine, 15, 211–213.

Donelson, R., Grant, W., Kamps, C. and Medcalf, R. (1991). Pain response to sagittal end range motion: a prospective, randomized, multi-centered trial. Spine, 16(Supplement), S206–S212.

Erhard, R., Delitto, A. and Cibulka, M. (1994). Relative effectiveness of an extension program and a combined program of manipulation and flexion and extension exercises in patients with acute low back pain syndrome. Physical Therapy, 74, 1093–1099.

Harms-Ringdahl, K. (1986). On assessment of shoulder exercise and load-elicited pain in the cervical spine. Biomechanical analysis of load–EMG–methodological studies of pain provoked by extreme position. Scandinavian Journal of Rehabilitation Medicine Supplement, 14, 1–40.

Karas, R., McKintosh, G., Hall, H. et al. (1997). The relationship between nonorganic signs and centralization of symptoms in the prediction of return to work for patients with low back pain. Physical Therapy, 77, 354–360.

Kellgren, J. (1977). The anatomical source of back pain. Rheumatology and Rehabilitation, 16, 3–12.

Kopp, J., Alexander, A. and Turocy, R. (1986). The use of lumbar extension in the evaluation and treatment of patients with acute herniated nucleus pulposus. A preliminary report. Clinical Orthopedics and Related Research, 202, 211–218.

Kuslich, S., Ulstram, C. and Michael, C. (1991). The tissue origin of low back pain and sciatica. A report of pain response to tissue stimulation during operations on the lumbar spine using local anaesthesia. Orthopedic Clinics of North America, 22, 181–187.

Long, A. (1995). The centralisation phenomenon: its usefulness as a predictor of outcome in conservative treatment of chronic low back pain (a pilot study). Spine, 20, 2513–2521.

McKenzie, R. (1979). Prophylaxis in recurrent low back pain. New Zealand Medical Journal, 627, 22–23.

McKenzie, R. (1981). The Lumbar Spine. Mechanical Diagnosis and Therapy. Lower Hutt, New Zealand: Spinal Publications.

Snook, S., Webster, B., McGorry, R. et al. (1998). The reduction of chronic nonspecific low back pain through the control of early morning lumbar flexion. Spine, 23, 2601–2607.

Sufka, A., Hauger, B., Trenary, M. et al. (1998). Centralization of low back pain and perceived functional outcome. Journal of Orthopedic and Sports Physical Therapy, 27, 205–212.

Werneke, M., Hart, D. and Cook, D. (1999). A descriptive study of centralization phenomenon. Spine, 24, 676–683.

Williams, M., Hawley, J., McKenzie, R. and van Wijmen, P. (1991). A comparison of the effects of two sitting postures on back pain and referred pain. Spine, 16, 1185–1191.

Wyke, B. (1980). Neurological aspects of low back pain. In The Lumbar Spine and Back Pain (M. Jayson, ed.) pp. 265–309. Tunbridge Wells, UK: Pitman Medical.

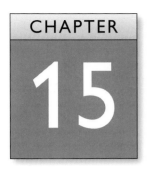

15

Craniovertebral dysfunction following a motor vehicle accident

Erl Pettman

SUBJECTIVE EXAMINATION

Amy, a 35-year-old full-time medical receptionist, presented with upper cervical pain and headaches of varying intensity. When asked to describe the headaches, she indicated they were most often bilateral over the suboccipital region. However, for the last 2 months there had been an increasing tendency for the pain to spread to behind the left eyeball when exacerbated (Fig. 15.1).

She had no other complaints of symptoms or physical dysfunction in any other areas. There had been no difficulties with speech or swallowing, and smell and taste were unaffected. Amy also denied any paraesthesia or numbness in the limbs, trunk, face or mouth or any dizziness, bladder problems, loss of balance, nausea, visual disturbances or hearing loss.

The primary aggravating factor was Amy's work, especially those tasks that involved looking down, such as typing and reading. She also reported that looking over her left shoulder while driving was particularly difficult. Turning her head to the right was very stiff but not painful. In the last month, she had noted that looking over her left shoulder while driving, if repeated frequently, could bring on her headache and left eye pain.

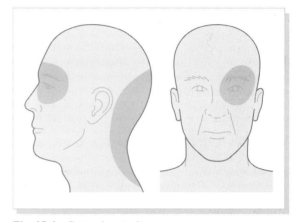

Fig. 15.1 Patient's pain diagram.

Pain could be slowly relieved by lying supine with no pillows. Early morning was considered the best time of the day. Invariably the pain would be minimal during the weekend, although it never abated completely. Amy felt that her analgesic medication had been helpful in reducing the pain, but the anti-inflammatory medication (naproxen), stopped because of stomach irritation, had not altered her symptoms.

REASONING DISCUSSION AND CLINICAL REASONING COMMENTARY

1 What were your initial thoughts about the source(s) of her symptoms? What evidence supported or negated your hypotheses?

■ Clinician's answer

Headaches can be caused by a huge mosaic of pathological conditions and physical dysfunctions. Much more detailed assessment is required (both in the history and the physical examination) to isolate the source(s). However, simply on the basis of the information thus far, we can begin to differentiate between some of the potential causes.

Cranial nerves. From the lack of immediate evidence of signs or symptoms of cranial nerve pathology (e.g. sensory disturbances; speech or swallowing problems; facial or oral paraesthesia or numbness; dizziness, loss of balance or nausea; facial paralysis; strabismus; pupil dilatation; etc.) it was unlikely there was a major problem with cranial nerve conduction.

Vertebrobasilar artery. Amy's denial of any dizziness, nausea, loss of balance or visual disturbances, as well as the apparent absence of dysarthria, made it unlikely that there was any involvement of the vertebrobasilar artery.

Meninges. The possibility of the upper cervical meninges being the pain generator was not ruled out at this stage. Flexed positions of the head aggravated the headache, particularly with the hips flexed in sitting, while it was relieved by lying supine with no pillow. The absence of any bilateral or quadrilateral paraesthesia or numbness and of significant night pain suggested that any meningeal involvement was probably not associated with a space-occupying lesion (e.g. tumour).

Temporomandibular joint. The symptoms may be caused by trigeminal reference as this nerve serves most of the head structures. Since observation and the history so far have not indicated a cranial nerve V dysfunction, other potential structures could include the temporomandibular joint (and related muscles) and the teeth. However, Amy did not refer to any dental discomfort or recent dentistry.

Middle ear. With the history of tinnitus, it was possible that a middle ear disorder might be involved; however the absence of any earache or loss of balance made the middle ear an unlikely candidate.

Cervical spine. Amy's account of the behaviour of the pain strongly suggested that the headaches were of cervical (musculoskeletal) origin because (i) the symptoms appeared to respond to mechanical changes, i.e. consistently worse with certain head/neck activities or postures; and (ii) the symptoms were consistently relieved by avoiding pain aggravating activities or postures during the days off work and following a night's rest.

Clinical reasoning commentary

Although the clinical evidence at this early stage suggests the cervical spine is the most likely source of the patient's symptoms, the clinician is obviously keeping an open mind to other possible sources. There is clearly a wide range of hypotheses considered in this category, including atypical manual therapy diagnoses such as meningeal tumours, vascular disorders and dental problems. This range of non-musculoskeletal potential sources highlights the breadth of propositional and non-propositional craft knowledge (i.e. clinical patterns) manual therapists must possess. By maintaining an open mind, the clinician is avoiding the common reasoning error of considering too few hypotheses, which may potentially bias the diagnostic decision-making process and related management decisions.

Another common reasoning error is to neglect negating features for hypotheses considered (confirmation bias). However, in this case, it is apparent that the clinician is alert to the absence of supportive findings (i.e. negative features) for some hypotheses and does not just weight the presence of supportive evidence (i.e. positive features). This requires substantial, reflective clinical experience to learn and be able to generate 'expected' cues or clinical findings associated with various patterns of presentation.

It is also of interest to note that even at this early stage of the clinical encounter the clinician feels he has sufficient information to begin to 'differentiate' between hypotheses as to the source of the pain. That is, as well as the obvious production of a good variety of hypotheses in this category, the reasoning process clearly also involves the ranking of hypotheses.

Amy had been involved in a rear-end motor vehicle accident 1 year previously. She was the driver of the car and was stationary at traffic lights with her head turned slightly to the right conversing with her passenger. She was hit without warning by a car about the same size as her own vehicle travelling at approximately 30 km/h. She stated that she was wearing a three-point seat belt and her head restraint was at her eye level, although she tended to drive with her back not in contact with the seat (i.e. leaning forward).

Amy denied any immediate pain or dizziness following impact and her head did not strike anything within the car. She remained conscious and alert.

Occipitofrontal headaches and tinnitus began within a few hours after the impact. Apart from temporary (1 month duration) lower neck and bilateral shoulder girdle pain, there were no other complaints following the accident. The headaches markedly decreased but did not disappear during a 2-week absence from work immediately after the accident. Upon returning to work, the headaches rapidly became worse, although the tinnitus had resolved completely

within 1 month. Initially, analgesics had little effect but anti-inflammatory medication relieved her symptoms sufficiently for her to be able to continue working. Amy had received high-velocity manipulative treatments from a chiropractor (2 months earlier) and also a physiotherapist (1 month earlier). On both occasions, the treatment had dramatically increased her symptoms and took several days to abate.

Amy reported a healthy childhood and there was no prior history of injury or disease, nor any relevant familial history. She had no current medical complaints. Presently she was unmarried and had no children.

REASONING DISCUSSION AND CLINICAL REASONING COMMENTARY

1 What did you think was the cause of the tinnitus?

Clinician's answer

Tinnitus can have a number of varying causes. These can be intracranial, such as an acoustic neuroma of cranial nerve VIII or damage to the cochleal nerve or organ of Corti (e.g. related to a fractured temporal bone). Tinnitus can also have extracranial causes and these fall into two categories: middle ear infections or damage to the tympanic membrane, and central excitation of the trigeminal nerve complex leading to hypertonus of the tensor tympani.

Amy denied any hearing loss, dizziness or loss of balance so this significantly decreases the likelihood of intracranial causes, middle ear infections or tympanic membrane damage.

The most likely cause would be central excitation from repetitive or unremitting input from a (damaged) structure within the trigeminal complex, with the tinnitus itself derived from hypertonus of the tensor tympani. Since Amy denied any head trauma and was not complaining of any jaw pain, toothache or earache, then the probable source of the tinnitus was the craniovertebral region (atlanto-occipital or atlantoaxial joints).

2 How did you interpret the unfavourable responses to the previous neck manipulations?

Clinician's answer

Exacerbation of symptoms can occur following manipulation when either there is tissue damage

present, which the manipulation increases, or the manipulation forces the joint to move into a hypermobile or segmentally unstable part of the range of motion. Since no recent trauma was reported, the most likely cause was that of an adaptively hypermobile or segmentally unstable joint. This will, of course, need to be confirmed later in the physical examination.

3 Given that she had now had constant headaches for 1 year and any soft tissue injury from the motor vehicle accident would have been expected to 'heal' in that time, what did you hypothesize was maintaining her headaches? Did you explore the possibility of any non-physical contributing factors?

Clinician's answer

The expectation of healing presupposes that the damage done to tissues leaves the potential for healing to occur. There are clear challenges to this supposition, amputation being the most obvious, but grade 3 ligamentous tears and untreated displaced fractures are further examples of tissue injuries that do not 'heal'. Of those that can heal, the most common type of healing in adults must be by 'second intention'.

Therefore, following traumatic arthritis, if one accepts that the capsule has been damaged then there will be generalized fibrosis throughout the capsular tissue, with resultant loss of motion and decreased sensitivity, i.e. ultimately a painless stiff joint. Habitual, functional movements that would normally require the lost motion of the damaged joint will determine any adaptation to this loss of motion. In the present case, the necessity for craniovertebral flexion, such as habitually looking down at work, would have demanded some compensatory movement in another craniovertebral joint. At the point that the compensating joint exhausts its adaptive potential, (trigeminal) pain will result.

Since this was an unsettled insurance claim, possible impending litigation was also an obvious factor. However, in the history, Amy detailed a very typical account of symptom delay followed by moderate head, neck and shoulder girdle pain that was relieved by rest from work for a short period of time. Upon return to work, despite an increase in symptoms, she remained at work and in addition admitted that within 2 weeks the lower neck pain, shoulder girdle pain and tinnitus were all totally relieved. Her current symptoms did not seem to be exaggerated, appeared to have a mechanical basis, and Amy readily admitted to being able to control them with rest. The consistent and non-exaggerated response to the physical assessment further supported the impression that there were no non-physical contributing factors.

◼ Clinical reasoning commentary

The responses to these questions show a progressive refinement of the primary diagnostic hypothesis, which incorporates consideration of both the structural source of the symptoms and the associated symptomatic and contributing impairments. The answer to Question 1 indicated the cervical spine was considered the most likely source of the patient's pain, but this hypothesis has clearly evolved with more clinical data. Consideration of the patient's tinnitus suggested the craniovertebral region in particular; the response to previous manipulation treatment raised the likelihood of a hypermobile joint; and finally the chronic nature of the problem and its mechanical behaviour suggested the presence of an adjacent hypomobile joint facilitating hypermobility of the symptomatic joint. The specificity of this hypothesis is typical of an expert clinician and the product of significant reflective practice.

While manual therapists are traditionally well aware of the importance of considering, assessing and managing physical contributing factors to patients' activity/participation restrictions, symptoms and impairments, as highlighted in Chapter 1, explicit attention to potential psychosocial contributing factors has historically been less formal, often a tacit impression gained through the course of other assessments. Psychosocial screening (e.g. patients' perspectives of their experiences, including their understanding, beliefs, feelings and attributions) is increasingly being recognized as an essential element of the manual therapist's assessment. The clinician's hypothesis in response to the second part of Question 3 (e.g. 'there were no non-physical contributing factors') illustrates his awareness and attention to this important area.

PHYSICAL EXAMINATION

Observation

Amy adopted an obvious forward head posture and this was brought to her attention. She stated that she had been made aware of this previously but that attempted correction of her posture had always led to increased headaches.

Cervical active movements

Gross movements were assessed:

◼ rotation to the right was limited 50% and painless on overpressure
◼ rotation to the left was full range and reproduced the suboccipital pain with overpressure

◼ gross flexion and extension appeared full range and was pain-free
◼ gross side bending appeared full range and was pain-free bilaterally.

On the basis of these findings, an assessment of range of motion was again performed, but with emphasis on localizing motion to the craniovertebral joints:

◼ from neutral (patient sitting up straight), craniovertebral flexion (chin to 'Adam's apple') was completely absent and overpressure reproduced the left-sided suboccipital pain
◼ craniovertebral extension was full range and pain-free

craniovertebral side bending to the left was 0 degrees and painless on overpressure, whereas right side bending appeared full range and was pain-free.

Compression and traction

Manual compression through the head did not alter Amy's symptoms, but sustained manual traction increased the suboccipital pain.

Neurological tests

Key upper limb muscle tests, skin sensation and reflexes were all normal. Lower limb reflexes, including clonus and Babinski, were all normal.

Neural mobility tests

The slump test was negative: although suboccipital pain could be reproduced by craniovertebral flexion this pain was not influenced by any lower limb motion. The suboccipital pain was also not influenced by performance of the upper limb neural tension/mobility test with the head maintained in craniovertebral flexion.

Passive intervertebral joint motion and stability tests

Passive range of motion was considered normal in all segments (C2–C3 to C7–T1). No instability was detected.

Craniovertebral joint stress tests

The following tests were performed on the craniovertebral joints:

- traction in craniovertebral flexion: craniovertebral flexion reproduced left suboccipital pain and traction further increased it
- anterior translation of occiput on fixed atlas did not reproduce symptoms
- lateral translation of the atlanto-axial joint did not reproduce symptoms
- anterior translation of atlas on fixed axis did not reproduce symptoms
- alar ligament tests (bilaterally tested in flexion, neutral and extension): craniovertebral

flexion reproduced left suboccipital pain; right-side bending motion increased this pain and other motions produced no change in the symptoms
- anterior translation of atlas and axis on a fixed occiput (posterior translation of atlanto-occipital joint) reproduced left suboccipital pain; if the stress was maintained, the left-sided retro-ocular pain was reproduced.

All tests were negative for instability. No cord or vertebrobasilar artery signs or symptoms were provoked.

Combined movement testing with overpressure

Rotation was again performed, this time in craniovertebral flexion (chin tuck) and then in craniovertebral extension (chin poke).

In craniovertebral flexion the left suboccipital pain was reproduced, but:

- with the addition of right rotation, there was a slight decrease in this pain and the limitation of right rotation (seen in neutral) increased to 75% (of left rotation in neutral); there was no increased pain with overpressure
- with the addition of rotation to the left, the left suboccipital pain gradually increased until Amy stopped moving, because of the pain, with a 10% loss of left rotation
- with the addition of overpressure to rotation to the left, a full range of motion was gained, with a significant increase in suboccipital pain; if performed slowly, the overpressure had a normal end-feel, but if performed more rapidly, an end-feel of spasm was evoked.

In craniovertebral extension, both rotation to the left and right were full range with no pain elicited on overpressure.

Isometric muscle tests

After overpressure of the combined active movements was released, isometric muscle resistance was given to the antagonistic (in relation to the movement) muscles while in their optimally lengthened position. Isometric muscle testing neither aggravated nor alleviated Amy's symptoms.

REASONING DISCUSSION AND CLINICAL REASONING COMMENTARY

1 Did the findings at this point suggest a clinical pattern that might implicate certain structures?

Clinician's answer

Restricted or painful neck movement can have several possible causes.

Zygapophyseal joint dysfunction. Although acute traumatic arthritis of a zygapophyseal joint might present with a significant loss of rotation, the loss of rotation is accommodated for within 3–6 months post-trauma, presumably by decompensation throughout the rest of the spine: that is, residual loss of rotation from a chronic zygapophyseal joint lesion is minimal ('decompensation' refers to neurophysiological and/or biomechanical strategies employed by the body to make itself more functionally efficient). Further, from clinical experience, the lesion would be associated with a significant loss of side bending that could never be compensated. There was no indication of a significant loss of side bending in this case.

Cervical spondylosis. Generalized degenerative changes will lead to a marked loss of rotation. However, the loss occurs as part of an articular pattern of restriction, which would involve an equal limitation of side bending. In addition, personal clinical observations indicate that restrictions of motion from degenerative spondylosis are more likely to be bilateral.

Muscle lesion. Since the limitation of right rotation motion was increased with craniovertebral flexion, the sternomastoid, trapezius or posterior suboccipital muscles could have been responsible. Because the isometric muscle tests were negative in terms of pain reproduction, one can assume that if muscle tissue were responsible it must be chronically scarred and contracted, given the time elapsed since the accident. If the offending muscle was shortened by scarring/fibrosis, the only detectable sign would be a loss of motion. The sternomastoid and trapezius muscles were unlikely culprits because there was no history of any pain in the anterolateral region of the neck. The degree and direction of lost motion suggested it would have to be a suboccipital muscle with a significant rotational line of force,

possibly either the left inferior oblique or the right superior oblique.

Upper cervical joints. The fact that head/neck motions reproduced or aggravated Amy's pain inculpates the neck. The upper three joints share a common sensory nerve supply from the cervical nucleus of the trigeminal complex. In particular, the gross unilateral loss of rotation suggested a craniovertebral joint dysfunction, as these joints are responsible for up to 50% of available head rotation (Dvorak et al., 1988). In this case, the magnitude of the rotational loss means that it could never be decompensated, no matter how chronic the injury.

Combined motions using flexion and extension may help to differentiate further the responsible craniovertebral joint. The reasoning behind this is that flexion and extension of the atlanto-occipital joint can also be viewed biomechanically as anterior roll with posterior glide (Fig. 15.2) and posterior roll with anterior

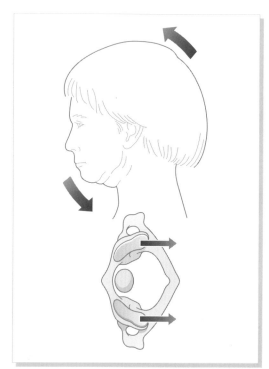

Fig. 15.2 During atlanto-occipital joint flexion, both condyles of the occiput glide posteriorly.

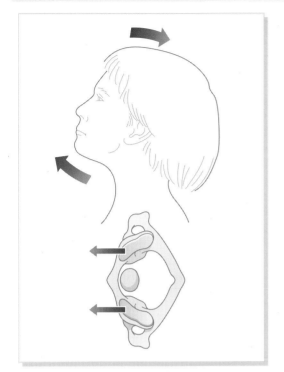

Fig. 15.3   During atlanto-occipital joint extension, both condyles of the occiput glide anteriorly.

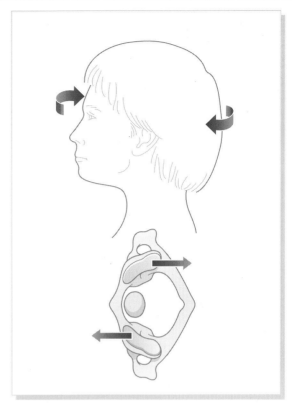

Fig. 15.4   At the atlanto-occipital joints during rotation of the head to the right, the right occipital condyle will glide posteriorly and the left occipital condyle will glide anteriorly.

glide (Fig. 15.3) respectively. Similarly, during right rotation, for example, there would be a corresponding anterior glide of the left occipital condyle and a posterior glide of the right occipital condyle (Fig. 15.4). By initiating the motion with flexion, some of the available posterior glide within both atlanto-occipital joints is taken up. If a restriction of posterior glide were to exist within the right joint, then right rotation, which utilizes further posterior gliding of the right occipital condyle, would appear to increase in its limitation.

However, flexion and extension of the atlanto-axial joint do not share any of the same biomechanical components as rotation of this joint. For example, right rotation occurs as a result of an anteroinferior glide of the left C1 condyle (on C2) and a simultaneous posteroinferior glide of the right C1 condyle (on C2). During flexion and extension, there is a bilateral and simultaneous anterior and posterior roll (respectively) only of the C1 condyles on the C2 condyles (reciprocally male/male) (Kapandji, 1974; Werne, 1958). Translation or gliding is normally prohibited by the dens/transverse ligament restraint mechanism (Fig. 15.5). Therefore, flexion and

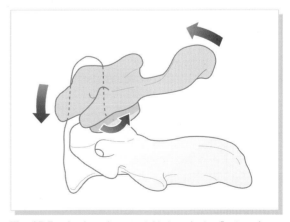

Fig. 15.5   At the atlanto-axial joints during flexion, the convex condyles of the atlas roll anteriorly. There is no significant anterior or posterior glide on the condyles of the axis.

extension can have no direct effect on rotation at the atlanto-axial joints.

Consequently, if there is an obvious change in the available rotation at the craniovertebral joints (either better or worse) when combined with flexion or extension, the restriction lies within an atlanto-occipital joint. If, however, the rotation range of motion does not alter during flexion or extension, then the restriction lies within an atlanto-axial joint.

Pain was also provoked during instability testing involving craniovertebral flexion, possibly suggesting inert tissue irritation. This response could have been coming from the atlanto-occipital and/or atlanto-axial joint capsules, the posterior atlanto-occipital ligament, the posterior atlanto-occipital membrane or the atlanto-axial joint ligamentum flavum.

■ Clinical reasoning commentary

A well-organized and accessible knowledge base is a vital element of the reasoning process and is especially applied by the expert in the recognition of clinical patterns and their associated actions. Clinical knowledge comprises both propositional and non-propositional information, the latter including professional craft or procedural knowledge and personal knowledge. The thinking evident in this answer provides a very good example of the seamless integration of propositional knowledge (e.g. biomechanics and structural anatomy of the cervical spine and related musculature) and professional craft knowledge (e.g. concept of decompensation and the application of combined movement examination findings) characteristic of the expert clinician.

Further examination

The information gained in the preliminary physical examination was extended by further passive tests.

Passive intervertebral motion tests for the craniovertebral joints

With the head positioned at the limit of flexion and right rotation:

- the right atlanto-occipital joint was tested with an anterior glide of the right condyle of the atlas: this was met with a firm, unyielding end-feel and was pain-free (Fig. 15.6)
- the atlanto-axial joints were tested with an antero-superior glide of the right condyle of the axis under a fixed atlas (Fig. 15.7), and an anteroinferior glide of the left condyle of the atlas on a fixed axis (Fig. 15.8): both showed normal available glide and were pain-free.

With the head positioned at the limit of left rotation in flexion:

- the left atlanto-occipital joint was tested with an anterior glide of the left condyle of the atlas, under a fixed occiput: there was some available glide before a firm end-feel was reached and Amy's

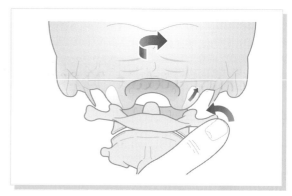

Fig. 15.6 Overpressure of right atlanto-occipital joint flexion is given by fixing the occiput at the limit of craniovertebral flexion and right rotation, and gliding the right condyle of the atlas anteriorly.

suboccipital pain was increased, with the retro-orbital pain also reproduced
- when the atlas was fixed and the left occipital condyle of the left atlanto-occipital joint was moved anteriorly, there was a marked decrease in Amy's pain
- the atlanto-axial joints were tested with an antero-superior glide of the left condyle of the axis under a fixed atlas, and an anteroinferior glide of the right condyle of the atlas on a fixed axis: both indicated a normal, firm end-feel with no reproduction of pain.

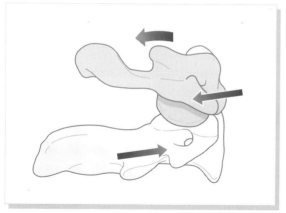

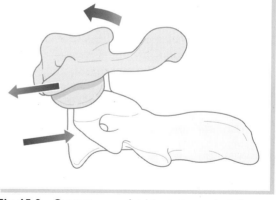

Fig. 15.7 Overpressure of right rotation at the right atlanto-axial joint is produced by fixing the atlas and gliding the right condyle of the axis anteriorly and superiorly.

Fig. 15.8 Overpressure of right rotation at the left atlanto-axial joint is produced by fixing the axis and gliding the left condyle of the atlas anteriorly and inferiorly.

Temporomandibular joint

Examination of the temporomandibular joint was not performed because at this stage Amy's symptoms were clearly induced or aggravated by motion of the head and neck.

 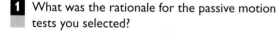

REASONING DISCUSSION AND CLINICAL REASONING COMMENTARY

1 What was the rationale for the passive motion tests you selected?

Clinician's answer

Flexion of the atlanto-occipital joint is produced by the simultaneous motions of an anterior roll (i.e. angular motion) and a posterior glide (i.e. linear motion). This combination of movements is stressed further in the right atlanto-occipital joint by combining flexion with right rotation. In this case, it was noted that the restriction of right rotation appeared to increase with the combination. The question was whether the restriction had an articular or extra-articular (e.g. muscle) cause. To answer this, Amy was asked to flex and rotate right to her barrier of motion. At that point, the head was fixed (occipital condyles) and the right condyle of the atlas was gently glided anteriorly (an anterior glide of the atlas under the occiput is the same as a posterior glide of the occiput on the atlas). The loss of joint glide at the point of motion restriction confirmed an articular hypomobility.

In the case of the atlanto-axial joint, the principles are basically the same. Amy was asked to move actively to her motion barrier (right rotation in flexion). Right rotation involves a simultaneous motion at the right and left joints. At the left atlanto-axial joint, the condyle of the atlas glides anteriorly and inferiorly on the C2 condyle, while at the right joint the right condyle of the atlas glides posteriorly and inferiorly. Therefore, the atlanto-axial joint's involvement in right rotation restriction may be tested by applying an anteroinferior glide of the left atlas condyle on a fixed C2, and then assessing the anterosuperior glide of the right C2 condyle under a fixed atlas (i.e. a relative posteroinferior glide of the right atlas condyle). If there is any motion available in these glides, which in this case there was, then the atlanto-axial joint tested is not responsible for the loss of active motion.

Similar glides to those detailed above may also be used to stress a joint's motion at the end of range to see whether the joint may be responsible for the pain. In this case, the head was actively rotated left to the end of range; the passive range of motion was considered normal but was painful. If the pain is coming from a joint then it follows that stressing the joint into its motion barrier will reproduce or aggravate the pain if that pain originates within the restraining structures of joint motion (in the absence of isometric muscle action): that is, the joint capsule and capsular ligaments.

2 What bearing did the physical examination findings have on your working hypothesis as to the source of the symptoms and physical impairments?

Clinician's answer

The passive movement tests confirmed that the cause of the motion restriction into right rotation, and right rotation in flexion, was an inability of the right atlanto-occipital joint to flex. The tests also confirmed that flexion of the left atlanto-occipital joint was the source of Amy's symptoms (i.e. posterior glide of the left occipital condyle occurring during flexion and left rotation of the head, exaggerated by anterior translation of the left condyle of the atlas). The findings, therefore, supported the working hypothesis of residual post-traumatic hypomobility of right atlanto-occipital joint flexion, with decompensatory, painful hypermobility of the left atlanto-occipital joint.

To explain this further, Amy has an atlanto-occipital joint that cannot flex. Initially her compensation will be to adopt a forward head posture; however, her job as a receptionist demands craniovertebral flexion. To decompensate for this dysfunction (i.e. to make flexion more functionally efficient), either the atlanto-axial joints or the contralateral (left) atlanto-occipital joint must adapt to this new biomechanical demand. It is uncertain why the left atlanto-occipital joint would have decompensated rather than the atlanto-axial joints.

Perhaps when the right atlanto-occipital joint became unable to flex or posteriorly glide, the atlas would have started to pivot around this new 'fixed point' (i.e. the fixated right atlanto-occipital joint), creating a new oblique axis of flexion/extension and leading to excessive posterior gliding of the left atlanto-occipital joint. This excessive posterior glide may have increased biomechanical stress on the joint capsule. Thus, muscle spasm was initiated during rapid motion to help to safeguard the anatomical integrity of the joint capsule and prevent subluxation.

This hypothesis of a reactive hypermobility was supported by the observation that during combined movement testing left rotation in flexion, although full range with slow overpressure, was painfully restricted actively. The fact that a spasm end-feel was encountered when rapid left rotation overpressure was attempted was an indication that the compensation was extremely irritable and possibly exceeding its adaptive potential.

Whatever the working hypothesis, it matters little since the key issue was that Amy's symptoms were reproduced by overpressure of left atlanto-occipital joint flexion (posterior glide) at the end of normal range. Since this accompanies the finding of a hypomobile right atlanto-occipital joint, logic would dictate a correction of this abnormal biomechanical state is needed, i.e. mobilize right atlanto-occipital joint flexion.

3 What were your thoughts regarding the mechanisms initially causing and subsequently perpetuating the patient's symptoms and physical impairments?

Clinician's answer

The onset involved a rear-end collision while stationary and with Amy caught unawares. The impact velocity of 30 km/h would have likely resulted in high acceleration forces. In addition, her head was rotated to the right and she habitually leaned forward when driving. The momentum may, therefore, have created a relative posterior translatory and right rotational force within segments of her neck. In particular, if Amy's head was positioned in flexion and right rotation at impact, the right atlanto-occipital joint may have been near the end of its range of motion, resulting in trauma to its capsule.

The most likely result of the injury was a post-traumatic arthritis of the right atlanto-occipital joint. This is supported by the fact that Amy could only get relief during periods away from work (when the need for craniovertebral flexion was reduced), when lying supine with no pillow, and by her adoption of a forward head posture (i.e. craniovertebral extension). Conversely, the symptoms were aggravated by head flexion postures at work. The initial relief afforded by anti-inflammatory medication further suggested a significant inflammatory response to an injury of the atlanto-occipital joint capsule.

Chronic post-inflammatory fibrosis of the right atlanto-occipital joint capsule probably limited its flexion. Because of the demands of her work, decompensation of this unilateral hypomobility likely involved the left atlanto-occipital joint. Eventually, the exhausted adaptive potential of the left atlanto-occipital joint may have given rise to worsening trigeminal symptoms (e.g. referred retro-orbital pain representative of the ophthalmic division of cranial nerve V). The extreme sensitivity (inflamed state) of the left atlanto-occipital joint was also evidenced by Amy's adverse reaction to manipulative treatment (usually targeted at the painful dysfunction) and by the onset of muscle spasm with combined movements in the physical assessment.

■ Clinical reasoning commentary

Clinical decisions should be based on the available evidence. However, because there are few research data on the sensitivity and specificity of most manual therapy assessment procedures, clinicians often must rely on extrapolation of biomedical theory (in this case, upper cervical joint kinematics) and logic (e.g. provocation of symptoms in a nociceptive dominant presentation implicating local joint structures as the source of the symptoms) in order to detect and judge the relevance of specific physical impairments. While some argue that theory is not evidence (e.g. Rothstein and Scalzitti, 1999), it is important not to down-play the value of using established theory to help to make sense of patient findings. As long as clinicians are critical of unvalidated assessment and management procedures, and are systematic and thorough in their application and reassessment of interventions, then clinical evidence should be accepted until such time as higher levels of evidence become available.

ᴍ Management

■ First treatment

The aim of management was to mobilize the right atlanto-occipital joint into flexion and restore normal posture. Following the physical assessment, the treatment plan was explained to the patient, especially the reasons why the 'wrong' joint would be treated.

The initial treatment then consisted of a sustained stretching mobilization of the right atlanto-occipital joint into the flexion barrier, using muscle assistance and levering indirectly through the right condyle of the atlas. For this technique, Amy was seated and slightly slouched so as to put the craniovertebral joints in a more neutral position. Amy's atlas was palpated with the left hand and the head was grasped with the right hand. She was asked to relax and the head was then passively guided through craniovertebral flexion until the atlas began to move, followed by right rotation until the atlas again began to move. At this point, the flexion/right rotation motion barrier of the right atlanto-occipital joint had been reached. The atlas was then gently secured with a lumbrical grip using the left thumb (posterior to the right transverse process of the atlas) and index finger (anterior to the left transverse process of the atlas) (Fig. 15.9).

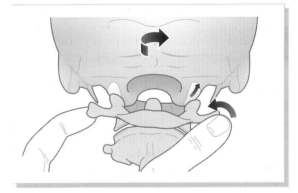

Fig. 15.9 During mobilization of flexion at the right atlanto-occipital joint, the occiput is fixed while the atlas is rotated to the left.

Next, Amy was asked to turn her head into the therapist's chest, which provided resistance to the movement, thus eliciting an isometric contraction. By reversing origin and insertion, the suboccipital muscles (mainly left superior oblique) will produce left rotation of the atlas under the occiput, that is relative right rotation of the occiput. After a 3 second hold, Amy was told to relax. Any subsequent slack occurring at the motion barrier was taken up by the therapist's left thumb pushing anteriorly on the right transverse process of the atlas. This was continued until no further slack was produced by the isometric contractions.

Upon reassessment of Amy's active motion, right rotation in flexion had increased by about 20 degrees. Craniovertebral flexion itself was less painful. Flexion and left rotation remained painful and slightly restricted.

In addition, Amy was instructed to exaggerate slightly the chin tuck action when bending forward, especially on lifting. After each treatment, exercises were also given aimed at improving the patient's craniovertebral movement and forward head posture.

Exercise 1 (atlanto-occipital flexion)

Amy was instructed how to produce craniovertebral flexion and right rotation in order to maintain and perhaps improve upon the motion gained by the mobilization.

Exercise 2 (passive upper thoracic extension)

Standing about 60 cm away from the corner of a room, the patient places their hands on adjacent sides of the corner, at about neck height. Keeping the chin gently tucked in, the patient leans forwards trying to place their chest into the corner.

The effect of this position is to extend the upper thoracic spine passively and stretch the pectoral muscles (especially pectoralis minor), which often become tight with a forward head posture. This position is held for 10 seconds and released. The exercise is repeated at least 10 times per session, three times a day. It is explained to the patient that they should make the exercise a habit whenever a flexed posture (e.g. deskwork) is adopted.

Exercise 3 (relaxed expiration with active upper thoracic extension)

The patient is seated on the edge of a treatment table with their feet supported on a stool. The therapist places a thumb and index finger in the patient's first intercostal space and pushes gently downwards. The following instruction is given: 'I want you to push your chest up against my fingers'. The patient will invariably comply by taking a deep breath in. This should be repeated a few times so that the patient gets the idea of pushing their chest upwards against the therapist's hand.

The therapist then continues: 'Now this time I want you take a breath in and then push up against my fingers as you breathe *out*'. Lower thoracic and lumbar spine 'trick' movements are easily corrected later by doing the exercise slouched in a chair. The important thing here is that the patient appreciates the idea of elevating the chest while breathing out. The patient is instructed to practise this exercise as often as possible during the day.

The exercise produces active extension of the upper thoracic spine and cervicothoracic junction and helps to regain/maintain craniovertebral flexion (with the aid of gravity).

■ Second treatment

In an attempt to desensitize the left atlanto-occipital joint, Amy was advised to take a week's leave of absence from work, during which time a second and similar mobilization treatment was given.

At the second visit, Amy demonstrated all home exercises well. It was decided to introduce further exercises, while continuing with the previous exercises.

Exercise 4 (active, resisted craniovertebral flexion)

Amy was positioned in supine lying, knees flexed over a pillow and with her head supported on a single, soft pillow of sufficient height for comfort. The therapist's fingers were placed under her occiput and she was instructed to gently move her chin towards her Adam's apple.

If the patient performs the motion correctly the therapist should feel a slight decrease in the weight of the patient's head, but the head should not lose contact with the therapist's hands. If contact is lost, then the patient is flexing lower down the neck. The therapist should also not feel any increased pressure or weight through their hands, as this would indicate the patient is using extensor muscles (probably thoracic).

Exercise 5 (resisted cervicothoracic and upper thoracic spine extension)

Continuing on from where the previous exercise ended (in craniovertebral flexion), Amy was instructed to gently push backwards against the therapist's fingers. Provided the patient's chin does not lift away from their throat, this exercise resists the upper thoracic extensor muscles. Amy was able to perform this exercise at home using a pillow for resistance.

Both exercises 4 and 5 were performed 10 times per set, three sets a day initially. As Amy felt stronger and less painful, the number of repetitions in a set was increased to the point of fatigue.

Subsequent treatments

Three more similar treatments were given, each a week apart, until the full range of right atlanto-occipital joint flexion was achieved. However, as this condition was one of chronic fibrotic hypomobility, regaining joint range of motion was largely dependent on Amy's home exercise and postural programme.

At the third treatment, Amy enquired about the possibility of joining a gym to regain her former (pre-accident) strength and fitness levels. This was encouraged but only after she was taken into the clinic's gym and taught how to use pulleys and weights without compromising the efficient and safe neck posture she had achieved. By the fifth and final treatment, she was participating in a 1 hour per day gym programme without any adverse effects and demonstrated a full range of flexion of the right atlanto-occipital joint. She had also been working full time for 2 weeks without any symptoms. Although the occipital pain could still be somewhat reproduced (4/10) with sustained overpressure of left atlanto-occipital joint flexion, treatment was ceased on the understanding that Amy would continue to self-manage her condition.

REASONING DISCUSSION AND CLINICAL REASONING COMMENTARY

1 What was the relationship between the patient's forward head posture and her clinical presentation?

Clinician's answer

When a forward head (poking chin) posture becomes chronic or habitual, it essentially becomes a respiratory dysfunction and must be treated accordingly to reverse its pathological changes. The accident may have elicited or contributed to the patient's habitual forward head posture; unless this was corrected, pathological sequelae were more than likely going to occur in the future.

The most immediate biomechanical effect of this posture is that the localized flexion of the upper thoracic segments will produce a depression of the first and second ribs anteriorly. This will effectively increase loading on the anterior chest, increasing the motor recruitment demands of the diaphragm, even during quiet respiration. The increased motor recruitment (tone) will resist complete expiration, maintaining the lower ribs in an elevated (inspiration) position. Eventually, without correction, this will lead to a 'barrel chest' and the onset of 'apical' breathing. It can also facilitate the development of degenerative changes in the lower cervical spine.

It was hypothesized that Amy was not going to get functionally better unless this dysfunction was treated, and it was expected the recovery period (of the postural dysfunction) would be measured in months. Although exercises were given primarily as a preventative measure, without correcting the posture it would have been impossible to regain full flexion of the craniovertebral region. The exercises also helped to strengthen the muscles necessary to maintain an optimally efficient posture.

2 What did you consider was the likely prognosis for this patient?

Clinician's answer

At the initial assessment, it was clear that the right atlanto-occipital joint was not going to start moving spontaneously and consequently the pain from the adapting left atlanto-occipital joint would have probably continued to worsen, especially if her work involving craniovertebral flexion was maintained. After such a protracted period of recovery, it was possible that the extreme of left atlanto-occipital joint flexion may have remained hypersensitive permanently. However, her rate of recovery, symptomatically and functionally, since having the cause of this secondary dysfunction corrected was rapid enough to indicate complete relief of symptoms was likely.

Amy's main struggle was to avoid returning to her habitual forward head posture, although her decision to take charge of her own recovery by joining a gym demonstrated a determination not to return to her former painful lifestyle. It was likely that after such a protracted recovery time there would always be some hypersensitivity of the left atlanto-occipital joint; however, short of further trauma, it did not appear that this would continue to be a symptomatic joint.

3 Did you consider treating the hypermobile left atlanto-occipital joint with a programme of muscle stabilization?

Clinician's answer

Muscle stabilization for treatment of cervical spine dysfunction is undertaken if there is an indication of segmental instability or obvious (rather than assumed) weakness of the cervical musculature that could predispose to segmental instability. In this case, Amy had a hypermobile joint, that is an abnormal increase in angular (physiological) motion, secondary to a hypomobile joint in the same kinetic chain. There were no indications of segmental instability in either the craniovertebral joints or in the middle to lower cervical spine. Indeed, the anatomical integrity of all structures tested was intact.

The treatment goal was to eliminate the left atlanto-occipital joint's need to adapt for a loss of motion within the kinetic chain (i.e. mobilize the stiff right atlanto-occipital joint). Nothing needed be done to the symptomatic left joint except for some palliative considerations (e.g. avoidance strategies). A muscular re-education programme was in fact initiated, but its

aim was to gain and maintain range of motion of the right joint.

Clinical reasoning commentary

The clinician, an expert in manual therapy, has demonstrated the importance of thinking beyond just the musculoskeletal system. The discussed potential interactions between the musculoskeletal and respiratory systems reflects a holistic approach to treatment and management. Consistent with this approach, the focus is not only on treating the present primary impairment (i.e. the hypomobile right atlanto-occipital joint), but also on the prevention of possible 'pathological sequelae' such as the development of a barrel chest and degenerative changes.

Making a decision about the prognosis of a problem is one of the most challenging tasks that the manual therapist faces. Patients inevitably wish to know whether full recovery is likely and, if so, the related timeframe and whether the problem will recur. To answer these questions, the expert clinician usually relies heavily on the process of pattern recognition, which is based on substantial experience with similar clinical presentations and their associated responses to intervention and paths to recovery. Nevertheless, the clinician in this case is clearly aware that each patient presentation is unique and any initial prognostic hypothesis must be tested by the application of findings from the interview and physical examination, as well as preliminary treatment. There is obvious evidence that prognostic indicators, both favourable (e.g. good response to manual therapy treatment) and unfavourable (e.g. chronicity of the problem), have been considered and weighted in the present case.

References

Dvorak, J., Penning, L., Hayek, J. et al. (1988). Functional diagnostics of the cervical spine using computer tomography. Neuroradiology, 30, 132–137.

Kapandji, I.A. (1974). Physiology of the Joints, 2nd edn: Vol. 3, Trunk and Vertebral Column. Edinburgh: Churchill Livingstone.

Rothstein, J.M. and Scalzitti, D.A. (1999). Commentary: physiotherapy quo vadis. Advances in Physiotherapy, 1, 9–12.

Werne, S. (1958). The possibilities of movement in the craniovertebral joints. Acta Orthopaedica Scandinavica, 28, 165–173.

CHAPTER 16

A judge's fractured radius with metal fixation following an accident

Robert Pfund in collaboration with Freddy Kaltenborn

SUBJECTIVE EXAMINATION

Ralf is a 54-year-old man who had fractured the distal part of his right radius in a motorcycle accident. No other significant injuries were sustained in the accident. He has been sent to our clinic for physiotherapy treatment 4 weeks after the injury. He has had an osteosynthetic procedure to stabilize the fracture with a permanent metal fixation, after which he was placed in a half-cast for 3 weeks. The cast has now been removed.

The accident did not involve another vehicle; rather, he was speeding and lost control, causing him to fall and slide off the roadway. There was not any significant damage to his motorbike and no involvement from the insurance company. Ralf works as a judge, lives alone and has a person who looks after the household. He generally appears happy, even when talking about the accident. His general health is good, with only slightly elevated blood pressure over the last 5 years; this is well controlled by beta-blockers.

Ralf appeared to be somewhat unfit and volunteered that because of his work he had little time for exercise. He reported being about 10 kg overweight and talked about doing some fitness training when he recovered.

There was no past history of any upper limb problems, although Ralf had experienced minor neck and low back problems over the previous 10 years. He stated that these never lasted more than 2 to 3 days and would always settle spontaneously without ever requiring treatment.

The distal part of the forearm and the wrist was swollen, with the skin slightly shiny. His distal forearm hair in this area was notably very dark compared

with the other side. No redness was present in the injured area.

At rest, Ralf described a feeling of swelling and slight soreness around his wrist, and increased sensitivity on the volar side of his second and third finger extending up the middle third of the radial side of his forearm. He had no complaints of any other symptoms in the arms, neck, face or trunk. All his symptoms were approximately 30% worse in the morning when he woke up, and then improved as he moved his wrist and hand during the first hours of the day. For the rest of the day, these symptoms stayed in a mild form just above his level of awareness. He did not have any night pain and could sleep without difficulty. Walking with his arm hanging for more than 30 minutes increased the feeling of swelling and changed his perception of temperature in the whole forearm (felt colder than the other side). Standing with a dependent arm did not produce the same symptoms, but he never stood for 30 minutes. When these sensations were present, the palmar side of his hand showed an increase in sweating that lasted for approximately 30 minutes after he stopped walking. While the dependent arm position produced changes in his feelings of swelling, temperature and sweating, it had no affect on his wrist soreness.

Using his hand during eating and any writing (he was right handed) immediately increased his resting symptoms around 10%, whereas more specific movements of his wrist produced a sharp pain (4–5/10 on a visual analogue scale), which eased immediately when the wrist was taken out of these positions. Ralf's main concern was his restricted and painful movement, especially the combined movement into dorsal flexion and radial abduction. Other screening questions about the influence of movements or fixed positions of the neck, thorax or shoulder complex showed no relation to Ralf's symptoms other than the effect of the dependent arm position already described.

REASONING DISCUSSION AND CLINICAL REASONING COMMENTARY

1 What were your initial impressions at this stage?

Clinicians' answer

The fracture was only of the radius with no involvement of the wrist joint or the distal radioulnar joint. Therefore we would not expect too much difficulty in restoring movement. Because of the time since the injury (4 weeks), we would take care in applying stress by active or passive manoeuvres directly to the stabilized radius. At this stage, his psychosocial status did not appear to be an issue (for example, there was no fear of losing his job), and he seemed to be coping well with his injury. His general health and fitness were not ideal, but these were not considered sufficiently compromised to affect significantly the healing of his injury. Overall, Ralf seemed to have a straightforward presentation with slight autonomic nervous system disturbance. We would place him into the normal range of patients with a fractured radius.

2 How did you interpret the specific nature of the increased sensitivity he reported? Similarly, what were your thoughts at this stage regarding the changes in swelling, temperature and sweating that he had noted when he was walking with his arm dependent? Did his report of these symptoms and symptom behaviour elicit any plans on your part for specific physical assessments?

Clinicians' answer

In patients with stabilized fractures, we commonly see symptoms suggestive of slight autonomic nervous system disturbance. These alterations mostly disappear when the stabilizing material is removed. Therefore, we would not use any specific assessment techniques at this stage but would take care not to raise his level of sympathetic activity any further. In particular, care was needed not to produce too much pain and to avoid making statements about possible impairments/disability, or any other comment that could increase his fear and uncertainty about the injury and his prognosis.

3 Could you comment on what potential sources you felt were implicated by his different symptoms?

Clinicians' answer

Disturbance of the *autonomic nervous system* could be the source of the:

- swelling of the distal part of the forearm and wrist
- shiny skin
- darker forearm hair
- swelling and slight soreness around his wrist at rest
- increased sensitivity on the fingers and radial side of his forearm
- feelings of swelling, temperature perception and sweating in the arm if it was dependent for more than 30 minutes while walking.

The continued presence of *inflammation* could cause the more severe symptoms to occur in the morning on awakening with improvement on movement of the wrist and hand, and continued mild symptoms through the rest of the day.

Irritation of the *median and the radial nerves* in the wrist area could cause the feeling of swelling and slight soreness around his wrist at rest and increased sensitivity on the fingers and radial side of his forearm. Altered sensitivity of the *central nervous system* could also give rise to these symptoms.

Damage to the *radiocarpal or intercarpal (radial and central column) joints* could give rise to the restricted and painful movement, especially the combined movement into dorsal flexion and radial abduction.

Clinical reasoning commentary

The clinicians' breadth of reasoning is evident through their answers here. Reference is made to considerations regarding the patient's psychosocial status, potential sources of the symptoms, pain mechanisms, tissue mechanisms, precautions and prognosis. Clearly, reasoning is taking place on multiple levels. While diagnostic reasoning with respect to possible sources and tissue mechanisms is obvious, the recognition that care is needed for the patient's understanding and feelings regarding the injury and prognosis also illustrates a broader consideration for the patient's psychosocial status and how this can influence the patient's symptoms. This sensitivity to the patient's 'pain experience' is a nice example of what was discussed as 'narrative reasoning' in Chapter 1.

PHYSICAL EXAMINATION

Screening examination

The screening examination was used to identify the area where it is possible to influence the patient's symptoms by alleviation and provocation. Based on these findings, the next more detailed part of the physical examination can be planned (Kaltenborn, 1999).

Using the painful combination of movement into dorsal flexion and radial abduction, differentiation of regional involvement between the wrist/hand complex, the elbow complex and neural structures was performed. To provoke the symptoms, Ralf's wrist was positioned just short of the onset of pain (P1). Ralf was then asked separately to move the elbow joint (flexion and extension), the shoulder girdle (elevation and depression) and the cervical spine (side bending left and right, flexion and extension) to determine if any of these movements provoked his symptoms. For the alleviation differentiation, Ralf's wrist was positioned in the same combined movement position, only this time just into pain, and the same movements of the elbow, shoulder girdle and cervical spine were used. None of the provocation differentiation manoeuvres elicited his symptoms and none of the alleviation manoeuvres eased them (Pfund and Zahnd, 2001).

Detailed examination

Angular (physiological) movements (active and passive) of the wrist

Active movement of Ralf's hand into dorsal flexion produced a sharp pain deep in the dorsal aspect of his wrist joint; whereas volar flexion gave a more superficial pulling over the dorsal part of the wrist joint. Ulnar abduction gave him a superficial pulling on the radial side of the joint; whereas radial abduction led to a sharp, more deeply located pain in the same area. Supination of the forearm was grossly restricted and painful in the radial and volar aspect of the wrist. Pronation was also restricted, but less so than supination, and elicited only a slight pain. When tested passively and compared with his active movements, each movement had slightly more available range but increased pain.

Translatory (passive accessory) movements

Translatory 'joint play' movements (i.e. traction, compression and gliding), assessing range and quality of movement, were performed in the resting position and then again just short of end-range (Kaltenborn, 1999). These tests are used to assess the arthrokinematics of the wrist complex and not the pain response.

Distal radioulnar joint. Passively gliding the radius in a dorsal and volar direction showed slightly more resistance than was seen on the other side. When pre-positioned just short of end-range, there was restricted dorsal gliding of the radius in supination, and restricted volar gliding in pronation. The resistance began very early in the range in both supination and pronation, although the pronation end-feel was harder compared with the other side.

Wrist joint. General translatory movements (i.e. traction and gliding in volar, dorsal, radial and ulnar directions) of the whole right wrist complex in the resting position showed less range and more resistance in each direction compared with the left wrist. Pre-positioned (short of end-range) traction into more resistance, in volar flexion and ulnar abduction, produced the same superficial pulling as described during the angular movements.

Intercarpal joints. Volar gliding of scaphoid on radius and of lunate on radius was restricted. The other intercarpal joints showed no movement alterations. Movement of lunate on radius was most restricted when the wrist was positioned in pure dorsal flexion; the movement of scaphoid on radius was most restricted when the wrist was pre-positioned in combined dorsal flexion and radial abduction (compared with the other side).

Isometric contraction

Because of the history, the results of the regional differentiation (i.e. moving the neck, shoulder and elbow with the wrist pre-positioned before and after P1) and the quality of the passive movements of the wrist (firmer end-feel compared with the other side), no isometric contraction tests were applied at this stage.

Specific provocation and alleviation tests

Additional provocation and alleviation differentiation tests are applied to gain more specific information about the area where the symptoms seem to be provoked. Through this testing, we try to answer the following questions:

- which joint out of a complex of joints, such as the distal radioulnar joint or the intercarpal joints, is the likely source of the patient's symptoms?
- which movement in the symptomatic joint provokes the patient's symptoms?
- what is the dominant provoking component (intra- versus extra-articular) of the painful movement?

Differentiation of distal radioulnar joint versus intercarpal joints

Provocation of pain in supination. With the forearm pre-positioned just short of pain, the radius was first moved into the volar and then into the dorsal direction while the ulna and the carpus were stabilized. Movement of the radius did not provoke any pain, whereas movement of the whole carpus into more supination (internal rotation while the radius was stabilized) reproduced Ralf's typical pain.

Alleviation of pain in supination. With the forearm pre-positioned just into pain, the radius was moved into the volar and then the dorsal direction while the ulna and the carpus were stabilized. Movement of the radius did not ease the pain, whereas movement of the whole carpus into more pronation (external rotation while the radius was stabilized) alleviated the pain.

Differentiation intra- versus extra-articular components

With the wrist pre-positioned into combined dorsal flexion and radial abduction just into pain, general traction and compression between the forearm and the carpus was applied. Traction immediately decreased the pain, whereas compression increased the pain.

Differentiation of intracarpal components

Provocation of pain in dorsal flexion and radial abduction. With the wrist pre-positioned just short of pain, the radial and central columns of the carpal complex were differentiated. The radial column was tested by stabilizing the radius and moving the scaphoid in a volar direction, followed by movement of both trapezii (os trapezium and os trapezoideum) in a dorsal direction while the scaphoid was stabilized. In testing the central column, the lunate was moved against the stabilized radius in a volar direction, followed by a volar movement of the capitatum against the stabilized lunate. Of all these tests, only movement of the scaphoid on radius in a volar direction reproduced Ralf's pain. None of the other movements produced any pain.

Alleviation of pain in dorsal flexion and radial abduction. With the wrist pre-positioned just into pain, the radial and central columns of the carpal complex were differentiated for pain relief. Based on a biomechanical rationale, the radial column was again tested by stabilizing the radius and moving the scaphoid, this time in a dorsal direction. Next, both trapezii were moved in a volar direction while the scaphoid was stabilized. In testing the central column, the lunatum was moved against the stabilized radius in the dorsal direction, followed by a dorsal movement of the capitatum against the stabilized lunatum. Of all these tests, only the movement of the scaphoid on radius in a dorsal direction alleviated Ralf's pain, while none of the other movements influenced the pain (Pfund and Zahnd, 2001).

Examination of adjacent joints and structures

Proximal radioulnar joint. Translatory testing of the proximal radioulnar joint showed a decreased gliding of the radius on ulna in an anterior direction.

Muscles of the forearm. Volar flexion of the wrist with fingers two to five fully flexed, and dorsal flexion of the wrist with these fingers fully extended were both restricted compared with the left side. With all fingers flexed, there was also less range in ulnar abduction, whereas radial abduction was the same as the uninvolved side. There was a firm elastic end-feel in each position.

Spinal assessment. Based on the neurological relationship of the cervical (C4–T1) and thoracic (T4–T8 sympathetic origin to upper extremity) spines to the wrist joint complex, spinal palpation was applied in prone lying to get a general idea about tissue texture abnormalities. Slight alterations of the soft tissue on the right side between C5 and C7, and stiffness and soft tissue changes between T5 and T8, were present. All changes were classified as minor tissue alterations from the situation on the other side.

REASONING DISCUSSION AND CLINICAL REASONING COMMENTARY

1 What was your hypothesis at this point regarding the dominant pain mechanism?

■ Clinicians' answer

The pain mechanisms (in order) considered most likely contributing to this patient's symptoms and disability were:

1. peripheral nociceptive (i.e. local wrist complex somatic tissues)
2. autonomic nervous system
3. central nervous system
4. peripheral neurogenic.

This order is proposed because of the direct trauma in the history, the length of the history and the clinical presentation. Present knowledge regarding pain mechanisms suggests that with trauma there is increased likelihood of pathobiological changes in the peripheral and central nervous systems. While central mechanisms were not strongly supported at this stage of our reasoning, they still must be considered. From the clinicians' clinical experiences, peripheral neurogenic mechanisms are often involved in patients with metal fixation at the wrist, likely caused by an irritation of local peripheral neural tissue (e.g. median nerve in the carpal tunnel).

2 Please comment on the hypotheses regarding potential sources and contributing factors that you were considering by the end of your physical examination. Include the supporting evidence, and also any negating evidence, from your examination for your hypotheses.

■ Clinicians' answer

At this stage, the primary potential source we hypothesized was a movement impairment of the wrist joint and the functionally connected structures, such as the muscles of the forearm, resulting from the fracture and the period of immobilization (hypothesis 1). Lack of mobility between the lunate and scaphoid on radius seemed to be the dominant cause of the restricted dorsal and volar flexion (hypothesis 2). Movement alterations of the radius on ulna in the distal radioulnar joint were likely responsible for the restriction in pronation and supination (hypothesis 3). The dominant contributing factor was considered to be a disturbance of the autonomic nervous system, the symptoms of which appeared to be neurophysiologically altering the sensitivity threshold of the local wrist structures (hypothesis 4). There were no negating features evident so far to differentiate these four hypotheses.

■ Clinical reasoning commentary

Two characteristics of expert reasoning evident in the clinical examination and the authors' answers is their use of differentiating procedures and their consideration of several potential sources operating simultaneously. Kleinmuntz (1968) introduced the concept of 'maximizing principles' to describe the clinical procedures and associated reasoning that experts use in order to narrow down competing hypotheses efficiently. The clinicians use of specific provoking and alleviating tests in this patient's physical examination represent a clear example of a 'maximizing principle' to enhance the efficiency and accuracy of their examination.

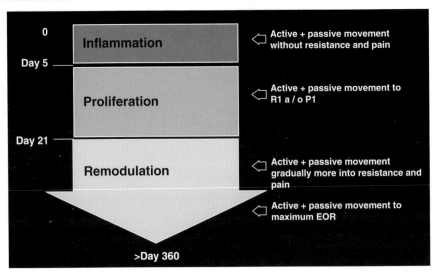

Fig. 16.1 Diagram of normal time for regular tissue healing. (Reproduced with kind permission of Thième, from van den Berg, 1999.)

Initial management

At the end of the initial session, the normal healing time after a fracture and the different stages of healing and their ability for loading was explained to Ralf. The model described in van den Berg (1999) was used as it provides a useful overview about the healing time and the ability of loading injured tissue with movement (Fig. 16.1). Because of the 3-week period of immobilization in the cast, a self-exercise programme was instituted. Ralf was instructed in regular pain-free and resistance-free movement into dorsal flexion and volar flexion, radial abduction and ulnar abduction, and pronation and supination, to be performed every hour for a total of 5 minutes. To explain the range of movement he should use, resistance-free movement was demonstrated on his left wrist.

Second visit

Two days after the initial session, Ralf returned for his next treatment and reported that his hand 'feels much better' and that the swelling and soreness had decreased around 15–20% compared with the initial session. When asked to demonstrate the self-exercises, he showed them correctly and appeared to have no fear moving his hand in the demonstrated range. No additional symptoms had developed since his first session. The sharp pain in dorsal flexion and radial abduction was unchanged.

Reassessment of the physical findings from the initial session revealed no change. The plan for the second session was to find techniques to increase further the range of motion (ROM) of the wrist joint, particularly dorsal flexion, with the aim of progressing into more resistance. Because of the metal fixation of the radius and the unknown ability of the fixation to withstand mechanical force, traction techniques were used initially to minimize the stress on the radius.

Treatment techniques

Translatory traction into resistance (i.e. end of grade II; Kaltenborn, 1999), was applied to the carpus with the forearm stabilized. This was carried out with the wrist in the resting position and then submaximally pre-positioned into dorsal flexion (Fig. 16.2), radial abduction, volar flexion, and then ulnar abduction (Kaltenborn, 1999). Retesting was applied after mobilizing (10 times for 10 seconds) in each position, with increases of the ROM in all directions. The same procedure was repeated and the result was similar, with further increase of ROM and a more comfortable feeling when moving his hand.

Self-exercise

Based on these results, Ralf was instructed in how to use a similar technique as part of his self-exercise

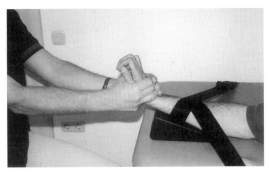

Fig. 16.2 Translatory traction into resistance applied to the carpus with the forearm stabilized (therapeutic technique).

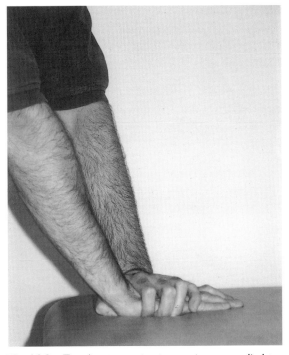

Fig. 16.3 Translatory traction into resistance applied to the carpus with the forearm stabilized (self-exercise).

programme. Specifically, he was shown how to pre-position his hand, stabilize this position and apply traction at the wrist joint (Pfund and Zahnd, 2001). He was advised to perform the self-traction exercise into resistance (end of grade II; Kaltenborn, 1999), in the same positions as the therapeutic technique (10 times for 10 seconds) every 2 hours (Fig. 16.3).

He was also advised to perform his angular self-exercises every hour, moving the hand without pain or resistance into dorsal flexion, volar flexion, radial abduction and ulnar abduction for a total of 5 minutes.

Third visit

Two days after the second session, Ralf returned with further improvement in his ROM (both physical find-ings and patient's comments), but with less gain in the swelling or the soreness. While there had been no additional symptoms, the sharp pain in dorsal flexion and radial abduction was unchanged. He was able to demonstrate his initial session and his second session self-exercises well.

The plan for the third session was first to increase the range of movement and reduce the pain produced dur-ing dorsal flexion and radial abduction. Initially, the translatory traction used in the previous session would be progressed and then, if this were unsuccessful, spe-cific mobilizations of the intercarpal bones would be tri-aled. After that, the plan was to test the influence of the shortened muscles on Ralf's movement impairment.

Treatment techniques

Distraction of the carpus on the stabilized forearm, pre-positioned in four submaximal positions (dorsal flexion, volar flexion, radial abduction and ulnar abduc-tion), was applied into more resistance (first to the end of grade II; Kaltenborn, 1999), then just into grade III ('just over the slack'; Kaltenborn, 1999). Retesting was performed after mobilizing (10 times for 10 sec-onds) in each position and showed a proportional increase of the ROM in all directions, as measured by simple observation of the movement. The same pro-cedure was repeated, resulting in further increases in the ROM and a more comfortable feeling for Ralf when moving his hand. The specific provocation and allevi-ation tests were unchanged from the initial visit. Even without specific treatment to the distal radioulnar joint, the supination movement improved (range and pain), whereas pronation was unchanged (i.e. restricted but no pain).

Stretching of the extensor and flexor muscles of the wrist into slight resistance was trialed next. The finger joints, the wrist joint and joints of the forearm were pre-positioned in their pain-free range and the stretch (five times 15 seconds) was applied by mov-ing the elbow into extension (Evjenth and Hamberg, 1984). Pulling in the stretched muscles was felt, and not the specific pain in his wrist, during this procedure. Retesting after stretching each position showed a slight increase in the ROM and a subjective improve-ment in the quality (ease) of moving the wrist.

Based on these results, Ralf was taught how to use a similar muscle-stretching technique as a self-exercise for the extensor and flexor muscles of the wrist (Evjenth and Hamberg, 1991). He was also shown how to apply self-traction in the pre-positioned hand in order to mobilize the wrist into more resistance.

The self-exercises to be performed at this stage were:

- every hour, moving the hand without pain or resistance into dorsal flexion, volar flexion, radial abduction and ulnar abduction for a total of 5 minutes
- every 2 hours, self-traction into resistance (i.e. just into grade III; Kaltenborn, 1999) in the same positions as the therapeutic technique (10 times for 10 seconds)
- stretching of the flexor and extensor muscles of the wrist joint into slight resistance four times a day, each muscle group five times for 15 seconds.

◼ Fourth visit

Three days later, the range of movement into volar flexion and ulnar abduction was much better, while only slight improvement was made into dorsal flexion and radial abduction. Despite the increase in ROM, the sharp pain at end of range was still unchanged. Supination and pronation ROM showed only a slight improvement; however, the pain with supination was reduced approximately 50%, while pronation was nearly pain-free. The 'autonomic' symptoms were unchanged. The specific provocation and alleviation tests showed the same pattern as at the initial assessment. Reassessment of muscle length revealed improvement in range and response but still an altered end-feel compared with the other side.

The plan for this treatment was to find techniques that were able to change the sharp pain in dorsal flexion and radial abduction. To achieve this, specific mobilization techniques for the restricted radiocarpal joints were trialed.

Treatment techniques

Translatory volar gliding of the scaphoid against the radius was applied just to the beginning of grade III (Kaltenborn, 1999) (five times, 10 seconds; Fig. 16.4). Retesting showed a direct reduction of the sharp pain and a slight improvement in the ROM into dorsal flexion and radial abduction. Translatory volar gliding of the lunatum against the radius was applied just to the beginning of grade III (five times, 10 seconds) (Kaltenborn, 1999). Retesting showed no reduction of

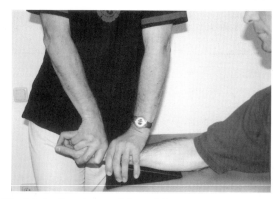

Fig. 16.4 Translatory gliding of the scaphoid against the radius (therapeutic technique).

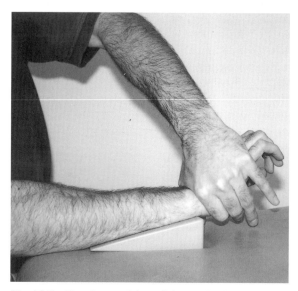

Fig. 16.5 Translatory gliding of the scaphoid against the radius (self-exercise).

the sharp pain and no improvement in the ROM. Based on these reassessments, mobilization of the scaphoid against the radius in the volar direction was continued in this session.

Self-exercise

In addition to the existing programme, Ralf was taught to apply a specific mobilization technique for the scaphoid against the radius (Fig. 16.5), to be performed every 2 hours (5–10 times for 10 seconds). The other self-exercises were unchanged, except he was instructed to take the muscle stretches into more resistance.

REASONING DISCUSSION AND CLINICAL REASONING COMMENTARY

1 Clearly you see patient understanding of tissue healing as important. Would you briefly highlight the key features of the van den Berg (1999) model of tissue healing and how you incorporate this into your management and prognostic decisions?

Clinicians' answer

The diagram for the normal time of regular tissue healing (Fig. 16.1; van den Berg, 1999) is clinically very useful in explaining to patients the different stages of healing. From a knowledge of these different stages, we can apply and progress our manual therapy treatment. In the inflammation phase (days 0 to 5), a fragile situation is dominant. New blood vessels are being built and the presentation is mostly irritable (i.e. pain is easily aggravated and does not settle quickly). Therefore, during this stage of healing our passive and active treatments are applied without provoking pain and without going into resistance. In the proliferation phase (days 6 to 21), only 20% of the normal loading ability of the injured tissue is restored (McGonigle and Matley, 1994) and, therefore, our active and passive movement is applied only to the begining of resistance and/or to the onset of pain. In the remodulation phase (after day 21), our treatment techniques will typically be taken more and more into resistance, gradually being progressed based on our ongoing reassessment. This model is purely focussed on tissue healing and should not be applied without consideration of the different pain mechanisms and altered healing capacities, such as in a systemic disease (e.g. rheumatoid arthritis). While being broadly guided by this model, our treatment progression is still largely informed by our continuous reassessment.

2 How did the reassessments and the patient's progress up to the fourth visit support, or not support, your previous hypotheses regarding the dominant pain mechanism, potential sources and contributing factors?

Clinicians' answer

There was no change in our hypotheses regarding pain mechanisms, except perhaps central and peripheral neurogenic pathological mechanisms were less likely; our evolving thoughts regarding sources and contributing factors were as follows.

Movement dysfunction of the wrist joint and functionally connected structures (hypothesis 1). The increase of ROM through local stretching techniques of the wrist joint and the forearm muscles supported this hypothesis.

Lack of mobility between lunate and scaphoid on radius as the dominant cause of the restricted dorsal and volar flexion (hypothesis 2). This hypothesis was not proven through specific treatment techniques at this stage.

Movement alterations of the radius on ulna in the distal radioulnar joint being responsible for the restriction in pronation and supination (hypothesis 3). This hypothesis was not proven through specific treatment techniques at this stage.

Autonomic nervous system disturbance (hypothesis 4). The reduction in swelling and soreness could be interpreted as decreased disturbance of the autonomic nervous system. Loss of fear about movement, a better understanding of the whole 'process of healing', and an improved blood supply through regular pain-free movement represented additional factors that had improved and which may have been contributing to his symptom presentation in their own right or as a manifestation of his autonomic disturbance.

Clinical reasoning commentary

The clinicians' treatment selection and progression in this case are based on a balance of biomedical (propositional) and clinical or craft (non-propositional) knowledge. While the biomedical principles of tissue healing will generally dictate similar treatment guidelines as the clinical presentation would suggest (such as avoiding much force in both the inflammatory stage and with an irritable presentation), the clinicians' flexibility in these judgments is evident by their caution that the above model must be considered within the broader picture of pain mechanisms and the patient's healing capacity. Biomedical principles clearly provide an initial framework within which management decisions are made, but the variability of presentations within this framework necessitates the flexibility of thinking shown here. That is, even within this biomedical model, treatment hypotheses are continually re-evaluated on the basis of ongoing clinical reassessment.

The clinicians' reasoning has been guided by the ongoing reassessment, which resulted in further, deeper understanding of the patient's presentation. Not being locked into their initial hypotheses, their thoughts have evolved with each visit and assessment, with some hypotheses supported while others were not. Treatment is clearly not the end of the decision-making process. Rather, treatment together with reassessment represent a form of hypothesis testing.

m | Subsequent management

Management continued over a further five visits (visits 5–10). The total ROM available at the wrist joint at the beginning of this stage (visit 5) was nearly unchanged from the previous session, but the sharp pain produced by dorsal flexion and radial abduction was reduced approximately 30%. Ralf's demonstration of the self-exercises was correct and no additional symptoms had developed since the last session.

During the next sessions, radiocarpal mobilization was continued. As the range increased, mobilization of the lunatum against the radius, in a volar direction particularly, reduced the sharp pain felt with the combined movement of dorsal flexion and radial abduction. The restricted and painful supination movement improved most with mobilization of the proximal and distal radioulnar joints, whereas pronation improved only slightly up to the seventh visit and then was unchanged. After the sixth visit, Ralf was introduced to the sequence training system (Gunnari et al., 1984) with the aims of improving general fitness and relearning to use the injured hand (Fig. 16.6). Care was taken that none of the exercises during the sequence training was performed within the painful ROM of the wrist. At this stage, the temperature changes and the swelling of the hand of the dependent arm when walking showed only slight change.

In addition to his hands-on treatment, Ralf trained four times a week for approximately 45 minutes with low resistance. The feelings of swelling and slight soreness around his wrist joint, and the hyperaesthesia on the volar side of his second and third fingers and the middle third of the radial side of his forearm, decreased steadily and after the tenth visit only minor sensations remained. Since he had started to do the sequence

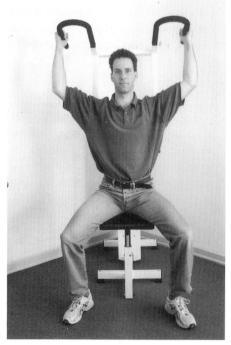
(a)

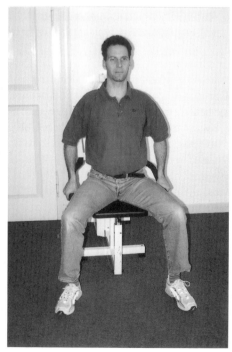
(b)

Fig. 16.6 Example of sequence training to improve general fitness and relearn use of the injured hand.

training, the swelling had lessened, and after he had done his daily 'workout' his hand felt nearly normal. Also the feeling of altered temperature in the whole forearm of the dependent arm during walking was nearly reduced by 100%. He described the overall dysfunction of his right arm to be approximately 20% compared with the other side.

REASONING DISCUSSION AND CLINICAL REASONING COMMENTARY

7 Could you explain your reasoning for introducing the sequence training at this stage, highlighting the particular features of his presentation and response to treatment that prompted its inclusion here?

doing uncontrolled movements is low, because of the stabilized position of the patient's body inside the sequence training machine.

Clinicians' answer

It is our clinical experience that patients with postsurgical problems, such as Ralf, achieve better results if improvement of general fitness and the integration of the involved body part (here the wrist) into total body movements is initiated than if local manoeuvres alone are used (e.g. mobilization). After the sixth treatment with passive and active movement, as well as self-exercise, we felt we had sufficient information regarding Ralf's attitude toward exercise and the ability of the injured tissue to tolerate mechanical load. The presentation seemed to be non-irritable and Ralf was able to demonstrate the selected exercise protocol correctly without fear of using the hand. The sequence training system is easy to teach and the potential for

Clinical reasoning commentary

The breadth of the clinicians' reasoning to include consideration of the patient's broader health/fitness status in its own right and with respect to how it may be contributing to the patient's current symptoms is again evident in this answer. Reflection is the means by which clinical patterns are discovered and clinically validated. While the clinicians' reflective experience has led them to incorporate their sequence training into the programme of such patients, the programme itself is not a set protocol or recipe. Rather, based on their consideration of the patient's understanding/attitude, as well as his specific physical presentation, they determined when best to commence his training and at what level.

Long-term management

At this stage, Ralf continued his regular sequence training and also received two treatment sessions per week for the next 2 weeks, mobilizing the hypomobile structures. Ralf resumed work 6 weeks after the injury, at which time treatment was reduced to only once a week. In addition to his normal work routine, he had to catch up with all the files he had not worked on during the last 6 weeks, necessitating a reduction in his training to two or three times a week. Then 2 weeks after starting work, he stopped the training completely. Following this, he started to get more soreness around the whole wrist joint and the swelling, morning stiffness and pain all increased; however, the temperature change and swelling feelings during walking did not return.

Because of his busy schedule, Ralf was unable to attend more than one treatment session per week and had lost his motivation for the self-exercise. He was increasingly frustrated with his difficulty getting caught up with his backlog of work and his lack of time and energy for his exercises. He thought he would never be the same person he was before. The pain in his hand was worse in the evening but settled when he relaxed at home watching TV or listened to music. No additional symptoms had appeared. While local treatment techniques (mobilization and stretching) could change the range and the pain response of the restricted movements, the improvement was only retained for 1 to 2 hours. Also, mobilization techniques applied to the cervical and the thoracic spines altered the sensitivity state of the hand for a short period of time, but this improvement did not last.

Six weeks after he started work, he described the overall dysfunction of the right arm to be more than 40%. Agreeing that manual techniques alone were not improving his situation, and since he felt he had no time to do regular exercises because of his busy work schedule, we decided to stop treatment for the next 6 weeks. Ralf was advised to perform his normal activity and resume the self-exercises at least once a day.

Ralf came back into our clinic 8 weeks later with nearly all symptoms reduced about 60%. There was still some morning stiffness and slight swelling, but he did not see this as abnormal. Ralf's wrist was still slightly restricted into dorsal flexion and radial abduction, but only minor pain was felt when his movements were taken to end-range. Pronation was the same as at the last visit, whereas the supination range was increased, with only minor restriction and no residual pain. Except for the restricted pronation, Ralf was able to move his hand pain-free with all his daily activities. He had done his muscle stretching and self-traction techniques every evening for the past 4 weeks. He seemed to be much more relaxed and did not mention his work at all. When he was asked about his work, he smiled and said that he was assigned a new assistant and was now able to catch up with all his old files. The presence of his new assistant significantly reduced his daily stress, and he consequently decided to take up the sequence training again on a regular basis three times per week. He had noted that this general exercise had helped him quite a lot. Because of the movement restrictions that still remained, an additional two treatments per week were recommended.

Four weeks later, the morning stiffness and swelling were absent, and dorsal flexion and radial abduction showed only slight restriction and minor discomfort at end-range. Supination was now normal, although the range of pronation was still unchanged, with end-range pain persisting. At this point, hands-on treatment was stopped and it was agreed that he would continue with his sequence training three times per week. Ten months after the accident, the metal fixation was removed. Ten days after the surgery, he described pronation as being much better than before the fixation was removed. Ralf resumed his sequence training a week after surgery and the wrist and forearm were again mobilized because of the restrictions in dorsal flexion, radial abduction and pronation that still remained. After six treatments, the wrist movement was pain-free and without restriction compared with the other side. Pronation and supination were without pain, but pronation still lacked 10 degrees of range. The mobilization treatment was again stopped because the hard and non-elastic end-feel of pronation indicated that further improvement would not be made with these techniques. Because of the general improvement in his overall fitness, Ralf has continued with his sequence training, attending our clinic two to three times per week. His wrist is now unrestricted during all his daily activities.

REASONING DISCUSSION AND CLINICAL REASONING COMMENTARY

1 To what did you attribute his deterioration in symptoms?

■ Clinicians' answer

Ralf's heavy workload and his frustration with the lack of help available to complete this work seemed to contribute to his reduced motivation to continue his self-exercise. We thought this affective state and the reduction of exercise were, together, the principal factors responsible for the deterioration of symptoms.

2 Could you comment on the reasoning for including the cervical and thoracic spines in your treatment at that stage?

■ Clinicians' answer

There were findings of tissue alterations in the cervical and thoracic spines early in the management, but the local findings were considered more significant and, therefore, local treatment was the first priority. Based on our clinical experience and the work of Vicenzino et al. (1996), we thought it possible to change the sensitivity of the periphery by applying manual techniques to related areas of the spine. The main reasoning for applying spinal mobilization techniques was to lower the sensitivity of the whole wrist complex.

3 Could you explain your reasoning regarding the value of breaks in hands-on treatment as used with this patient?

Clinicians' answer

After Ralf came back to our clinic, local mobilization techniques restored all movements, except pronation. Pronation was still restricted, but pain-free. Based on our clinical experience, a hard non-elastic end-feel indicates that no further improvement is likely to be gained with mobilization techniques. Earlier in the course of treatment, we stopped hands-on intervention because there was only slight improvement, which was not sustained after the treatment. As this observation was consistent over several treatment sessions, we stopped passive mobilization techniques and used a more active approach (i.e. sequence training).

4 Was the year that this problem took to resolve consistent with your initial prognosis? Please explain why you think it ultimately took this long and in hindsight whether there are any aspects of this patient's management that you would approach differently given the same presentation.

Clinicians' answer

The initial prognosis was for a straightforward presentation with local tissue changes and what was hypothesized to be a dominant peripheral nociceptive pain mechanism. However, the presentation turned out to have significant contributing central and affective components to the symptoms and associated pain behaviours/attitude. We think it took so long to resolve largely because the impact of the overwork situation was underestimated and not addressed.

In hindsight, it is probable that further probing about his working situation and his associated feelings, and addressing this in our management, may have allowed us to obtain the same outcome in a shorter timeframe. Had we been able to encourage him to find help much earlier and had we integrated the philosophy of training not only into the special exercises but also into his work, this too may have assisted in bringing about a quicker recovery.

Clinical reasoning commentary

The clinicians can be seen here to be drawing on an organized knowledge base that combines knowledge derived from similar clinical cases and also from relevant research. Their interventions and associated reassessments again illustrate hypothesis testing that continues to occur throughout the ongoing management.

The clinicians' critical appraisal of improvement made and sustained allowed them to progress their management from one of hands-on mobilization and self-mobilizing exercise to the more general exercise/fitness-based approach. It is common that the full picture of a patient's psychosocial status does not emerge at the start. As such, the concept of psychosocial screening questions, analogous to screening questions for additional symptoms or general health, can assist in identifying pertinent psychosocial factors. Manual therapists' overt assessment of psychosocial 'yellow, black and blue flags' (Kendall and Watson, 2000; Main and Burton, 2000; Watson, 2000; Watson and Kendall, 2000) is still relatively new, and greater attention to these factors should strengthen the thoroughness of our reasoning and management. The clinicians' generous sharing of their reflections on how they may have obtained their final outcome sooner had they probed this area of the patient's presentation further from the start is testament to the self-criticism and willingness to continue to learn that is characteristic of experts.

References

Evjenth, O. and Hamberg, J. (1984). Muscle Stretching in Manual Therapy. Alfta, Sweden: Alfta Rehab.

Evjenth, O. and Hamberg, J. (1991). Autostreching: The Complete Manual of Specific Stretching. Alfta, Sweden: Alfta Rehab.

Gunnari, H., Evjenth, O. and Brady, M. (1984). Sequence Training. Oslo: Dreyers.

Kaltenborn, F. (1999). Manual Mobilisation of the Extremity Joints. Oslo: Olaf Norlis Bokhandel.

Kendall, N. and Watson, P. (2000). Identifying psychosocial yellow flags and modifying management, In Topical Issues in Pain 2. Biopsychosocial Assessment and Management. Relationships and Pain (Gifford, L. ed.) pp. 131–139. Falmouth, UK: CNS Press.

Kleinmuntz, B. (1968). The processing of clinical information by man and machine. In The Formal Representation of Human Judgment (B. Kleinmuntz, ed.) pp. 149–186. Chichester, UK: Wiley.

Main, C.J. and Burton, A.K. (2000). Economic and occupational influences on pain and disability. In Pain Management: An Interdisciplinary

Approach (C.J. Main and C.C. Spanswick, eds.) pp. 63–87. Edinburgh: Churchill Livingstone.

McGonigle, T. and Matley, K.W. (1994). Soft tissue treatment and muscle stretching. Journal of Manual and Manipulative Therapy, 2, 55–62.

Pfund, R. and Zahnd, F. (2001). Leitsymptom Schmerz: Differenzierte manualtherapeutische Untersuchung und Therapie bei Bewegungsstörungen—Kopf, HWS, Brustkorb, Arme. Stuttgart, Germany: Thième.

van den Berg, F. (1999). Angewandte Physiologie: Das Bindegewebe des Bewegungsapparates verstehen und beeinflussen. Stuttgart, Germany: Thième.

Vicenzino, B., Collins, D. and Wright, A. (1996). The initial effect of a cervical spine manipulative physiotherapy treatment on the pain and dysfunction of lateral epicondylalgia. Pain, 68, 69–74.

Watson, P. (2000). Psychosocial predictors of outcome from low back pain, In Topical Issues in Pain 2. Biopsychosocial Assessment and Management. Relationships and Pain (Gifford, L. ed.) pp. 85–109. Falmouth, UK: CNS Press.

Watson, P. and Kendall, N. (2000). Assessing psychosocial yellow flags, In Topical Issues in Pain 2. Biopsychosocial Assessment and Management. Relationships and Pain (Gifford, L. ed.) pp. 111–129. Falmouth, UK: CNS Press.

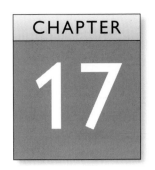

17

A university student with chronic facial pain

Mariano Rocabado

SUBJECTIVE EXAMINATION

Pamela, an 18-year-old girl in her first year at university, presented with a complaint of chronic right facial pain that had been present for 2 years and treated unsuccessfully by an interocclusal orthopaedic appliance (IOA, i.e. a splint) administered by a dental professional. The symptoms had developed spontaneously without any history of macrotrauma. Her pain was localized on the right mandibular ramus without any radiation of pain to the cranium or neck areas (Fig. 17.1). She also noted occasional earache and bilateral temporal headaches. The facial pain was constant, sharp and had been increasing in intensity. Further screening revealed no overt neurological symptoms or any other areas of symptoms.

The pain was mostly felt with attempted opening of the mouth and was associated with a loud snapping sound. Her symptoms were only felt during the day and there was no report of symptoms affecting her sleep. However, in the morning she noted an increased limitation of mouth opening, with increased deflection of the mandible to the right side. Mastication was limited by increased pain associated with the biting forces. Any parafunctional activity, such as nail biting, pencil biting and gum chewing, produced a grinding sensation and pain. Her pain significantly affected her life, interfering with her university work and social activities. She acknowledged the stress this created and could see the interconnection between her pain, this stress and her biting parafunctional activities.

None of Pamela's signs and symptoms had been alleviated at any point by her previous treatment with

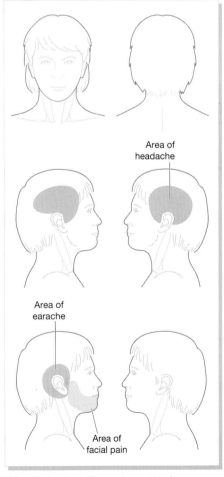

Fig. 17.1 Body chart illustrating patient's symptoms.

the IOA. She reported that she used the IOA for a period of 2 years; however, this had not reduced her pain or improved her mandibular functional capacity. On the contrary, using the device on a daily basis had increased her facial pain and precipitated her headaches, which had not been present prior to the dental craniomandibular orthopaedic treatment. Pamela's parents decided to seek a second opinion from another specialist because of this lack of improvement.

 ## REASONING DISCUSSION AND CLINICAL REASONING COMMENTARY

1 Given the symptom area and the behaviour and history of the symptoms, what were your thoughts at this stage regarding possible sources and contributing factors for her symptoms?

■ Clinician's answer

Given her area of symptoms and that the factors aggravating her symptoms were related to masticating, the structures I considered as possible sources at this stage included the temporomandibular joint (TMJ), local muscles and nerves, as well as referral from upper cervical spine structures, although I felt spinal referral was less likely given she had no spinal symptoms. In particular, I suspected a disc subluxation disorder, with severe intracapsular involvement, including posterior ligament irritation and synovitis secondary to overloading of the condyle. The most likely contributing factors predisposing to and maintaining her symptoms were her parafunctional bad habits (involving gliding with load) over a poorly balanced occlusion, and stress, which she acknowledged aggravated her symptoms.

2 At this stage, did you feel psychosocial factors may be relevant to her presentation?

■ Clinician's answer

I felt that her frustration with the failure of the splint to relieve her condition for so long had likely contributed to her problem. Stress and associated negative feelings are often manifest by abnormal parafunctional activity, such as clenching and grinding, which are difficult for patients to avoid even when they are aware of them. The clenching and grinding then further contribute to the problem both by perpetuating and further increasing craniomandibular muscle activity and by becoming annoying symptoms in themselves.

I suspected that they added to Pamela's frustration and interferred with her social life. In addition to the obvious need to explain these relationships, management is also going to require advice to minimize further irritation. For example, diet modification to soft foods and care to avoid excessive opening beyond 25 mm will be important (e.g. only small bites and little kisses allowed).

3 Please comment on your thoughts regarding the worsening of this patient's symptoms (i.e. increasing in intensity) over the past 2 years.

■ Clinician's answer

The worsening of Pamela's symptoms over the past 2 years was likely the result of an increase in the intra-joint pressure caused by overloading through continued eating of hard foods and her clenching habits. These forces are sufficient alone to create symptoms for some patients; when present together with a disc subluxation disorder, as I felt Pamela had, a story of worsening symptoms is common.

■ Clinical reasoning commentary

The clinician's answers to the above questions reflect the dynamic nature of clinical reasoning. Consistent with expert reasoning, he clearly formulates hypotheses across a range of both physical and psychosocial issues, illustrating both diagnostic and narrative reasoning. There is evidence that even at this early stage hypotheses are being considered with respect to sources of the symptoms (e.g. TMJ), factors contributing to the maintenance of the problem (e.g. clenching habits), activity/participation restrictions (e.g. social life), pathobiological mechanisms (e.g. disc subluxation) and management (e.g. advice).

PHYSICAL EXAMINATION

Posture assessment

Pamela showed good head, neck and shoulder girdle alignment, with no structural changes that may have contributed to her facial pain condition.

Neurological examination

All neurological tests were negative. Cotton tip applicators were used to compare light touch discrimination between the right and left maxillary, ophthalmic and mandibular branches of the trigeminal nerve. Facial sensitivity was normal. Gross hearing was evaluated by rubbing a strand of hair between the index finger and thumb near the patient's ear with no difference noted between right and left hearing sensitivities.

Cervical spine examination

Upper cervical mobility testing. Upper cervical physiological and accessory joint mobility (i.e. C0–C1, C1–C2 and C2–C3) testing was asymptomatic and revealed no abnormality of movement.

Palpation of suboccipital triangle. Abnormality of soft tissue can be manifest by its texture (e.g. hardness) and sensitivity or reproduction of symptoms with palpation. The occiput–atlas space was evaluated by palpation, following a line of palpation from the centre of the occiput to the transverse process of the atlas. Similarly, the atlas–axis space was palpated following a line from the transverse process of the atlas to the spinous process of the axis. With Pamela, the suboccipital tissues, specifically the deep suboccipital rectus capitis, posterior minor, major and left inferior obliquus muscles, were tender to palpation.

Instability tests for upper cervical region. While stabilizing C2 posteriorly in full available upper cervical flexion, a posterior cranial translation was induced. The same test was then performed stabilizing the cranium and inducing a ventral glide of C2. No displacement was perceived or symptoms provoked with either of these two tests for antero-posterior transverse ligament instability. Atlas–axis range of movement was then assessed by having the patient assume full flexion of the head and neck and then assessing the range of rotation movement to the right and left (45 degrees each way is considered normal). Her mobility was approximately 45 degrees bilaterally and did not elicit any symptoms.

Upper cervical provocation-alleviation pain tests. Compression, distraction and gliding of the O–C1–C2 region were all asymptomatic and judged to be of normal mobility.

Muscle function assessment

Gross mandibular motor function was tested by having the patient clench while palpating masseter, temporalis and digastric muscles. Local muscle pain was reproduced bilaterally from contraction of the posterior and anterior temporal muscles and the right digastric muscle.

The hyoid region muscle function was normal. There was no discomfort elicited by palpation of the inferior border of the mandible, the hyoid bone and the infrahyoid region to the sternum. Lateral manual displacement of the thyroid cartilage was possible with crepitation. This is a common finding where limited movement is indicative of abnormality of the infrahyoid musculature.

Isometric muscle contraction of the neck flexors, including the suprahyoid and infrahyoid muscles, did not elicit any discomfort. There was also no restriction of cervical movement caused by muscle tightness or hyperactivity in the suboccipital or cervicothoracic regions.

Motor control

Motor control was very good, as assessed by the patient's ability to maintain good upper and lower quarter postural alignment during functional tasks such as sitting, sitting to standing, walking and carrying loads.

 REASONING DISCUSSION AND CLINICAL REASONING COMMENTARY

 1 When looking for specific clinical patterns associated with the TMJ itself, what local tissues do you consider as potential sources for a painful TMJ?

Clinician's answer

Several local tissues can be a source of pain since they are highly innervated and vascularized.

- Synovial membrane is a highly vascularized connective tissue producing synovial fluid to lubricate the articular surfaces.
- Inferior, anterior or posterior synovial tissues can be painful as a result of compression of the condyle when functioning towards anterior or posterior extreme articular positions.
- Anterior, posterior or superior synovial tissues can become painful when the anterior or posterior dense edges of the disc press against the upper joint space. The disc translates anteriorly or posteriorly along the temporal eminence during functional movements. During protrusive and opening movements, the anterior thick portion of the disc encroaches upon the anterosuperior synovial pouch, potentially inducing anterosuperior joint pain. The same situation occurs with posterior translation of the disc and encroachment of the posterosuperior dense portion of the disc into the posterosuperior synovial pouch during closure with load or during clenching, resulting in posterosuperior joint pain.
- The articular ligaments and capsule that contribute to limiting articular movement are often painful as a result of distension secondary to repeated microtrauma (e.g. parafunctional habits), macrotrauma (e.g. blow to the jaw, prolonged opening as with a lengthy dental procedure) or high-velocity trauma such as a motor vehicle accident.

2 Could you comment on the ability to differentiate specific tissue involvement through clinical examination?

Clinician's answer

Of course, specific tissue differentiation by clinical examination is not an exact science. However, I have developed what I call a 'pain map evaluation' whereby TMJ articular tissue pain sensitivity and joint mobility are assessed by eight specific tests to incriminate specific tissues. These tests and this patient's findings are described below.

Clinical reasoning commentary

Expertise in clinical reasoning is closely linked to the clinician's organization of knowledge. As evident in the above answer, this knowledge includes both propositional (e.g. research-validated biomedical facts) and non-propositional (e.g. experience-validated professional opinion) components. Skilled manual therapy requires a specialized and rich store of both these forms of knowledge, organized in an integrated manner as clinical schema or patterns. Knowledge and recognition of a wide range of often subtly different patterns of clinical presentation—such as those highlighted in the answer to question 1 above—allows the expert practitioner to reach diagnostic and other clinical decisions more efficiently and accurately than the novice. This knowledge of clinical patterns is usually associated with principles that guide actions to facilitate maximally efficient testing of the hypothesis formed and also to suggest intervention strategies frequently found effective for that disorder.

Evaluation of the temporomandibular joint

Pain evaluation

The synovial TMJ pain map shown in (Fig. 17.2) illustrates the specific tissues examined through the eight tests described below. The first step is to locate the mandibular condyle lateral pole. Then, applying gentle pressure, the therapist places an index finger under the patient's zygomatic arch and requests mandibular protrusion until the condyle's anterior pole can be felt. Next, the patient is asked to maintain that contact position while opening their mouth 10 mm. While maintaining this initial evaluation position, the therapist locates the specific areas of soft tissue tenderness under assessment. The therapist instructs the patient to raise their hand as a visual signal if pain is experienced when the specific procedures described below are performed (Fig. 17.3).

1. *Anteroinferior synovial membrane palpation.*
   The anteroinferior synovial tissue is palpated with the index finger just inferior to the anterior pole

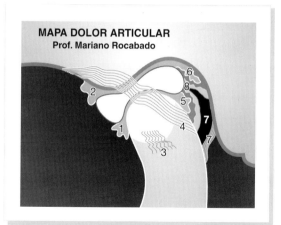

Fig. 17.2 Synovial temporomandibular joint pain map illustrating specific tissues that can be assessed. 1, Anteroinferior synovial membrane; 2, anterosuperior synovial membrane; 3, lateral collateral ligament; 4, temporomandibular ligament; 5, posteroinferior synovial membrane; 6, posterosuperior synovial membrane; 7, posterior ligament (disc bilaminar zone); 8, retrodiscal tissue insertion.

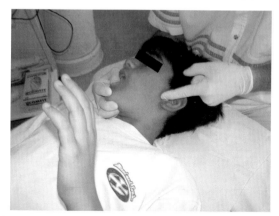

Fig. 17.3 Illustrating patient's hand signal to indicate pain during the temporomandibular articular soft tissue pain sensitivity evaluation.

of the condyle. Hard and abnormally sensitive soft tissue is indicative of the initial phase of anterior condylar hypermobility, as occurs with repetitive protrusive mandibular activity (e.g. oral bad habits such as nail biting, nocturnal bruxism, etc.) or exaggerated mouth opening, both of which result in the condyle compressing the anteroinferior synovial membrane.

2. *Anterosuperior synovial membrane palpation.* While keeping the anterior pole of the condyle in contact with the index finger, the therapist smoothly moves it upwards until the condyle's anterosuperior edge can be palpated adjacent to the inferior edge of the articular eminence. Soft tissue abnormality detected here is present in patients who have excessive condylar movement beyond the inferior edge of the articular eminence. When this occurs, the dense anterior edge of the disc compresses the anterosuperior synovial membrane, while the excessive condylar translation eventually leads to lengthening/hypermobility of the articular capsule.

3. *Lateral collateral ligament palpation.* Maintaining finger contact on the lateral pole, the therapist then requests the patient to open their mouth. Normally during condylar movement below the articular eminence inferior edge, the disc moves medially, allowing direct superolateral palpation of the lateral collateral ligament, which in the mouth-open position is under slight distension. Abnormality on palpation of the lateral collateral ligament is one feature of a medially subluxed disc. This implies lateral instability of the disc attachment at the lateral pole of the condyle, which, when present, facilitates medial disc displacement.

4. *Temporomandibular ligament assessment.* Gripping the mandible with the thumb placed intraorally at the premolar level and the remaining fingers inferiorly under the mandible, the therapist gently moves the mandible in an anteroposterior direction until the articular capsule is felt to 'loosen' or 'relax'. Here, finesse is the key! Once a relaxed position is achieved, the therapist passively glides the mandible (and hence the condyle) posteroinferiorly. This movement is normally limited by tension in the temporomandibular ligament. Pain elicited by this manoeuvre implies posteroinferior condyle–disc initial displacement. This initial biomechanical displacement of the condyle on the posterior dense portion of the disc is usually caused by occlusal interferences. If this test is positive, the therapist must immediately contact the patient's dentist and communicate this condition as there is a high risk that it may progress to an anterior disc displacement on the temporal eminence (based on the concept that the condyle subluxes on the disc and the disc subluxes on the temporal eminence).

5. *Posteroinferior synovial membrane palpation.* With the patient's mouth halfway open, or in slight

lateral excursion to the opposite side until condylar movement is felt, the lateral pole of the condyle is identified. The therapist then moves the palpating finger posteroinferiorly as far as the neck of the condyle and assesses for any soft tissue abnormality. When pain is elicited, it implies that either the condyle is in an excessively distal (dorsal) position during maximum intercuspation, and hence irritating these posteroinferior tissues, or that repeated posterior microtrauma has occurred, possibly as a result of repeated intercuspidal interference during function, causing repetitive mechanical pivoting and abnormal condylar posteroinferior displacement.

6. *Posterosuperior synovial membrane palpation.* The posterosuperior synovial membrane can be palpated with the patient's mouth open. Starting at the posterior edge of the condyle, the therapist moves the palpating finger towards the cranium to the top of the temporal cavity, where the posterosuperior edge of the condyle can be felt. Abnormal soft tissue sensitivity at this point suggests the condyle is beginning to adopt a posterosuperior position without disc subluxation at the maximum angular position of full opening. A patient with hyperactivity of the powerful mandibular elevators will also present with reduced vertical dimensions (i.e. posterosuperior displacement of the condyle) and sensitivity to palpation.

7. *Posterior ligament (disc bilaminar zone).* The mandible is again grasped with the therapist's thumb placed intraorally at the premolar level and the remaining fingers inferiorly under the mandible. The condyle is initially moved slightly in a distal (dorsal) direction. If pain is not elicited, pressure is then applied through the body of the mandible towards the cranium. If this is provocative, the most probable situation is that there is an intracapsular injury with an anterior displacement of the disc on the eminence and a displacement of the condyle posterosuperiorly.

8. *Retrodiscal tissue insertion.* The procedure for test number 7 to evaluate the posterior ligament is repeated taking the condyle toward the posterior and superior zones. This retrodiscal region is highly vascular and, therefore, vulnerable to inflammation and bleeding if traumatized. Maintaining the cranial pressure, the mandible is then translated anteriorly. If condylar displacement with cranial pressure increases pain, then retrodiscitis, plus or minus retrodiscal bleeding, is implicated.

Severe disc subluxation is associated with a posterior condyle–disc subluxation and an anterior disc articular eminence subluxation. In more chronic conditions, it is also commonly associated with lateral disc displacement and, less commonly, medial disc displacement.

Summary of pain map findings

Pamela's right TMJ was painful to tests 2, 5, 6, 7 and 8, characteristic of both condyle–disc and disc–temporal bone subluxations. Her left TMJ was painful to tests 1, 2 and 3, characteristic of condyle hypermobility with excessive anterior translation.

Active physiological movement testing

Protrusion. This occurred to 6 mm at the left TMJ but was limited to 3 mm at the right TMJ with deflection to the right (normal protrusion is 10 mm).

Right lateral deviation. This was 6 mm and painful at the right TMJ (normal lateral deviation is 10–12 mm), reproducing posterior joint pain consistent with posterior ligament pain as per test 7 of the pain map evaluation on the right side. This fits with the presentation for posterior displacement of the condyle.

Left lateral deviation. This was 3 mm and painful at the right TMJ, corresponding to pain map tests 7 and 8 and characteristic of retrodiscitis caused by compression of the condyle on the posterior band of the disc.

Opening. There was limited opening, to 18 mm, with pain reproduced at the end of the movement. The opening end-feel was 3 mm with an increase in right TMJ pain (normal end-feel is 1–3 mm).

Passive accessory movement testing

Lateral, medial and anteroposterior passive accessory glides of the right TMJ were limited by pain from compression of the posterior ligament of the right TMJ. The end-feel was soft for the lateral and medial glides and the anteroposterior glide was extremely limited by pain. Long-axis distraction was asymptomatic with normal range of accessory movement. All left TMJ passive accessory glides were asymptomatic with normal range of movement.

REASONING DISCUSSION AND CLINICAL REASONING COMMENTARY

1 Please comment on how your physical/clinical examination findings contributed to your evolving thoughts regarding this lady's problem.

Clinician's answer

While minor signs of suboccipital muscle sensitivity were evident, the evidence overwhelmingly supported a local TMJ problem. Her good posture and lack of any impairment in cervical joints, cervical muscle function or general motor control led me to the conclusion that she had no cervical or muscular component to her presentation.

The TMJ examination was very straightforward in revealing a clinical pattern of a right posterosuperior condyle–disc displacement and an anterior disc–temporal component subluxation. The condyle was able to reduce on the disc, but the disc was not able to reduce on the eminence. This resulted in retrodiscitis, associated with a painful posterior ligament. The sound (click) in the joint present with opening, protrusion and contralateral movement of the mandible was related to a reduction of the displaced disc. During the process of closure, retraction or deviation of the mandible to the same side, the disc would then re-sublux.

Clinical reasoning commentary

Perhaps most evident in this answer is the clinician's skill in pattern recognition. Competing hypotheses (e.g cervical joint impairment) are considered and ruled out on the basis of insufficient evidence; a dominant pattern of impairment with associated structures involved and pathophysiology is recognized.

Diagnostic imaging

As a result of the chronic facial pain and functional limitation of the TMJs, a therapeutic dynamic magnetic resonance imaging (TDMRI) procedure (Fig. 17.4) was performed. I developed the TDMRI protocol myself in order to enhance clinical examination of TMJ problems. The TDMRI findings further substantiate the clinical pattern suspected through the interview and physical examination and can also assist the manual therapist's determination of treatment procedures.

The TDMRI protocol was carried out with the patient lying in a supine examination position with her cranium fastened to limit movement. A sagittal view was obtained in a position of teeth contact in maximum intercuspation, firstly without the IOA in the mouth but later with the appliance in position between the teeth. The TDMRI revealed a right posterior condyle–disc subluxation and an anterior disc–temporal bone subluxation (i.e. condyle subluxed posteriorly in relation to the disc and disc subluxed anteriorly in relation to its normal temporal position).

After performing the MRI procedure with the teeth in maximum intercuspation, the procedure is repeated with a mouth opening dynamic examination. Here the right TMJ was reduced in the sagittal plane at

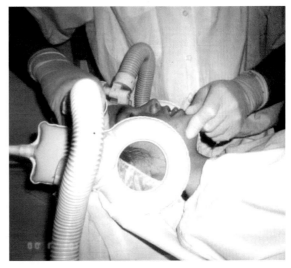

Fig. 17.4 Therapeutic dynamic magnetic resonance imaging (TDMRI) procedure.

20 mm of opening and was painful at 30 mm of opening (as signalled by the patient pressing the panic button). However, when performing active protrusive and retrusive movements, the posterior condyle–disc subluxation was not reduced.

REASONING DISCUSSION AND CLINICAL REASONING COMMENTARY

1 Please briefly discuss your interpretation of how the TDMRI results correlated with your findings from the clinical (physical) examination and how together they guided your management decisions.

Clinician's answer

The TDMRI correlated well with the clinical examination findings in that they supported a chronically subluxed disc. The painful reduction that occurred with the mouth opening during dynamic examination, and the lack of reduction when performing active protrusive and retrusive movements, demonstrated that any previous therapeutic reduction procedure which the patient had received had, in fact, increased her discal subluxation, causing increased condylar compression of the retrodiscal tissues and thereby making her intra-articular condition more severe.

Since the TMJ is a three-dimensional complex joint, reduction of the subluxation must also be three dimensional. When observing the TDMRI, the joint was reduced at the limit of full opening only when the patient gave a strong active extra effort to open further in the sagittal plane. During the coronal plane study of the right joint, it was possible to reduce the disc without effort in lateral excursion to the opposite side. This reduction in the contralateral movement to the left may be used to guide the construction of a reduction splint in left lateral deviation of 2.5 mm. The protrusive (horizontal plane) TDMRI assessment showed no reduction of the condyle–disc subluxation. In this situation, long-axis caudal distraction is essential prior to any manual reduction procedure in order to stretch the capsule and allow the condyle to glide over the posterior dense portion of the disc, thereby achieving reduction without intra-articular irritation (non-forceful reduction).

Following the TDMRI examination, it was decided that her IOA would need to be redesigned. The examination findings and recommended management were then discussed with the patient and her doctor. This is critical to facilitate consensus in understanding and compliance in self-management.

2 Please elaborate on the significance of the reduction during the TDMRI procedure being achieved with opening but not with the protrusive movements.

Clinician's answer

A reduction of the disc in opening and not by protrusion reflects the extent of her subluxation, and hence posterior ligamentous lengthening. A more minor subluxation will reduce with protrusion. Pamela clearly had a significant subluxation that required full opening to reduce, a much more forceful activity than protrusion. Therefore, it was essential that reduction in protrusion was achieved to avoid further displacement of the disc and further trauma to the posterior ligament.

It is also favourable if the reduction occurs during lateral excursion to the opposite side as this is far less traumatic than a reduction in opening. The pattern of reduction during the TDMRI strongly suggests an excentric splint requirement of 2.5 mm to the left in order to achieve reduction.

Clinical reasoning commentary

Manual therapists must continually search for objective outcome measures to validate their clinical impressions and monitor their clinical efficacy. Impressively, this expert has devised his own advanced radiological assessment to correlate with his clinical examination and assist in guiding his treatment selection and progression. As commented on above, this provides another excellent example of the importance of professional craft knowledge in its own right and as a precursor to the discovery of new biomedical knowledge.

---

m Management

As a consequence of the posterior condyle–disc subluxation evident on the TDMRI, a decision was made to take Pamela out of the imaging resonator and have her undergo a manual discal reduction treatment immediately. The technique performed was a manual condylar distraction in the long axis of the joint, followed by anterior and contralateral condylar movement. In performing this, it is important to maintain good immobilization of the patient's head to avoid altering the preset position of the resonator, which had already calculated the long axis of the condyle during the previous TDMRI procedure. This reduction test under MRI is a sophisticated procedure and expensive, because of the extremely long time (up to 2 hours) required for the whole process, which includes initial observations of the MRI, assessment of images on the screen, bringing the patient out of the resonator to perform the manual therapy procedure, and then placing the patient back in the resonator for additional imaging to reassess the effect of the manual technique on the condyle–disc relation. Further manual distraction may be required at this point. My decision to try and reduce the disc was primarily guided by the coronal image of lateral excursion to the opposite side, which showed a good condyle–disc reduction without effort, and by the lack of anterior reduction in protrusion.

Manual distraction technique

Distraction in the longitudinal axis is performed with the patient lying in a supine position and the head stabilized; the therapist's thumb is introduced at the right premolar–molar mandibular level and the mandibular body is held with the rest of the hand (Fig. 17.5). Caudal pressure is applied at the molar level with simultaneous cranially directed pressure given at the mandibular level.

Pamela was comfortable during the mobilization phase of treatment and no pain was reproduced.

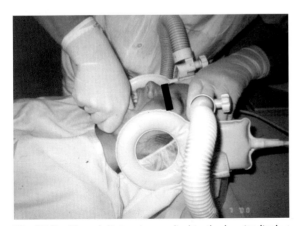

Fig. 17.5 Manual distraction applied in the longitudinal axis during the therapeutic dynamic magnetic resonance imaging procedure.

It was then decided to continue with the second reducing trial using a condylar lateral and medial mobilization. In order to reduce the disc, a three-dimensional combined movement mobilization had to be performed to prepare the soft tissues in the three planes of space. Chronic subluxated conditions such as this usually produce static or hypomobile disc positions, so lateral and medial glides are necessary to liberate the disc in all planes. This mobilization was performed by means of lateral pressure applied at the level of the lingual molar surfaces, with digital medial pressure applied at the external condylar neck of the right TMJ. The technique was applied on an intermittent basis for 30 seconds. The patient should not feel any pain, as indeed Pamela did not. Next, a strong longitudinal distraction technique with mandibular condyle contralateral and anterior mobilization was performed on the right TMJ for 30 seconds. Total procedure time for the reduction was 5 minutes. After the procedure, Pamela could perform protrusive condylar movement without pain, and there was an increase in her mouth opening from the protruded position, which suggested disc reduction had been achieved.

Pamela was then informed that the complete TDMRI procedure would be performed again to confirm the effect of the manual reduction technique. This is necessary in order to determine the progression of treatment. Pamela was again placed into the magnetic resonator and the sagittal study was repeated. The mandibular dynamics were reassessed, revealing an increase in proportional lateral excursive and protrusive movements without any deflections. Her opening was now full with no pain and only right facial muscle fatigue. Good anterior disc–condyle reduction was observed, thus showing that longitudinal distraction and condyle mobilization are of vital importance for the preparation of a joint affected by discal subluxation before trying reduction (Fig. 17.6).

The TDMRI is completed with dynamic frontal cuts performed with the patient in maximum intercuspation and maximum right and left lateral mandibular positions. It can be observed that a significant distracter effect of the right TMJ condyle is produced with left laterality (i.e. active lateral deviation to the left), as well as a right condyle–disc reduction effect (Fig. 17.6b). Lateral excursion to the opposite side showed very clearly the caudal distraction position of the condyle, with a central reduction of the disc over the condylar head. This reduction condition suggests that, for Pamela, the reduction position is in

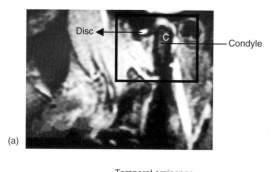

(a)

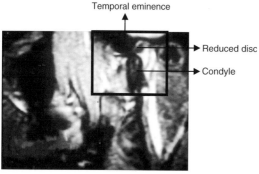

(b)

Fig. 17.6 Therapeutic dynamic magnetic resonance imaging illustrating right temporomandibular joint protrusion before (a) and after (b) reduction treatment.

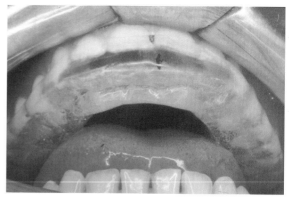

Fig. 17.7 Interocclusal orthopaedic appliance (splint) showing a 2.5 mm lateral mandibular deviation to the left in maximum intercuspation.

longitudinal distraction and contralateral mandibular laterality. Therefore, the disc must be reduced sagittally and coronally; otherwise the disc is only partially reduced in the sagittal plane and is not coronally reduced. Once discal reduction has been achieved, a new IOA is required. This consisted of an upper element with even point-shaped occlusal contacts in the maximal intercuspation position and with a left 2.5 mm eccentric relation of contact (Fig. 17.7).

REASONING DISCUSSION AND CLINICAL REASONING COMMENTARY

1 Could you elaborate on the procedural considerations when performing the manual distraction technique?

Clinician's answer

The initial capsular elongation (i.e. distraction) for reduction purposes is performed while maintaining the patient's head in a stabilized position; this avoids interferring with the MRI technique. Care is needed to avoid exceeding the patient's pain limit because if this happens muscle guarding can occur, which interferes with the distraction effect. If the procedure is painful, distraction is performed for 1 second and repeated six times. The aim here is to mobilize the capsule so that the distraction reduction can then be achieved without increasing intra-articular pressure. If the distraction technique is not painful, distraction is begun as a sustained longitudinal-type reduction manoeuvre performed from maximum articular capsular distension

(i.e. at the end of available mouth opening) as a grade II or III (Kaltenborn, 1999) mobilization short of pain. The sustained distraction is then maintained for 6 seconds and is repeated six times. A minimum of 30 seconds is necessary in order to achieve a physiological capsular elongation. If distraction is painful, a very gentle intermittent distraction is performed short of any resistance/stretching (i.e. grade I) and without provoking any pain.

2 Please discuss your use of reassessment in general and your interpretation of these clinical and TDMRI reassessments in particular.

Clinician's answer

It is critical always to reassess the patient's movements and symptom response following a treatment procedure; this ascertains the treatment effect and, in this case, whether a reduction was achieved. Range of movement alone is not sufficient to indicate normality of the TMJ. A disc can be totally subluxed and still have normal patterns of movement.

The TDMRI reassessment in this case indicated a positive reduction effect of the technique. The TMJ normally functions in a 4:1 ratio; that is, 1 mm of lateral and protrusive excursions should give rise to 4 mm of opening. Following Pamela's manual reduction procedure, her movements were then consistent with these proportions and within the expected normal ranges, indicating a successful reduction had been achieved.

3 Please explain how 2.5 mm was arrived at as the amount of left laterality required for correction in the IOA.

Clinician's answer

The eccentric condition was determined by the fact that a discal reduction was observed at 10 mm of opening after the TDMRI reduction phase. Therefore, if we take into consideration that mandibular opening and laterality normally maintains a proportional relation of 4:1 (Farrar and McCarty, 1983), it means that 2.5 mm of interincisal mandibular deviation was the necessary laterality required to reduce the disc without excessive internal articular pressure or intracapsular irritation.

Clinical reasoning commentary

As discussed in Chapter 1, manual therapists' craft knowledge informs their 'procedural reasoning'. The level of expert craft knowledge and procedural reasoning reflected in the above answers evolves through years of experience with managing these types of problem. This evolutionary process is, by necessity, facilitated by reflection upon individual clinical experiences and by the maintenance of an open-minded but critical approach to clinical practice. While broad guidelines, such as direction and length of mobilization procedures, are established, application of these guidelines are then tailored to the individual patient presentation.

Treatment selection and progression must be guided by the clinician's assessment and ongoing reassessment, as is the case here. Clinical measures such as range of movement will not always be reliable or valid indicators of impairment or improvement, and as such must be correlated with other outcome measures such as pain, functional change, quality of life or, in this case, TDMRI assessment. Reassessment also provides confirmation (or otherwise) of hypotheses and, therefore, facilitates the acquisition of new, or refinement of, existing clinical patterns and associated actions.

m Staging management based on outcomes

From my experience, while reassessment of the effects of specific interventions guides progression of treatment, there are specific outcomes that, when achieved in a particular order, result in the most efficient and effective final outcome. Therefore, the management for this patient could be described as progressing through seven stages.

Stage 1

For Pamela, the diagnostic and therapeutic TDMRI were performed on the same day. The result was that the disc could be reduced without pain in both protrusion and lateral deviation to the opposite side after manual therapy. This represents the first stage of management. Further treatment was then needed to improve the capsular flexibility and motor control in order to maintain this disc reduction.

Stage 2

This stage of management for disc subluxation involved a combination of manual procedures, self-exercise and splint usage, all with the aim of reaffirming the condyle–disc position and the posterior disc's new relation in the fossa. The splint maintained this relation in a reduced, stabilized position. The initial time frame for this particular patient was that, after her first appointment, she was treated (mobilization, laser and motor retraining) daily for five sessions to optimize her ability to wear the IOA. Pamela was also initially seen daily for treatment consisting of manual therapy and laser directed to the retrodiscal tissues in order to accelerate the healing process of these soft tissues. In addition, motor retraining was utilized via a 'roll back technique' (described below) to optimize her flexibility, muscular balance/control/relaxation and disc remodelling in order to maximize the effectiveness of the splint. She was also instructed to wear the splint day and night (i.e. 24 hours) during these 5 days of daily treatment. Following this, treatment continued (mobilization, laser, motor control), along with continued use of the splint, for a further 5 weeks. The following procedures and advice were given over these initial 6 weeks of treatment.

1. Infrared laser was used on the right TMJ with the points of application determined by the TMJ pain map (Fig. 17.2). Points 1 (lower anterior synovium), 3 (lateral collateral ligament), 7 (posterior ligament or bilaminar zone) and 8 (retrodiscal tissue) were treated.
2. Longitudinal distraction was applied to the right TMJ. For this procedure, Pamela had her mouth half-opened without provocation of pain. A thumb was then introduced at the right lower molar level and the mandibular body was held with the rest of

the hand. The maximum painless capsular relaxation position was sought by means of small and gentle anteroposterior movements of the mandible, while maintaining midway opening of the mouth. Longitudinal grade I distraction of the mandibular condyle was then performed in the relaxed capsular (i.e. loose-packed) position. The next step was to perform a gradually increasing longitudinal distraction in a pain-free manner, in order to realign the collagenous fibres of the articular capsule and thereby allowing sufficient condyle joint space for the discal reduction.

3. Retraining of the articular rest position was carried out by instructing Pamela in pure condylar rotation, performed with superior lingual placing (i.e. tongue on the roof of her mouth) and up to 10 mm of opening.

REASONING DISCUSSION

1 Please elaborate on the 'retraining' component of your management. What was the basis of the guidelines as to the extent of movement you requested of her (i.e. up to 10 mm)?

Clinician's answer

The active movement of 10 mm of interincisal opening was chosen as it was at this point during the TDMRI that the anterior condylar rotation was associated with a posterior disc condyle rotation and successful disc reduction.

Pamela was instructed to produce the pure condylar rotation initially from the midline position and then

from the eccentric position of left canine–canine contact. It was in this position of left canine–canine contact that the disc was seen to reduce on the TDMRI. Therefore, Pamela was coached in opening and closure movements not exceeding 10 mm. Once the movement was learned, a light resistance was added to the opening in order to reduce hyperactivity of the elevator muscles, which often occurs. This elevator inhibiting action is critical because, during the use of the IOA, the elevator masticatory musculature, particularly the middle and anterior temporalis, is affected as it is subject to a forced mandibular position. This action could be defined as an expected muscular parafunction.

By the end of the 6 weeks Pamela was asymptomatic and had regained normal, functional range of movement. At that point, it was decided to modify the splint to bring it back to skeletal midline (centre midline of the maxilla aligned with the centre midline of the mandible). The decision to modify Pamela's splint was based on the fact that in her present off-midline splint position she was not in a completely normalized condyle–disc relation position. The reduced condyle was slightly anteriomedial while the contralateral side was slightly posterior, placing that joint at risk of

posterior condyle–disc subluxation. Therefore, once the right joint was reduced and clinically stable, splint modification aimed at returning her to midline was considered necessary in order to maintain equal reduction in both joints. After this, Pamela was seen twice a week for a further 5 weeks. She was instructed to wear her IOA during the night and for 4 hours (on an even basis) throughout the day.

Pamela reported having had temporal headaches during the use of the splint, which was most likely a result of the change of mandibular alignment and the muscle adaptation associated with her new mandibular position. As her headaches were judged to be the result of overactivity of the mandibular muscles, they were treated with a combination of mandibular muscular rest, by means of the lingual rest position, and by temporal muscle soft tissue management.

Use of the hyperboloid to promote discal remodelling

The hyperboloid is a device made out of silicone that resembles the shape and size of a disc. It comes in five different sizes, numbered from 1 to 5, number 5 being the smallest (Fig. 17.8). Keeping the hyperboloid between the upper and lower incisors, Pamela was instructed to perform lateral mandibular movements to the left, which is the position where a disc reduction was seen to occur with the TDMRI. While in maximum active laterality, Pamela was instructed to perform a 6 second sustained biting compression against the hyperboloid. This action should be absolutely pain-free. The aim of this exercise was to use active compression to promote remodelling of the reduced disc. After 6 seconds of biting she was instructed to relax, releasing the pressure on the hyperboloid, and then return to the midline without biting down. This sequence was then repeated six times and was also performed with and without the IOA in the mouth. This exercise was continued as self-management for 2 to 3 days until the next appointment. If the patient performs the exercise

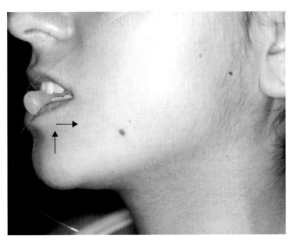

Fig. 17.8 Hyperboloid used in an interincisal position while the patient actively performs the reduction 'roll back exercise' to promote discal remodelling.

without pain, as Pamela was able to do, treatment is then progressed to the next stage.

■ Stage 3

The aim of stage 3 management is to continue with the mobilization and hyperboloid exercises in order to optimize the disc mobility and remodelling and ensure that the condyle is functioning normally on the concave joint surface of the disc. The following procedures were used.

1. Longitudinal distraction was performed with the capsule in a relaxed position. The distraction was sustained for 6 seconds and repeated six times, taking care to avoid any provocation of pain.
2. Longitudinal distraction was performed from a protrusive and maximally opened position without provocation of pain. In this position, maximum tension is placed on the capsule and collateral ligaments. This elongation of the articular capsule causes, in turn, a distraction of the upper articular compartment (disc follows condyle in this case). Distraction is held for 6 seconds and repeated six times.
3. Mandibular relaxation was facilitated by means of the lingual rest position with condyle rotation (six times), which also enhances articular surface lubrication.
4. Gentle anteroposterior passive gliding oscillations were performed from the protrusive mid-opening position. Following 2 years of an immobilized, subluxed disc, Pamela required these accessory glides in order to mobilize her disc on the temporal eminence.
5. Biting on the hyperboloid to facilitate disc remodelling was progressed from size 1 hyperboloid to size 2 or 3, depending on the pain reaction to hyperboloid biting (i.e. compression) between the upper and lower incisors. This time, hyperboloid biting was performed from a position of maximum mandibular protrusion. If this exercise is well tolerated by the patient, it supports the hypothesis that the condyle is pressing over the disc articular surface (a non-painful condition). (Fig. 17.9) illustrates the hyperboloid biting 'roll back' exercise; this example demonstrating retrusion performed from a protruded position while biting the hyperboloid. Fig. 17.10 shows TDMRI images of the right TMJ in protrusion, protrusion with biting, and retrusion with biting taken after 10 days of treatment.

6. Hyperboloid biting was progressed to being performed strongly in protrusion, then retrusion and finally in the incisal position (biting sustained for 6 seconds in each position and repeated six times). This represents the first stage of posterior discal condylar reduction. (Fig. 17.10c) demonstrates Pamela's posteriorly placed disc on the articular eminence. Attention should be paid to teeth sensitivity. If odontalgia (teeth discomfort) occurs, the procedure should only be repeated three times and then gradually increased to six times as the

sensitivity lessens. Once reduction has been achieved, muscular stabilization exercises should then continue for at least a further 6 months.

Stage 4

The aim of stage 4 management was to release the disc from the temporal eminence. Most chronic disc subluxations are in a state of hypomobility, or are actually static on the articular eminence. The following procedures were used.

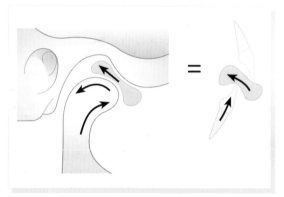

Fig. 17.9 Schematic diagram illustrating proper disc position (i.e. reduction achieved) during the hyperboloid biting exercise performed in protrusion. The arrows illustrate how the condyle and disc simultaneously move posteriorly when retrusion with biting is then performed from this protruded position.

1. Distraction was performed with capsular relaxation and mouth opened. This procedure is important as it provides an active disc–condyle reduction with maximum tension on the collateral ligaments, both medial and lateral, allowing the disc to accompany the condyle. It also produces a significant effect on the upper compartment, resulting in a separation of the articular surfaces between the disc and the temporal eminence. This enhances articular gliding and upper synovial articular compartment lubrication, thereby facilitating posterior disc–temporal bone reduction.

2. Hyperboloid biting for disc remodelling was continued with hyperboloids 2 and 3 as tolerated. Biting was performed from a position of left contralateral mandibular deviation, followed by strong biting from midline. If this hyperboloid exercise can

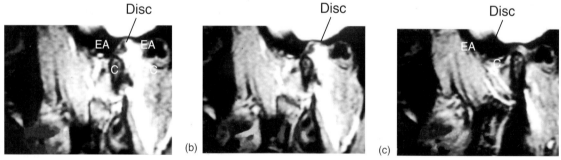

Fig. 17.10 Therapeutic dynamic magnetic resonance image illustrating right temporomandibular joint (TMJ) protrusion. (a) Right protrusion where the condyle (C) reduces the disc with a good convex–concave relation and a stable joint surface relation. (b) Right TMJ protrusion with vertical bite (while performing the biting 'roll back' exercise) where the condyle increases pressure over the concave surface of the disc, remodelling the posterior dens portion of the disc, which is now thicker and slightly more posterior. This effect is necessary to facilitate posterior glide of the disc over the articular eminence (EA) when performing retrusion with biting from a protruded position. (c) Right retrusion while performing the biting 'roll back' exercise, where disc reduction has occurred. A new relation between condyle–disc-fossa is observed. The condyle is now functioning slightly on the posterior dens portion of the disc, but the disc is in a normal position with respect to the articular eminence and mandibular fossa. The final proper condyle–disc-fossa relation will be obtained with final orthodontic treatment.

be performed successfully without discomfort, the patient can then normally progress to the next hyperboloid exercise. Pain at this point is the only reference that we have as to whether the patient is performing the reduction procedure correctly and in the reduced condyle–disc position. If the patient experiences pain during the protrusive reduction exercise, the therapist must stop the exercise, use distraction to ease the pain and then start again by trying lateral excursion to the opposite side and biting. If these procedures are asymptomatic, they should be continued until the next appointment. It is important to keep in mind that the disc is subluxed three-dimensionally and each exercise (hyperboloid biting in different positions) can alter the disc position. Therefore, there is no recipe for treatment. Rather, the TDMRI will provide evidence of the disc subluxation and requirements for splint correction, and then the various exercises must be trialed and progressed according to each patient's individual response and the results of continual reassessment. The aim is to be able to perform all exercises without pain, which should correlate with disc reduction as confirmed by TDMRI.

3. The hyperboloid protrusion, biting, then retrusion only to edge-to-edge anterior incisor relation exercise was carried out. If there is no loss of the condyle–disc relation and no pain, the biting should be sustained while a 2 mm retrusive movement is performed, followed by a return to the interincisal position. Extreme caution is required with this procedure, with the movements and biting force progressed slowly so as to avoid a possible posterior condyle–disc resubluxation. The strong forces placed on the posterior ligament with this exercise can cause severe local pain or pain radiating to the ear region if progressed too quickly. It is of vital importance to keep a finger on the lateral pole of the condyle of the joint being treated in order to detect quickly if a discal subluxation is occurring during this exercise.

▮ Stage 5

Stage 5, like the other stages, is guided by TDMRI reassessment. In the present case, the TDMRI reassessment and progression of procedures through stage 5 were as follows.

1. When the TDMRI was reassessed with the patient in a protrusive position while biting on the hyperboloid, a hypomobile disc in an anterior disc–temporal bone position was observed. This situation suggested that the protrusive movement with biting would result in an excessive compression of the disc against the articular eminence. Such compression could have been interfering with the synovial lubrication of the articular surface and, as such, may have compromised the posterior disc–temporal bone reduction process. Fig. 17.6b shows the condyle–disc reduced position. Biting in that position can produce a hypomobile disc relation.

2. As a consequence of the disc hypomobility, the distraction mobilization was continued in the open mouth position. After this, anterior and posterior glides of the condyle with the disc were performed in order to lubricate the disc–eminence joint surface. This technique was achieved by grasping the patient's mandible and, while providing cranial pressure in mid-opening, performing small oscillatory anterior and posterior glides. This procedure facilitates the ability of the disc to reduce posteriorly on the eminence and fossa, while the roll back technique with the hyperboloid device moves the disc backwards on the articular eminence.

3. Protrusive and retrusive movements were next performed while maintaining light biting on the hyperboloid in order to maintain the newly achieved condyle–disc and disc–temporal bone relations. This also helps to maintain normal lubrication at the disc–eminence joint surface, which facilitates reduction of the disc by normal posterior sliding.

4. Reassessment of the IOA revealed that the eccentric position (normal condyle–disc–eminence relationship) was maintained. However, as a result of disc hypomobility and the patient's tendency to have temporal headaches, it was decided to add an anterior guidance and a canine desocclusion guidance to the IOA. Anterior guidance is a protective mechanism for the TMJ that reduces the intra-articular pressure which can occur with desocclusion. A canine guidance is an articular protection modification. When the lateral deviation movement against the canine guidance is performed, a contralateral articular distraction effect occurs. Together, the anterior guidance and canine guidance provide protection against excessive compressive forces (Fig. 17.11). This protective function is particularly important during parafunctional behaviours, such as grinding/bruxing of teeth when sleeping.

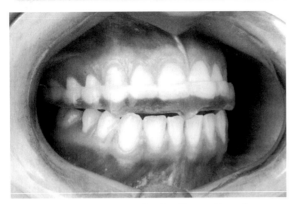

Fig. 17.11 Upper interocclusal orthopaedic appliance with anterior and canine guidance.

Every new stage of progression of treatment was based on continual reassessment of the intra-articular condition and referred patterns of pain.

Stage 6

The aim of stage six of management was to address further the temporal component of the disc derangement through exercises designed to facilitate good cranial position in a horizontal position in space and in relation to the rest of the body. An orthostatic rest position was sought where the head maintains a vertical alignment with the shoulder girdle. The progression of therapeutic procedures (tailored to the patient's individual presentation) used in stage 6 was as follows.

1. The patient begins with anterior rotation of the occipitalatlantoid joints (i.e. upper cervical flexion or nodding). This action also promotes anterior rotation of the mandible and disc–condyle anterior rotation.
2. Longitudinal distraction with the mouth open and capsular relaxation was continued on a concomitant basis with disc–condyle mobilization in order to facilitate supradiscal articular surface lubrication and mobility.
3. Posterior discal self-mobilization with the hyperboloid continued with increases in hyperboloid diameter (progressing from size 1 to 5), provided the disc remained reduced and the patient was able to tolerate greater muscular contraction over the disc without joint pain.
4. Postural correction of the cranium, neck and shoulder girdle was instigated to improve the muscular rest relation of the mandibular–cranial–cervical functional unit.

 REASONING DISCUSSION

1 Previously you had noted in your physical examination that the patient 'showed good head, neck and shoulder girdle alignment, with no structural changes that may have contributed to her facial pain condition'. Could you elaborate on the need for postural correction to improve the muscular rest relation of the mandibular–cranial–cervical functional unit?

Clinician's answer

Even though this patient did not have poor alignment of the craniocervical region, to maintain a rest position of the mandible with normal function of the inframandibular musculature, it was necessary to use patterns of movements that would promote a shorter distance between the mandibular symphysis and the sternum. This postural correction assists in reducing hyoid musculature activity, thereby avoiding excessive inferoposterior muscle forces on the mandible. It should be kept in mind that the mandible has a supramandibular muscular relation with the cranium by means of temporalis, masseter and pterygoid muscles, and an inframandibular relation with the shoulder girdle by means of the mylohyoid, geniohyoid and anterior digastric muscles. This inferior muscular relation is continued down to the shoulder girdle through the sternohyoid and omohyoid muscles. Consequently, changes in the position of the head and anterior neck increase mandibular descending activity; simultaneously, there is reciprocal mandibular elevation (i.e. an opposed action). This favours the elevator muscle parafunction and, consequently, teeth contact (normally there should be no teeth contact at rest). This parafunctional action increases articular internal pressure, thus altering the expected mandibular rest position.

The postural alignment should not interfere with the active joint reduction process. As many patients have poor compliance with postural exercises, it was important that their purpose was explained and understood and that the patient was assisted to appreciate the need for this more holistic approach. While postural exercises are important, they were not mandatory for this particular patient given that her posture was quite good and hence the abnormal mandibular force was less significant in her presentation.

Stage 7 (3 month reassessment and progression of treatment)

After 3 months, a new TDMRI was performed to evaluate the effects of the IOA, manual therapy and self-management exercises. The TDMRI revealed good reduction of the disc–condyle and disc–eminence (Fig. 17.12).

The following procedures were used.

1. The IOA was modified to achieve interincisal midline alignment with anterior and canine guidance (skeletal midlines aligned). After using the splint, the IOA is modified to set the mandibulae back to midline once the condyle–disc–eminence reduction is achieved. Pamela was advised that this appliance, realigned on the midline, was to be used on a continual basis, 24 hours a day and only removed for hygiene purposes. This schedule of usage was to be maintained for a period of 6 months.

2. Neuromuscular and articular eminence–disc–condyle relation stabilization was continued. In a position of 10 mm of interincisal opening and in midline, Pamela was instructed in self-resisted exercises consisting of light isometric muscle contractions (held for 6 seconds) for each of the agonistic and antagonistic muscle groups. This involved intermittent pressure given over the lateral aspect of the condyle and anteroposterior resistance to protraction and retraction, while taking care to avoid resistance of the elevator muscles. Isometrically delivered resistance to the depressor muscles was used to induce relaxation of the elevator muscles.

3. After 6 months of stabilization in the reduced condition and reassessment of the TMJ pain map twice a month, Pamela had maintained the normal arthrokinematic pain-free 4:1 ratio for mandibular patterns of protrusion, lateral excursion and opening. Adaptation of joint surfaces and collagen realignment to the reduced position was anticipated to take a further 2 to 3 years.

Outcome

Pamela has since reported by telephone that she has remained asymptomatic with no mandibular limitations of motion.

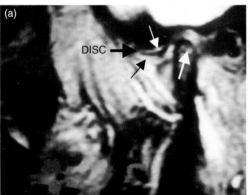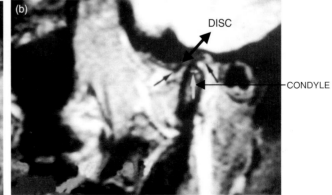

Fig. 17.12 Therapeutic dynamic magnetic resonance image of the right temporomandibular joint. (a) Pretreatment image taken in retrusion while biting and illustrating a subluxed disc. (b) Image at 3 months demonstrating the reduced disc during retrusion with biting. In this position final stabilization is maintained through continued exercise, splint therapy and orthodontics.

References

Farrar, W. and McCarty, M. (1983). A Clinical Outline of Temporomandibular Joint Diagnosis and Treatment. Montgomery, CA Walker Printing.

Kaltenborn, F. (1999). Manual Mobilisation of the Extremity Joints. CA: Walker Printing.

Suggested reading

Palacios, E., Valvassori, G.E., Shannon, M. and Reed, C.F. (1990). Magnetic Resonance of the Temporomandibular Joint. New York: Thième.

CHAPTER 18

Adolescent hip pain

Shirley Sahrmann

SUBJECTIVE EXAMINATION

Steven is a 14-year-old white male with an 18-month history of severe bilateral groin pain; he was referred to physical therapy on his mother's insistence. His initial visit was to his family physician, with subsequent referral to an orthopaedic surgeon in his home town. The radiological studies performed by the orthopaedist were negative for hip or pelvic lesions. Steven was then referred to a paediatric orthopaedic surgeon at a leading medical centre for further diagnostic testing. The paediatric orthopaedic surgeon was unable to diagnose Steven's problem and advised him to avoid activity and just to take it easy. Steven had complied with these recommendations for over a year, but his condition was not improving.

Prior to the severe onset, Steven had been experiencing only occasional pain in his groin, mostly on the right side. At that time, the pain was not present during activity and did not interfere with activities such as walking, running or sports. Then about 20 months prior to his referral, the family experienced a tragedy involving another sibling. Because of the tragedy, Steven did not participate in his primary sport, karate, for 1 month. In fact, the impact of the tragedy on the family had been so severe that Steven ceased all forms of sports-related activities. His resultant inactivity had made coping with the loss even more difficult because he was deprived of an outlet for his feelings. The mother also stated that being unable to find any treatment to resolve her son's problem was adding to her distress. At the time of his withdrawal from participation, Steven had been a karate champion and was particularly well known for his kicks. His karate classes were held three to four times per week.

As Steven began to resume participation in karate, the previous pain that he had noted occasionally in his right groin returned, gradually intensified, and progressed to involve the left groin. The pain in the right groin was more intense than that in his left groin but the symptoms on both sides were severe enough to interfere with his activities. The intensity continued to increase until he had pain when walking for 15 minutes at a normal speed, so he had to walk slowly. He also had pain when attempting to lift either his left or right thigh (bringing his knee toward his chest) or when squatting. After 20 minutes of standing, he developed bilateral groin pain. When his symptoms were at their worst, he rated them 8–9/10, and at their least they were 2/10. Once the severe pain developed it took 30–40 minutes to subside to the lower level. Steven did not have pain when sitting or when in the recumbent position. He occasionally experienced pain when rolling or coming to a standing position from sitting. Any activity that involved the upright position or flexion of the hips to more than 100 degrees caused symptoms.

When Steven and his mother were asked about any visceral or health problems, they indicated that he did not have any complaints except for the groin pain and that his physician had performed a thorough physical examination and ordered other tests that had ruled out any type of systemic, visceral, or genitourinary disease. Steven had been in good health with just the usual childhood diseases.

Steven had been a good student who enjoyed school and was popular with his classmates. He was quiet and did not volunteer any information that was not requested but answered all questions directly and clearly.

REASONING DISCUSSION AND CLINICAL REASONING COMMENTARY

1 Please discuss your thoughts at this stage regarding possible sources and contributing factors to this patient's groin pain.

Clinician's answer

Physical therapy treatment of patients with hip pain presents a particular challenge because clinical information that is available about the causes and characteristics of dysfunction is minimal. The prevailing source of hip pain in patients referred to physical therapy is degenerative hip joint disease. Degenerative hip joint disease is present in older not younger individuals. Few sources of hip or groin pain in the younger individual have been identified. Therefore, once systemic and severe musculoskeletal conditions have been excluded, formulating a tentative diagnosis is difficult. Potential local sources of pain include muscle strain or injury to the areas of muscle attachment, such as iliopsoas tendinopathy, rectus femoris muscle avulsion, adductor muscle strain, and internal oblique avulsion, as well as pubalgia, osteitis pubis, bursitis and local peripheral nerves (e.g. iliohypogastric nerve, ilioinguinal nerve, femoral nerve, genitofemoral nerve) (Adkins and Figler, 2000; Meyes et al., 2000; O'Kane, 1999; Polglase et al., 1991; Taylor et al., 1991). Pain can be referred into the pelvic girdle area from a wide variety of regions, including the low back and pelvic organs, and by a variety of systemic diseases. Systemic causes of hip pain, such as spinal cord tumours, ureteral pain, ascites, gastro-intestinal bleeding associated with haemophilia and abdominal aortic aneurysm, must also be considered (Fagerson, 1998; Goodman and Snyder, 2000). Musculoskeletal causes of groin pain that require immediate medical attention include hip avascular necrosis, hemiarthrosis, slipped capital femoral epiphysis, femoral neck fractures (Clement et al., 1993; Goodman and Snyder, 2000; Jones and Erhard, 1996) and stress fractures of the lesser trochanter and medial femur (Adkins and Figler, 2000).

Two main factors support the belief that Steven's pain was not the result of systemic disease or severe musculoskeletal pathology. First, his symptoms had been present for more than a year; if a serious medical problem was present, it would be obvious by now. Secondly, Steven had been thoroughly examined, including extensive laboratory and radiological testing, by his physician and two orthopaedic surgeons. Therefore, the most likely source of Steven's problem was soft tissue, with ongoing persistent irritation by daily activities, minimal as they were; otherwise the tissues would have healed in the significant time since the onset of the symptoms.

In a young patient with groin pain who is an athlete, consideration must be given as to how participation in a particular sport can lead to the problem (Wilkerson, 1997). Because of the persistence of the pain after ceasing participation, trauma to the tissues during the sport is not an adequate explanation. Instead, the sport must have induced changes in neuromuscular control resulting in alteration of the precision of movement of the hip joint. Such changes are identified as muscle and movement impairments. Though identifying the specific tissues that have become painful may be useful, it does not address the reason these tissues have become symptomatic unless the presumption is that pure overuse is the cause, which is not likely. The negative examination by the orthopaedic surgeons for skeletal or soft tissue lesions suggests that the problem must have a more dynamic cause, such as a movement impairment that causes repeated microtrauma to the joint tissues, rather than a severe static lesion of tissues, which would be evident by radiological examination.

One clinical theory is that repeated movements and sustained postures alter tissues that control the characteristics of movement, thus causing movement impairments (Sahrmann, 2001). We have described the signs and symptoms of movement impairment syndromes and contributing factors, based on the findings of clinical examinations of individuals with groin pain without systemic or serious musculoskeletal pathology. Two main categories of movement impairment syndromes have been described. One category is based on impairments in accessory motions of the hip joint and the other on impairments in physiological movements. *Femoral syndromes* are believed to be impairments of the accessory motions, which cause irritation of tissues about the joint. *Hip syndromes* are impairments of physiological motions, which produce pain in muscles associated with the movement. The femoral syndromes are named for the accessory motion that is believed to be impaired, either because the motion is excessive or because the motion is occurring when it should not be. The movement impairment, the diagnosis, is attributed to the joint developing a particular susceptibility to movement in a specific direction. Specific sports and activities are believed to contribute to particular syndromes (Stricevic et al., 1983). The therapist can formulate a tentative diagnosis based on how well the history corresponds to the signs and symptoms associated with a specific diagnosis. The results of the examination will either confirm or exclude the tentative diagnosis. Similarly, the physician examining a patient who is obese, over 40 years of age, complaining of polyuria, polydyspia, and polyphagia, knows the most likely diagnosis is diabetes, and his examination will, therefore, focus on confirming or excluding this tentative diagnosis.

2 Given the tragedy that occurred within Steven's family, did you feel his psychosocial status may have been contributing to his presentation?

Clinician's answer

No, I did not. My impression was that this was a very nice, well-adjusted young boy, who was dealing as well as possible with both the loss of his brother and the upset associated with his undiagnosed pain problem, which had not improved in 1 year in spite of his efforts to follow medical recommendations. The characteristics of Steven's symptoms and his intense participation in karate were consistent with a femoral movement impairment diagnosis. Furthermore, he attempted to participate in activities such as paintball, which did not require running. He was not having any trouble in school and was socially active. Therefore, there was nothing to suggest that psychological problems were contributing to his condition. I prefer to conduct my examination and relate

the pattern and consistency of the results with the tentative diagnosis. If the results are not consistent and no pattern of signs or symptoms is present, then I am more likely to move on to consider a psychological problem.

Steven did not either verbally or physically manifest any anxiety, impatience or fear about his symptoms or enforced inactivity, nor did he seem withdrawn. This behaviour is in contrast to that of other young individuals whom I have seen, in whom depression was a contributing factor. Steven was not using his pain to avoid school or any other responsibilities and was continuing to participate in social activities. Therefore, I had no reason to believe that either central pain mechanisms or an emotional component were factors in his problem.

■ Clinical reasoning commentary

While experts are able to recognize quickly the most likely clinical pattern through the process of inductive reasoning, they also are thorough in their deliberations, using deductive reasoning to rule out alternative patterns, especially those of a more serious nature. This is evident here in the clinician's consideration of a broad range of possible sources, including local tissues, tissues capable of referring pain to the groin area and more sinister pathologies. As the clinician highlights, consideration of specific sources is important, but given the lack of definitive diagnostic criteria, particularly for the various soft tissue sources of groin pain, reasoning must then focus on patterns of impairments associated with the pain state. The source of the symptoms can and should still be hypothesized, but as soft tissue sources are often unable to be confirmed, management directed to impairments substantiated through subjective and physical evidence (combined with reassessment of interventions directed to the hypothesized impairment) is arguably more valid. The hypothesis category 'contributing factors' also features strongly in the clinician's reasoning. Using knowledge of tissue healing and questioning that revealed that the patient's symptoms persisted even when sport had been stopped, the clinician has deduced that other factors are likely to be contributing to the persistent irritation of the symptomatic tissues. In this case, possibly altered neuromuscular control resulting in muscle and movement impairments about the hip.

In addition to this biomedical, 'diagnostic reasoning', the clinician also reveals her biopsychosocial, 'narrative reasoning' through her attention to, and analysis of, potential psychosocial factors. This hypothesis is then linked to the likely pain mechanisms, which are considered to be nociceptive and not central.

 ## PHYSICAL EXAMINATION

The examination to identify movement impairment syndromes is a combined examination where a number of positive findings are necessary to confirm the diagnosis. The examination assesses the effects of movements and joint positions on symptoms, and the presence of neuromuscular and movement impairments. The examination includes assessment of:

- alignment
- movement patterns
- muscle length
- muscle strength
- muscle stiffness
- pattern of recruitment
- presence of a joint's susceptibility to movement in a specific direction.

At the time of his physical therapy examination, Steven was 1.78 metres tall, with the last 5 cm added during the past year. He was slender but well proportioned, with well-developed thigh and gluteal musculature. The tests are described below and their implications are discussed at the end of the set of tests in the Reasoning discussion.

Standing tests

1. *Alignment.* Thoracic and lumbar spinal curves were normal. The iliac crests were level, without pelvic rotation or pelvic tilt. The patient stood in bilateral hip abduction and slight lateral rotation.

2. *Forward bending.* Motion occurred primarily in the lumbar spine with hip flexion limited to 60 degrees. Even with instruction to bend his knees and manual assistance in trying to flex his hips during forward bending, his hip flexion range of motion did not increase. There was no pain during this movement.

3. *Side bending and rotation of the trunk with the pelvis stabilized.* Neither of these motions elicited symptoms and no asymmetries were observed. Lumbar extension was not examined,

primarily because it is not part of my routine examination but also because if extension is a cause of the symptoms, they are usually present in standing. Several other tests may help in assessing whether lumbar extension is a cause of symptoms.

4. *Single-leg standing.* The patient stands on one leg while flexing the contralateral hip to about 90 degrees and allowing the knee to flex as the knee is brought toward the pelvis. There was no obvious hip drop, but when standing on the right foot, the hip medially rotated, which could be observed in a posterior view of the knee. The same observation was made when Steven stood on the left foot to a lesser degree.

Supine tests

5. *Hip flexor length test.* With the hip in neutral in the frontal plane, the right hip was 25 degrees short of full extension and painless. When the hip was allowed to abduct, the hip extended completely. The left hip was 20 degrees short of full extension until abduction was permitted, and then the hip extended completely. There was no anterior pelvic tilt during the test.

6. *Passive hip and knee flexion.* At 90 degrees of hip flexion on both the right and left sides, Steven experienced pain in the groin. Marked resistance to hip flexion was noted at 90 degrees but there was no posterior pelvic tilt with lumbar flexion. Passively laterally rotating the hip and applying pressure on the femur in a posterior direction increased the range of hip flexion by 10 degrees before Steven experienced pain in the groin. Steven was instructed to remain completely relaxed during the passive hip and knee flexion. When he did remain relaxed, the pain-free range into hip flexion increased by 10 degrees. There was slightly less resistance to hip flexion on the left than on the right side, but Steven still experienced pain at 90 degrees of flexion.

7. *Active hip and knee flexion.* Steven experienced pain in the groin at 80 degrees of flexion of both the right and left hips. The pelvis did not rotate at all during the movement.

8. *Straight-leg raise.* When performed passively, the range was limited to 50 degrees bilaterally and no symptoms were provoked. Monitoring of the greater trochanter during the movement indicated the trochanter followed an antero-medial path rather than maintaining a constant position. When pressure was applied at the inguinal crease to prevent the anteromedial path of the greater trochanter, there was marked resistance to hip flexion (Fig. 18.1).

9. *Iliopsoas muscle test.* The test position of hip flexion, abduction and lateral rotation with the knee extended (Kendall et al., 1993) was used to assess the performance of the iliopsoas muscle. Steven had difficulty maintaining the position, though he did not have pain.

10. *The FABER test.* This test is also known as Patrick's test position and comprises hip abduction/external rotation with the hip and knee flexed (Fagerson, 1998). Steven's range of motion was within normal limits. He did experience pain in the groin at the end of the range for either hip. No pelvic rotation was evident during this motion with either the right or left lower extremity.

11. *Abdominal muscle testing.* The upper abdominals (internal obliques and rectus abdominis) were tested using the method described by Kendall et al. (1993). Steven was able to complete the trunk curl-sit up with his arms folded on his chest, which is an 80% or 4/5 grade. The lower abdominals (external obliques and rectus abdominis) were tested with the method described by Sahrmann (2001). From the supine position with his hips and knees extended, he was able to flex and extend his hips and knees bilaterally, by holding them off the supporting surface and without pelvic tilt. This is consistent with grade 4/5. No pain was reported during the testing.

Side-lying tests

12. *Hip lateral rotation from hip and knee flexion.* From the position of 45 degrees of hip and knee flexion, Steven performed the motion by movement at the hip and without associated pelvic rotation.

13. *Posterior gluteus medius muscle function.* This tested 3/5 on the right side and 3+/5 on the left (Kendall et al., 1993; manual muscle testing method) (Fig. 18.2). These grades mean that Steven was unable to maintain the test position, which is against gravity. When the hip was

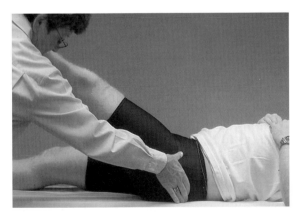

Fig. 18.1 Hamstring shortness contributing to the anteriomedial path of the greater trochanter during the straight-leg raise. When the therapist applies pressure at the inguinal crease to maintain precise movement of the femur during the passive straight-leg raise, marked resistance from the hamstrings is evident that was not present without the control of the proximal femoral motion.

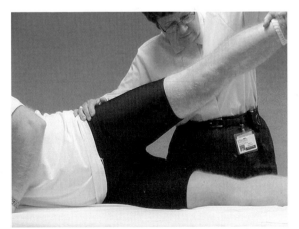

Fig. 18.2 Manual muscle test of the posterior gluteus medius muscle. When the patient attempted to resist the pressure applied by the therapist during the muscle test, the hip medially rotated and flexed. The patient was unable to hold his hip in the correct position of extension and lateral rotation.

placed in flexion, medial rotation and abduction, his muscles tested 5/5. The Ober test was positive, with the hip remaining in 10 degrees of abduction. During the return from hip abduction, Steven medially rotated his hip to achieve hip adduction.

Prone

14. *Passive knee flexion with the hip abducted.* No motion of the pelvis was noted and the test was painless.
15. *Hip rotation.* Lateral rotation of both the right and left hips was 75 degrees. Medial rotation range of motion was 10 degrees.
16. *Active hip extension with the knee extended.* The hamstring muscle was observed to change its contour before the gluteus maximus, and the hip extended 10 degrees before there was a notable change in the contour of the gluteus maximus. Monitoring of the greater trochanter of the femur indicated that it moved anteriorly and medially. However, it should be noted that normal reliability studies of assessing the path of the greater trochanter during hip extension or flexion have not been performed. To be considered clinically important, the movement of the trochanter must be at least 1 cm. Van Dillen et al. (1998) have reported that 1 cm variations can be reliably detected by trained clinicians when examining pelvic motion and contours of the lumbar spine. Furthermore, there are few reliability studies of manual muscle testing, although Florence et al. (1992) have demonstrated reliability in patients with muscular dystrophy. The validity of these tests has not been examined.
17. *Gluteus maximus manual muscle test.* The patient is in the prone position with the knee flexed. The hip is passively extended to 10 degrees and the patient is asked to hold that position while resistance is applied to the thigh and the pelvis is passively stabilized by the examiner (Kendall et al., 1993). The left and right gluteus maximus muscles both tested 4−/5.

Quadruped

18. *Preferred position.* Steven's preferred position was with lumbar spine in flexion and hips in less than 70 degrees of flexion. With verbal and manual cues, the alignment of Steven's lumbar spine and hips could be corrected so that the hips were flexed to 90 degrees.
19. *Rocking backward.* When Steven rocked backward, his lumbar spine flexed but not his hips. If the pelvis was controlled by the therapist, preventing the lumbar flexion, this forced the hips to flex a few degrees. Approximately 10 to 15 repetitions of rocking backward were performed, with each repetition resulting in a few more degrees of hip flexion. Upon completion of the repetitions, Steven's hips flexed to almost 110 degrees without pain in the groin.

Sitting tests

20. *Knee extension.* As Steven extended his knee in sitting, his hip medially rotated. This rotation is best assessed when the examiner places his hands on the thigh while the patient extends his knee. Knee extension was −30 degrees of extension bilaterally; when the hip medial rotation was prevented, the range was −35 degrees of extension. The lumbar spine flexed during knee extension, but no symptoms were elicited.
21. *Iliopsoas manual muscle test.* To perform this test, the hip is passively flexed as much as possible to eliminate the participation of the hip flexors that attach in the area of the anterior iliac spine (Kendall et al., 1993). The passive range into hip flexion was limited because of pain in the groin and by resistance to flexion. Both the right and left iliopsoas muscles tested 3+/5.
22. *Hip rotation.* Hip lateral rotation range of motion was 70 degrees bilaterally. Hip medial rotation range of motion was 15 degrees for both the right and left hips.
23. *Hip lateral rotator manual muscle test.* The hip lateral rotators are tested with the hip positioned at the end of the range to be tested and resistance is applied to the ankle in the appropriate direction while the distal thigh is stabilized (Kendall et al., 1993). Both the left and right hip lateral rotator muscles tested 4−/5.

REASONING DISCUSSION AND CLINICAL REASONING COMMENTARY

1 How did each test to identify movement impairments suggest the principal source or impairment?

Clinician's answer

1. *Alignment.* In patients with the femoral anterior glide syndrome, most typically the hip is extended by a combination of posterior pelvic tilt and hyperextension of the knees. In the syndrome without rotation, and in the medial rotation subcategory, pain occurs during hip flexion usually at about 90 degrees. In the femoral anterior glide syndrome with medial rotation, the hips are often medially rotated in standing. In the lateral rotation subcategory, the hips are often laterally rotated and the pain usually occurs during hip extension when walking. In this patient the pain was most notable during hip flexion.

2. *Forward bending.* If the pain was from his lumbar spine and occurred during forward bending in which excessive lumbar flexion was present, a possible diagnosis would be lumbar flexion syndrome. Because susceptibility to rotation is usually present in patients with low back-related pain, a tentative diagnosis of flexion–rotation would be the one to confirm or disconfirm. However, because Steven did not have symptoms when bending forward, although he had excessive lumbar flexion motion, this suggests the spine is not the site producing the symptoms, but rather the most likely site is the hip. The limited range of hip flexion is one of the signs of the femoral anterior glide syndrome.

3. *Side bending and rotation of the trunk with the pelvis stabilized.* The failure of these to elicit symptoms was additional support that the lumbar spine is not the site eliciting the pain.

4. *Single-leg standing.* The anterior glide syndrome with medial rotation was supported, indicating that the intrinsic hip lateral rotators (obturators, gemelli, quadratus femoris and piriformis) could be weak or long or both.

5. *Hip flexor length test.* The results indicated marked shortness of tensor fascia lata (TFL)–iliotibial band (ITB). This is a positive finding for the femoral anterior glide syndrome, particularly when present without shortness of the iliopsoas muscle. The lack of anterior pelvic tilt, which would indicate a compensatory motion of the lumbar spine, further supports the hypothesis that the spine is not the site causing the pain. As none of the test movements were painful a local neurogenic source (e.g. iliohypogastric nerve, ilioinguinal nerve, femoral nerve, genitofemoral nerve) was considered unlikely.

6. *Passive hip and knee flexion.* These findings are consistent with the femoral anterior glide syndrome. The passive lateral rotation reduces the stretch of the lateral rotator muscles, reducing the posterior stiffness and restriction to posterior glide. The pressure on the femur in a posterior direction increases the posterior glide, and the subsequent increased range before onset of symptoms is consistent with insufficient posterior glide contributing to the symptoms. The reduction in symptoms and increase in range of motion when Steven was relaxed (i.e. completely passive hip flexion) occurred because contraction of the two-joint hip flexors (rectus femoris, TFL and sartorius) tends to contribute to anterior gliding.

7. *Active hip and knee flexion.* Increased symptoms with active hip and knee flexion is consistent with the anterior glide syndrome. The TFL, rectus femoris and sartorius muscles are believed to be the dominant hip flexors and not iliopsoas. The result is insufficient depression of the femoral head. The lack of femoral head depression causes the femur to impinge on the anterior joint capsule tissues. The lack of lumbopelvic rotation during the motion is consistent with the hypothesis that the lumbar spine is not the site eliciting the symptoms.

8. *Straight-leg raise.* The painless limitation in range of hip flexion observed is consistent with hamstring muscle shortness. The anteromedial deviation of the greater trochanter during the straight-leg raise is a key sign of the anterior glide syndrome. The alteration in the path of the greater trochanter is believed to occur because of the lack of posterior glide of the femur during the flexion motion and because of slight medial rotation of the femur. The medial rotation of the femur during hip

flexion suggests that the dominant hip flexor or flexors must be the TFL and possibly the anterior gluteus medius and gluteus minimus muscles and not the iliopsoas, which would laterally rotate the hip.

9. *Iliopsoas muscle test.* A positive test for diminished performance of iliopsoas is a key sign of the anterior glide syndrome.

10. *FABER test.* Pain in the groin with this test is considered a sign of hip joint dysfunction. Radiological studies had ruled out degenerative joint disease, but the presence of symptoms could indicate joint capsule irritation. The same motion of hip abduction/external rotation with the hip and knee flexed can be accompanied by pelvic rotation, which is a sign of a lumbar movement impairment syndrome. The absence of pelvic rotation during the movement further supports the hypothesis that the spine is not the site of the symptoms, but that the hip joint is probably responsible.

11. *Abdominal muscle testing.* These tests provide information about the musculature that controls pelvic tilt and rotation. These findings do not contribute to the diagnosis but to the understanding of contributing factors. The abdominal muscles were tested, because the TFL–ITB muscles were short. Because these muscles were short, motions such as walking (when the hip has to rotate laterally and extend) would be restricted and compensatory motions would be likely to occur. The compensatory motions would be lumbopelvic rotation, lumbar extension or anterior glide at the hip joint. The strength of the abdominals and the lack of symptoms during testing suggest that the lumbar spine is not the site of compensation or the source of symptoms. When the lumbar spine is the source of symptoms, a strong contraction of the iliopsoas muscle usually produces symptoms, probably because of the anterior shear and compression forces.

12. *Hip lateral rotation from hip and knee flexion.* Because Steven preferentially moved the hip and did not demonstrate pelvic rotation, this supported the hypothesis that the lumbar spine was not the source of the symptoms.

13. *The posterior gluteus medius muscle.* The marked weakness of the posterior gluteus medius is a contributing factor to the femoral anterior glide syndrome with medial rotation.

The normal strength of the hip abductor, medial rotator and flexor muscles is consistent with the dominant hip abductors being the anterior gluteus medius, gluteus minimus and TFL, and with an evident imbalance in hip musculature. The positive Ober test (the hip does not adduct 10 degrees from neutral) indicates that the flexor/medial rotator/abductors are short and that the compensatory motion is hip medial rotation and flexion.

14. *Passive knee flexion with the hip abducted.* Passive flexion of the knee stretches the TFL and the rectus femoris, while also indirectly placing tension on the femoral nerve through its fascial interface. Abduction of the hip indicates that shortness of the TFL–ITB caused compensatory motion of the hip but not of the pelvis. This provides further support that the pain is from hip dysfunction and not lumbar spine dysfunction.

15. *Hip rotation.* The surprising finding was the extreme range of hip lateral rotation, particularly with shortness of the TFL–ITB, which is a hip medial rotator muscle. The extreme range of hip lateral rotation and the bilateral presentation suggests possible retrotorsion of the femur.

16. *Active hip extension with the knee extended.* The dominant performance of the hamstring muscles and the delayed onset of the gluteus maximus muscle is another indication that the musculature that controls the proximal end of the femur is not functioning optimally. Because the hamstring muscle attaches to the ischial tuberosity and to the tibia, the distal end of the femur can move posteriorly without the proximal end of the femur maintaining a constant position. The anterior/medial motion of the greater trochanter supports the hypothesis that the hip musculature controlling the proximal end of the femur (the gluteus maximus, piriformis and lateral rotator muscles) is not participating optimally and is permitting inappropriate motion of the proximal femur.

17. *Gluteus maximus manual muscle test.* The finding of gluteus maximus muscle weakness indicates that the pattern of muscle participation during hip extension with the knee extended is consistent with weakness of gluteus maximus.

18. *Preferred position.* The assumed position of lumbar flexion and less than 70 degrees of hip

flexion is consistent with resistance to posterior glide of the femur and that the lumbar spine flexes more easily than the hips. This is also a common finding in the lumbar flexion syndrome and is, therefore, not specific to the femoral anterior glide syndrome.

19. *Rocking backward.* These results are a key sign of the femoral anterior glide syndrome. The resistance to hip flexion is attributed to stiffness of the posterior structures of the hip. In the quadruped position, the weight of the pelvis and thorax helps to bring the acetabulum down over the femoral head, which is not possible when the patient is in the supine position and flexing his hip. The greater range obtained without groin pain indicates that when the femur does posteriorly glide, the symptoms are reduced.

20. *Knee extension.* The medial rotation of the hip during knee extension is another indication of the dominance of the hip medial rotators. When the medial rotation was prevented, the knee extension range of motion was decreased. Consequently, another factor contributing to the rotation was that the medial hamstrings were shorter than the lateral hamstrings. However, both the medial and lateral hamstrings were short, as indicated by the limited knee extension range of motion. Though the lumbar spine flexed during knee extension, Steven did not experience any symptoms, indicating that the lumbar spine was probably not the site of his symptoms.

21. *Iliopsoas manual muscle test.* Weakness of iliopsoas is a key sign of the femoral anterior glide syndrome. The compromised performance of the iliopsoas muscle is another factor contributing to the diminished control of muscles attaching close to the axis of rotation and that stabilize the femoral head in the acetabulum and prevent medial rotation. The iliopsoas muscle, through its attachment to the lesser trochanter and the path of its muscle fibres over the femoral head, contributes to stabilizing the head and laterally rotating the femur. In contrast, the other hip flexors (rectus femoris, TFL and sartorius) attach to the anterior iliac spines of the pelvis and to the tibia via tendons and fascia. Therefore, these muscles, which attach at a distance from the axis of rotation of the hip joint,

cannot provide fine control of femoral head motion nor can they stabilize the femoral head in the acetabulum.

22. *Hip rotation.* The excessive hip lateral rotation and limited medial rotation range are present in the extended hip position and in the flexed hip position; this suggested that Steven had retrotorsion of both hips. According to a study of hip antetorsion by Gelberman and Hekkar (1987), marked asymmetry of medial versus lateral hip rotation ranges of motion, with either the hip extended or flexed, indicates hip anteversion. By inference, an asymmetry of greater hip lateral rotation versus hip medial rotation in the hip flexed and extended positions would also support the presence of hip retrotorsion.

23. *Hip lateral rotator manual muscle test.* Weakness of the hip lateral rotator muscles is consistent with the medial rotation pattern of the hip.

2 Please summarize your principal diagnosis at the end of the physical examination.

Clinician's answer

The findings of the examination are consistent with a diagnosis of femoral anterior glide syndrome with medial rotation. In this syndrome, the pain in the groin is believed to be caused by the head of the femur failing to glide posteriorly during flexion and during medial rotation, and thus impinging on the anterior joint capsule tissues. The syndrome develops because of the repeated movement of hip flexion/medial rotation. The repeated movement increases the performance and thus the dominance of the TFL and other medial rotators. The muscles that attach close to the axis of rotation, such as iliopsoas, gluteus maximus and the hip lateral rotators (including piriformis, the gemelli, the obturators and quadrus femoris), become weakened and/or lengthened and, therefore, fail to maintain precise control of the femoral head. An additional contributing factor in Steven was structural hip retrotorsion, which limited the normal range of medial rotation. An activity that required hip medial rotation, such as the kick in karate, required an abnormal range of hip motion for this patient, thus predisposing him to the syndrome.

The findings consistent with the diagnosis were:

- pain with passive hip flexion at 90–100 degrees
- decreased pain with increased range of passive hip flexion if the hip is laterally rotated and pressure is exerted on the femur in a posterior direction
- anteromedial deviation of the greater trochanter during hip flexion; increased resistance to hip flexion if the axis of rotation is maintained by passive pressure exerted by the examiner
- shortness of the hamstrings
- short TFL–ITB, weakness of the iliopsoas muscle
- weak posterior gluteus medius muscle and strong hip abductor/medial rotator muscles
- stiffness of the TFL, which caused the hips to abduct when the knee was flexed while the patient was in the prone position
- excessive hip lateral rotation, which indicated the patient had retrotorsion of the femur
- gluteus maximus muscle weakness
- dominance of hamstring muscles during hip extension
- limited hip flexion in the quadruped position that improved (increased hip flexion range of motion without symptoms) with the examiner assisting repeated attempts to rock backward to ensure that the hips were flexing and not the lumbar spine
- hip medial rotation during knee extension
- weak hip lateral rotators.
- hip retrotorsion, which is a pathologic decrease in the normal 14 degree anteriorly directed angle of the head and neck of the femur with respect to the transverse axis of the femoral condyles
- anterior movement of the greater trochanter during hip extension (the greater trochanter should remain constant or move slightly posteriorly as the gluteus maximus and piriformis muscles control its position and prevent the medial rotation or anterior glide of the femoral head): when an abnormal pattern of recruitment and muscle performance is present, the motion of the femur is similar to a see-saw, with the proximal end moving in an anterior direction and the distal end moving in a posterior direction.

The torsion of the femur cannot be seen on standard radiographs and requires computer tomography scans or other types of special radiological tests for detection. It is established by 6–8 years of age. Wide variations in femoral torsion have been reported, and conservative measures to modify torsion have not been effective (Kling and Hensinger, 1983; Staheli et al., 1985). The condition has not been shown to result in hip joint disease and, consequently, is not considered to be of importance except in extreme cases. Steven was a karate champion with particular skill in the kick. The karate kick involves hip medial rotation and because Steven had structural hip retrotorsion, the repeated rotations altered the muscular control and presumably the precision of femoral accessory motion. These presumptions are based on the results of the examination that has been described. Once the pattern of femoral motion has become abnormal, with anterior glide in the direction of motion that is the path of least resistance, the anterior joint capsule tissues are subjected to repeated microtrauma and thus injury.

Additional contributing factors that were explored after the initial examination supported the diagnosis. Steven slept on his side with his hip adducted and medially rotated. He also sat with his legs crossed so that the ankle of one lower extremity was on the thigh of the other lower extremity. Even though this is lateral rotation, the accessory motion is anterior glide. Therefore, even this position is contributing to the anterior glide of the femoral head. When sitting, he did not have his hips flexed to 90 degrees but was always in a slumped, slouched position with only about 60 degrees of hip flexion.

■ Clinical reasoning commentary

Having been asked to comment on how each of the above tests specifically supported or did not support her principal hypothesis regarding the most likely source of pain and dysfunction or impairment, the clinician has nicely demonstrated the evolving nature of her reasoning. That is, while the femoral anterior glide syndrome was noted as the most likely impairment based on the subjective examination, each test of the physical examination was then interpreted with respect to whether it did or did not support this hypothesis. Reasoning can be seen to occur with every examination procedure, in this case reinforcing the principal hypothesis. A secondary hypothesis of lumbar spine impairment was also being simultaneously tested, indicating that the clinician was open to other potential explanations for the patient's presentation.

Experts in all professions possess a rich store of patterns within their area of expertise, which form prototypes of frequently experienced situations. These are used to recognize, interpret and respond to other situations. In physiotherapy, patterns exist in classic diagnostic syndromes, in associated management strategies, in pathobiological mechanisms associated with those syndromes, and in the physical, environmental, psychosocial, behavioural and cultural factors that contribute to the development and maintenance of patients' problems. Here the clinician has outlined an extensive list of physical examination findings associated with her principal diagnostic hypothesis. The process is almost made to look simple, where in reality there is much overlap between the features of different clinical patterns; distinguishing between competing patterns requires thorough and systematic examination, treatment and reassessment. Being the first to identify a clinical pattern, as this expert can be credited with, requires more than just years of experience. Such a contribution to the profession requires skilled, reflective clinical reasoning.

m Management

The movement impairment diagnosis directs the treatment because it identifies the movement direction that must be corrected. Therefore, the main goal of the management programme was to improve the posterior glide of the femoral head, prevent excessive anterior glide, eliminate the excessive medial rotation, and restore the correct pattern of muscle length, strength, and participation. In order to achieve these goals, the home exercise programme included performing the test movements that were positive. The movement patterns and postures used in daily activities that contributed to the development of the syndrome also needed to be corrected. A particularly important exercise was rocking backward in the quadruped position with the motion occurring in the hips and not in the lumbar spine. This exercise forces the femur to move in a posterior glide by stretching the stiff and/or shortened posterior structures. Another important exercise was hip abduction with lateral rotation performed in the side-lying position. Once Steven had at least 115 degrees of hip flexion without pain, he would begin exercises to strengthen the iliopsoas muscle specifically.

At the time of his initial visit Steven was instructed in the following exercises.

1. Quadruped rocking backward with emphasis on hip flexion and avoiding lumbar flexion. Steven rocked backward to the point of pain in the groin. He then rocked back to the starting position and repeated the exercise.

2. Hip extension in prone. Steven lay with two pillows under his abdomen so his hips were flexed. He then performed hip extension with his knee extended and with the emphasis on initiating the motion with the gluteus maximus muscle. He was taught to monitor the path of the greater trochanter and not to attempt more than 10 degrees of motion.

3. Gluteus medius muscle. Steven was positioned in side lying with two pillows between his knees and thighs (so that his hip was in abduction and slight lateral rotation) and with his knee flexed to approximately 30 degrees. He was taught to palpate the gluteus medius muscle belly and to be sure he could feel it become firm when he attempted to abduct and laterally rotate his hip.

4. Knee extension in sitting. This was performed while maintaining slight hip lateral rotation. He was instructed to 'think about only using a few fibres of his quadriceps' to extend his knee. This direction was given to prevent exaggerated use of the dominant rectus femoris and TFL muscles.

5. Hip flexion. While still sitting: he was instructed to use both hands to lift passively his hip into flexion but to stop if he felt pain in his groin.

6. He was shown how to use a lightweight stretch cord for resistance to hip lateral rotation while sitting.

7. Actively contracting the muscles in the gluteal area to prevent hip medial rotation while standing on a single leg.

All exercises were to be performed 8–10 times twice a day. In addition, Steven was instructed to sit with his hips flexed to 80–90 degrees and to avoid crossing his legs. When sitting he could lean forward by flexing his hips if he pushed his trunk forward with his hands. If he slept on his side, he had to use two pillows between his knees.

Visit 2

Reassessment

Steven returned in 2 weeks for assessment of his progress and progression of his programme. At that time, he did not have any pain in his right hip but did develop pain in his left groin after walking for more than 30 minutes. His pain did not reach the previous level of 8–9/10, but only became 2–3/10 after standing or walking. At the time of his visit, he did not have any pain in either groin. Test results were as follows:

- hip flexor length: without hip abduction the right and left hips extended to within 10 degrees of complete extension
- passive hip flexion was 125 degrees without symptoms on the right side and 115 degrees with slight pain on the left
- hip flexion with lateral rotation of the hip and posteriorly directed pressure into the hip joint: symptom-free hip flexion range improved by 5 degrees
- posterior gluteus medius manual muscle test: 4/5 bilaterally
- gluteus maximus manual muscle test: 4/5 bilaterally
- iliopsoas manual muscle test: 4−/5 with some pain
- quadruped: Steven could rock back to 125 degrees of hip flexion without pain and without a tendency to flex his lumbar spine
- knee extension in sitting: no longer associated with hip medial rotation and was full range of motion.

The assessment indicated that Steven had made good progress, as evident by the marked decrease in the severity and frequency of his pain. This is the first period in which he had an improvement in his condition in the past 18 months.

Programme modification

The programme was then modified:

- increasing the resistance for the hip lateral rotator exercises

- performing forward bending when standing by flexing the knees and hips and not the lumbar spine, while supporting the upper body on a counter; the return to the upright position should be achieved by making a conscious effort to contract the gluteus maximus muscles
- performing hip abduction with the hip and knee extended while side lying; in addition, performing hip adduction with the bottom lower extremity
- instructions in walking to take a slightly longer stride, using contraction of the gluteal muscles of the stance leg at heel strike; the push-off should begin at the end of mid-stance phase
- walking should be progressively increased to 5 km, provided no pain developed in his groin
- other exercises were to be continued and increased to 10–15 repetitions twice daily.

Steven's return appointment was set for 2 weeks.

Visit 3

Steven reported continued improvement in his condition. He was able to walk for 5 km but did develop slight pain in his left groin about halfway. The pain gradually increased during the remainder of the walk; however it subsided almost immediately upon cessation. Steven was pain-free with all of his exercises, including active and passive hip flexion to 135 degrees. Active and passive straight-leg raising was to 80 degrees, with both the right and left greater trochanters maintained in a constant position. In the prone position, the greater trochanter also maintained a constant position during hip extension. All muscles tested 5/5 except for the iliopsoas, which tested 4+/5 bilaterally.

Steven was told he could start alternately running for 1 minute and walking for 1 minute for a total of 30 minutes every other day for 1 week. If he remained pain-free, he could increase the running to 2 minutes. He was asked to call me in 3 weeks to report his progress.

When Steven called 3 weeks later, he said he was able to run for a total of 5 km every other day. He was given permission to return to karate so long as he maintained his exercise programme and performed the exercises after the karate session.

Steven's mother called a month later and indicated that her son was doing very well and had resumed his karate without experiencing a recurrence of his symptoms.

REASONING DISCUSSION AND CLINICAL REASONING COMMENTARY

1 Did you expect such rapid and complete recovery given the chronicity of the disorder and failure of previous medical intervention?

Clinician's answer

Based on my experience with other patients with this syndrome, I did expect a good recovery and pain elimination within 4 weeks. The patient's clinical findings were so consistent with those of the syndrome, that I did expect the condition to resolve quickly. My major concern was that because the patient lived so far away and return visits to physical therapy could not be frequent, his correct performance of the exercises was essential. I usually do not see patients more than once a week, but knew that this type of frequency for appointments over an extended period would not be possible. The patient's motivation and participation were enhanced by learning about the obvious muscle and movement impairments that were present, how his symptoms could be changed, and that the condition was known to me. He had specific performance problems to correct, which aided his motivation and understanding of what was to be achieved. The opportunity to be 'in charge' of his condition had been absent during the past year. He had been unable to do anything but wait and hope. The patient was bright, was an athlete, knew his body and wanted to be active. The combination of all these factors certainly provided optimal conditions for the necessary participation by the patient.

I believe that the rate and extent of the patient's recovery supports the belief that presence of the impaired movement pattern was the cause of the tissue irritation. I believe that, all too often, therapists assume that they have to provide pain-relieving modalities or 'calm tissues down' before beginning exercises. I consider this a misdirection, because my experience has been that correcting the movement impairment and the contributing factors is necessary to alleviate the pain. This does not mean that acute injuries should not be treated with appropriate modalities, but certainly not chronic conditions that have had suitable time for tissue repair. This syndrome also illustrates the critical importance of precision in kinesiological observation and in the

development and instruction in therapeutic exercises. There is a prevailing belief that strengthening exercises are the key to tissue recovery, but that is only true if the underlying movement pattern and muscle participation is precise.

Painful conditions of the hip are of particular interest to me, because medical interventions have been limited. Surgical treatment has been for hip joint replacement, which of course is limited to the elderly when clear signs of degeneration are present. More recently, labral tears have been identified in younger individuals and now surgeons are debriding (repairing this) these tears, believing this will address the patient's pain. The question has to be asked, what caused the tear? Debriding the tear without addressing the movement impairments that I believe cause the tear is only partial treatment. Unfortunately, surgeons are not aware of the kinesiological movement impairments or that therapists can effectively treat these problems; therefore, too few patients with these problems are referred to therapists. Medical intervention for musculoskeletal problems is limited to medication that reduces inflammation and pain or to surgery for damaged tissues. Neither of these treatments addresses the causes of mechanical musculoskeletal pain problems. That is why, as physical therapists, we must describe the syndromes requiring our intervention, so that patients, referral sources and therapists become aware of our professional expertise in diagnosis and treatment of these conditions.

Clinical reasoning commentary

With a clear link of management to examination findings, the clinician's collaborative reasoning stands out through her involvement of the patient in self-management. Patient learning (i.e. altered understanding/beliefs, feelings, behaviours and neuromuscular control or motor programmes) is the primary outcome sought in the collaborative reasoning approach. Rather than being passive recipients of health care, and manual therapy in particular, patients are taught, counselled and coached so as to enable them to construct a new perspective and, as for Steven, a new motor programme; these hopefully allow them to maintain the improvement achieved and to minimize the risk of recurrence. This level of learning and responsibility for self-management requires shared decision-making. Exercises need to be understood, accepted and progressed from a cognitive awareness of the control required to automatic functional execution. A written text of selected exercises, as provided here, can never fully capture the teaching and collaborative reasoning skills that underlie successful attainment of this outcome. Propositional knowledge of learning and motor control theory, professional craft knowledge, skills in teaching and motor retraining strategies, and personal knowledge from life experiences to establish rapport with and motivate the patient represent some of the prerequisites for success with complex clinical presentations.

References

Adkins, S.B. and Figler, R.A. (2000). Hip pain in athletes. American Family Physician, 61, 2109–2118.

Clement, D.B., Ammann, W., Taunton, J.E. et al. (1993). Exercise-induced stress injuries to the femur. International Journal of Sports Medicine, 14, 347–352.

Fagerson, T.L. (1998). The Hip Handbook. Oxford: Butterworth-Heinemann.

Florence, J., Pandya, S., King, W. et al. (1992). Intrarater reliability of manual muscle test (Medical Research Council Scale) grades in Duchenne's muscular dystrophy. Physical Therapy, 72, 115–122.

Gelberman, R. and Hekhar, S. (1987). Femoral anteversion. Journal of Bone and Joint Surgery, 69B, 75–79.

Goodman, C.C. and Snyder, T.C. (2000). Differential Diagnosis in Physical Therapy. London: Saunders.

Jones, D.L. and Erhard, R.E. (1996). Differential diagnosis with serious pathology: a case report. Physical Therapy, 76, S89–S90.

Kendall, F., McCreary, E. and Provance, P. (1993). Muscles Testing and Function. London: Williams & Wilkins.

Kling, T. and Hensinger, R. (1983). Angular and Torsional Deformities of the Lower Limbs in Children. Clinical Orthopedics and Related Research, 176, 136–147.

Meyers, W.C., Folely, D.P., Garrett, W.E.J., Lohnes, J.H. and Mandlebaum, B.R. (2000). Management of severe lower abdominal or inguinal pain in high-performance athletes. American Journal of Sports Medicine, 28, 2–8.

O'Kane, J.W. (1999). Anterior hip pain. American Family Physician, 60, 1687–1696.

Polglase, A.L., Frydman, G.M. and Farmer, K.C. (1991). Inguinal surgery for debilitating chronic groin pain in athletes. Medical Journal of Australia, 155, 674–677.

Sahrmann, S.A. (2001). Diagnosis and Treatment of Movement Impairment Syndromes. London: Mosby.

Staheli, L., Corbett, M., Wyss, C. and King, H. (1985). Lower-extremity rotational problems in children. Journal of Bone and Joint Surgery, 67A, 39–47.

Stricevic, M.V., Pael, M.R., Okazaki, T. and Swain, B.K. (1983). Karate: historical perspective and injuries sustained in national and international tournament competitions. American Journal of Sports Medicine, 11, 320–324.

Taylor, D.C., Meyers, W.C., Moylan, J.A., Lohnes, J., Bassett, F.H. and Garrett, W.E.J. (1991). Abdominal musculature abnormalities as a cause of groin pain in athletes. Inguinal hernias and pubalgia. American Journal of Sports Medicine, 19, 239–242.

van Dillen, L., Sahrmann, S., Norton, B. et al. (1998). Reliability of physical examination items used for classification of patients with low back pain. Physical Therapy, 78, 979–988.

Wilkerson, L.A. (1997). Martial arts injuries. Journal of the American Osteopathic Association, 97, 221–226.

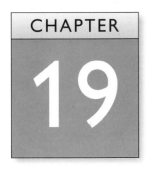

A software programmer and sportsman with low back pain and sciatica

Tom Arild Torstensen

SUBJECTIVE EXAMINATION

Olav is a 48-year-old married male with two sons, aged 21 and 24, from a prior marriage. He is of average height for his weight, being 164 cm tall and weighing 75 kg. Olav is a non-smoker and has a normal intake of alcohol. In his free time, he is a keen soccer player and is still on his company's soccer team. His sons also participate in sport, with one a contender for the national cross-country ski team. When possible, Olav likes to join his sons in their sports. However, his physical activity level has decreased significantly over the last few years, both from the pressures of his work and because of his recurrent back problems.

Olav enjoys his work as a senior computer software programmer with an international company. At the time of his initial consultation he was having to travel quite a lot between Oslo and Copenhagen, which is approximately 1 hour by air. His work is very stressful with constant pressure to meet company deadlines. He has a typical computer workplace and uses both a desktop personal computer and a laptop. During a typical working day, he spends most of his time sitting in front of his computer or in meetings.

Past medical history

Ten years ago, Olav experienced acute back pain when lifting a computer. He was off work for 1 month with back pain, which developed into classic S1 sciatica, and was bedridden most of the time 'eating' painkillers. When symptoms were resolving, he started slowly increasing his activity level, until he finally got back to

work. He also resumed other activities such as soccer, jogging and other sports. However, after this episode of sciatica, he never fully recovered and continued to experience relapses, with back pain, buttock pain and some leg pain, mostly on his left side but sometimes also on his right side. He reported that over the last few years he could 'feel' his back most days, and he always had to be careful with what he was doing. Except for painkillers and non-steroidal anti-inflammatory drugs (NSAIDs), he had never had any treatment for his back problem. Lying down and resting the back eased the symptoms, while sitting and being too physically active increased the symptoms. His twin brother had had low back surgery because of sciatica and two uncles had also undergone surgery for low back problems. The operations were initially successful, with an improvement in symptoms and function, but all three have had repeated relapses with back pain and some leg pain. His twin brother was working full-time running a travel agency and his uncles also returned to full-time work before they retired due to age.

Present medical history

Olav was 'referred' to physiotherapy by a co-worker who had been a patient of mine for some time. He walked into the treatment room with a slightly flexed posture and using short steps. While waiting outside, he preferred not to sit but varied his posture between standing still and walking. He told me that his back pain now was much worse than in the past and that

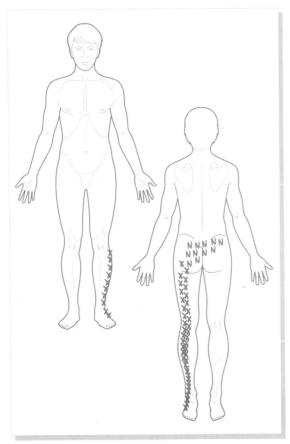

Fig. 19.1 Body chart illustrating patient's symptoms.

required him to sit. He was also afraid that he would not be able to travel by air because of his difficulty with prolonged sitting. Olav had now been on sick leave for 2 weeks, although during the last week he had been at work for short periods to catch up with his projects. He was also frustrated because he now realized that the symptoms recurred fairly quickly whenever he started to load his back during ordinary daily activities. He expressed concern that he might end up lying in bed for a month or two as he did 10 years ago. The treatment so far had consisted of painkillers only (NSAIDs), easing the symptoms slightly.

Because of the increased symptoms, he had to lie down during the middle of the day. His symptoms changed with biomechanical factors such as loading of the spine, as well as with positions of the spine, such as flexion versus extension. When he was in a weight-bearing position or a sitting position, the pain in his back and the lower extremity increased. When lying down, the pain generally decreased and after lying for a couple of hours he could be close to being pain-free. His pain was 8–9/10 in a standing or sitting position and 2–3/10 in a lying position. Walking could relieve his symptoms for a short while, but walking for longer than 30 minutes increased the symptoms. During a typical day, there were nearly no symptoms when waking up in the morning. On getting out of bed, he was a little bit stiff in the back, but the pain was basically gone. The stiffness disappeared after moving around for 10–20 minutes. When weight bearing during the day, the pain in the back and leg reappeared and he had to lie down in the middle of the day to ease the symptoms. In the afternoon, the pain was quite marked if he had pushed himself earlier by doing a lot of sitting and standing. After a good night's sleep he felt fine, the next morning being again basically symptom free. Going to the toilet was problematic, especially when having to 'push'. Also coughing increased the symptoms.

during the last 2 weeks he had been regularly lying down to ease the back and leg pain (Fig.19.1). He felt his most recent relapse 3 weeks ago was probably the result of a lot of lifting when moving some furniture. Over the next 48 hours the pain had increased slowly, until it was unbearable and he had to lie down. Sitting was not possible and he was now quite frustrated because he was busy at work and some of his work

REASONING DISCUSSION AND CLINICAL REASONING COMMENTARY

1 Please highlight what you considered to be the key information that had come out at this stage of the initial examination and briefly comment on your hypotheses regarding this information.

■ Clinician's answer

I tend to get 70–80% of the information I need to design a treatment programme from most patients through the conversation (past and present medical history). This applies especially for patients with long-lasting chronic pain. This view is supported by a research study showing that for new patients 76% of diagnoses was based on patient history, with 12% based on physical examination and 11% on laboratory investigation (Hamton et al., 1975; Peterson et al., 1992).

From talking with Olav I felt that he was an active coper, being able to deal with his problems in a healthy way. It was a good sign that for many years he had dealt with his back problem himself rather than run from one health professional to another. He was not afraid of using his back even though he had back pain, and he was not afraid of testing out and pushing himself with his recurrent back problem. However, he probably needed some support regarding 'phasing', particularly in relation to how much he should push himself. In addition to this, he enjoyed his work and tried within his capability to get back to work as quickly as possible. So psychosocial issues, such as negative fear-avoidance beliefs or believing that physical activity and going back to work would be dangerous, were not likely to feature. He was coping in a normal way to his pain experience. I considered that I was dealing with a patient who was now suffering from quite a lot of pain caused by straightforward tissue pathology: an inflammatory process from a possible prolapsed intervertebral disc (IVD) causing sciatica. The history supported this view: sitting increasing the symptoms, lying down easing the symptoms, feeling well in the morning but both back pain and leg pain increasing as the day progressed and the back was loaded in weight-bearing positions. He also had a recognizable 24-hour symptom pattern. I have found there are three different categories of 24-hour symptom pattern, which are very useful as a predictor for outcome and for responsiveness to exercise therapy (Faugli, personal communication, 1986):

Pattern 1.   The patient wakes up in the morning because of pain and morning stiffness. This eases with rising and starting to move and the patient is basically symptom free during the day. The more the patient moves the better the back gets. The signs and symptoms are typically joint related, similar to those associated with an arthritic hip joint. Most of these patients respond very positively to active graded exercise therapy like the medical exercise therapy (MET) approach.

Pattern 2.   The patient is close to symptom free in the morning, but the pain and stiffness return as the patient moves around and bears weight. During the day, the patient has to rest in a supine position,

which relieves the symptoms. This is typical of a possible inflammatory process, for example as can occur with a disorder of the IVD.

Pattern 3.   The main symptom is morning stiffness with pain, which decreases as the patient starts to move. However, after weight bearing for a couple of hours the symptoms reappear and may even start to increase. Now the patient often has to lie down to rest the back in order to ease the symptoms. For the rest of the day the patient has back pain, with or without leg pain, but is able to keep going by having short rest periods in a supine position. This patient has a pattern of symptoms associated with impairment of both the disc and the facet joints, but the disc is probably the main organic structure from which the symptoms are coming.

Patterns 2 and 3 usually take longer to treat and are generally more complicated/difficult to manage. Olav has a typical pattern 2 presentation, where both the distribution and the pattern of pain indicate a prolapsed disc with an inflamed sciatic nerve. This is especially supported by the fact that sitting was difficult and painful. It is one of Olav's major concerns because his job requires him to sit for long periods of time, which results in a pain in both the back and the leg. His work situation with constant deadlines makes it difficult to avoid sitting and yet he has to take time off work to lie supine at home. I note that I will need to advise Olav that he will need to change position at work as much as possible, avoiding positions that are really painful and make him worse. If necessary, he must also try to find time to lie down for short periods at work. When at home in the evening or during weekends he must again try to stay in comfortable positions, avoiding the 'pain'. This means that he must stay in a comfortable, close to pain-free, supine position until he is experiencing symptom control and is able to sit for longer periods. This approach is very important during the first early stage of the treatment. I also think that MET will be appropriate to begin to load the body and the back in a controlled environment using comfortable starting positions, such as lying and standing deloaded positions. If this proves effective in decreasing his symptoms, the programme could then be progressed to exercises in sitting and standing to condition his tolerance to spinal loading further.

2 Could you elaborate on this impression that Olav was an 'active coper' and was likely to be suffering from genuine tissue pathology? That is, if this hypothesis is to be supported, what would you expect from your physical examination and how does this issue influence your management?

Clinician's answer

Coping has been described as 'An individual's efforts to master demands (conditions of harm, threat, or challenge) that are appraised (or perceived) as exceeding or taxing his or her resources' (Monat and Lazarus, 1991, p. 5).

Stress, coping and physical illness can be closely linked. Holroyd and Lazarus (1982) suggest three main ways in which stress might lead to somatic illness:

- by disrupting tissue function through neuro-humeral influences under stress (e.g. hormones causing increased heart beat, trembling)
- engaging in coping activities that are damaging to health (e.g. a pressured style of life, type A behaviour): taking minimal rest, poor diet, heavy use of tobacco or alcohol
- minimizing the significance of symptoms or failing to comply with treatment as a result of psychological and/or sociological factors.

In this context, an active coper is a person who is able to deal with stress in a positive way, who handles the stress and finds positive, constructive solutions to the stressor(s).

As a clinician, I often find that patients with normal positive active coping strategies most often present suffering from genuine tissue pathology and with normal pain behaviour, which was the case for Olav. I also hypothesized at this early stage of the examination that Olav's presentation was consistent with the source of his symptoms as a recognizable pathology in the musculoskeletal system. This would need to be tested further in the physical examination and the response to treatment. In this context, I have found it useful to broadly classify patient presentations into three categories (type I, type II and type III presentations) with respect to the symptoms and pain behaviour; this assists me in determining the appropriate approach to management (De Clerck, 1998, 1999; Torstensen and De Clerk, 2001).

Type I. This group have normal pain behaviour, identifiable tissues at fault, local or recognizable pain patterns and reproducible signs. The pain distribution is usually in a well-known pattern and signs and symptoms are consistently reproduced by clinical tests. For a type I presentation, it may be possible to make a straightforward diagnosis by recognizing the tissue at fault which is causing the symptoms.

Type II. This presentation is somewhere between types I and III; there is close to normal pain behaviour, but it is difficult to relate signs and symptoms directly to a tissue at fault. A type II patient presentation may lean more towards type I or type III, depending on the unique characteristics of their presentation; this can change over time and with treatment. An example of this is the patient who starts with a local problem (e.g. lumbar pain with sciatica) that changes to a more diffuse presentation where some signs can be reproduced and others cannot. The pain pattern may also have changed over time to larger anatomical areas in the trunk and lower extremities, not typical for straightforward sciatica. The majority of patients in my practice fall into this category.

Type III. This presentation has abnormal pain behaviour with major psychosocial stressors, non-specific/diffuse pain, and the signs and symptoms are non-reproducible. It is difficult to reproduce symptoms consistently when repeating tests, and on the pain drawing the patient may mark the pain outside the body or over large anatomical areas that do not coincide with 'normal' pain patterns related to dermatomes, myotomes and sclerotomes.

Through the course of management, a patient can stay in the same presentation or can move from type III to type II or from type II to type I. In my clinic, I probably see approximately 20–25% type I, 10–15% type III and 60–70% type II presentations

A type I presentation is usually easy and straightforward to treat using well-known methods in manual therapy. Here pain can be a guide to treatment, using a pain contingent treatment approach. The treatment is aimed primarily at physiological effects (locally), symptom control, and promoting healing and recovery. Signs and symptoms can guide the treatment and different manual therapy approaches may be effective. This patient presentation category is typically covered by the traditional courses and seminars in manual therapy and is described in clinical textbooks. The clinical presentation is easily recognized by clinicians.

For a type II presentation, I would initially treat the patient similar to a type III presentation. Then, depending on their response over the next few sessions, the treatment will either change to a type I approach or continue with a type III approach. After dealing with psychological issues like pain behaviour, it may become clearer for the therapist which presentation is dominant.

A type III presentation is more difficult to treat in that treatment is primarily aimed at changing behaviour (globally), focussing on slow, progressive functional recovery with a clear understanding of mal-adaptive pain. For a type III presentation, pain may be an unreliable guide for treatment; therefore, a quota-based exercise programme may be used. In addition, the treatment should include intensive education using cognitive–behaviour techniques (Keefe et al., 1992, 1996), with emphasis on clear realistic goals using appropriate phasing skills (Bassett and Petrie, 1999; Wayanda et al., 1998). For a type III presentation, a non-pain contingent approach should be used, or a so-called time contingent approach, where the patient's pain is not used as the guide for treatment. Further, traditional manual therapy methods, where the aim is to decrease pain, may make the patient worse by increasing the illness/pain behaviour.

This classification of patient presentations in relation to their pain behaviour also has implications for determining the type of exercise, the grading and dosage of exercises, the loading of each exercise and if the exercises should have a global, semi-global or local focus to normalize function:

- *global exercises* involve using exercise equipment such as a rowing machine, stepping machine, stationary bike, treadmill, which work the whole body
- *semi-global exercises* are exercises using the MET pulleys or free exercises working against gravity, where only a part of the musculoskeletal system is activated
- *local exercises* are exercises using the MET pulleys and other MET equipment where the exercises are even more localized to a few segments of the back; a typical local exercise would be to try to activate transversus abdominis in four-point kneeling or supine lying.

For example, for type III presentations, a MET programme could consist of four global exercises and four semi-global exercises, where the most comfortable exercise is repeated twice. Global and semi-global exercises are performed alternatively.

I classified Olav, based on our conversation, as a type I presentation. I thought that exercises would need to be carried out initially using comfortable, close to pain-free starting positions performed within his comfortable range of motion. It could be counterproductive to ask him to ignore his pain by treating him as a type III presentation and making him exercise

with pain, as with an operant cognitive–behavioural approach. Further, simple grading of exercises will enable his treatment to be close to pain-free anyway, an experience that is positively motivating for patients with pain and decreased function. Most of the exercises chosen for Olav were semi-global and global. In the early phase, the exercises chosen focussed on stability, using primarily semi-global and local exercises. Later, when the treatment progressed, more global exercises were introduced.

I also knew from experience that if Olav was able to avoid any flare-ups and slowly increase his tolerance for loading through a graded exercise programme, he should recover within 2 to 3 months. To reach this goal, I felt it was of the utmost importance that he understood what was going on and what type of pain he had and where the pain was coming from. If he appreciated this information, it would be easier to modify, in a very structured way, his daily activities so that he achieved symptom control. Because his history indicated a fairly straightforward organic dysfunction, with a possible prolapsed disc and an inflamed S1 nerve root, I felt it was important to explain that for now he had to try to avoid biomechanical positions that gave or increased his pain. Already, I was thinking of what comfortable exercises to choose, comfortable starting positions, range of motion to work in and the loading of the exercises. It was clear that comfortable starting positions for the exercises probably would be a combination of lying and standing deloaded. The aim of the active exercise therapy was to take away any fear and anxiety that physical activity would increase the symptoms. MET should act as a positive coping strategy, easing symptoms as well as the distress and anxiety he was experiencing. By designing an exercise programme that is comfortable for him to do, he will be put in a position where he again is in control of his own body, that is, controlling the situation of having back pain with sciatica. Consequently, I felt quite early that it was important to minimize any psychological issues of the pain experience and thereby gain the patient's trust from the start. In addition to the positive psychological effects of exercise there are also the additional physiological and neurological benefits. Graded exercise is a common sense approach to regain motor control, muscle balance and coordination. The exercise will also have positive physiological effects on muscle, collagen and bony tissue. It was important that all these positive aspects were explained to the patient in detail to optimize his understanding and return to normal function.

In addition to the pain distribution, the 24-hour pain pattern was also typical for a patient with a prolapsed disc experiencing sciatica. One hypothesis is that during the night Olav felt fine because the disc was not being compressed and the nociceptive activation was consequently decreased. Weight bearing when getting up in the morning and throughout the day then compresses the disc, resulting in increased nociceptive activity, likely as a result of the inflammatory process, with the end result being an increase in symptoms. When lying down, Olav effectively decreased the loading on the spine and the disc, resulting in less pain/ symptoms.

◼ Clinical reasoning commentary

Chapter 1 discussed the need for clinicians to be able to understand the 'person' and the 'problem'. This requires skills in narrative and physical diagnostic reasoning; a highly developed organization of bio-psychosocial knowledge; professional craft knowledge of manual therapy advice, active and passive procedures; and communication skills to clarify the patient's pain experience (effects on life, understanding, beliefs and coping). It also requires a collaborative effort with the patient to determine and carry out appropriate management. All of these aspects of clinical reasoning theory are evident in this clinician's patient enquiries and the answers to the questions. He clearly takes a broad biopsychosocial approach to his patients and endeavours to understand both the person and the problem, importantly also tailoring his management to his assessment of presenting psychosocial and physical issues. Pattern recognition, acquired through a combination of research and reflective experience-based evidence, is a central, but not limiting, feature in his reasoning. That is, through a combination of prior education, personal experience and familiarity with current research, he has constructed a personal organization of knowledge comprising recognizable patterns in presentations from common variations of the 24-hour pattern to his classification of three broad presentations and his hypotheses regarding specific sources or pathology implicated. These are not simply patterns of academic interest, rather they are each clearly linked to issues of treatment selection and prognosis. In addition, consistent with clinical reasoning research, recognition of these patterns and their associated thoughts and actions occurred 'from the first moments' of the interview.

While pattern recognition is a characteristic of expertise in all domains, it is also one of the greatest sources of error in clinical reasoning. It is critical that clinicians are not locked into their own clinical patterns but use processes of reassessment and reflection to reappraise constantly their clinical patterns in general and their prior judgments regarding a particular patient's presenting patterns. This continual reassessment of the patient's dominant pattern is evident here in the clinician's type II presentation, which lies somewhere between types I and III and only really becomes clearer through attention and reflection on the patient's response to the evolving management. Similarly, the clinician has specific patterns of pathology such as disc and nerve root that are recognized, yet these hypotheses do not dictate recipe treatments, rather they provide a basis for explanation and communication; treatment itself is guided more by the presenting disability and impairments. This, we believe, is a critical distinction as our clinical hypotheses on pathology are often not validated and as such must remain as hypotheses. In contrast, as discussed in Chapter 1, decision making based on disabilities and impairments (with careful consideration of pathology) is arguably more accurate, more patient centred and, from the perspective of the biopsychosocial model of health and disability, less likely to encourage pathology-focussed unhelpful thinking on the part of the patient.

 ## PHYSICAL EXAMINATION

Undressing

Olav found it difficult to take off his shoes, trousers and shirt. It was obviously painful to move and bend the spine while undressing.

Neurological assessment

Olav had no problems with regular walking or with walking on his heels or toes. He was able to do 28 heel rises on the right leg and 19 on the left side, indicating that there was some weakness in the left calf muscle (supplied by S1/S2). He had a positive sciatic nerve stretch test in a standing weight-bearing position, reproducing his symptoms down the back of his left leg when passively flexing the hip above 45 degrees. In sitting, he also had a positive slump test on the left side, with provocation of a deep burning pain in the posterior part of his thigh and down the back of his calf to the ankle. The patellar reflex was similar and normal bilaterally. In supine lying, he also had a positive straight leg raise test on the left side at 45 degrees, with the same pain pattern as was produced with the slump test and the weight-bearing sciatic nerve stretch test. The Achilles reflex on the left side was slightly decreased compared with the right. During sensibility testing, the patient reported slightly decreased skin sensation laterally on the left leg (S1 dermatome). All other nerve provocation tests were negative including prone knee bend (femoral nerve stretch test). Except for the area mentioned above, he had normal skin sensitivity with no paraesthesia or anaesthesia. No other lower limb weakness was detected and there were no cord or cauda equina symptoms or signs.

Posture

In the standing position, Olav demonstrated a slight lateral deviation/shift of the spine, with a convex scoliosis to the right in the lumbar spine and a compensatory scoliosis convex to the left in the mid-thoracic spine. When he looked in the mirror over the last 2 weeks, Olav had noted that his trunk was deviating to the right. The height of the iliac crests were equal bilaterally and so were the anterior superior and posterior superior iliac spines. He also had a straightened lumbar spine with a loss of the normal lordosis.

Global mobility tests of the spine and pelvis

Active movement testing of the spine in the standing (weight-bearing) position revealed that Olav kept his lumbar spine straight when bending forward. He was able to touch the middle of his lower leg with his fingers, but further movement was limited by an increase in back and leg pain. Lumbar extension was reduced by increased pain in the back and down the leg. Extending the spine in a cranial–caudal direction

(the extension movement starts by extending the head and neck and then the extension movement moves caudally, finally extending the lower lumbar segments) caused pain in the back and the lower extremity. When moving the back the other way, in a caudal–cranial direction (the extension movement starts by rotating the pelvis ventrally moving the lower lumbar segments into extension in a caudal–cranial direction), pain was felt in the back and the lower extremity. The symptoms were reproduced and increased at end-range when the tests were repeated. Pain in the back only was also increased when side flexing the lumbar spine to either side, but more so to the left than to the right, causing a limitation in the range of movement both ways. My general impression was that Olav was hesitant to move his spine too far in any direction because of his fear of increased pain.

Local segmental mobility tests of the spine

Testing of passive physiological intervertebral movement for extension/flexion, side flexion and rotation segmental hyper/hypo/normal mobility of the lumbar spine in side lying revealed a distinct resistance to movement (Evjenth and Hamberg, 1988; Kaltenborn, 1989; Norske Fysioterapeuters Forbund, 1998). Olav resisted the movement because of pain and probably because of his fear of increased pain with movement. As a result, Olav had decreased local segmental mobility of all lumbar segments. This was also the case in the thoracolumbar junction and the middle and lower thoracic spine.

The hip

Active and passive flexion and extension movements of the hip joints bilaterally were full range but were giving pain and discomfort in the lower lumbar spine when the movements were taken to the end of range. For example, when Olav was lying supine and the hip joints were passively flexed above 90 degrees, there was an accessory posterior rotation of the pelvis with accompanying flexion of the lumbar spine, the movement of the spine giving pain in the lower back. Rotations, abduction and adduction of the hips were full range and symptom free.

The pelvis and the iliosacral joints

No dysfunction was found of the pelvis when tests were performed in standing (weight-bearing) or lying (non-weight-bearing) positions. Forward bending test, ipsilateral kinetic tests in standing, arthrokinematic tests of craniocaudal translation, anteroposterior translation in lying of the sacroiliac joints (Lee, 1994) and gapping tests of the iliosacral joints bilaterally were all normal. Again, tests of the pelvis and the the iliosacral joints resulted in movements of the lower lumbar area, thus provoking pain in the lumbar area with some radiating pain down the posterior left thigh.

Provocation tests

The 'spurling test' for the lower back, combining rotation and side flexion to the left in extension with some compression (pressing caudally on his shoulders), reproduced and increased his symptoms in the back and the left leg when performed in either sitting or standing. In prone lying, Olav found the springing test over the spinous processes uncomfortable, especially at the lower three lumbar segments, where pain in the buttock was reproduced with only gentle rhythmic pressures performed in time with the patient's breathing pattern. Compression of the sacrum, including nutation and counter-nutation, was also painful. When performing the provocation tests of the spine and sacrum, there was a general impression of hypomobility of the lumbar segments, with firm resistance felt when performing the rhythmic mobility tests (i.e. posteroanterior intervertebral movements). However, it was not possible to determine the cause of the hypomobility because of Olav's inability to relax fully when experiencing pain.

Manual traction

Deloading of the lumbar spine through manual traction in sitting and in supine lying eased the symptoms in the leg and the lower back.

Mechanical positioning of the spine

When side gliding (in both directions, extension/side flexion) was applied in standing and in prone lying in an attempt to centralize the symptoms, the patient instead experienced increased pain and discomfort down the leg. This test was repeated several times with no change in symptoms. However, the symptoms were eased when he lay down in the psoas position (supine lying with hips and knees flexed to 90 degrees while resting the lower legs on a square bolster). Sitting or leaning forward increased the symptoms in his back and down his left leg.

Palpation of soft tissue

Palpation of soft tissue, including the back muscles, was also painful, especially in the lower lumbar spine. On his left side, his gluteus medius and minimus had distinct trigger points and produced referred pain into the posterior and posterolateral parts of the thigh when palpated and massaged.

Elongation of soft tissue/muscle length

The patient had shortened iliopsoas and quadriceps muscles, although both tests reproduced his back pain, making it difficult to evaluate the true length of the muscles.

Radiological findings

Radiographs revealed normal bony structure of the lumbar spine and normal height between each of the three lower vertebrae. However, there was a 'normal' spina bifida anomaly of L5. Computed tomography (CT) scanning revealed a mid- to left-sided prolapse of the L4 IVD (Fig. 19.2).

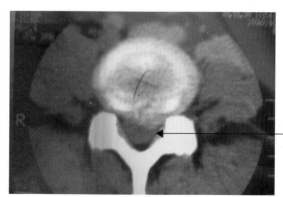

Fig. 19.2 Computed tomography illustrating mid- to left-sided prolapse of the L5 intervertebral disc.

REASONING DISCUSSION AND CLINICAL REASONING COMMENTARY

1 Please discuss your reasoning following the physical examination using the hypothesis categories: pain mechanisms, principal physical impairments identified, source of the symptoms, precautions to management, and the management considered appropriate.

Clinician's answer

Pain mechanisms

Pain mechanisms can be divided into five categories:

- sensory
- neurogenic (sciatica)
- central pain mechanisms (neural plasticity)
- affective (psychosocial elements, such as psychological stressors and social interaction)
- autonomic and motor.

The most relevant pain mechanisms for Olav were sensory and neurogenic (Olmarker and Rydevik, 1992). My working hypothesis was that nociceptive activation with a possible inflammatory reaction at the outer/lateral IVD and an inflamed nerve root caused the signs and symptoms. Findings from the patient history (e.g. area, behaviour and history of symptoms) and the physical examination (e.g. posture and posture correction, provocation tests, segmental mobility assessment and neurological tests) supported these pain mechanisms. They were further supported by the CT scan showing a prolapsed L5 disc.

Principal physical impairments

One of the main impairments was Olav's extremely stiff spine, or rather the decreased range of motion in all directions. This was also evident when specifically testing flexion, extension, side flexion and rotation mobility of the L5, L4, L3 and L2 segments (Evjenth and Hamberg, 1988; Kaltenborn, 1989). The decreased mobility was probably a secondary reaction to the pain provocation and will normalize when the pain decreases. Similarly, his postural impairment had likely developed, at least in part, as a means to avoid pain. The decreased range of motion and neural function were probably also a result of the pain and nociceptive activation, possibly through an L5 IVD prolapse provoking an inflammatory reaction of the S1 nerve root.

Source of the symptoms

While I feel consideration of the source of the symptoms is important, I also believe that some clinicians overly focus on organic tissue structures and pathology in the structures. Research has shown that there is very little correlation between a patient's pain level, impairments and disability (Waddell et al., 1982; Waddell, 1987). Therefore, in practical work with individual patients, this means that some patients will have been on long-term sick leave with minimal symptoms/impairments, while other patients will function quite well (even working) with significant pain and pathology. To confuse the matter even more, research has also documented that increased strength and endurance of the back muscles after 3 months rehabilitation programme with exercise therapy (Mannion et al., 1999) could not be explained by morphological changes in the back muscles (changes in fibre proportion and fibre size; Kaser et al., 2001). Rather, significant changes in muscle performance after such active rehabilitation appeared to be mainly a consequence of changes in neural activation (neuromuscular adaptations) of the lumbar muscles and psychological changes such as increased motivation to tolerate pain (Mannion et al., 2001). The practical implication is that there is little or no correlation between changes in organic tissue structures, symptoms and function.

Regarding a structural change like a prolapsed IVD, some patients will become symptom free through treatment or natural resolution even if there is confirmed pathology such as IVD prolapse, because prolapse and bulging discs are also a normal phenomenon among asymptomatic individuals (Jensen et al., 1994), making the assessment and interpretation of clinical findings more important than imaging studies (Khan et al., 1998). Yet other patients will have structural changes and clinical findings that do correlate with their functional status. I felt that Olav's symptoms did correlate with a structural change like a disc prolapse, an impression supported by his CT scan findings (Kuslich et al., 1991). However, even if there were no positive findings on the CT scan, I still would treat him with a similar approach, because it is possible to have sciatica even when there is no verified prolapse. Olmarker and Rydevik (1992) have hypothesized that it is possible to have cracks in the IVD and that material from the nucleus pulposus can slip through these 'cracks' eliciting an autoimmune reaction when nuclear material makes contact with the outside tissue. The end result is an inflammatory process affecting the nerve root and resulting in sciatic pain. Such a hypothesis has been confirmed in animal studies (Olmarker and Rydevik, 1992), which demonstrated that tissue from the nucleus pulposus provoked a strong inflammatory reaction when placed in contact with the sciatic nerve in pigs. However, because it is so difficult to make a 'tissue at fault' diagnosis in humans, and the fact that structural changes of tissue do not necessarily correlate with symptoms and function, it is the patient's reaction/pain behaviour which is the most important finding to screen regarding choice of treatment strategy (Khan et al., 1998; Main and Booker, 2000). Traditional tests from orthopaedic medicine/manual therapy are still important but secondary to the patient's pain behaviour.

Regarding the issue of structure versus function, if there is an objective finding on CT scan at the right level and side, it is easy to focus on the structural change and believe that the only thing that might help is surgery (e.g. taking the prolapse out). What I try to explain to my patients, and this was also the case with Olav, is that as much as 50% of the population without any pain have bulging discs and prolapses (Jensen et al., 1994). Further, when the patient becomes symptom free through treatment and the body's own self-healing mechanisms, the prolapse is probably still there and it may take a good time before it partly dries up.

For Olav, the findings from clinical tests (physical examination) supported his reported history. Different clinical tests reproduced his symptoms and the symptoms appeared in well-recognizable anatomical areas and dermatomes in the back and lower extremity. All this supported the view that Olav had a type I presentation with straightforward sciatica possibly caused by a prolapsed L5 IVD. The clinical findings supported the original working hypotheses generated from the medical history. The positive findings from the nerve stretch tests, such as the slump test and the straight leg raise test, indicated that there was an inflammatory process involving the S1 nerve root. This was also supported by the diagnosed prolapse of the L5 IVD evident on the CT scan.

Precautions to management

There were no serious precautions to treatment. Active graded exercise therapy such as the MET approach is probably one of the safest treatment approaches available for treating patients with sciatica. However, care should be taken so that the exercises do not significantly increase the patient's pain. Close communication with the patient regarding the symptoms experienced during the exercises, and whether they increase, is important for the management to be successful.

Appropriate management

The key findings range from impairments like pain and decreased range of motion of the spine to disabilities in different daily activities. MET is appropriate for managing all these impairments and disabilities. It is the aim of MET to treat both signs and symptoms (impairments), in addition to improving function on both an individual level (disability) and a societal level (handicap).

▌ Clinical reasoning commentary

Here the clinician explicitly shares his philosophy in that, while he hypothesizes about pathology and clearly screens for serious pathology (e.g. spinal cord, neurological and cauda equina tests), his management is based on the patient's presenting disabilities (i.e. activity and participation restrictions) and impairments. Rather than selectively using evidence from the literature, as occurs when someone wants to argue their favourite hypothesis (see errors of reasoning discussed in Ch. 26), here the clinician cites evidence substantiating processes whereby IVD pathology can be symptomatic on its own and irritative of adjacent neural tissue while also reporting the literature that documents not all pathology is symptomatic. This is precisely the sort of critical and open-minded reasoning we expect from an expert clinician. While he has clear views, he is also unmistakably reflective and open to changing those views, personality and reasoning attributes that lead to continued learning regardless of years of experience or status. Chapter 1 claims that manual therapists' thinking and judgments extend over a range of interrelated areas, which were called hypothesis categories. This is evident here in the clinician's reasoning regarding pain mechanisms, physical impairments, sources of the symptoms, precautions to management and management itself.

Explanation of intended management

Treatment commenced as I went through the assessment in that my assessment is a part of the treatment and the actual treatment is a part of a continuous assessment. However, after finishing the assessment I sat down with Olav and attempted to explain my findings, how they could be interpreted, and what treatment I would suggest for managing his pain and disability.

First of all, I spent some time explaining what pain is: notably that pain is a multidimensional experience, primarily with a sensory and discriminative dimension but also with a cognitive and evaluative dimension and a motivational and affective dimension. I also explained that with time the sensory dimensions becomes less important and the cognitive and emotional dimensions of pain become more involved (Main et al., 2000a,b; Main and Brooker, 2000). The explanation I provided was essentially as follows:

Your back and leg pain are probably caused by an inflammatory reaction in your back irritating the sciatic nerve. Structures in the far low back, such as the intervertebral disc at either the L4 or L5 level, are to blame. However I am not quite sure if you have a prolapsed intervertebral disc. If you do not have one, it is still possible to have the same symptoms as if you did have a prolapse. It is not dangerous to have sciatica, and it is not dangerous to have a possible prolapsed disc. What we have to deal with and treat are the impairments such as pain, stiffness and decreased range of motion. Research has shown that as much as 50% of the general population have a bulging or prolapsed disc and no symptoms, so such structural changes are normal. However, we do not really know why some people get back pain and sciatica while others do not. It may be hereditary, where some people have a narrower spinal canal and are more prone to inflammatory processes. In your case, the lifting work you did in your cellar may have overloaded tissues in your lower lumbar spine and discs, causing an inflammatory reaction. The pain you now experience will also influence you psychologically. Because the methods you tried earlier to get rid of the pain are not working now, it is quite normal to get frustrated and scared. The pain is still there and you are worried about your work and what to do to get better. You have experienced that sitting at work makes you worse, and that the best position to ease the pain is lying down. But I understand that you cannot lie down forever, and you have also tried this; when you then get up and start to move, the pain is back to the same level as before. This is a frustrating situation. What we have to try is to get you active, but at a level that is acceptable for you. Proper pacing is the key issue, both when you come for treatment and when you are at home or at work. I am going to put you immediately into an exercise programme, using starting postural positions that you find comfortable, such as lying and standing, which are known as deloaded or non-weight-bearing positions. With a deloaded exercise, I mean that through the exercise some of the weight is taken off your spine. One way of deloading the back at home is to grasp the top of a door with both hands and then hang by your arms, which will take some of the weight off your back. It is important that the treatment is comfortable and does not significantly increase the symptoms. We have to concentrate on what increases the symptoms and what eases the symptoms, and it is important to find the exercises that ease the symptoms, choosing starting positions that give you as little back pain as possible. This is done by trial and error and it is important that we find an acceptable level of loading for your back, otherwise you will not get the expected improvement and may end up with long-lasting back pain and disability. However, your prognosis is good and within 2 to 3 months you should be significantly better. My suggestions are threefold: first, what to do at home, secondly, what to do at work, and finally, what to do at the clinic.

Treatment at the clinic. Lets look at the last point first and what to do here. I would like to put you into a graded exercise programme, which we call medical exercise therapy or MET, ideally using seven to nine exercises, and doing three sets of 30 repetitions within the range of motion that is comfortable and close to pain free. The aims of the exercises are to decrease the pain you experience, help you to become more flexible and generally to improve your function, thus increasing your tolerance for physical loading and psychological stress. I want you to attend three times a week and the exercises will take approximately

1 hour each time. Later, when you start to improve, the programme will take 1½ hours including a warm up. The exercise programme will consist of exercises that are comfortable to perform, thus avoiding stimulation of the pain receptors or so-called nociceptive receptors, but rather stimulating mechanoreceptors from muscles, tendons and joints resulting in a 'blocking' of the pain. The exercises will also increase the circulation to muscles, tendons, joints and the bony structures of the spine. There is also some evidence that the intervertebral disc itself reacts positively to an appropriate physical loading. We will test out three different exercises today.

What to do at home. Try to stay active, but lie down when symptoms are increasing. Even though you may feel better on some days, I do not think lifting or heavy physical work is a good thing at the moment. The important thing now

is to reduce the inflammatory process, hence you should not do things that will maintain or increase the pain you feel. At this stage, I do not want you to do any home exercises, because if you should get worse we will not know what made you worse. That is, whether it was the exercises here, the home exercises or something else. When you have control over the symptoms I will give you plenty of exercises to do at home.

What to do at work. Try to sit as little as possible. We know that sitting will increase your symptoms, so try to alternate between standing and lying. Stay at work for only a few hours. When travelling to and from work take a taxi so that you can lie down in the back seat, thus not having to sit in the uncomfortable flexed sitting position that increases your pain. If extending your spine feels comfortable try to stay in that position.

REASONING DISCUSSION AND CLINICAL REASONING COMMENTARY

1 Changing patients' understanding and feelings that you judge to be 'impaired', unhealthy or represent potential obstacles to their recovery is obviously important to you. However, this can also be very difficult to achieve, especially for patients whose perceptions and beliefs are well established. Can you comment on the strategies you use to assist patients in changing their perceptions?

■ Clinician's answer

I agree that changing patient's perceptions and beliefs may be difficult. Some of the basic criteria that must be fulfilled to be able to change negative perceptions and beliefs are to have close and effective communication with the patient, being able to listen to the patient, and providing explanation using plain simple language. When you are with a patient over a period of time, it is important to try various ways of explaining, with the theory you want to get across linked with clear practical examples. By repeating this explanation and the changes you want to see, you increase the likelihood of the patient grasping the message. Shared decision making and empowerment is a must, with the patient slowly becoming more and more in charge of the treatment and focussing on what he can do instead of

on what he cannot. Manual therapists have a golden opportunity to work on these matters because we spend so much time together with the patient. So as a specialist in manual therapy, I utilize cognitive–behavioural therapy in the exercise room, spending at least 1 hour with the patient two to three times a week.

When MET is used as an operant cognitive–behavioural approach, the focus is on treating pain behaviour and disability rather than focussing primarily on impairments (Keefe et al., 1992, 1996). This is a great challenge, especially in manual therapy, where we have been taught to look for impairments and deal with specific movement disorders to normalize function (Gifford and Butler, 1997; Zussman, 1997, 1998). The question is when to treat local impairments and when to go global and 'treat' behaviour. For patients with chronic long-lasting pain, a quota-based exercise programme with a time-contingent approach may be applied, focussing on improvement in function instead of on symptoms only. However, for other patients, who have normal pain behaviour with pain in a well-known and relevant anatomic area, where symptoms can be reproduced and where it is possible to diagnose an organic tissue structure at fault, the approach is fairly straightforward, applying a pain-contingent approach with comfortable close to pain-free exercises working through comfortable ranges of motion normalizing both function as well as the structure at fault (Torstensen, 1990, 1993; Torstensen et al., 1994). I feel it is important to be able to use both time- and pain-contingent treatment approaches and to choose the right approach in relation to the patient's pain behaviour and presentation of signs and symptoms. In Olav's case a pain-contingent approach was used.

The aim of the treatment is to deal with any negative perceptions and beliefs about back pain, changing them to something positive. Because patients vary in the degree to which they are ready to engage in new adaptive behaviours, I have found the following model (Prochaska and DiClemente, 1982; Prochaska et al., 1994) useful as a broad guide for my interaction and communication with my patients.

1. *Pre-contemplation:* raise doubt, increase patient's perception of the risks and problems associated with their current behaviour.
2. *Contemplation:* tip the balance, evoke reasons to change, emphasize the risk of not changing, strengthen the patient's self-efficacy for change of current behaviour.
3. *Preparation:* help the patient to determine the best course to take in seeking change.
4. *Action:* help the patient to take steps toward change.
5. *Maintenance:* review the progress; renew motivation and commitment as needed.
6. *Relapse:* help the patient to review the processes of contemplation, determination and action, without becoming stuck and demoralized because of relapse.

To have successful communication with patients, the therapist must express empathy and avoid argument ('roll' with resistance). It is important to provide information while giving the patient options and choices.

Over the years I have become more aware of patients' different belief systems and how their beliefs can influence the treatment outcome negatively. Patients' beliefs have emerged from talking with family, friends, health workers of different categories and reading popular articles in the media or watching health programmes on television. Common examples of statements that often reflect unhelpful beliefs or personal perspectives that may be counterproductive to the patient's recovery include 'My pain is in the L5 facet joint on the right side', 'That prolapsed disc must be taken out because it is pressing on my nerve', 'Rotation is dangerous for my back because I have a prolapse'. There are many more such beliefs.

Changing patients' negative beliefs about their back pain is often critical to successful management. Helping them to understand that the pain is not dangerous and that it is not dangerous to move the back and to become more physically active so that they can return to work, even though they believe that work is dangerous for their back, is often very difficult and probably the biggest challenge we have as manual therapists. It is also important to make the patient aware that to achieve this will take some time, at least 2 to 3 months to begin with, and that the first period will in many ways be painful for the patient and a struggle for both the patient and the therapist.

My most important job as a manual therapist is, therefore, to motivate the patient, supporting the patient while the patient is exercising. Through my behaviour working with the patient in the exercise room, I am hoping to achieve some kind of bonding between myself and the patient, making the patient understand and believe in what I am saying and doing. Uvnäs-Moberg (1998, pp. 819–820) says:

> ... positive social interactions and emotions are associated with an unified pattern of physiological and behavioral events ... lead to physiological adaptations necessary for relaxation, digestion, anabolic metabolism, growth and healing. The corresponding mental states associated with positive social interactions include calmness and openness to social engagement. In the context of positive social interactions and emotions, one neuropeptide system containing oxytocin has emerged as a common regulatory element. Oxytocin coordinates both causes and effects of positive social interactions.

To be able to achieve a positive social interaction with patients being treated with exercise therapy in the exercise room, it is essential for the therapist to be present with the patient, an important and fundamental element from the criteria for the MET approach. These criteria are discussed in detail in the section below describing the MET regimen. A fundamental element of MET is the presence of the therapist in the exercise room constantly monitoring the patients while exercising. For many years I have been in the exercise room every second hour during my working day having a MET group consisting of up to five patients with different movement disorders ranging from orthopaedic to vascular to neurological problems. In the hour between each group, I either assess a new patient or have two separate individual treatments each of 30 minutes. After the assessment of a new patient, I often bring that patient straight into the exercise room to start designing/testing out an exercise programme. The organization of my working day makes it easier to combine active exercise therapy with any other method in physiotherapy.

As mentioned above, my role in the exercise room is to motivate the patient and provide positive feedback, giving the patient a new and positive experience regarding his/her own body, while at the same time addressing any fear-avoidance beliefs regarding physical activity and work that may exist. If the patient experiences increased pain from the exercise therapy, there is always the risk that they may drop out of treatment. This risk is minimized when patients are helped to understand the purpose and planned progression of the exercises and that a degree of discomfort in the early stage is common. Being present with the patient stimulates compliance and empowerment and not dependence. Being present makes it possible to grade the exercises optimally for the patient to get physiological effects from the training, resulting in improved fitness and improved tolerance for loading.

However, making the patient motivated is fundamental for being successful, and to motivate a patient with a type II and III presentation I use the following checklist while working with the patient in the exercise room:

- patient sets baseline of the exercise programme (manageable, almost easy level)
- for a type II and type III presentation, progression is quota based rather than pain based
- providing immediate positive reinforcement
- ignore pain behaviour (roll with resistance)
- patient in charge of charting programmes
- good communication style, dealing with any negative beliefs and negative perceptions about exercise and dealing with movement in a positive and, if possible, humorous way.

If the patient experiences increased pain:

- acknowledge the fact that the patient is worse
- reassure, providing clear guidance that it is normal to get increased pain and that it will level off after a few days
- offer a number of suggestions to ease the increase in symptoms from which the patient can choose; for example, heat and cold contrast baths, hot packs/ice packs to be used at home, warm/cold

shower, and the use of low-grade global exercises like just walking for 30 to 45 minutes.

For a patient with a type I presentation, a pain-contingent treatment approach is used, where the exercises are graded according to the patient's pain experience working close to pain-free, within the comfortable range of motion.

■ Clinical reasoning commentary

Expertise in manual therapy requires much more than advanced biomedical knowledge and manual skills. Successfully understanding and managing the diverse range of patient presentations that regularly confront manual therapists also requires advanced psychosocial knowledge and communication skills. Chapter 1 presents a model of clinical reasoning in manual therapy, linked to a model of health and disability, which highlights the importance of having a number of different but related clinical reasoning strategies to be able to understand and 'manage' both the person and the problem. While diagnostic reasoning is explicit in most therapists' reasoning for patient's activity/participation restrictions, physical and psychosocial impairments, pathobiological mechanisms, sources of symptoms and contributing factors, other reasoning strategies such as narrative reasoning, interactive reasoning, collaborative reasoning and teaching are often less-developed or tacit skills. The explanation provided to this patient and the clinician's answers to this reasoning question are excellent examples of these strategies in practice.

Narrative reasoning refers to therapists' enquiries directed toward understanding the patient's personal story/narrative or the context of the problem beyond the mere chronological sequence of events. It requires trying to understand the patient as a person, including their perspective of the problem (e.g. understanding, beliefs, desires, motivations, emotions), the basis of their perspectives and how the problem is affecting their life. Interactive reasoning relates to the thinking and actions that underpin the rapport and confidence therapists establish with their patients (Jones et al., 2002). While socializing with patients is not typically considered a purposeful act of cognition or reasoning, often therapists must be strategic and purposeful in these interactions, which then constitute a strategy of reasoning, perhaps accounting for more of the successful outcome than has been generally appreciated. Collaborative reasoning relates to the consensual approach between therapist and patient towards the interpretation of examination findings, the setting of goals and priorities, and the implementation and progression of treatment. Reasoning should also guide our teaching of patients in that there is no single approach to teaching that will be effective for all patients. Skilled therapists have learned how to modify their teaching for individual patients and reassess the effectiveness of their efforts with the same critique they give their physical interventions. Importantly, these various aspects of our reasoning occur throughout both our examination and treatment of patients. There is not an artificial division between one form of reasoning and another as understanding the person requires understanding the problem and vice versa. Similarly, our communicative management directed toward assisting patients to acquire healthier, more constructive perspectives and health behaviours does not necessarily occur separate from other management interventions. Rather, as highlighted by the clinician here, therapists will continue to 'get to know' their patients throughout their ongoing management, often integrating their psychosocially directed management with their physical treatment.

The medical exercise therapy approach

Odddvar Holten, who developed MET during the early 1960s, was also one of the founders of manual therapy in Norway (Torstensen et al., 1999). MET is 'an exercise approach where the patient performs exercises in specially designed apparatus, without manual assistance, but being constantly monitored by the physiotherapist' (Holten, 1968). The programme has a number of specific criteria:

- the apparatus must be designed for optimal stimulation of the relevant functional quality in question: neuromuscular, arthrogenous, circulatory and respiratory
- the effect is obtained by the patient carrying out the exercises from a defined starting position, in a specific range of motion, against a graded load
- there is a minimum of 1 hour effective treatment (excluding dressing and undressing, shower/bath etc.)
- prior to treatment a thorough assessment is carried out based on:
  — muscle tests
  — specific joint tests
  — functional tests
- diagnosis is determined from the patient's history and assessment and an optimal treatment is established
- the exercise programme is reassessed and adjusted when required
- a maximum of five patients in a group setting are treated for 1 hour.

These criteria for MET treating/exercising patients were sanctioned in March 1967 by the Norwegian Health Authorities as a special therapeutic system, code C32, for Norwegian physiotherapists. The criteria are fundamental to the organization of the workplace and workday to allow exercise therapy to be used efficiently to help patients to change towards a more healthy belief system promoting recovery. Consequently, one of the most fundamental elements of the MET criteria is the therapist being present in the exercise room constantly monitoring the patients while exercising.

MET and manual therapy have been closely linked for many years (Holten, 1968, 1976; Holten and Faugli, 1993; Holten and Torstensen, 1991; Jacobsen et al., 1992). This has been a very positive and creative 'marriage' but may also be one of the reasons why many over the years have misunderstood the MET concept, believing that it is the design of a finely tuned/ graded exercise programme for patients using pulleys and other exercise equipment specifically to stimulate tissue structures locally. This is only a part of the MET approach; some other fundamental prerequisites must be fulfilled to be able to apply graded exercises efficiently. One of these is the criteria mentioned above of being with patients the whole time they are exercising: supporting, motivating, ensuring that the patient is coping with the exercising and dealing with kinetic phobia. Unfortunately, many have focussed too much on being 'specific' and in doing so have missing out on the importance of being present to motivate the patient; consequently, these therapists do not organize their working day and exercise room so that they can work efficiently with graded exercises as a treatment. Being present with the patient in the exercise room also allows the exercises to be graded according to the patient's needs and expectations and ensures that the quality of the performance of the exercises is optimal in relation to the patient's resources.

Other elements from the MET criteria are having five patients in a group setting and the therapist being in the exercise room for 1 hour, making MET both an efficient and cost-effective approach. The presence of the therapist for the whole hour is important to ensure that the patient is exercising with the right dosage and that the patient performs the exercises correctly for maximal stimulation of the desired functional qualities, such as stability, mobility and coordination/kinetic control.

MET exercises

The MET exercises range from free exercises on a mat working against gravity only to exercises with elastic bands, sling exercise therapy, exercises with dumbbells and barbells, to the use of weight cuffs. Aerobic exercise equipment is the backbone of the MET approach, using global exercise equipment like treadmills, step machines, rowing machines, different types of stationary bicycle, arm ergometers and cross-training machines. The aerobic exercise equipment is used for warm-up, where patients work for 15–20 minutes before the 1 hour of the treatment required by the criteria. However, global aerobic exercises can also be integrated into the treatment, more so for patients with chronic pain who are dealing with pain behaviour. To be able to grade exercises more locally and to be able to choose comfortable starting positions, the MET exercise equipment comprises different types of bench (multiple purpose, angle and mobilizing benchs) and pulley (single, double, speed and lateral pulleys).

The smallest resistance using the pulley is 500 g, making it possible to start exercising at a very early stage. The weight from the lateral pulley and the single pulleys can be used in the early stage of the rehabilitation to deload the body or a part of the body in order to stimulate movement, normalize function and assist the patient to cope and actively handle their dysfunction. The principle of deloading is an important feature of MET that makes it possible to start exercising at an early stage of treatment using a high number of repetitions in sets working through the comfortable available range of motion.

Methodology for assessing the exercises

It is an important part of the MET approach that the therapist is present while the exercises are being carried out and that the exercises of the treatment programme are reassessed for appropriateness and starting level (position, weight and repetitions). The reassessment has four steps.

1. *Explanation.* First I explain the reason for each exercise and then show the patient how to perform the exercise.

2. *Assessing repetition load.* Next I ask the patient to do as many repetitions as he can manage, working dynamically approximately one repetition every 2 seconds. The patient is told to stop if he is getting really tired or if the exercise increases the symptoms. If I see that the patient is starting to work in an unco-ordinated manner, I stop the assessment. I also ask the patient to count and to indicate when he reaches six to seven repetitions if he thinks he would be able to manage to continue to at least 40 repetitions. If he answers, 'Yes, I think so but I'll have to try', he is asked to do as many repetitions as he can manage beyond 40. If he answers, 'This is too easy or too light … no problem, I can certainly do more than 40', I increase the loading of the particular exercise. If he answers, 'No, this is too heavy and uncomfortable', I change either the starting position (choose another exercise) or just change the grading of the exercise.

3. *Setting a repetition level.* I deduct 20% from the patient's number of repetitions (for type I presentation) and then round this to an easy number to remember (e.g. if the maximum is 40 repetitions, 20% is deducted, which is eight, giving 32, which is then down to 30). For treatment purposes, the patient is then instructed to do three sets of 30 repetitions with a 30-second break between each set, using the principle of interval training. For a type III presentation, 50% is deducted from the test (40 then becomes 20).

4. *Avoiding overloading.* If patient manages to do more than 40 repetitions (e.g. 50–60), I would probably still want the patient to do only three sets of 30 repetitions, consciously undergrading to make sure that the patient receives a positive experience from the exercises. Later I would increase the weight resistance for that particular exercise, making the loading more optimal while still keeping it at three sets of 30 repetitions. If the patient is only able to do 10–15 repetitions during the assessment, it suggests that I have probably chosen the wrong exercise or wrong weight resistance. In that case, I would reassess that exercise the next time the patient came for treatment. If the patient can only do 15 repetitions

with the easiest exercise available and with the lowest weight resistance available, I would then start the patient on three sets of 10 repetitions, with a goal to increase the number of repetitions until the patient could do three sets of 30 repetitions.

The methodology for evaluating the exercises can be varied. For example, to make sure that the patient copes with the exercise, the starting point can be calculated by reducing the 'maximum' number of repetitions by 50%, instead of by 20%. This is a type of behavioural therapy focussing on what the patient can perform. Another way of grading the exercises is to ask the patient just to work for a certain time period; for example Olav was asked to do exercise 1 (see below) for 5 minutes continuously repeated three times with a 30–60 second break.

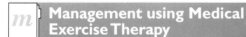

Management using Medical Exercise Therapy

For Olav, the aim of the treatment in the early phase was to apply graded exercises to treat impairments like pain and decreased range of motion, normalize kinetic control, and increase muscle strength and endurance using comfortable starting positions in lying and standing deloaded postures. As Olav's signs and symptoms improved, the exercises could be regraded and made more functional by using starting positions in weight bearing (i.e. sitting and standing). To achieve this, an exercise programme was designed consisting of eight to ten exercises doing three sets of 30 repetitions of each exercise with 30 seconds break between each. The treatment also aimed at increasing the tolerance for loading so that Olav would be physically and psychologically stronger compared with when the treatment began. Through the high number of exercises, repetitions and sets in different starting positions, muscle imbalances and kinetic control can be improved and hopefully normalized. An important goal is to regain task-specific motor improvements and regeneration of tissue structures through neural adaptations. The grading of the exercises makes it possible to load affected tissues optimally in the 'optimal load zone' as well as to exercise the tissue with an optimal volume of training within that zone, resulting in regeneration of the tissue (Kelsey and Tyson, 1994; Torstensen et al., 1994).

Initial assessment

The assessment and treatment of Olav overlapped in that the muscle/motor control assessment was performed in the exercise room, initially evaluating Olav's control with three different exercises (exercises 1–3, see

Box 19.1   Exercise 1 Global stabilizing exercise: standing deloaded squatting

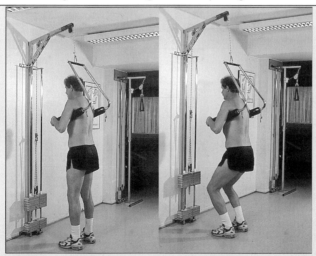

Fig. 19.3   Exercise 1.

■ This exercise is often used when treating patients with back pain where the patient finds that deloading the spine is comfortable and decreases the symptoms. By attaching a deloading frame to the lateral pulley, the weight from the pulley pulls up the deloading frame, effectively deloading the patient holding on to the frame (Fig. 19.3). © Holten Institute and Tom Arild Torstensen, with permission.

Boxes 19.1–19.3). Not surprisingly, pain influenced his ability to perform the exercises. By testing these exercises, Olav's fear-avoidance beliefs in relation to physical activity (as hypothesized earlier) could be evaluated together with his movement strategies in relation to his back pain/sciatica. The starting point for the exercises in terms of weights was defined at this point too.

At this early stage, the focus was on stability and awareness of how to stabilize the lower back, while at the same time working the upper and lower extremities.

Box 19.2   Exercise 2 Semi-global stabilizing exercise: supine lying alternate arm swing out

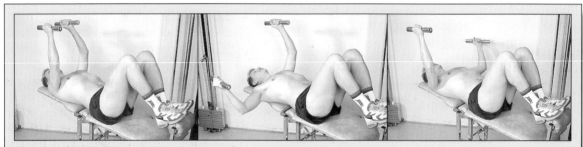

Fig. 19.4   Exercise 2.

■ The starting position of this exercise is in a comfortable supine-lying position. The patient is taught how to stabilize the back by pulling in the stomach (by thinking of having a pair of trousers that are too tight and having to 'draw-in' the lower abdominal area to button the trousers). A comfortable firm pillow can be put under the patient's back in the lumbar area to provide support and something to push against. Holding one dumbbell in each hand, the patient alternates swinging out the arms, resulting in a rotational moment of the trunk. To avoid any movement or rolling off the angle bench, the patient must stabilize the back, causing the muscles around the torso to work (Fig. 19.4). When swinging the right arm, the patient is at the same time pushing the right leg down into the surface to give a counterforce to aid in further stabilization of the back. © Holten Institute and Tom Arild Torstensen, with permission.

Box 19.3   Exercise 3 Local stabilizing exercise: four-point kneeling abdominal 'drawing-in action'

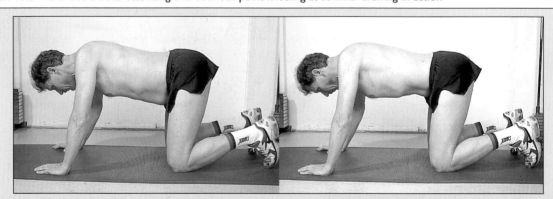

Fig. 19.5   Exercise 3.

■ This exercise is used as awareness training for activation of the abdominal muscles and, in particular, the transversus abdominis (Fig. 19.5). The patient focusses mentally on the area around the pelvis and the lower abdomen, hopefully facilitating the back stabilizers, performing three sets of 30 repetitions (Richardson et al., 1999a). © Holten Institute and Tom Arild Torstensen, with permission.

Stage 1

The first stage of Olav's exercises was carried out in six treatments over 2 weeks using exercises 1–3 (Boxes 19.1–19.3). Table 19.1 shows the format that this

Table 19.1 Exercise chart for stage 1 of the medical exercise therapy treatment programme

Exercise	Format[a]	Full description of exercise
1	25 kg, 3 sets of 5 min	Box 19.1
2	Two 2 kg dumbbells, 3 sets of 30	Box 19.2
1 repeated	25 kg, 5 min	Box 19.1
3	3 sets of 30	Box 19.3
1 repeated	25 kg, 5 min	Box 19.1

[a]Each exercise is done with a 30 second break between sets.

programme took. The treatment time to complete these exercises was approximately 30 minutes. The initial assessment defined the weights that Olav should use initially in each exercise (see Table 19.1). Exercise 1 was so comfortable for Olav that he was able to do it continuously for 5 minutes. When doing this exercise Olav felt that his back and leg pain decreased significantly. Exercise 2 started with 2 kg dumbbells and progressed later to 3 kg.

Stage 2

The second stage of Olav's treatment programme was carried out in 10 treatments over 4 weeks (Table 19.2). After the first 3 weeks, Olav was better able to tolerate the loading from the exercises and consequently three additional exercises were introduced (exercises 4–6; Boxes 19.4–19.6) using comfortable starting positions in both standing (deloaded) and lying. Exercise 4 started with 10 kg and progressed to 25 kg. Over the

Box 19.4 Exercise 4 Global stabilizing exercise: standing pull down behind the neck

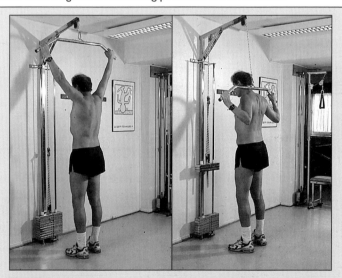

Fig. 19.6 Exercise 4.

■ This is another stabilizing exercise for the lumbar spine. The back is kept in a comfortable and stable position by applying the 'drawing-in action' of the lower abdominal area and tightening the gluteal muscles. Working the arms by pulling down behind the neck requires both back and abdominal muscles to work together in synergy (Fig. 19.6). The exercise stimulates normal muscle balance and kinetic/motor control in working the arms and the lower extremity together with the muscles stabilizing the back. Pulling down behind the neck and contracting the extensor muscles of the back results in co-contractions of the abdominal and pelvic floor muscles, giving a normal stimulus in a functional starting position to all structures stabilizing the spine. By working in a standing starting position, the lower extremity is also integrated as an important factor in retraining stability of the lower back. © Holten Institute and Tom Arild Torstensen, with permission.

Table 19.2 Exercise chart for stage 2 of the medical exercise therapy treatment programme

Exercise	Format	Full description of exercise
1 repeated with less weight	20 kg, 5 min	Box 19.1
2 progressed	Two 3 kg dumbbells, 3 sets of 30	Box 19.2
1 repeated with less weight	20 kg, 5 min	Box 19.1
3 repeated	3 sets of 30	Box 19.3
4 added	10 kg, 3 sets of 30	Box 19.4
5 added	11 kg, 3 sets of 30	Box 19.5
6 added	2 kg, 3 sets of 30	Box 19.6
1 repeated with less weight	20 kg, 5 min	Box 19.1

[a]Each exercise is done with a 30 second break between sets.

Box 19.5 Exercise 5 Semi-global stabilizing exercise: prone lying rowing (double elbow flexion/extension)

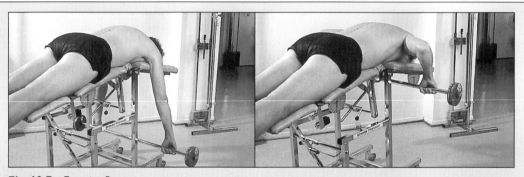

Fig. 19.7 Exercise 5.

■ The patient lies prone on the angle bench and performs rowing action, extending the shoulders/arms while holding onto a barbell. By working the upper extremities in extending the shoulders, muscles in the upper extremity, shoulder girdle and upper trunk are all working, giving a stimulus for extension of the whole trunk and activating the back extension muscles (Fig. 19.7). © Holten Institute and Tom Arild Torstensen, with permission.

Box 19.6 Exercise 6 Semi-global stabilizing exercise: supine lying, arm swing back behind the head and back up

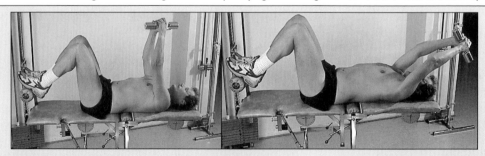

Fig. 19.8 Exercise 6.

■ The patient is lying supine on the angle bench, applying the 'drawing-in action', to stabilize the lower back. By swinging both arms backwards, a movement is initiated 'rotating' the trunk backwards into extension. However, at the same time the abdominal muscles are tightened to counteract the momentum into extension, thus stabilizing the lumbar spine (Fig. 19.8). To progress the exercise, the arms are moved with a higher speed down and back up. © Holten Institute and Tom Arild Torstensen, with permission.

following 4 weeks, Olav had 10 treatments (two or three a week), each treatment lasting approximately 1 hour. He was now also breaking a sweat during the treatment. Olav still continued with the original three exercises, two of which were regraded: exercise 1 was deloaded from 25 kg to 20 kg and the dumbbell weights

for exercise 2 were increased from 2 kg to 3 kg. In this second phase of exercises, Olav started with 5–10 minutes work on a stationary bike, where he was beginning to break a sweat. In addition to this, Olav was doing eight exercises and the total treatment time was approximately 1 hour and 10 minutes (Table 19.2).

REASONING DISCUSSION AND CLINICAL REASONING COMMENTARY

1 Please discuss briefly your reasoning behind the specific exercises chosen, including the starting positions used and the dosage prescribed.

Clinician's answer

Because Olav had what I judged to be a type I presentation, the exercises were chosen in relation to a pain-contingent treatment approach, exercising in comfortable close to pain-free starting positions. My selection of starting positions for Olav was based on my earlier experience with similar patients and, of course, information obtained from Olav through both the subjective interview and the physical assessment. The exercises were chosen by asking simple questions such as what positions and activities ease your back and leg pain and what positions and activities increase your symptoms?

The exercises chosen are a combination of global, semi-global, and local exercises based on a very simplistic philosophy that the back and trunk link the upper and lower extremities together. During locomotion, we use the lower extremity to move from point A to point B, and the upper extremity to perform a desired task with the hands. The upper and lower extremities work together with the trunk in complicated kinetic chains/patterns when performing normal functional activities, all in accordance with known physiology for motor control (Richardson et al., 1999a,b; Shumway-Cook and Woollacott, 2001a,b).

The exercise programme is also based on the knowledge that the deep abdominal and multifidus muscles are important stabilizing structures of the back. Results from research suggest that the central nervous system stabilizes the spine by contraction of the abdominal and multifidus muscles in anticipation of reactive forces produced by limb movements (Hodges and Richardson, 1997). However, in an investigation of the contribution of transversus abdominis to spinal stability during limb movements (Hodges et al., 1996),

a clinical test of the function of the deep abdominal muscles using an air-filled pressure bag (Stabilizer, Chattanooga, Australia) did not correlate with electromyography (considered the 'gold standard' of laboratory assessment). It is also still unclear how changes in these local muscles correlate with the patients' pain experience or with improvements of function for activities of daily living and returning to work.

In fact, we do not completely understand what 'stability' of the back is nor do we have any valid or reliable measurements for 'back stability'. Panjabi (1992a) has suggested three systems for spinal stability: a control system (neural), a passive subsystem (spinal column) and an active system (spinal muscles). Panjabi (1992b, p. 394) has defined clinical instability as, 'A significant decrease in the capacity of the stabilizing system of the spine to maintain the intervertebral neutral zones within physiological limits, which results in pain and disability'. This is still a working hypothesis because we have no objective, valid or reliable way of measuring the neutral zone in vivo. Consequently, the neutral zone and stability/instability itself become abstract phenomena. A fundamental question in relation to this is how stability/instability correlates with a patient's pain experience and function. Do these clinical changes really change with improved back stability? We do not know, but I believe that, if we could measure stability/instability objectively, one would probably find that the correlation is very weak, supporting other research findings that there is little or no correlation between organic tissue structures, pain, impairments and activities of daily living (Kaser et al., 2001; Mannion et al., 2001; Waddell, 1987; Waddell et al., 1982). Therefore, stability/instability would be an impairment finding meaning that some patients would probably become pain free with normal function still having an 'unstable' back/spine.

However, we all do agree that it is important to have a strong and stable back, and that a normalization of the stability of the back through exercise therapy is an important part of the treatment for patients with low back pain; this is the MET approach.

The choice of exercises and their grading in MET is also based on research regarding the force closure of the sacroiliac joint and its importance for stabilizing the back and pelvis. In this regard, four muscles are believed to be especially important: the erector spinae, gluteus maximus, latissimus dorsi and biceps femoris. It is proposed that knowledge of the coupling mechanisms between the spine, pelvis, legs and arms is essential to understand dysfunction of the human locomotor system, particularly the lower back, where three muscle slings (a longitudinal and two oblique) can be activated for optimal stability (Snijders et al., 1993; Vleeming et al., 1997).

From the information above, one can conclude that it is just as important to involve the upper extremity as it is the transversus abdominis muscle locally, and it is just as important to involve the lower extremity as it is the multifidus muscles locally when designing an exercise programme for a patient with low back pain/dysfunction. According to theories in movement science, the human body organizes all movement patterns in relation to task-specific activities and moves in complex kinetic patterns involving complex muscle synergies. The aim of the exercise programme is to make the back as 'functional' as possible, ultimately doing functional activities like lifting, pushing and pulling.

While simple questions such as 'What positions increase or decrease your symptoms?' and 'What is your preferred direction of movement?' assist in determining appropriate starting positions, finding the specific dosage is based on trial and error from earlier experience with using this method, and trial and error with each individual patient. The method of assessing the appropriateness and starting level (position, weight and repetitions) for each exercise is described in detail above, under Methodology for assessing the exercises (p. 290). In general, the aim is to end up with seven to nine exercises, but this may take 2 to 3 weeks to achieve for some patients. In the early phase, the aim is to familiarize the patient with the exercises while working on any negative perceptions and beliefs about dysfunction in relation to physical activity. The early phase, therefore, for most patients involves behavioural therapy. Later, the grading is increased according to ordinary exercise principles described in the work physiology literature.

One exception is the deloaded squatting exercise, where the patient tries the exercise initially for 1 minute, then for 2–5 minutes and then if possible for 10 minutes. This is trial and error; if the patient tolerates doing standing deloaded squatting for 10 minutes, and it is easing the back and leg pain, the stimulus from the exercise is considered appropriate and typically contributes to normalizing function. One can hypothesize that during the deloaded squatting exercise intermittent compression is occurring in the lumbar spine, thereby increasing circulation to all structures, including those causing the pain. Another possible mechanism that may contribute to the easing of symptoms is the stimulation of mechanoreceptors in muscles, tendons, joints and other structures in the upper extremities, the trunk and the lower extremities. Psychologically, when the patient finds the exercise comfortable and easing symptoms, there will probably also be a cognitive reaction to the pain stimulus, resulting in a further decrease in the pain experienced.

In this early phase of the treatment, the focus was on stability of the lumbar spine, regardless of the starting position, with the aim of stimulating the stabilizing structures around the back. The dosage chosen (Table 19.2) is usually enough for many patients to break a sweat, working the upper extremity together with the lower extremity and stimulating core stabilization of the spine, thus normalizing kinetic control. Another reason for focussing on stability at this stage for Olav is that mobilizing will usually increase symptoms. When focussing on stability, I can only use my eyes to evaluate the quality of the performance of the exercise and palpating fingers to make sure that the patient is keeping the back stable and not moving it. Then, one must still assume that the muscles and ligaments keeping the back stable are working as they should do. However, research has shown that it is difficult to palpate the contraction of the transversus abdominis and that there is poor correlation between palpation and the gold standard of real-time ultrasound imaging (Haug Dahl, 2000).

The philosophy is that there is not one specific exercise that is on its own sufficient, rather it is the sum of all the exercises and all the repetitions performed that is important. In fact, I could probably have chosen three or even four other stabilizing exercises, so this is a pragmatic approach, not dogmatic, where the only limitation is the therapist's experience and imagination.

▮ Clinical reasoning commentary

Manual therapists are rightfully being increasingly challenged as to whether their practice is 'evidence based'. This is also a requirement of skilled clinical reasoning. However, this does not mean that therapists should be restricted to only using what has been 'proven' through randomized controlled trials, as to suggest this would not only leave us with little to use but also limit our discovery of new and better approaches. Manual therapists must draw on the full range of available evidence from clinical trials and the associated systematic reviews through to experience-based evidence, providing the experience

is based on skilled, critical and reflective reasoning. The reasoning of this expert clinician is clearly based on both research-based and experience-based evidence. The broader experimental evidence, basic science muscle work/physiology evidence, prior clinical experience and this patient's particular presentation have all guided his logical strategies for selection, dosage and progression of exercises.

Assessing early progression

During the first week of the treatment, only three out of the six exercises were introduced (exercises 1–3, with three repeats of exercise 1; Table 19.1). These three exercises were the most comfortable for Olav. The aim of the exercises was to get symptom control with the loading induced through the exercises. To meet this aim, comfortable starting positions were chosen, working through a comfortable range of motion, and with either gravity assistance/resistance or with weights resisting or assisting the movement.

Following close communication with the patient, more exercises were introduced over the next 2 weeks

so that after 4 weeks Olav was doing all six different exercises with progression (i.e. regrading) of two exercises (Table 19.2). The exercises were evaluated using the methods described above under Methodology for assessing the exercises (p. 290). All eight exercises performed by Olav focussed on dynamic muscular work, doing one repetition every 2 seconds, and using starting positions that were comfortable by unloading the spine. The emphasis was on coordination and stability of the lumbar spine. By working the upper extremity together with the trunk and the lower extremity, normal muscle balance is induced, facilitating overflow to the core-stabilizing muscles of the trunk and lower back.

REASONING DISCUSSION AND CLINICAL REASONING COMMENTARY

1 The number of repetitions of exercises you use are greater than what some therapists would generally prescribe. Can you discuss the physiological and psychological basis underpinning these large numbers of repetitions?

Clinician's answer

The main aim at this early stage was to make exercising a positive experience for Olav, and to motivate him to start exercising and stay active. Consequently, undergrading was employed to help to ensure that exercising was a positive experience and useful as a positive coping strategy. Undergrading at the beginning of the treatment also allows a higher number of repetitions, which can produce increased circulation to all tissues and structures; enhance local and general endurance; facilitate neuromuscular adaptations (Sale, 1988, 1992), kinetic/motor control and muscle balance; and modify the patient's pain.

However, there is today no hard scientific evidence regarding what type of exercise or dosage is best for managing back pain (Faas, 1996; van Tulder et al., 2000). There is an increasing body of knowledge that indicates aerobic exercise is associated with better clinical results (Mannion et al., 1999) and that, given the general lack of treatment specificity with aerobic exercise, the main effects are likely the result of some 'central' modulation, perhaps caused by changing the patient's perceptions and beliefs (Mannion et al., 1999). The Cochrane Collaboration Back Review Group (van Tulder et al., 2000, p. 2795) concluded that there is really no documentation that exercise therapy is any better than traditional physiotherapy:

> There is strong evidence that exercise therapy is more effective than usual care by General Practitioners (GPs) and that exercise therapy and conventional physiotherapy (consisting of hot packs, massage, traction, mobilisation, shortwave diathermy, ultrasound, stretching, flexibility

and co-ordination exercises, electrotherapy) are equally effective. However, it still is unclear whether exercise therapy is more effective than inactive treatment for chronic low back pain, and it also remains unclear whether any specific type of exercise (flexion, extension, or strengthening exercises) is more effective than another.

Randomized controlled trials have shown that MET is effective for patients with chronic low back pain (Torstensen et al., 1998) and for patients after discectomy (Danielsen et al., 2000). Even though there are divergent opinions about what exercises to choose, when working with patients on an individual level, efficacy has been demonstrated with local specific exercises (e.g. O'Sullivan et al., 1997) and when a combination of local, semi-global and global exercises are used (Torstensen, 1993, 1998; Torstensen et al., 1999).

The theoretical rationale for asking Olav to use a high number of exercises and a high number of repetitions in sets is that it will provide a good stimulus to normalize function on an organic level (of different tissue structures), increase range of motion and muscle strength (normalize function on an impairment level), normalize function in relation to different daily activities (on an individual level, i.e. disability), and, finally, help him to participate in different social activities, which is fundamental for living a whole life (function on a societal level, i.e. handicap; Wood, 1980).

The following physiological, neurophysiological and psychosocial goals are sought through this level of exercise therapy:

- physiological goals:
  — decrease pain
  — decrease swelling
  — stimulate regeneration of tissue structures
  — increase range of motion
  — increase local and global endurance
  — increase local and global muscle strength
  — increase the physiological tolerance for loading (local and global)
  — make the patient sweat, stimulating the body's own pain-inhibiting substances (e.g. endorphins)
- neurophysiological goals:
  — decrease pain
  — improve coordination, motor control/kinetic control
  — improve stability
  — increase muscle strength (neuromuscular adaptations)

- psychosocial goals:
  — stimulate an active coping strategy
  — stimulate empowerment
  — decrease fear-avoidance beliefs regarding physical activity
  — decrease anxiety and depression
  — improve sleep patterns
  — return to work
  — give a new understanding regarding what can be done to improve the condition
  — promote patient responsibility for management and personal health
  — decrease reliance on medication.

Through the application of a high number of varied exercises, one of the aims is to increase local and general endurance (stimulate the cardiovascular system), as well as increase muscle strength. Muscle strength will increase when the pain decreases and the patient is less scared and more motivated to do stronger muscular contractions.

Over the years I have met many therapists through courses/seminars where I have been teaching MET. At the start of the course, I often ask the participants how many exercises, sets and number of repetitions in each set they apply to increase muscle strength in patients with pain and movement dysfunction. The answer I get most times is 7–10 repetitions, two sets and four to six exercises. This is very interesting as it is, of course, true for healthy individuals. However, it also shows that we do not take into consideration the fact that patients have pain, decreased range of motion, and maybe a fear of moving, and that we have to deal with these issues before we can put a patient straight into a typical strength training programme. In fact, we cannot train muscle strength in patients who experience pain, and it is only when they are symptom free with normal function that this becomes possible. The effect of pain and swelling on muscular function is well documented (Ben-Yishay et al., 1994; Brox et al., 1995; Røe, 2000; Solem-Bertoft et al., 1996; Stokes and Young, 1984), but such knowledge is often not fully integrated into the teaching of exercise therapy in manual therapy and other courses. Consequently, therapists think they can put patients with pain and dysfunction into a straightforward exercise programme with few repetitions; this may be one reason why the number of repetitions of exercises used in MET is greater than some therapists would generally prescribe.

Muscle strength is an abstract phenomenon influenced by the patient's motivation to contract his/her muscles with the possible result of increased pain and injury to tissue structures. Further, when testing muscle function/strength in a Cybex/Biodex machine, the numbers coming out of the machine are not an objective measure of muscle strength, peak torque, total work, or whatever muscle function we want to measure; rather, they are an integrated measure of pain, motivation, coping, somatization, anxiety, depression, fear-avoidance beliefs, kinetic phobia, and the effect these variables have on an individual's willingness to perform. This view has been promulgated by Newton et al. (1993), who conclude that 'isokinetic testing of patients with chronic low back pain should be regarded as an indicator of the level of performance at the time of testing and more as a psycho-physical test than as a valid test or measure of true muscle capacity'.

Another reason for Olav performing the high number of sets and repetitions is to stimulate improved neuromuscular control (coordination, kinetic control). This is achieved by activating neuromuscular adaptations (Moritani, 1992; Sale, 1988, 1992; Staron et al., 1994) such as:

- increased activity in the central nervous system
- improved synchronization of motor units
- decrease of neurological inhibiting reflexes
- inhibition of Golgi tendon organs
- increased inhibition of antagonist muscles
- increased activation of synergy muscles
- improved interplay (co-contractions) of synergy muscles
- inhibition of neurological protective mechanisms
- more effective neurological recruitment patterns
- improved motor neuron activation level.

There is also evidence that the increase in muscle strength during the first 4–6 weeks of exercising in untrained individuals is mainly a result of these neuromuscular adapations. An increase in muscle fibre diameter as the reason for increased muscle strength occurs later. In MET, an endurance stimulus with at least 1000 repetitions performed during each treatment gives an increase in muscle strength through a decrease in pain; an increase in motivation to contract the muscles, generating a greater force; and stimulation and normalization of neuromuscular adaptations. Later, when the patient becomes symptom free, a straightforward strength training programme with less repetitions (six to nine

repetitions) in sets must be used to increase muscle strength further.

An important aim of the exercise programme for Olav was also to obtain regeneration of different tissue structures. There is good evidence that loading through exercises is the optimal stimulus for regeneration of muscle, bone, fascia, tendons and nerves (Bailey and McCulloch, 1990; Hendricks, 1995; Järvinen and Lehto, 1993; Kannus et al., 1992a,b; Maffulli and King, 1992; Moltz et al., 1993; Tipton et al., 1975). The exercises make the tissues stronger, increasing their tolerance for loading, and condition the person with back pain to perform, or at least cope better with, heavy work such as lifting, pushing and pulling different objects. Through the exercises and repetitions, the tissues are biomechanically loaded, stimulating regeneration in the stress lines of the loading. Thus the regeneration of the tissue is functional because it happens within normal movement patterns performed in a coordinated manner (Kelsey and Tyson, 1994; Torstensen et al., 1994).

The MET programme for Olav was also designed to increase local endurance and more global endurance. Increased local and global endurance is important in that as it improves there is generally a corresponding decrease in the pain experienced, an increased range of motion, an increase in general and local circulation (thus increasing metabolism and regeneration and increasing local concentrations of effectors such as bradykinin) and a positive effect on psychological/cognitive components; the last follows with the positive experience of being able to do so many exercises and so many repetitions and breaking a sweat, something many patients never experience. Increasing the endurance and exercising to the point of breaking a sweat during the treatment will hopefully also release endorphins.

The high number of exercises in sets, ending up with more than 1000 repetitions during each treatment, was also aimed at decreasing Olav's pain as stimulating mechanical receptors in muscles, tendons, joint capsules and many other tissue structures can block off the 'pain gate'.

Positive psychological reactions (i.e. Olav experiencing that he actually can use his body and that he in fact can do quite a lot) decrease the fear of moving/loading the spine and the body. There is also the potential for pain to decrease as a result of the increased knowledge gained from experiencing what exercises are comfortable, what ranges of motion are acceptable to work in and that a patient is able to break a sweat when the exercises are appropriately graded according to signs and symptoms. By having a range of exercises with comfortable starting positions, working coordinated through the comfortable range of motion, with a high number of repetitions in sets (more than a 1000 repetitions in total), the stabilizing and dynamic structures of the back plus the upper and lower extremities are worked.

Through the limbic system, the patient may also experience less pain through the security and motivation provided by the therapist's presence and support. It is important that patients are comfortable about doing the right thing and feel that the reactions from exercising are not dangerous but normal.

Olav had a decreased range of motion and another goal with the MET programme was to normalize this impairment. Range of motion should increase as pain and fear of moving decreases. This increase in range probably results from both neuromuscular variables (e.g. normalizing the interplay between agonist and antagonist—muscle synergies in kinetic chains) and physiological variables (e.g. stretching effect on muscular tissue/collagen). The exercises are a form of ballistic movements, stimulating increased range of motion. Through the exercises, coordination and kinetic control is improved, which also stimulates increased range of motion. Muscle strength and endurance are also improved through the exercises. Muscle strength generally increases as the pain decreases and the patient becomes less afraid of actively contracting the muscles. The increase in muscle strength and endurance, in turn, further enhances the gains in range of motion.

Hopefully all these different effects of MET will assist Olav to resume normal daily activities as he improves. With this improvement, the exercise starting positions are changed to more functional positions in sitting and standing weight-bearing positions. According to theories of movement science, daily activities should be improved by working in functional and varied starting positions and movement patterns.

The MET programme will increase Olav's physical and psychological tolerance for loading—his back will become 'stronger' and more 'durable'—so that he is better able to tolerate his work and daily demands. He should become more coordinated, improving his lifting techniques and other relevant working techniques,

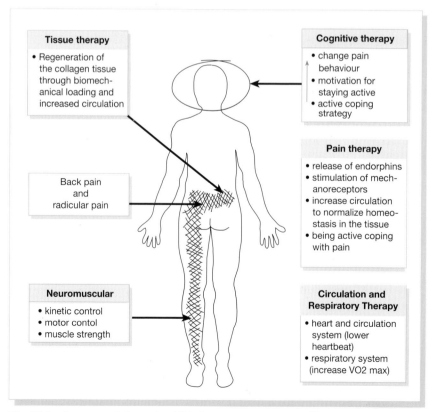

Fig. 19.9 Summary of the goals of Olav's exercise programme. The aim was to act as 'tissue therapy', 'neuromuscular therapy' and 'cognitive therapy'.

which will reduce the risk of further back pain. Hopefully, the exercise programme will give Olav a new and better understanding of what back pain is and what he himself can do to function normally in life. Maybe he will be better able to see the connection between work, rest and physical activity. These changes may be important regarding return to work, but other factors may well be more important, such as work satisfaction, control of own work situation, relationship with employer and colleagues at work, content of work, work load, etc. (Torstensen, 2001). However, Olav, as with each patient, must be individually screened and assessed in relation to all the different variables, ranging from physical to psychosocial, in relation to return to work. A summary of the goals of Olav's exercise programme is illustrated in Figure 19.9.

■ Clinical reasoning commentary

Procedural reasoning to select and progress manual therapy treatment should be based on a combi-

nation of propositional research-validated evidence and the clinician's personal craft knowledge, linked to what is 'known' from the available research but instantiated through critical reflective reasoning from prior clinical experience. Where the novice is likely to be overly biased by either unproven claims of other professionals or the latest research findings, experts will operate on a higher level, weighing all forms of evidence. Importantly, as illustrated here, the expert will also recognize the limitations of available evidence, applying (physiologically and cognitive–behaviourally) what evidence is available with consideration for each patient's individual presentation and not just as a recipe. This is impressively demonstrated here with the clinician's use of physiological, neurophysiological and psychosocial evidence combined with his own reflective experience-based evidence to effect a broad range of changes through his treatment.

m ■ Subsequent management

After 4 weeks, and a total of 12 treatments, Olav had started to improve. His pain decreased and he tolerated a greater loading both at work and at home. The MET programme was also changed accordingly, by increasing the loading and also by changing the starting positions from standing deloaded and lying, to standing loaded and sitting starting positions.

■ Stage 3

The third progression of Olav's exercises was carried out in 16 treatments over 7 weeks (Table 19.3). The aim of this third progression was to increase further Olav's tolerance for loading and working the spine in flexion and extension. Rotational exercises were also introduced, working in a cranial to caudal direction of the spine. These new exercises, 7–13, are described in Boxes 19.7–19.13. In the MET approach, trunk

Table 19.3 Exercise chart for stage 3 of the medical exercise therapy treatment programme

Exercise	Format[a]	Full description of exercise
1 repeated	20 kg, 5 min; increased over 4 weeks to 15 kg, 5 min	Box 19.1
7 added	3 sets of 15; increased over 4 weeks to 3 sets of 25	Box 19.7
4 progressed	20 kg, 3 sets of 30; increased over 4 weeks to 25 kg, 3 sets of 30	Box 19.4
8 added (progressed to exercise 9)	3 sets of 15; increased over 4 weeks to 3 sets of 25	Boxes 19.8 and 19.9
10 added	15 kg, 3 sets of 30; increased over 4 weeks to 20 kg, 3 sets of 30	Box 19.10
11 added	4 kg, 3 sets of 30; increased over 4 weeks to 6 kg, 3 sets of 30 (no rest between 30 rotations to left and 30 to right)	Box 19.11
12 added	2 kg, 3 sets of 30; increased over 4 weeks to 4 kg, 3 sets of 30	Box 19.12
13 added	4 kg, 3 sets of 30; increased over 4 weeks to 6 kg, 3 sets of 30	Box 19.13

[a]Each exercise is done with a 30 second break between sets.

Box 19.7 Exercise 7 Semi-global exercise: mobilizing in a cranial–caudal direction

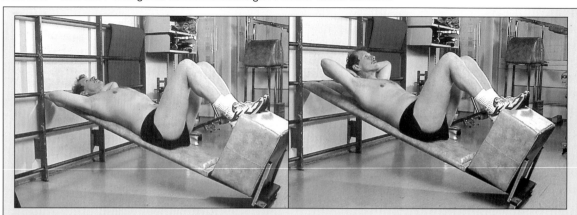

Fig. 19.10 Exercise 7.

■ This abdominal exercise is easier to do lying at an incline than lying horizontal (Fig. 19.10). However, if the incline is increased too much, so that the patient is moving towards a sitting position, symptoms usually increase. The exercise is started by applying the 'drawing-in action' of the lower abdominal wall, thus stabilizing the back, and then flexing the trunk in a cranial–caudal direction, working through a comfortable range of motion. In the early phase it is important to rest completely between each repetition. © Holten Institute and Tom Arild Torstensen, with permission.

Box 19.8 Exercise 8 Semi-global stabilizing and mobilizing exercises: prone-lying trunk extension

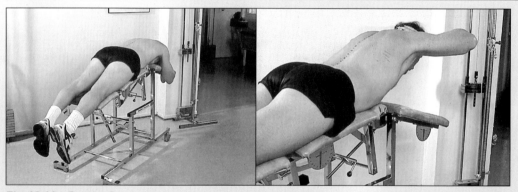

Fig. 19.11 Exercise 8.

■ Prone-lying trunk extension is a progression from exercise 5. By lying further back on the angle bench, less of the upper trunk is lifted against gravity (smaller lever arm) (Fig. 19.11). Also, range of motion (extension/flexion of the trunk) is graded based on the patient's available range of comfortable movement. The top part of the angle bench can be angled to accommodate for this range of motion. Again, the lower back is kept stable during the exercise, while working the trunk in a cranial–caudal direction. The patient fully relaxes between each repetition. This exercise also serve to mobilize the thoracic spine while partly stabilizing the lumbar spine. © Holten Institute and Tom Arild Torstensen, with permission.

rotation exercises can be performed in lying, standing and sitting starting positions (Torstensen, 1998). The deloaded squatting exercises were regraded in that the weight from the latissimus pulley was decreased, until finally Olav was doing squatting exercises against gravity with an additional weight from a barbell (Exercise 14, see below). Again all the new exercises were assessed to determine the correct starting weight for the patient and this weight was later re-assessed (for Stage 4).

Box 19.9 Exercise 9 Semi-global stabilizing and mobilizing exercises: prone lying on extension stool

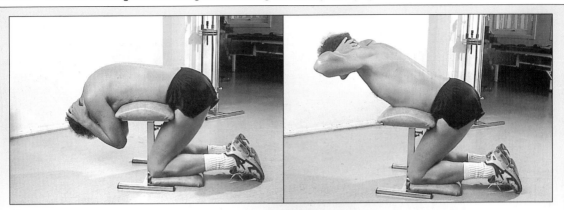

Fig. 19.12 Exercise 9.

■ Exercise 9 (Fig. 19.12) is an extension of exercise 8 using a new starting position. Trunk extension is performed while lying prone on the extension stool with flexed hips and knees. This exercise also serves to mobilize the thoracic spine while partly stabilizing the lumbar spine. © Holten Institute and Tom Arild Torstensen, with permission.

Box 19.10 Exercise 10 Global stabilizing exercise: walk–standing pull down to chest

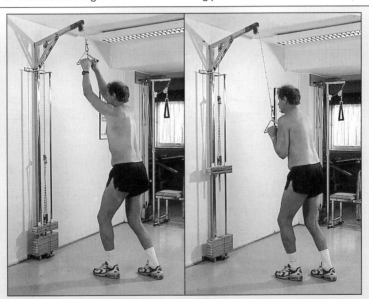

Fig. 19.13 Exercise 10.

■ The aim of this particular exercise is to stimulate structures that are stabilizing the back. The patient is instructed to flex the knees and hips slightly, performing the draw-in action of the abdominal muscles (transversus abdominis) while performing the walk–standing pull down to his chest and back up (Fig. 19.13). To find a comfortable starting position, the patient has to move and position the pelvis and lumbar spine into such a position before stabilizing. The loading on the stabilizing structures is increased if the speed of the pull down and letting up is increased. © Holten Institute and Tom Arild Torstensen, with permission.

Box 19.11 Exercise 11 Semi-global mobilizing exercise: sitting with back supported forward trunk rotation

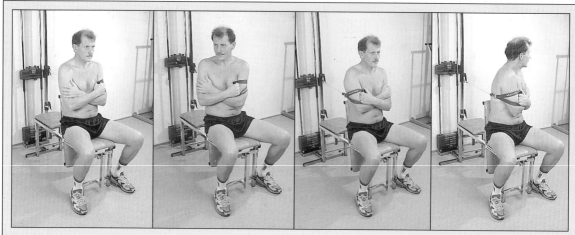

Fig. 19.14 Exercise 11.

■ This exercise activates the spinotransversal system, with emphasis on the abdominal and back muscles working in a cranial–caudal direction (Fig. 19.14). The exercise also has a mobilizing effect in a cranial–caudal direction, where the patient rotates the trunk within a comfortable range. The angle and pull from the pulley rope determines the localization of resistance. For example, if the rope comes from above, the resistance is biased to the oblique abdominal muscles. To obtain the 'drawing-in action' of the lower abdominal area, the instructions are as follows: 'Tighten your abdominal muscles (or "suck in your abdomen and pull the naval in and up") and sit against the back support putting your lower back in a stable starting position. Then turn your head to the right and rotate the trunk.' For treatment purposes, the trunk rotation exercises are done consecutively with no rest: first 30 repetitions to the right, then 30 repetitions to the left, doing a total of six sets alternating to left and right. © Holten Institute and Tom Arild Torstensen, with permission.

To progress the stabilization of his lumbar spine further, exercise 4 (Box 19.4) had been introduced at Stage 2 with a weight of 10 kg; during Stage 3, the weight was progressed to 20 kg and then to 25 kg over 4 weeks. The muscles of the upper extremity, shoulder and shoulder girdle, the interscapular muscles and other back muscles extending the spine are activated by this exercise. Also, the abdominal muscles are activated to counterbalance the activation of the posterior trunk muscles.

In this third phase of exercises, Olav continued to start with the stationary bike, increasing his riding time from 10 minutes to 15–20 minutes. The total number of exercises was eight and the total treatment time was now approximately 1½ hours (Table 19.3).

The introduction of global aerobic exercise

After approximately 3 to 4 weeks, when Olav was able to sit for short periods without increasing his symptoms, he started the MET treatment with 5–10 minutes and later with 15–20 minutes warm-up on an ergometer cycle before commencing the other exercises. While this was only a warm-up, it was sufficient for Olav to break a sweat.

However, everything did not go as smoothly as anticipated. After 6 weeks of treatment Olav was getting a little bit too motivated and increased the weight on some exercises without conferring with me. The increased loading resulted in a setback, with increased pain in the back and in his left foot. This experience made it clear to Olav the importance of proper pacing and that increased loading with the exercises has to be done in a stepwise manner within his tolerance for loading. This aggravation of symptoms settled after the exercises were paced back and Olav then continued his programme successfully for another 8 weeks.

■ Stage 4

The fourth progression of Olav's exercises was carried out in 15 treatments over 8 weeks (Table 19.4).

Box 19.12 Exercise 12 Global stabilizing exercise: stride side-standing two-arm pull from one side to the other (short range)

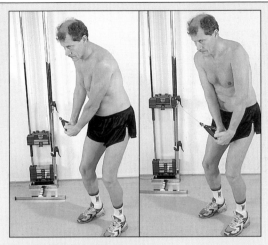

Fig. 19.15 Exercise 12.

■ Exercise 12 is a stabilizing exercise for the lumbar spine, producing a rotational stimulus where both arms and upper trunk are required to work against a graded resistance from the pulley apparatus, as if making a golf put (Fig. 19.15). Here it is important to keep the lumbar spine stable, avoiding any rotation in the lower lumbar area, applying the 'drawing-in action' of the lower abdominal wall. The instructions to the patient are: 'slightly flex your knees and hips, draw in your lower abdominal area stabilizing your back. Now, keep you arms straight with the elbows slightly flexed and move them together laterally, first slowly and then faster. Alternate between the two sides, doing first 30 repetitions to the left, then turn around and do 30 repetitions to the right for a total of six sets (three to right and three to left).' © Holten Institute and Tom Arild Torstensen, with permission.

Box 19.13 Exercise 13 Semi-global (mobilizing in a caudal–cranial direction) exercise: front sitting trunk rotation

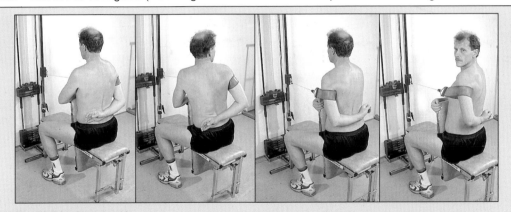

Fig. 19.16 Exercise 13.

■ Exercise 13 activates the transversospinal system, now with a greater emphasis on the posterior back muscles, the abdominal muscles and the muscles of the shoulder girdle (Fig. 19.16). The movement also mobilizes the spine working in a cranial–caudal direction, where rotation and side flexion are in opposite directions in extension (i.e. rotation to the right will be accompanied by side flexion to the left in extension). Thus, the movement stimulates the normal biomechanics of the spine, enhancing motor control/kinetic control of the complicated muscle synergies of the trunk. Many patients with back pain find it difficult to sit for long periods of time and, therefore, it may be difficult to begin with this starting position in the early phase of the treatment. However, later, when the patient tolerates exercising in sitting, this is a very important exercise. © Holten Institute and Tom Arild Torstensen, with permission.

Table 19.4   Exercise chart for stage 4 of the medical exercise therapy treatment programme

Exercise	Format	Full description of exercise
4 repeated	25 kg, 3 sets of 30 maintained over 8 weeks	Box 19.4
7 progressed	3 sets of 30 maintained over 8 weeks	Box 19.7
14 added	7 kg, 3 sets of 30; increased over 8 weeks to 16 kg, 3 sets of 30	Box 19.14
11 progressed	8 kg, 3 sets of 30; increased over 8 weeks to 10 kg, 3 sets of 30	Box 19.11
9 repeated	3 sets of 20 maintained over 8 weeks	Box 19.9
12 progressed	5 kg, 3 sets of 30; increased over 8 weeks to 6 kg, 3 sets of 30	Box 19.12
10 progressed	20 kg, 3 sets of 30; increased over 8 weeks to 25 kg, 3 sets of 30	Box 19.10
13 progressed	7 kg, 3 sets of 30; increased over 8 weeks to 8 kg, 3 sets of 30	Box 19.13
15 added	4 kg, 3 sets of 30; increased over 8 weeks to 6 kg, 3 sets of 30	Box 19.15

[a]Each exercise is done as three sets of 30 repetitions with a 30 second break between sets.

Box 19.14   Exercise 14 Global stabilizing exercise: stride standing–knee bending to stoop knee standing (squatting)

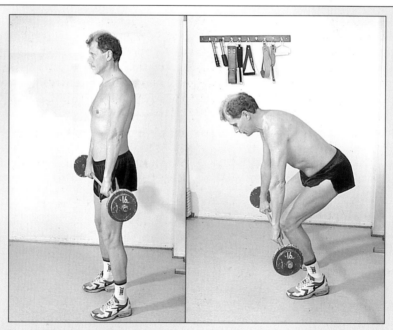

Fig. 19.17   Exercise 14.

■ This is another stabilizing exercise for the lumbar spine, where the patient is instructed to keep the lumbar spine in a neutral comfortable position while performing a squatting exercise (Fig. 19.17). As in prior exercises, the patient needs to apply the 'drawing-in action' of the lower abdominal wall. Together with the stabilizing structures of the back, both upper and lower extremities are involved with this exercise. The exercise is also important, as it is more functional in relation to daily activities. © Holten Institute and Tom Arild Torstensen, with permission.

Box 19.15   Exercise 15 Global stabilizing exercise: lifting exercise

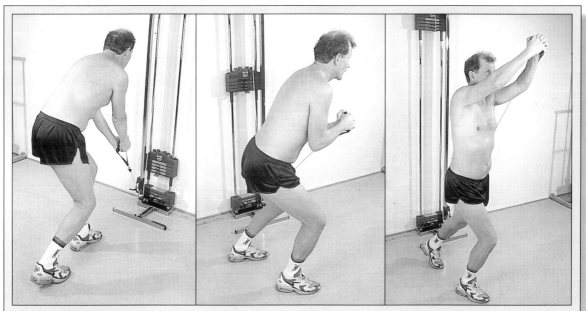

Fig. 19.18   Exercise 15.

■ With this exercise, the patient stands sideways pulling the weight using trunk rotation from the feet and weight transference, with muscular effort moving from the midline towards the periphery (Fig. 19.18). Emphasis here is on stabilization, weight transference and coordination/kinetic control. The lower lumbar spine is again positioned comfortably and then kept stable during the movement. A set of 30 repetitions is split into 15 to the right and then 15 to the left; this set is then repeated. © Holten Institute and Tom Arild Torstensen, with permission.

In this fourth phase of exercises, Olav maintained his 15–20 minute warm-up with the stationary bike, still breaking a sweat as with the other phases of his progression. Two new exercises were added (exercises 14 and 15, described in Boxes 19.14 and 19.15). The total number of exercises in this progression was nine and the total treatment time was approximately 1½ hours.

REASONING DISCUSSION

1 In addition to monitoring the patient's pain and performance with the exercises themselves, can you discuss any other outcome measures you re-assessed?

■ Clinician's answer

For clinical use, I apply an objective measure of subjective variables using a 10 box scale for both pain and different activities of daily living (functional activities) where 10 is the level of pain or dysfunction the patient is experiencing when starting treatment and 0 is symptom-free or normal function. Sometimes I use a visual analogue scale (VAS) for measuring pain and the Oswestry Low Back Disability Scale for function. For Olav I used the 10 box scale for both pain and function, because my experience is that in a busy outpatient clinic working with individual patients, a simple 10 box scale is easier to use than a more abstract VAS and the Oswestry Low Back Pain Disability Scale. The latter outcome measures are more valid doing outcome research comparing differences between large patient groups (Torstensen et al., 1998). Olav's condition did not really change much the first 3–4 weeks, but then pain started to decrease in the leg and the back and function improved correspondingly. His straight leg raise and slump test signs disappeared and the range of motion of his back in all movement directions improved significantly. These variables were indirectly re-assessed through the progression of his management. Another sign of improvement was the markedly increased load he could tolerate during the exercises, and weight resistance was increased from 50% to 150% for most of the exercises. In addition, improvement was indicated by the fact that he managed to exercise in starting positions that earlier were unbearable because of the pain, such as sitting starts and also squatting exercises flexing the trunk forward. In the clinical setting, by contrast with the research setting, it is important to use outcome measures that are patient friendly and understandable for the patient (Torstensen et al., 1998). Pointing out to the patient what they can do now compared with earlier is for most patients very motivating, giving them an understanding that they are actually treating themselves and through that action they will get better. An exercise card is used to document objectively the progressions of the treatment. The name of the exercise, weight resistance, and the number of sets and repetitions is recorded on the exercise card. Through highlighting the progressions on the exercise card, I focus on what the patient can do and what they have achieved, thus adapting cognitive–behavioural therapy for the exercise room.

2 Please comment on your prognosis for Olav and the key criteria you consider in making this judgment.

Clinician's answer

I consider the following five elements are important to predicting outcome:

- how the patient presents himself/herself at the assessment, i.e. a positive outcome is often related

to the patient having a firm and definite handshake, whether the patient looks into the therapist's eyes when shaking hands, and whether the patient states a definite treatment aim (e.g. that within a certain time period they will be back working and doing ordinary activities as before)
- what thoughts the patient has about their symptoms and how quickly they can return to work and normal activities of daily living with the present symptoms
- how motivated the patient is engaging in an active exercise-based treatment
- the patient's pain pattern and pain behaviour
- the time the patient has been on sick leave/unemployed/off work: there is scientific evidence that length of time away from work is a negative predictor for returning to work.

The treatment is usually fairly straightforward when one can reproduce symptoms and if the symptoms can be related to an organic structure. Olav had a firm handshake, was not on sick leave, enjoyed his work and hoped that, within the not too distant future, he would be much better and working normally. I also judged that he had a type I presentation with a symptom pattern in a recognizable dermatome and did not present as having any type of abnormal pain behaviour. Other relevant information indicating a positive outcome included the fact that Olav was normally fairly physically active and enjoyed exercising. Therefore, introducing an active treatment from day one consisting of graded exercises was likely to be well accepted by Olav. In many ways, I would categorize Olav as an 'easy' patient where single discipline therapy, like MET, would be sufficient to decrease symptoms and normalize function. Today, when I get similar patients, as well as other symptom patterns that are typical of type I patients, I feel confident in offering them a positive outcome. However, a positive outcome is dependent on the patient being motivated to performing the supervised graded exercises two to three times a week for a period of at least 2–3 months.

Outcome

After a total of 24 weeks of treatment and a total of 47 treatments (1½ hours exercise therapy two

to three times a week), Olav was symptom free and able to engage in any daily activity. The final test that he had recovered was a trip with his two sons to Svalbard 5 months after he finished the treatment.

Svalbard is an island far north towards the North Pole. During the 1 week trip in the wilderness they did a lot of cross-country skiing with heavy back packing, as well as driving scooters with pronounced vibration. Olav managed well and never experienced any back or leg pain.

References

Bailey, D.A. and McCulloch, R.G. (1990). Bone tissue and physical activity. Canadian Journal of Sport Science, 15, 229–239.

Bassett, S. and Petrie, K. (1999). The effect of treatment goals on patient compliance with physiotherapy exercise programmes. Physiotherapy, 85, 130–137.

Ben-Yishay, A., Zuckerman, J.D., Gallagher, M. and Cuomo, F. (1994). Pain inhibition of shoulder strength in patients with impingement syndrome. Orthopedics, 17, 685–688.

Brox, J.I., Holm, I., Ludvigsen, P. and Steen, H. (1995). Pain influence on isokinetic shoulder muscle strength in patients with rotator tendinosis (impingement syndrome stage II). European Journal of Physical Medicine Rehabilitation, 5, 196–199.

Danielsen, J.M., Johnsen, R., Kibsgaard, S.K. and Hellevik, E. (2000). Early aggressive exercise for postoperative rehabilitation after disectomy. Spine, 25, 1015–1020.

De Clerck, P. (1999). Clinical reasoning for directing treatment for patients with low back problems. In Medical Exercise Therapy: The Theoretical Basis (T. Torstensen, ed.) pp. 67–90. Stockholm, Sweden: Holten Institute (www.holteninstitute.com).

Evjenth, O. and Hamberg, J. (1988). Muscle Stretching in Manual Therapy, Vol. 2: A Clinical Manual. The spinal column and the TM-joint, 2nd edn. Alfta, Sweden: Alfta Rehab.

Faas, A. (1996). Exercises: which ones are worth trying, for which patients, and when? Spine 21, 2874–2879.

Gifford, L. and Butler, D. (1997). The integration of pain science into clinical practice. Journal of Hand Therapy, 10, 86–95.

Hamton, J.R., Harrison, M.J., Mitchell, J.R., Prichard, J.S. and Seymour, C. (1975). Relative contributions of history-taking, physical examination, and laboratory investigation to diagnosis and management of medical outpatients. British Medical Journal, ii, 486–489.

Haug Dahl, H. (2000). Palpation and Ultrasound Imaging of Contraction of Deep Abdominal Muscles. A Descriptive, Exploratory Study of Concurrent Validity. MSc Thesis, Division of Physiotherapy Science, University of Bergen.

Hendricks, T. (1995). The effects of immobilization on connective tissue. Journal of Manipulative Therapy, 3, 98–103.

Hodges, P.W. and Richardson, C.A. (1997). Contraction of the abdominal muscles associated with movement of the lower limb. Physical Therapy, 77, 132–144.

Hodges, P., Richardson, C. and Jull, G. (1996). Evaluation of the relationship between laboratory and clinical tests of transversus abdominis function. Physiotherapy Research International, 1, 30–40.

Holroyd, K.A. and Lazarus, R.S. (1982). Stress, coping and somatic adaptation. In Handbook of Stress: Theoretical and Clinical Aspects (L. Goldberger and S Breznitz, eds.) pp. 21–35. New York: Free Press.

Holten, O. (1968). Treningsterapi. Fysioterapeuten, 35, 236–240.

Holten, O. (1976). Medisinsk treningsterapi. Fysioterapeuten, 43, 9–14.

Holten, O. and Faugli, H.P. (1993). Medisinsk treningsterapi, Oslo: Universitetsforlaget.

Holten, O. and Torstensen, T.A. (1991). Medical exercise therapy: the basic principles. Fysioterapeuten, 58, 27–32.

Jacobsen, F., Holten, O., Faugli H.P. and Leirvik R. (1992). Medical exercise therapy. Fysioterapeuten, 59, 19–22.

Järvinen, M.J. and Lehto, M.U.K. (1993). The effects of early immobilization and remobilization on the healing process following muscle injuries. Sports Medicine, 15, 78–89.

Jensen, M.C., Brant-Zawadzki, M.N., Obuchowski, N., Modic, M.T., Malkasian, D. and Ross, J.S. (1994). Magnetic resonance imaging of the lumbar spine in people without back pain. New England Journal of Medicine, 331, 69–73.

Jones, M.A., Edwards, I. and Gifford, L. (2002). Conceptual models for implementing biopsychosocial theory in clinical practice. Manual Therapy, 7, 2–9.

Kaltenborn, F.M. (1989). Manuell mobilisering av ryggraden. Oslo: Olaf Norlis Bokhandel.

Kannus, P., Jozsa, L., Renström, P. et al. (1992a). The effects of training, immobilization and remobilization on musculoskeletal tissue. 1: Training and immobilization. Scandinavian Journal of Medicine and Science in Sports, 2, 100–118.

Kannus, P., Jozsa, L., Renström, P. et al. (1992b). The effects of training, immobilization and remobilization on musculoskeletal tissue. 2: Remobilization and prevention of immobilization atrophy. Scandinavian Journal of Medicine and Science in Sports, 2, 164–176.

Kaser, L., Mannion, A.F., Rhyner, A. et al. (2001). Active therapy for chronic low back pain. Part II. Effects on paraspinal muscle cross-sectional area, fiber type size, and distribution. Spine, 26, 909–918.

Keefe, F.J., Dunsmore, J., Burnett, R. (1992). Behavioural and cognitive behavioural approaches to chronic pain. Recent advances and future directions. Journal of Consulting and Clinical Psychology, 60, 528–536.

Keefe, F.J., Kashikar-Zuck, S., Opiteck, J. et al. (1996). Pain in arthritis and musculoskeletal disorders: the role of coping skills training and exercise interventions. Journal of Orthopedic and Sports Physical Therapy, 24, 279–290.

Kelsey, D.D. and Tyson, E. (1994). A new method of training the lower extremity using unloading. Journal of Orthopedics and Sports Physical Therapy, 19, 218–233.

Khan, K.M., Tress, B.W., Hare, W.S.C. et al. (1998). Treat the patient, not the

X-ray: advances in diagnostic imaging do not replace the need for clinical interpretation. Clinical Journal of Sports Medicine, 8, 1–4.

Kuslich, S.D., Ulstrom, C.L., Michael, C.J. (1991). The tissue origin of low back pain and sciatica: a report of pain response to tissue stimulation during operations on the lumbar spine using local anesthesia. Orthopedic Clinics of North America, 22, 181–187.

Lee, D.G. (1994). Clinical manifestations of pelvic girdle dysfunction. In Grieve's Modern Manual Therapy, 2nd edn (J.D. Boyling and N. Palastanga, eds.) pp. 453–462. London: Churchill Livingstone.

Maffulli, N. and King, J.B. (1992). Effects of physical activity on some components of the skeletal system. Sports Medicine, 13, 393–407.

Main, C.J. and Booker, C.K. (2000). The nature of psychological factors. In Pain management. An Interdisciplinary Approach (C.J. Main and C.C. Spanswick, eds.) pp. 19–42. Edinburgh: Churchill Livingstone.

Main, C.J., Spanswick, C.J. and Watson, P. (2000a). The nature of disability. In Pain management. An Interdisciplinary Approach (C.J. Main and C.C. Spanswick, eds.) pp. 89–106. Edinburgh: Churchill Livingstone.

Main, C.J., Spanswick, C.J. and Watson, P. (2000b). Models of pain. In Pain management. An Interdisciplinary Approach (C.J. Main and C.C. Spanswick, eds.) pp. 3–18. Edinburgh: Churchill Livingstone.

Mannion, A.F., Muntener, M., Taimela, S., Dvorak, J. (1999). A randomized clinical trial of the active therapies for chronic low back pain. Spine, 24, 2435–2488.

Mannion, A.F., Taimela, S., Muntener, M. et al. (2001). Active therapy for chronic low back pain Part I. Effects on back muscle activation, fatigability, and strength. Spine, 26, 897–908.

Moltz, A.B., Heyduck, B., Lill, H. and Spanuth, E. et al. (1993). The effect of different exercise intensities on the fibrinolytic system. European Journal of Applied Physiology, 67, 298–304.

Monat, L. and Lazarus, R.S. (1991). Introduction: stress and coping—some current issues and controversies. In Stress and Coping. An Anthology,

3rd edn (L. Monat and R.S. Lazarus, eds.) p. 5. New York: Columbia University Press.

Moritani, T. (1992). Time course of adaptations during strength and power training. In Strength and Power in Sports (P.V. Komi, ed.) pp. 266–278. London: Blackwell Scientific.

Newton, M., Thow, M. and Somerville, D. et al. (1993). Trunk strength testing with iso-machines. Part 2: Experimental evaluation of the Cybex II back testing system in normal subjects and patients with chronic low back pain. Spine, 18, 812–824.

Norske Fysioterapeuters Forbund (1998). Standard for undersøkelsesprosedyrer i manuell terapi., Oslo: Utgave 1, Norske Fysioterapeuters Forbund.

Olmarker, K. and Rydevik, B. (1992). Pathophysiology of sciatica. Orthopaedic Clinics of North America, 22, 223–235.

Panjabi, P. (1992a). The stabilising system of the spine. Part 1. Function, dysfunction, adaptation, and enhancement. Journal of Spinal Disorders, 5, 383–389.

Panjabi, P. (1992b). The stabilising system of the spine. Part II. Neutral zone and stability hypothesis. Journal of Spinal Disorders, 5, 390–397.

Peterson, M.C., Holbrook, J.H. and von Hales, D. et al. (1992). Contribution of the history, physical examination, and laboratory investigation in making medical diagnoses. Western Journal of Medicine, 156, 163–165.

Prochaska, J.O. and DiClemente, C.C. (1982). Transtheoretical theory toward a more integrative model of change. Psychotherapy: Therapy and Practice, 19, 276–287.

Prochaska, J.O., Norcross, J.C. and DiClemente, C.C. (1994). Changing for good. New York: William Morrow.

Richardson, C., Jull, G., Hodges, P., Hides, J. (1999a). Clinical testing of the local muscles: practical examination of motor skill. In Therapeutic Exercise for Spinal Segmental Stabilization in Low Back Pain (C. Richardson, G. Jull, P. Hodges and J. Hides, eds.) pp. 105–123. Edinburgh: Churchill Livingstone.

Richardson, C., Jull, G., Hodges, P. and Hides, J. (1999b). Traditional views of the function of the muscles of the local stabilizing system of the spine. In

Therapeutic Exercise for Spinal Segmental Stabilization in Low Back Pain (C. Richardson, G. Jull, P. Hodges and J. Hides, eds.) pp. 21–40. Edinburgh: Churchill Livingstone.

Røe, C. (2000). Interaction between Pain and Muscle Activation in Chronic Shoulder Pain. PhD Thesis, Department of Physiology, National Institute of Occupational Health, Section for Health Sciences, Faculty of Medicine, University of Oslo.

Sale, D.G. (1988). Neural adaptations to resistance training. Medical Science in Sports and Exercise. 20, S135–S142.

Sale, D.G. (1992). Neural adaptations to strength training. Time course of adaptations during strength and power training. In Strength and Power in Sports (P.V. Komi, ed.), pp. 249–265. London: Blackwell Scientific.

Shumway-Cook, A. and Woollacott, M.J. (2001a). Physiology of motor control. In Motor Control Theory and Practical Applications (A. Shumway-Cook and M.J. Woollacott, eds.) pp. 50–90. Philadelphia, PA: Lippincott, Williams & Wilkins.

Shumway-Cook, A. and Woollacott, M.J. (2001b). Physiological Basis of Motor Learning and Recovery of Function. In Motor Control Theory and Practical Applications (A. Shumway-Cook and M.J. Woollacott, eds.) pp. 91–126, Philadelphia: Lippincott Williams & Wilkins.

Snijders, C.J., Vleeming, A. and Stoeckart, R. (1993). Transfer of lumbosacral load to iliac bones and legs. Part 1: Biomechanics of self-bracing of the sacroiliac joints and its significance for treatment and exercise. Journal of Clinical Biomechanics, 8, 285–294.

Solem-Bertoft, E., Lundh, I. and Westerberg, C.E. (1996). Pain is a major determinant of impaired performance in standardized active motor tests. A study in patients with fracture of the proximal humerus. Scandinavian Journal of Rehabilitation, 28, 71–78.

Staron, R.S., Karapondo, D.L., Kraemer, W.J. et al. (1994). Skeletal muscle adaptations during the early phase of heavy resistance training in men and women. Journal of Applied Physiology, 76, 1247–1254.

Stokes, M. and Young, A. (1984). The contribution of reflex inhibition to arthrogenous weakness. Clinical Science, 76, 7–14.

Tipton, C.M., Matthes, R.D., Maynard, J.A. and Carcy, R.A. (1975). The influence of physical activity on ligaments and tendons. Medicine and Science in Sports, 7, 165–175.

Torstensen, T.A. (1990). Medisinsk treningsterapi og manuell terapi. Fysioterapeuten, 57, 16–19.

Torstensen, T.A. (1993). Medisinsk treningsterapi etter ryggoperasjon. Fysioterapeuten, 60, 319–327.

Torstensen, T.A. (1998). Medical Exercise Therapy. Exercise Manual for Thoracic and Low Back Pain. Stockholm, Sweden: Holten Institute (www.holteninstitute.com).

Torstensen, T.A. (2001). Methodological considerations of clinical studies on low back pain. MSc Thesis, Division of Physiotherapy Science, University of Bergen.

Torstensen, T.A. and De Clerck, P. (2001). Upper extremity dysfunction. a pragmatic approach. In Upper Extremity Dysfunction—A Pragmatic Treatment Approach (T.A. Torstensen and P. De Clerck, eds.) pp. 7–101. Stockholm, Sweden: Holten Institute (www.holteninstitute.com).

Torstensen, T.A., Meen, H.D.M. and Stiris, M. (1994). The effect of medical exercise therapy on a patient with chronic supraspinatus tendinitis. Diagnostic ultrasound—tissue regeneration: A case study. Journal of Orthopedics and Sports Physical Therapy, 20, 319–327.

Torstensen, T.A., Ljunggren, A.E. and Meen, H.D. et al. (1998). Efficiency and costs of medical exercise therapy, conventional physiotherapy, and self exercises in patients with chronic low back pain: a pragmatic, randomized, single-blinded, controlled trial with 1-year follow-up. Spine, 23, 2616–2624.

Torstensen, T.A., Nielsen, L.L. and Jensen, R. et al. (1999). Fysioterapi som manuell terapi. Tidsskr Nor Lægeforen, 119, 2059–2063.

Uvnäs-Moberg, K. (1998). Oxytocin may mediate the benefits of positive social interaction and emotions. Psychoneuroendocrinology, 23, 819–835.

van Tulder, M.W., Malmivarra, A., Esmail, R. and Koes, B.W. (2000). Exercise therapy for low back pain: a systematic review within the framework of the Cochrane Collaboration Back Review Group. Spine, 25, 2784–2796.

Vleeming, A., Snijders, C.J., Stoeckart, R. and Mens, J.M.A. (1997). The role of the sacroiliac joints in coupling between spine, pelvis, legs and arms. In Movement, Stability and Low Back Pain. The Essential Role of the Pelvis (A. Vleeming, V. Mooney, T. Dorman, C. Snijders and R. Stoeckart, eds.) pp. 53–71. London: Churchill Livingstone.

Waddell, G. (1987). Clinical assessment of lumbar impairment. Clinical Orthopedics and Related Research, 221, 110–120.

Waddell, G., Main, C.J. and Morris, E.W. et al. (1982). Normality and reliability in the clinical assessment of backache. British Medical Journal, 284, 1519.

Wayanda, V.K., Armenth-Brothers, F., Boyce, A. (1998). Goal setting: a key to injury rehabilitation. Athletic Therapy Today, Jan, 21–25.

Wood, P.H.N. (1980). The language of disablement: a glossary relating to disease and its consequences. International Rehabilitation Medicine, 2, 86–92.

Zusman, M. (1997). Instigators of activity intolerance: review article. Manual Therapy, 2, 75–86.

Zusman, M. (1998). Structure oriented beliefs and disability due to back pain. Physiotherapy, 44, 13–20.

An elderly woman 'trapped within her own home' by groin pain

Patricia Trott and Geoffrey Maitland

SUBJECTIVE EXAMINATION

Moya is an 83-year-old woman who had been recommended for physiotherapy by her general practitioner (GP). She has intermittent right groin pain that is consistently brought on by standing for 10–15 minutes and walking for 15–20 minutes. She also experiences a sharp catching pain in her groin that is inconsistently associated with standing up from sitting and lifting her right leg to get into a car or to put on her shoe.

At night she was unable to lie supine with one pillow because of the groin pain and found most relief in the half-lying supine position on three pillows. At times she also needed a pillow under her right knee. She reported no pain or stiffness first thing in the morning. Her groin pain was worse towards the end of the day and some nights she slept poorly because of the pain. Sometimes this was when she had slipped off the pillows into a more horizontal position, but at other times it was not related to position. She could sleep on her sides, propped on three pillows, but if pain developed then she had to return to the half-lying supine position and this would ease the groin pain within a few minutes. The number of times she woke per night was variable and was not related to her daily activities. Sitting eased both her day and night pain within 5 minutes.

Other activities that might implicate the hip joint as the source of pain (e.g. crossing the right knee over the left in sitting and squatting) were negative. Similarly, there was no pain with activities performed in trunk flexion, such as cleaning the bath and gardening.

General screening questions

Moya reported good general health, no gastrointestinal or gynaecological complaints or relevant history, no weight loss, and no symptoms of spinal cord or cauda equina irritation/compression. She takes analgesics (two disprin, one or two nights per week) if unable to sleep because of groin pain but has no history of taking steroids or anticoagulants. She has had no radiographs or other tests recently.

Present history

Over the last 3 months, Moya experienced a gradual onset of right groin pain for no known reason. There was no trauma or change in routine activities at or around the time of onset. She had to give up swimming three times per week and working as a volunteer in a hospice 2 days per week because of her inability to stand and walk. Because of this, she acknowledged feeling very frustrated and 'trapped within her own home'. Further questioning revealed that she was a widow who lived alone in a roomy unit. Her two children lived within 10 km and contacted and visited her regularly. She had worked as a private secretary until aged 70 years and since then had trained as a counsellor for the dying and for bereaved families and friends. She had good insight into her own feelings of being confined to her home and to loss of her hospice work. There were no indications of depression. The groin pain was worsening in both intensity (could reach

8–9/10) and frequency with more activities bringing on the pain.

Past history

There was no past history of back or leg symptoms. Moya had experienced many years of occipital headaches, which were helped by physiotherapy treatment to the cervical spine. In the last year, she reported having occasional central low cervical aching associated with sustained flexion. There had been no treatment for this low cervical problem and no history of trauma to the neck.

REASONING DISCUSSION AND CLINICAL REASONING COMMENTARY

1 What were your thoughts regarding this lady and her problem? From your comment regarding activities implicating the hip, you were clearly considering this as a likely source of her symptoms. Could you briefly highlight the clues from her presentation that supported this hypothesis, as well as any that perhaps did not fit?

Clinicians' answer

It was intuitively felt that this elderly woman was able to give an accurate description of her symptoms and their behaviour. Moya was quite clear regarding the consistent aggravating effect of standing and walking and the easing effect of sitting and supine lying on three pillows. Her difficulty in relating the pain's behaviour with other activities seemed more related to their variable effect than to her vagueness.

The early hypotheses regarding the source(s) of right groin pain, and the associated evidence, were:

- lumbar spine
  - spinal canal stenosis: supported by the pain being worse with standing and walking and eased by sitting and half-lying supine; the former narrows the spinal canal, while sitting and half-lying supine flexes and so widens the canal
  - upper or lower lumbar zygapophyseal joints, which can refer pain to the groin: aggravating and easing effects of standing and sitting (half-lying), respectively, are more commonly associated with zygapophyseal joint problems than with a discogenic source

- hip joint (anterior structures): pain felt in weight-bearing positions of standing, walking, moving from sitting to standing or lifting the leg to get into a car; degenerative hip disease is a common source of groin pain in patients of this age group, but the inconsistent effects of hip movements did not support the hip joint as a source of pain
- bursae and local muscles in the groin area: pain associated with hip movements such as walking and lifting the leg to get into a car; however, these movements did not consistently cause pain
- neural sources (ilioinguinal nerve and femoral branch of the genitofemoral nerve): inability to lie flat in supine, which can apply tension to the ilioinguinal nerve as it pierces the anterior abdominal wall, and pain in hip extension, which tensions the femoral branch of the genitofemoral nerve that pierces the psoas major
- gastroenterological and gynaecological disorders: can refer pain to the groin (considered unlikely).

The condition appeared to be:

- mechanical (pain worse with postures and movements, though the latter showed some inconsistencies)
- non-inflammatory (no morning stiffness, no resting symptoms)
- non-irritable (eased after 5 minutes of sitting or half-lying supine)
- peripherally neurogenic or nociceptive (pain mechanisms).

2 Could you comment on your thoughts regarding the onset and progression of this lady's symptoms?

■ Clinicians' answer

The insidious onset supports a degenerative process leading to lumbar spinal canal stenosis and/or osteoarthrosis of the zygapophyseal joints or hip joint. It does not support groin tissues as the source of pain as one would expect a history of some incident or trauma.

The central low cervical aching associated with sustained neck flexion was not attended to at this stage.

The worsening in intensity and frequency of the groin pain, despite a reduction in activities involving standing and walking, suggests that there may be other pathology, which needs further investigation by the GP. Computed axial tomography (CAT) or magnetic resonance imaging (MRI) would best demonstrate both the bony and soft tissues of the spine and the spinal canal itself.

The feelings of frustration (not depression) seemed appropriate for this woman, who had led an active life. She kept up her general fitness by swimming three times per week and gainfully employed her mind by doing 2 days of voluntary work. She was now confined to her home and spent most of her time sitting.

■ Clinical reasoning commentary

Intuition, as referred to in the clinicians' first response, is a well-recognized feature of expert thinking. It typically occurs at what might be called a subconscious level, based on a general impression from a combination of patient responses and even more subtle cues conveyed in the tone of the patient's answers, demeanor and behaviour. Reflecting on such subtle patterns can be helpful to recognize and critique one's own reasoning and is critical when attempting to teach reasoning to others, as is discussed in Section 3.

The significance of any finding, whether it is a subjective feature or a physical sign, is a difficult judgment, one that often leads less-experienced therapists astray in their reasoning and management. Here the clinicians recognize quite early in the patient interview that, while local hip joint and surrounding soft tissues are incriminated by the area of symptoms and pattern of aggravation, inconsistencies in this pattern are apparent (e.g. degenerative hip joint disease, which is common in patients of this age group, is more likely to be associated with difficulties crossing the legs and squatting). Attending to features that do *not* fit the typical pattern is a characteristic of expertise. Here, even experts will proceed with a deductive or backward approach to reasoning whereby further information (subjective and physical) will be sought to test competing hypotheses while still remaining open minded to the possibility that the patient may have an atypical variation of a common disorder. The clinicians' account of this case reveals the breadth of their reasoning. Their diagnostic reasoning to determine whether manual therapy is appropriate, and if so where should treatment be directed, is obvious. However, attention is also given to the context of the patient's problem, including the effect the problem is having on her life, her understanding and feelings: what has been called her 'illness or pain experience'. This was discussed in Chapter 1 as narrative reasoning.

The other significant feature of expert reasoning evident in the clinicians' answer is their early recognition and concern regarding the worsening nature of the problem. Here, consideration to the boundaries of manual therapy intervention are starting to be formulated such that, even though the disorder presents as being mechanical and non-irritable and screening questions for red flags were negative, thought is already being given to the possible need for further medical consultation and investigation.

PHYSICAL EXAMINATION

Posture

Moya had very pronated flat feet, worse on the left side; equal leg length; protruding abdomen; forward head posture.

Functional tests

Sitting, hip flexion to remove a shoe, and sitting to standing produced no pain. In the simulated getting into the left side of a car, lifting and abducting the right leg gave a sharp catch of groin pain, but was not consistently repeatable.

Lumbar spine active movements

There was excellent lumbar mobility. Flexion (hands flat on floor) showed good spinal and hip movement and there was no pain with addition of cervical flexion. Extension had a good range but the low lumbar spine was slightly stiff; extension reproduced her right groin pain (unaltered by varying weight through the right leg). Both lateral flexions and rotations were full range and pain-free, with good intersegmental movement.

Lumbar spine passive movements

Passive intersegmental testing revealed some hypomobility but no symptom reproduction at L2–L3, L3–L4 and L4–L5 with central posteroanterior passive accessory intervertebral movement (PAIVM) testing. Unilateral posteroanterior PAIVMs on the left and right from L2 to L4 were hypomobile and on the right produced local pain only. It was considered that the PAIVM tests gave sufficient information to justify excluding passive physiological intervertebral movement tests at this stage.

Neural mobility

Straight leg raise (right and left to 90 degrees) and passive neck flexion were all pain-free; prone knee bend (PKB) on the left produced no pain (135 degrees) but on the right reproduced the groin pain and an anterior thigh pulling sensation (120 degrees).

Right hip movements

Moya was bilaterally very mobile for her age. Right hip extension was 25 degrees and reproduced her groin pain at end of range. Other active movements and combined movements were full range and pain-free.

Joint mobility

Moya's wrists, elbows, hips and knees all showed generalized joint hypermobility.

Motor control

Lumbopelvic and hip motor control, as assessed by Moya's ability to find neutral postures and control neutral while loading and dissociating limb movement, was quite good. Similarly, her ability to move her lumbar spine and hips through range and through functional tasks revealed good motor control.

Muscles

The low abdominals and hip adductors muscles were pain-free on resisted static contraction and they had full extensibility.

REASONING DISCUSSION AND CLINICAL REASONING COMMENTARY

1 Please discuss your reasoning after the physical examination with respect to the most significant physical impairments identified, sources, contributing factors and dominant pain mechanisms you hypothesized at this stage.

■ Clinicians' answer

Moya's key physical impairments were:

- hypomobility of low lumbar extension, which reproduced her right groin pain
- bilateral hypomobility of unilateral posteroanterior PAIVM tests from L2 to L4 with local pain on the right

- extreme range of extension of the right hip, which reproduced her groin pain
- right PKB was limited and reproduced her groin pain.

Hypothesized sources of the impairments were:

- lumbar spine canal stenosis involving the nerve roots in the cauda equina
- degenerative changes in the zygapophyseal joints
- hip
- neural tissues

If lumbar spine canal stenosis was occurring in the cauda equina (L1–L2 being possibilities), extension could cause groin pain by narrowing the canal of the lumbar spine and further compromising the L1–L2 nerve roots. The finding that other active movements of the lumbar spine were full and pain-free would also support the presence of canal stenosis.

Unilateral posteroanterior PAIVM tests have a more direct effect on the zygapophyseal joints than central tests. The bilateral hypomobility at L2 to L4 levels is consistent with degenerative changes in the zygapophyseal joints. Reproduction of only local pain on the right side was not consistent with the intensity or frequency of groin pain experienced by Moya when standing, walking or lying flat supine; we would have expected this test to reproduce her groin pain if the zygapophyseal joints were the source. It was hypothesized that one or two treatments applied to the right-sided joints would clarify this issue, as passive mobilization would be expected to change these joints sufficiently to cause a change in the groin pain if the pain was somatically referred from these joints.

Reproduction of Moya's groin pain by the extreme range of hip extension could implicate both the hip and neural tissues as the source of impairment, but the inconsistency of groin pain with functional movements of the hip and the lack of other hip signs suggests that the hip is a less likely source. There was a similar lack of signs in the muscles and soft tissues in the groin.

At this stage of the examination, the neural tissues were considered the likely source of this impairment. Neural movement is the likely source of limited right PKB and the reproduction of groin pain. PKB indirectly places tension on the femoral nerve (L2 to L4 spinal nerves/nerve roots), which anatomically can cause groin pain.

Contributing factors

Several factors could be contributory to Moya's problem:

- generalized peripheral joint hypermobility
- degenerative changes in the zygapophyseal joints of the lumbar spine, which contribute to spinal canal stenosis
- psychosocial issues: these were considered unlikely.

Generalized peripheral joint hypermobility requires effective muscle/motor control and while Moya's

lumbar-pelvic-hip motor control appeared to be quite good, it still may have contributed to irritation of spinal and hip structures.

Degenerative changes in the zygapophyseal joints of the lumbar spine may contribute to spinal canal stenosis. Upright activities (involving standing or walking) would further narrow the spinal canal, as would lying flat in bed.

It was considered unlikely that psychosocial issues affected her symptoms significantly. Moya was not depressed and was able to present her case in a straightforward manner without outward signs of emotion or use of exaggerated language.

Dominant pain mechanisms

The mechanisms considered likely were:

- peripheral neurogenic (L1, L2 spinal nerves) activity secondary to spinal canal stenosis
- Nociceptive stimuli related to right L2–L3, L3–L4 and L4–L5 zygapophyseal joint pathology
- central processing deficit, as indicated by inconsistent mechanical responses.

2 Were you at all surprised by the lack of any marked physical impairment in this lady's spine and hips given the degree of disability she was experiencing?

■ Clinicians' answer

More definite signs in the lumbar spine had been expected, for example a greater limitation of extension and easy reproduction of right groin pain using PAIVM tests. Such signs would have been consistent with the painful restriction of standing, walking and lying flat supine.

The lack of physical impairments, in the face of Moya's disability, in both the somatic tissues underlying the area of groin pain and in the spinal tissues that can somatically refer to the groin led to the consideration of more serious pathology within the spinal canal or a central pain mechanism.

■ Clinical reasoning commentary

As discussed in Chapter 1, clinical reasoning throughout the physical examination should be an extension of the reasoning undertaken during the subjective examination or interview. Specific impairments and structures hypothesized as possibly being involved are tested further during the routine assessments of posture; active, passive and resistive movement; and neural and motor control. In this case, inconsistencies noted during the subjective examination are evident in the physical examination. While this has not resulted in complete rejection of the structures initially postulated as possibly being involved, it has strengthened the previous concerns regarding more serious pathology and elicited a reconsideration of the dominant pain mechanism. The clinicians' reference to 'expected' findings reflects their testing of hypotheses, an example of 'reflection-in-action', a recognized attribute of experts (Schön, 1983, 1987). Hypothesis testing is also seen to continue throughout the management, as evident here in the practitioners' plans to treat and reassess the effect of zygapophyseal joint mobilization. The evolving nature of expert reasoning is clearly evident.

Initial management

Initial treatment was carried out at three visits over 6 days.

Treatment (day 1)

Passive mobilization (right and left unilateral posteroanterior PAIVMs (grades IV and III) was used to mobilize L2–L5 but not to produce any referred groin pain (Maitland, 1986). Following this, there was increased low lumbar movement on active extension but the groin pain provoked was unchanged, as it also was on active hip extension and PKB.

Treatment 2 (day 3)

Subjective examination reassessment

There was no flare in symptoms after treatment. Her symptoms and functional activities were unaltered.

Physical examination reassessment

There continued to be no difficulty with sitting to standing but sitting hip flexion to take off her shoe caused a catch of sharp groin pain (not repeatable). The range of active lumbar extension was maintained. Lumbar intersegmental tests still revealed hypomobility of right L2–L5 zygapophyseal joints, with only local pain produced on firm stretching. Right hip extension and PKB were unaltered.

Intervention

Lumbar rotary mobilization was applied to both sides as a mixture of grades III and IV. Following this, the right zygapophyseal joints were more mobile on PAIVM testing. This was further improved with two applications for 45 seconds of right unilateral posteroanterior PAIVMs grade IV− and IV+, which produced only local pain (Maitland, 1986). Hip extension and PKB remained unaltered.

Treatment 3 (day 6)

Subjective examination reassessment

Moya reported a good day following the last treatment: less catching groin pain with daily activities. However, standing and walking were unchanged, as were her symptoms subsequently.

Physical examination reassessment

Lumbar extension, plus combinations of extension, lateral flexion and rotation, no longer caused groin pain. Intersegmental PAIVM tests were the same on both sides. Hip extension and PKB remained unaltered.

Intervention

In prone lying, three applications of hip extension (grade IV+ as a strong, sustained (60 seconds) stretch) were applied and provoked a moderate degree of groin pain. Knee flexion was kept at 90 degrees during the procedure. Following this, the range of hip extension increased from 25 to 35 degrees with only a pulling feeling in the groin. PKB increased slightly (125 degrees) but this still reproduced anterior thigh pulling and groin pain; through-range resistance was greater than on the left side.

REASONING DISCUSSION AND CLINICAL REASONING COMMENTARY

1 Were you at all concerned about using strong mobilization in an elderly lady, with respect to osteoporosis and an unknown, potentially serious, spinal pathology that may involve canal narrowing?

■ Clinicians' answer

No. Moya showed no obvious signs of osteoporosis such as upper thoracic kyphosis, and the general screening questions were negative.

The rotary mobilization was performed carefully to limit the movement to the lumbar spine and to place minimal stress on the thoracic spine: that is, the thoracic spine was stabilized in a neutral position. The unilateral posteroanterior mobilization was performed to stretch the hypomobile zygapophyseal joints on the right side. While these mobilizations were firmly applied, they were not vigorous and the symptomatic response during application was continuously monitored.

It was important to produce sufficient change in the range and pain response of the lumbar intervertebral joints to establish whether they were a source of groin pain and whether an increased range of lumbar extension would increase Moya's ability to stand and walk for a longer time. These answers were needed as quickly as possible because of the worsening symptoms. Should manual therapy not be useful, then further investigations would be needed.

2 Please discuss briefly what prompted you to change your treatment from techniques directed to the lumbar spine to those directed to the hip, commenting on what you were aiming to achieve.

■ Clinicians' answer

The aims of treatment were to confirm the source(s) of the groin pain and, if possible, to treat it mechanically.

At first, passive mobilization of the lumbar spine, using central and unilateral (on both sides) posteroanterior techniques, was aimed at improving the range of lumbar extension so that there would be more extension range available for standing, walking and flat supine lying. This treatment effected an increase in the pain-free range of lumbar extension.

The next treatment, using rotary mobilization and right-sided unilateral posteroanterior pressures, was directed at improving the pain-free range of the right L2–L3, L3–L4 and L4–L5 zygapophyseal joints. This resulted in full-range pain-free lumbar extension.

These results were considered sufficient to demonstrate definite changes in the groin pain and to determine whether the hip extension and PKB signs were related to the lumbar spine. After 3 days, there was no significant change in the latter parameters; therefore, treatment next involved hip extension stretches. By stretching the hip into extension, it was intended to confirm that the hip joint was not the source of groin pain and to demonstrate any relationship between the hip joint and the range and pain response of the PKB test of neural mobility.

■ Clinical reasoning commentary

While the body of research-based evidence regarding validation of musculoskeletal clinical patterns is limited, the research-based evidence regarding treatment progression is virtually non-existent. Therefore, manual therapists must rely more on empirical experience-based evidence to guide these judgments. Treatment procedures must have clear aims and reassessment must be thorough and regular for definitive decisions to be reached. In this case, the clinicians describe the progression of mobilization being made with care (i.e. awareness of relevant precautions and selection of a procedure that was judged to be safe) and with the specific aim of determining the relevance of the spinal findings to the patient's groin pain, hip signs and neural signs. All treatment interventions, including hands-on manual therapy, have both physical and psychological influences. Nevertheless, when performed with awareness of the broader psychosocial presentation, specific procedures delivered and reassessed for a specific purpose (e.g. increased local segmental mobility and decreased local mechanical sensitivity) enable clinicians to gauge the 'mechanical' nature of the problem and the appropriateness of continuing such treatment.

Reassessment and further treatment

Treatment 4 (day 9)

Subjective examination reassessment

Moya reported some improvement in her groin pain, but overall it was unchanged, especially with standing and walking. On further questioning, she said she could not alter her groin pain by varying her standing posture or varying her stride length.

Physical examination reassessment

Functional tests revealed sharp groin pain with standing from sitting and abduction of the right hip, but these were not repeatable. The extreme range of hip extension caused groin pain, as did PKB at 125 degrees.

Interventions

The first intervention was right hip extension with firm stretching (as a grade IV+ and IV−) and then repeated with the addition of abduction and then adduction (Maitland, 1991). This restored full-range painless passive hip extension but PKB was unchanged.

The second intervention was a right PKB applied as a grade III− large-amplitude oscillatory mobilization without, and then with, 20 degrees of hip extension (Maitland, 1991). On both occasions, strong groin pain ('her pain') was produced. Retesting PKB showed a slight increase in range from 125 degrees to 135 degrees, with groin pain and anterior thigh pulling reproduced through the last 15 degrees. Tissue resistance was unchanged, being first felt at 110 degrees.

Treatment 5 (day 11)

Subjective examination reassessment

There was no change in symptoms associated with standing and walking and the symptoms still eased within 5 minutes with sitting. However, catches of sharp groin pain were definitely less frequent.

Physical examination reassessment

Right hip extension was full range with a slight pull in the groin. Right PKB was tight from 110 to 130 degrees with groin pain unchanged (120–130 degrees).

Intervention

With the right hip in full extension, five large-amplitude strong PKB (grade III+) stretches were applied. Strong groin pain was produced with each stretch and afterwards there was a constant ache in the groin. PKB increased to 140 degrees with minimal pain (now equal to the left side) but tissue resistance was only minimally changed. PKB was not altered by cervical flexion or extension.

Moya was asked to cease treatment for 2 weeks (unless her symptoms worsened) to allow the effect of treatment to be assessed.

Treatment 6 (day 25)

Subjective examination reassessment

This was also a retrospective assessment. Moya considered her right groin pain to be unchanged since before commencing treatment. Her ability to stand remained at 10–15 minutes before she needed to sit to relieve her pain. Walking was the same (15–20 minutes) and she still needed three pillows in order to remain pain-free during the night. The sharp catches of groin pain were about 30% better since treatment, but she could not specifically attribute this to treatment of the lumbar spine, hip joint or neural structures.

Physical examination reassessment

Active lumbar spine extension was full range and painless and intersegmental PAIVM testing revealed similar mobility on both the left and right sides. Right hip extension was full range and pain-free on overpressure. Right PKB remained tight (110–125 degrees) and still reproduced her groin pain.

Intervention

We explained to Moya that the examination had found insufficient abnormalities to account for the disability caused by her right groin pain. Stiffness of her low back joints and right hip extension had been significantly improved by manual therapy but these changes had not resulted in improvement in her ability to stand, walk or to lie flat in supine. Treatment had not improved the tightness in the neural tissues to the right leg. It was noted that no radiographs had been taken to date and that these might prove helpful in diagnosing her problem.

It was agreed that a letter would be sent to her GP suggesting further investigations. This letter outlined the lack of examination findings and that treatment directed to the lumbar spine, right hip and right-sided neural structures had not significantly altered her symptoms. Further investigations were suggested. A follow-up telephone call was made to the GP a week later. The GP agreed with the need for further investigations and said that he had referred Moya to an orthopaedic surgeon. The GP also said he would report on the findings and future management.

REASONING DISCUSSION AND CLINICAL REASONING COMMENTARY

1 Determining how much change is sufficient to warrant continued treatment must be one of the most difficult reasoning decisions manual therapists must make. Would you briefly discuss, in the context of Moya's response to your various treatments, the key features that led you to discontinue treatment and seek further investigations at this stage?

determining whether a decision could be made regarding the cessation of manual therapy and referral back to her GP. With Moya, there was no definite change in the groin pain associated with the functional activities despite a marked improvement in lumbar and hip signs. Of more significance was the lack of improvement in the range of motion and through-range resistance of the PKB test despite strong stretching. It could be hypothesized that the tethering of the neural tissue was elsewhere along the neuraxis.

■ Clinicians' answer

From the initial examination, the worsening of the right groin pain (despite Moya decreasing activities that provoked the pain) was a source of concern. Lumbar spinal canal stenosis was hypothesized and it was considered that a CAT scan or MRI scan would likely be needed to establish the pathology.

It was, therefore, planned to establish as quickly as possible whether manual therapy could effect a change in the consistent functional aggravating factors of standing, walking and certain sleeping postures.

Screening questions provided no contraindications to treatment; however, the lack of radiological examination of the lumbar spine, pelvis and hip was kept in mind. Therefore, so long as her symptoms were not worsened by treatment, it was planned to use techniques to effect sufficient change in the lumbar signs to be able to expect a definite change in standing, walking and sleeping postures, and to demonstrate any relationship with the hip extension and PKB test findings.

It was the extent of change in the lumbar signs (intersegmental mobility/pain response), hip signs and neural signs, rather than the rate or extent of change in the functional activities listed above, which guided the time spent in treating the various areas and

■ Clinical reasoning commentary

Strategic use of a break from treatment (2 weeks in this case) and careful subjective and physical examination and retrospective reassessment enabled the clinicians to confirm their earlier suspicion/hypothesis that the patient's symptoms and activity/participation restrictions were not caused by straightforward impairment in the lumbar spine or hip tissues. Importantly, treatments provided during the first five visits, while performed with care, were definitive, allowing the final decision regarding further medical consultation and investigation to be reached as quickly as possible. Trial treatments of this nature are critical to determine the appropriateness of continued manual therapy and to be able to inform the referring doctor so that further medical interventions can proceed with confidence and the knowledge that a simpler musculoskeletal source of the symptoms has been eliminated. This course of action may contrast with that undertaken by a less-expert clinician, who is more likely to persist with manual treatment on the basis of improved lumbar signs, with undesirable consequences of delayed appropriate management.

Assessment by medical practitioner

The GP telephoned to report that he had sent Moya to two orthopaedic surgeons. The first had plain radiographs taken of her lumbar spine, pelvis and hips and a CAT scan of her lumbar spine. The radiographs showed advanced arthritic changes bilaterally of her mid/low lumbar zygapophyseal joints and that both hips were reported as having minor degenerative changes. The CAT scan showed only minor narrowing of the spinal canal. The surgeon gave her an epidural injection that afforded no relief of symptoms. He advised that nothing further should be done; however, Moya wanted the matter explored further.

The second orthopaedic surgeon injected Moya's right L2–L3, L3–L4 and L4–L5 zygapophyseal joints with steroids, following which she had a reduction in the right groin pain for 3 days only; repeat injections 6 weeks later were of no benefit.

It was agreed that no further treatment be given at this stage and that both the GP and Moya should monitor her symptoms.

REASONING DISCUSSION

1 How did you interpret her lack of any lasting change from the surgeons' injections?

Clinicians' answer

If indeed, there was only minor narrowing of the lumbar spinal canal, then an epidural injection might not be expected to relieve her symptoms. The clinical pattern was highly suggestive of spinal canal stenosis, which is the likely reason why an epidural injection was given.

The short-term relief from intra-articular injections into the L2–L3, L3–L4 and L4–L5 zygapophyseal joints may have resulted from the effect of the local anaesthetic, which is incorporated with the steroid, or it may have been a short-term placebo effect. The lack of a lasting improvement also may reflect that the source of her pain was not within the lumbar spinal canal or zygapophyseal joints.

Re-presentation for treatment

Moya referred herself for more treatment 7 months later. She corroborated the details in her GP's report of the investigations and outcomes of treatment by the two orthopaedic surgeons.

Moya reported that for the last 5 months she had experienced more constant right groin pain with the same pattern as before, namely a marked increase with standing more than 10 minutes or walking for 15 minutes. Sitting still eased the pain within a few minutes. Then last week, suddenly for no apparent reason, the pain became bilateral and spread to the anteromedial aspects of both thighs and to the shin on the left when severe.

When questioned, she also experienced deep central aching in the low cervical, low thoracic and low back areas, which she described as minor compared with her groin pains. She had no other leg symptoms and bladder and bowel functions were normal.

Functionally, her groin pains interfered with her sleep and her GP had prescribed analgesics and a sleeping tablet. She slept in the sitting position with three pillows; supine lying was more comfortable than on her sides. To get out of bed on the left side to go to the toilet was extremely painful in both groins, left more than right. She was unable to stand erect for more than 5–10 minutes because of bilateral groin pain and a dull low back ache. Sitting eased the pain in less than 5 minutes and she spent most of the day sitting in an armchair. Standing was worse first thing in the morning (but with no stiffness) and in the evenings, and she tended to be bent forward for the first few steps.

The groin pain seemed unrelated to her hip movements.

REASONING DISCUSSION AND CLINICAL REASONING COMMENTARY

1 What was your interpretation of the worsening nature of her symptoms and disability?

Clinicians' answer

The sudden worsening of symptoms was most concerning regarding the likely pathology. It was decided to perform a thorough physical examination, being careful not to provoke her groin/anterior thigh pain and to ask Moya to bring her radiographs and reports at the next visit. The provision of manual therapy treatment would be governed by these findings and a discussion with her GP.

Moya's responses to the subjective examination suggested a spinal canal source as indicated by:

- the change to a bilateral problem, now worse on the opposite side
- the distribution of pain, which was consistent with a L2–L4 neurogenic source (but with no bladder/bowel changes at this stage)
- unilateral movements of the left hip causing bilateral groin pain
- the unchanging behaviour of symptoms, that is, consistent with changes in anteroposterior diameter of the spinal canal
- the sudden onset of symptoms for no apparent reason, which does not support the joints/muscles of the legs as the cause

- concomitant low cervical, low thoracic and low lumbar aching, which may suggest pathology affecting the structures and contents of the spinal canal anywhere from the cervical spine to the lumbar spine regions.

The pain mechanism was strongly neurogenic with a mixture of central and peripheral symptoms, the former accounting for a less clear picture of cause and response to mechanical stimuli.

Clinical reasoning commentary

With recognition of a worsening problem and potentially significant if not sinister pathology, the decision was made to make a further thorough physical examination, to correlate with the now consistent subjective pattern of presentation. The potential seriousness of the disorder has been respected and will guide the care planned for the physical testing. No assumptions have been made that the physical findings will necessarily be the same after 7 months; their careful reassessment will provide a fuller picture of any physical impairments that may be present, including any relationship to the original and new symptoms. In this way, more informed decisions regarding the appropriateness of further rehabilitation (via manual therapy or other means) and medical investigation can be made.

PHYSICAL EXAMINATION

Standing from sitting caused bilateral groin pain, which was unaltered by the degree of weight-bearing through each leg or by altering hip rotation.

Lumbar spine active movements

Flexion and flexion plus cervical flexion were full range and did not alter the groin pains. Extension and both lateral flexions were full range and caused a low back ache centrally. There was no groin or anterior thigh pain with passive overpressure added. Passive intersegmental PAIVM testing showed no focal

hypomobility or pain, but rather generalized hypomobility from L2 to L5.

Left and right hip movements

Left and right hip movements were full range and pain-free.

Neurological examination

No abnormality was detected in neural conduction of the lower limbs. There was no ankle clonus, hypertonicity or hyperreflexia, and plantar responses were normal.

Neural mobility

Left and right straight leg raises were 80 degrees with no pain provoked, including with the addition of passive neck flexion, ankle plantarflexion/inversion or ankle dorsiflexion. PKB on the left was 100 degrees and produced a pulling feeling on the anterior thigh with groin pain. Right PKB was 120 degrees with an anterior thigh pulling sensation and abnormal resistance to movement between 100 and 120 degrees.

Slump testing

Slump testing caused severe anterior neck pain with the addition of cervical flexion to trunk flexion, so cervical flexion was released short of pain provocation. Left knee extension lacked 10 degrees but produced no pain, and added left ankle dorsiflexion was full range and painless. Right leg testing was normal.

Effect of examination

Afterwards Moya reported that she felt dizzy and unwell. Further examination, especially of the cervical spine, was considered contraindicated in the light of the unknown and worsening pathology. After 30 minutes of resting in the half-lying supine position, her dizziness and unwell feeling had settled and she went home. She was asked to bring her radiographs at the next treatment.

■ Further examination

Moya returned 2 days later for a further examination.

Subjective examination reassessment

Moya reported feeling disorientated and had tachycardia for the rest of the day following the previous examination; the next day she felt unwell and lethargic. On detailed questioning, she admitted having had this feeling several times in the last 2 months, including a feeling of poor balance. She had not experienced the anterior neck pain before or since the last appointment. Because of her past experience of a feeling of poor balance, detailed questioning of the presence and behaviour of upper quarter symptoms was conducted. She

described bilateral numbness in her hands and difficulty with fine finger movements such as doing up buttons and tying shoelaces. These symptoms had come on for no known reason in the last 3 months; she felt these symptoms were slowly worsening but had not consulted her GP. Moya reported that she did not have her radiographs and that they were held at the GP's clinic.

Physical examination reassessment

It was decided to undertake a neurological examination of the upper and lower extremities as a priority.

Neurological examination of the upper extremities

There was loss of sensation to light touch over the whole of both hands, but sensation to pinprick was variable: diminished in some areas and hypersensitive in other parts of the hands. Upper limb reflexes were exaggerated. Asterognosis (loss of ability to recognize shapes when held) was present in both hands. There was no increased tonus, but there was weakness of all muscles in both her arms.

Neurological examination of the lower extremities

No abnormality was detected.

Intervention

At this point, it was obvious that Moya should receive urgent medical investigation of her neurological status. No further examination was undertaken; this included reassessment of the lumbar and neural mobility signs and examination of the cervical spine as the findings were unlikely to shed light on the likely pathology or alter the need for urgent medical investigation and management.

An explanation was given to Moya that she had symptoms and signs of 'nerve involvement' in her arms that could be originating from her cervical spine, and that there could be a connection between this and her groin/thigh pains. Further medical investigations were needed and an appointment was made for her to see her GP that day. Moya took a letter for the GP that outlined the examination findings.

REASONING DISCUSSION AND CLINICAL REASONING COMMENTARY

1 What was your interpretation of the severe reaction to the slump test?

Clinicians' answer

At the time of performing the slump test, the production of severe anterior neck pain could not be definitively interpreted. However, because of the worsening symptoms and signs in the presence of unknown pathology, it was not considered prudent to repeat the test but rather to lessen the cervical flexion so that the effect of caudal mobility tests on the neural tissues could be explored.

At the second appointment, the matter was explored further. The presence of what sounded like cervical spinal cord symptoms felt bilaterally in the upper limbs strengthened the likely relationship between cervical spinal cord pathology and pain felt on the addition of cervical flexion to the slump test.

2 What was your interpretation of these most recent neurological findings?

Clinicians' answer

The neurological examination confirmed a bilateral pattern of cervical spinal cord compressive signs that extended from C4 to T1. This suggested a lesion somewhere in the vicinity of C4 that involved both sensory and motor tracts to the upper limbs but spared those to the lower limbs.

Clinical reasoning commentary

As we have seen in other cases in this book, an important decision clinicians face is whether further manual therapy management is warranted. Here the neurological findings combined with the worsening nature of the symptoms dictated the decision to initiate further medical consultation and not recommence any physical rehabilitation at this stage. Red flags (Roberts, 2000) and their associated implications are an essential part of a manual therapist's knowledge base.

Outcome

Moya was referred to a neurologist who diagnosed C3–C4 myelopathy and subsequent MRI confirmed a huge osteophyte protruding from the posterior aspect of C4 and indenting the spinal cord by more than 50% (Fig. 20.1). Degenerative changes were present in the cord at this level. Similar, but less-marked changes were noted at C5–C6. A neurosurgeon removed the osteophytes and fused both areas.

Six months after the cervical fusion, the neurologist referred Moya for assistance with poor balance on walking. He noted that her neurological deficit was stable, but that without the surgery she would have become a quadriplegic.

Of special interest was the fact that Moya had experienced no further groin or anteromedial thigh pain immediately following the surgery. On examination, PKB on both sides was 140 degrees with only anterior thigh stretching felt and the through-range resistance previously felt was no longer present.

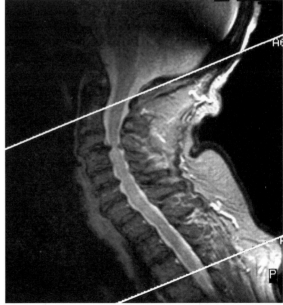

Fig. 20.1 Magnetic resonance image demonstrating a large osteophyte protruding from the posterior aspect of C4 into the spinal canal and indenting the spinal cord.

Moya remains free of groin and thigh symptoms. She presents every 6 months or so for treatment for her occipitofrontal headaches, which are mostly occipitoatlantal joint in origin.

REASONING DISCUSSION AND CLINICAL REASONING COMMENTARY

1 With the advantage of hindsight, do you consider there were any features of this lady's presentation when she initially presented to you that you may have over- or underweighted?

▇ Clinicians' answer

Yes, with hindsight, by the fourth visit more weight should have been placed on the role of a central pain mechanism for her groin pain. The focus was more on the consistent effects of standing, walking and half-lying supine, and to a lesser extent on the many times in the day that she inconsistently felt sharp groin pain with activities. The significance of the fact that the range and through-range resistance of PKB changed very little, even with strong stretching, was also undervalued. It should have flagged the need to consider tethering of neural tissues at a more proximal site.

Also, reflection on the MRI scan results and finding at surgery provided a likely explanation for the severe pain experienced with the slump test. During flexion, the contents of the spinal canal are drawn more tightly against the vertebral column and, therefore, against the protruding large osteophyte at C3–C4 (Grieve, 1981).

2 Could you discuss your thoughts on why this patient had relevant cervical pathology but no upper quarter symptoms until the last 3 to 4 months? Also, why do you think some early treatments produced changes in her groin symptoms and signs if the source was in fact cervical pathology?

▇ Clinicians' answer

Degenerative changes per se need not cause local or referred symptoms. In contrast with the lumbar spine, the cervical spinal canal is relatively large and can, therefore, accommodate osteophytes from the zygapophyseal joints or vertebral bodies (Grieve, 1981). In Moya's case, the posterior osteophytes were midline and, therefore, did not impinge upon or irritate more laterally placed nerve roots.

Improved range of the lumbar zygapophyseal joints and the hip joint was an expected outcome of end-range passive mobilization; however, there was no consistent improvement in groin pain associated with daily activities. The lack of consistent response was most likely a consequence of a dominant central pain mechanism related to cervical myelopathy.

▇ Clinical reasoning commentary

Reflection, as generously shared here, is the means by which manual therapists learn from their own experiences. It is easy to assume that the expert, being an 'expert', does not make 'errors' and resolves all patients' problems. As all the experts contributing cases to this book will acknowledge, this is far from the truth. Experts, like everyone, do make errors. The difference perhaps is their ability to learn from their errors, which we believe is closely linked to their metacognitive skills, be they deliberate or intuitive. It is through this process of continual reflection and critique that experts modify their future interpretations, acquire new patterns and develop variations of management strategies.

▇ References

Grieve, G.P. (1981). Common Vertebral Joint Problems, Edinburgh: Churchill Livingstone.

Maitland, G.D. (1986). Vertebral Manipulation, 5th edn. Oxford: Butterworths.

Maitland, G.D. (1991). Peripheral Manipulation, 3rd edn. Oxford: Butterworths.

Roberts, L. (2000). Flagging the danger signs of low back pain. In Topical Issues of Pain 2. Biopsychosocial Assessment. Relationships and Pain (L. Gifford, ed.) pp. 69–83. Falmouth,

MA: CNS Press.

Schön, D. (1983). The Reflective Practitioner: How Professionals Think in Action. New York: Basic Books.

Schön, D. (1987). Educating the Reflective Practitioner. San Francisco, CA: Jossey-Bass.

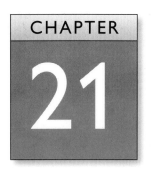

CHAPTER

21

Chronic peripartum pelvic pain

John van der Meij,
Andry Vleeming and Jan Mens

 SUBJECTIVE EXAMINATION

Maree, aged 34 years, was referred to the outpatient clinic at the Spine and Joint Centre (SJC) in Rotterdam, the Netherlands. She complained of persistent, deep pelvic pain described as stabbing, pressing and burning. The pain was worse over the left posterior superior iliac spine (PSIS) and gluteal region, with some pain left of the pubic symphysis and coccyx. There was pain referred into the ventral and dorsal aspects of the left leg as far as the knee joint. The pain was accompanied by a tingling sensation throughout the entire left leg (Fig. 21.1).

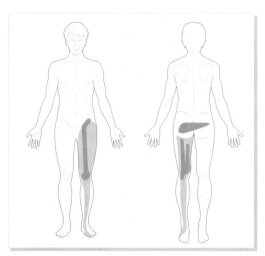

Fig. 21.1 Map of the patient's symptoms. The darker shaded areas represent pain and the lighter shaded areas represent the tingling sensation.

Her complaints were provoked by turning in bed, sitting (particularly in a flexed lumbar spine position), moving from sitting to standing, standing for longer than 4 minutes, and walking or lying supine for more than 10 minutes. Changing position gave partial relief for a short time. Maree slept, on average, only 2 hours per night because of the pain. There was no particular time of the day when the complaints were worse. However, in the week prior to menstruation her pain increased and her stamina decreased. Maree took sleep medication and occasionally paracetamol to relieve the pain. There were no problems with her general health, including no current or past history of gastroenterological or gynaecological conditions. In addition, there was no current or past history of fractures, neoplasms, inflammatory disease, or previous surgery or problems of the lumbar spine or pelvis.

Maree's complaints began in the fifth month of her first pregnancy, slowly increased until she gave birth 6 months prior to the interview, and continued to persist, with an exacerbation whilst attending a symposium 2 months earlier that involved prolonged sitting. She had been seen by numerous individual healthcare practitioners. From these practitioners, she received conflicting suggestions and information concerning treatment and explanations for her symptoms. Although her response to passive treatment was variable, no single treatment was consistently effective.

REASONING DISCUSSION AND CLINICAL REASONING COMMENTARY

1 What were your first impressions of Maree's presentation, with respect to both biomedical and psychosocial considerations?

Clinicians' answer

The first impression was that Maree was desperate and that she had used all her energy to escape from her situation. The more she fought, the worse she was trapped in a vicious cycle of physical dysfunction, pain, fatigue, and depression.

The relationship of the onset of her pain with her pregnancy was also considered important. Pain in the lumbar spine and pelvic region is a common complication of pregnancy and delivery, with the reported 9-month prevalence rate during pregnancy ranging from 48 to 56% (Berg et al., 1988; Fast et al., 1987; Östgaard et al., 1991). In studies of young and middle-aged women with chronic low back pain, 10–28% state that their first episode of back pain occurred during pregnancy (Svensson et al., 1990).

2 How did the conflicting messages that the patient had received from the various individual health-care practitioners influence her behaviour, particularly with regard to a potential collaborative approach to her problems?

Clinicians' answer

She was greatly disturbed by the lack of clarity from the various health-care services, including a lack of a distinct diagnosis. In general, the conflicting messages tended to worsen the prognosis and complicate the situation, particularly as Maree was greatly distressed. For instance, advice to rest in bed gave her some temporary relief from pain but probably increased her muscle weakness. In contrast, performing prescribed exercises sometimes resulted in more pain in the short term but likely improved her muscle strength. However, by alternating between bedrest and exercise, the end result may well have been both increased muscle weakness and increased pain, in combination with physical and psychological exhaustion.

A consistent, collaborative approach was considered more desirable. At the SJC we specialize in the multidisciplinary management of chronic low back and posterior pelvic pain (PPP) starting during pregnancy or within 6 weeks after delivery, and with a duration of more than 6 months. The patients we see have been treated elsewhere predominantly with structure-directed therapies that have failed, such as in the case of Maree. We overcome the issue of conflicting messages by employing a multifactorial and integrated treatment approach, and by attempting to make sense of seemingly non-related complaints. Our approach can be described as follows (Vleeming, 1998).

> In medicine there is generally an evolutionary pattern that starts with the study of symptoms and signs. From that level, it becomes feasible to analyse the relations between symptoms and to describe a syndrome. With advancing knowledge, a more causal pathophysiological explanation can be found that describes the underlying mechanism.
>
> The physical path predominantly taken to study the locomotor system is mainly based on topographic anatomy that reduces systems into simple parts. Structures such as bones, muscles, nerves, etc. are studied in isolation, which does not allow sufficient insight into the complexities of the function of the human locomotor system. The practical consequence for patients often is that kinematic systems are analysed and diagnosed at tissue level, using increasingly sophisticated technology to search for quantifiable physical impairments, mainly producing a description of symptoms. Frequently, this search does not aim to reach a specific diagnosis but to exclude serious causes of lumbopelvic pain. If the 'impaired' structure can be identified, predominantly single modality treatment is indicated to solve the problem, without sufficient consideration of the consequences for the kinematic system as a whole. If structural identification fails, patients are easily classified as suffering from non-specific low back pain or a psychosomatic problem.

The above quotation emphasizes that single modality approaches based on limited or restricted theoretical constructs do not provide an ideal means of management for patients with chronic lumbopelvic pain. Pelvic pain comprises physiological, psychological and behavioural dimensions, which inter-relate with one another. Patients with pelvic pain, such as Maree, require an integrated multifactorial approach in which one of the main goals is to restore the patient's control over his or her own body and life. Both practitioners and patients may need to participate in a paradigm shift from a medical model to a self-healing model in which a 'hands-off' approach involving self-management and education is essential, rather than the practitioner actually 'solving' the patient's problem (McIndoe, 1995).

Patients with chronic pelvic pain are restricted in daily activities as a result of persisting dysfunctions in the human locomotor system combined with psychosocial factors (e.g. counterproductive beliefs, inadequate coping strategies and dysfunctional social interactions). Because of the chronicity and complexity of the pelvic problems of patients who present to the SJC, a biopsychosocial approach offers the best possibility for recovery. This certainly seems to be the case for Maree.

Clinical reasoning commentary

It is apparent that the initial clinical reasoning evident in these responses is very broad and beyond just the typical diagnostic/structural reasoning likely to have been applied to Maree's problems in the past. Indeed, there is obvious confidence that considering the patient's activity/participation capabilities/restrictions, in addition to the factors that have contributed to the maintenance of her problems, will result in a more complete and holistic understanding of the patient's presentation and will likely lead to an optimal resolution. From previous clinical experience and from the literature—that is, non-propositional knowledge and propositional knowledge—the errors associated with only employing diagnostically driven clinical reasoning with such a complex presentation are avoided. It is also quite clear that there has already been some consideration given to the management strategies to be employed, including the addressing of psychological impairments through education and empowerment, as well as specific physical impairments.

PHYSICAL EXAMINATION

Biomedical evaluation

Routine blood and urine tests were negative.

Neurological examination

There were no signs indicating radiculopathy (e.g. asymmetric tendon reflexes, altered sensation in a radicular pattern).

Load transfer

The active straight leg raise (SLR) test was used to assess instability caused by a disturbed load transfer from the trunk to the legs (Mens et al., 1997, 1999). The test is carried out with the patient in supine lying. The patient is asked to lift one leg so that the heel lies 20 cm above the couch. The active SLR test is positive for disturbed load transfer if the patient is unable to lift the leg or if the patient experiences diminished strength. The test is repeated while the patient is wearing a pelvic belt, which has been shown to have a stabilizing effect on the pelvis (Mens et al., 1997, 1999; Vleeming et al., 1995)

(Fig. 21.2). In the case of impairment of the self-bracing mechanism, it will be easier to lift the leg while wearing the belt. Maree was unable to perform a left active SLR because of weakness but application of a pelvic belt partially restored her strength.

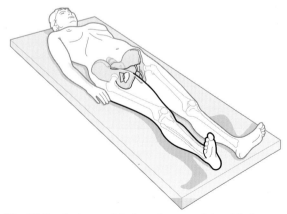

Fig. 21.2 Active straight leg raise test of the right leg. The OS pubis on the right is located a few mm lower than the left.

For patients with pain in the pelvic region, contraction of the hip abductor and adductor muscles is also often painful and weak. In healthy women, the mean adduction force is 214 N, compared with 117 N in the PPP patients of the SJC, while the mean abduction forces are 284 N and 184 N, respectively. The forces are measured with a small device (Microfet, Hoggan Health Industries Inc., Draper, UT, USA) that digitally displays peak force (van Meeteren et al., 1997). In this case, isometric hip adduction was measured maximally at 57 N and caused pain in the pubic symphysis region. Isometric hip abduction was measured maximally at 146 N.

Pain provocation tests

Attempts have been made to assess impairment of pelvic joints in an objective manner, but manual mobility tests tend to lack intertester and intratester reliability (Mens et al., 1999; Potter and Rothstein, 1985). The most popular measurements in clinical back and pelvic pain research are pain provocation tests. These tests determine the degree of irritation of ligaments in the pelvic girdle and the lumbosacral region. Two of the best validated provocation tests are the PPP provocation test (PPPP test) (Östgaard et al., 1994; Potter and Rothstein, 1985) and the tenderness test for the long dorsal sacroiliac ligament (LDL) (Vleeming et al., 1998).

The PPPP test is performed with the patient supine and her hip flexed to 90 degrees. The patient's femur is gently pressed posteriorly by the examiner (Fig. 21.3). The test is positive when the patient feels pain in the posterior part of the pelvis. Examination of Maree revealed that the PPPP test was positive on the left side. Palpation of the LDL was painful at its PSIS attachment.

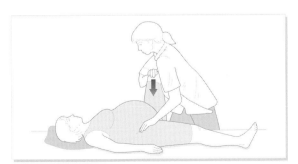

Fig. 21.3 The posterior pelvic pain provocation test. (From Östgaard et al., 1994, p. 258. Reproduced with kind permission of the publishers.)

Active movements

Lumbar spine flexion demonstrated loss of range of motion of about 20 degrees, possibly caused by severe pain in the left PSIS. Lumbar spine extension showed a slight loss of range of motion, with pain provoked in the left gluteal region. Passive left hip flexion and external rotation were decreased approximately 5–10 degrees in comparison with the right side, possibly because of left-sided pubic symphysis and pelvic pain.

Hypertonia of the left hip adductors was detected. This was found by passively moving the leg into abduction: tension of the adductors could be seen and felt as soon as the movement was initiated. However, when Maree was asked to relax her muscles and the movement was performed gently it was possible to gain almost full range.

Muscle assessment

Poor recruitment of the transversus abdominis muscle was detected. This was found by instructing the patient to perform abdominal hollowing in the supine lying position. During this action, the tone of the muscle was palpated near its insertion to the ilium (Jull et al., 1998; Richardson and Jull, 1995).

Assessment of functional capacity of the trunk and pelvis was performed with the Isostation B-200 (Isotechnologies Inc., Hillsborough, NC, USA) (Gomez et al., 1991) and by the use of video analysis (van Wingerden et al., 1995). The B-200 records data on the mobility of the low back in three directions of movement, and also on isometric forces of the trunk and pelvis. In order to record lumbar and pelvic motion, infrared markers and video cameras are used. Preliminary research results at the SJC show a distinct lumbopelvic rhythm, which differs between healthy subjects and patients with low back pain.

In a study of 57 healthy male and female subjects, the relative contributions of the lumbar spine and hip joint to forward bending were measured using the video analysis method (van Wingerden et al., 1997). The results showed a significant homogeneous motion pattern. In the initial part of forward bending, the lumbar spine is responsible, on average, for 66% of the motion, compared with 34% for flexion of the hip joint. This indicates that in this phase of motion the angular displacement of the lumbar spine is almost twice as fast as the angular rotation of the hip joint. In the middle part of the motion, the lumbar spine slows down while the hip joint increases its angular speed. In the final phase of forward bending, lumbar motion constitutes 27% of the movement, compared with 73% for hip motion. From the erect posture to maximal forward bending, the ranges of motion of the lumbar spine and hip joint are 58 and 54 degrees, respectively.

In an additional study (J.P. van Wingerden, A. Vleeming, G.J. Kleinrensink and R. Stoeckart, unpublished data) of 31 patients with chronic low back pain, the contribution of the lumbar spine during the first phase of foward bending was decreased (55%), whereas the contribution in the final phase was increased (37%). In this group, the ranges of motion of the lumbar spine and hip joint from the erect posture to maximal forward bending were 45 and 52 degrees, respectively.

For Maree, the isometric torque strength of the spinal and pelvic musculature measured using the Isostation B-200 showed homogeneous but very weak muscles during flexion, extension, side bending and rotation. The values of the isometric torque strength for Maree were 45–69% below the acceptable level (i.e. 10th percentile of the value for healthy women).

Passive movement testing

There was reduced general mobility and increased muscular tension of the upper cervical spine, cervicothoracic junction, mid-thoracic spine, lower lumbar spine and left sacroiliac joint (SIJ). When performing these general passive accessory and physiological mobility tests, Maree reacted with pain and anxiety.

REASONING DISCUSSION AND CLINICAL REASONING COMMENTARY

1 What were your thoughts regarding the findings from the physical examination?

Clinicians' answer

The information found up to this point supported what was already hypothesized from the interview. That is, there was probably:

- no major pathology responsible for Maree's symptoms
- a lot of fear about the problem
- fear of movement and associated pain
- insufficient and inadequate use of muscles.

2 What was your interpretation of this patient's active SLR response?

Clinicians' answer

Impairment of active SLR correlates highly with mobility of the pelvic joints in patients with peripartum pelvic girdle pain (Mens et al., 1999). During raising of the leg, the hip bone on the tested side is forced to rotate anteriorly about a horizontal axis near the SIJ (counter-nutation). In the case of Maree, the test was positive on the left side, so it may be concluded that the mobility of the left hip bone during anterior rotation (and thus the SIJ) was increased.

Raising of the leg was easier to perform with a belt fastened around the pelvic girdle; this confirms that the weakness was not caused by insufficient hip flexor muscle action but rather by increased mobility of the pelvic joints. Importantly, this test is both reliable (intratester 0.83–0.87, intertester 0.77–0.78) and valid (sensitivity 0.87, specificity 0.94) (Mens et al., 2001).

Clinical reasoning commentary

Physical examination procedures have been applied judiciously to test hypotheses relating to physical impairments (e.g. inadequate muscle action) and patient perceptions (e.g. fear of movement), in addition to precautions and contraindications to management (e.g. no major pathology). These tests (e.g. active SLR) appear to have been selected on the basis of maximizing principles, in that they provide a large pay off in terms of information relating to hypotheses (impairments, management, etc.) for a relatively small cost in terms of time and effort. The high reliability and validity of these tests, such as the active SLR, is important because it reduces the likelihood of reasoning errors and thus enhances accuracy in clinical decision making. Efficient and accurate clinical reasoning, such as demonstrated here, is typical of the expert practitioner.

Further investigations

Current radiographic report

In 1930, Chamberlain introduced a method to visualize SIJ mobility radiographically. He showed that small rotatory displacements of the pelvic bones about a transverse axis are not demonstrated on anteroposterior roentgenograms. He described how movement of the SIJ is best determined by measuring the movement between the pubic bones with alternation of weight bearing from one leg to the other. Later, Berezin (1954) compared women in the puerperium with and without pelvic pain complaints. He measured a shift between the pubic bones of 5.9 ± 3.3 mm in women with complaints and 1.9 ± 2.2 mm in those without.

The radiographic report for Maree stated that the pubic symphysis showed smooth delineation of the joint surfaces, with a joint width of 4 mm. There was sclerotic subchondral bone on the left pubis. When standing on the left leg with the right leg hanging, the left and right pubic bone heights were symmetrical. When standing on the right leg with the left leg hanging, the left pubic bone was 2 mm lower than the right (Fig. 21.4). While standing on both legs, there was no 'step' between the pubic bones, but the right femoral head was 4 mm lower than the left. The SIJs, lumbar spine and hips showed no abnormalities.

Lumbopelvic rhythm

Video analysis (van Wingerden et al., 1995) in the standing position revealed an anterior pelvic tilt with increased thoracolumbar lordosis. During forward bending, the average contribution of the lumbar spine during the first phase was 61%, which is slightly less than that found in the healthy population. In the final phase, however, the contribution was 47%, which is markedly greater than the 27% contribution shown in the healthy population. The ranges of motion of the lumbar spine and hip joint from the erect posture to maximal forward bending was 68 and 49 degrees, respectively, which indicates a relatively mobile lumbar spine but diminished hip mobility.

Psychosocial evaluation

Maree presented as a tense, emotionally sensitive woman who felt she could not 'cope any more' and was simply overwhelmed. Her anxiety and inability to cope was further aggravated by the failure of previous single-modality treatments, the recent exacerbation of her pain and her inability to work as a make-up artist. She avoided activities or situations that might cause pain, that is her pain was related to fear. With her gradual withdrawal from social activities, she began to feel increasingly helpless and hopeless.

Since the onset of pain, she had not been able to have sexual contact with her husband. Because of renovations at her home that took longer than planned, Maree was obliged to move house several times, which caused her considerable stress and, in turn, intensified her symptoms. Maree paid for household help for 4 hours a week.

Pain related to fear of movement

Excessive pain-related fear of movement was measured with the Tampa Scale for Kinesiophobia (TSK) (Kori et al., 1990; Vlaeyen et al., 1995). The degree of functional restriction is described in terms of experienced physical injury, fear of injury, fear of re-injury, importance of mobility and the degree of measured physical activity. The TSK score of 51 indicated intense pain was related to fear of certain movements.

Psychological testing for maladjustment

The presence of psychopathology was evaluated with the Symptom Check List 90 (SCL-90). This is a multidimensional complaint list that describes the presence and degree of eight psychological dimensions (e.g. fear, depression, hostility, etc.), as well as providing a total score that describes the general psychoneurotic parameters (Arindell and Ettema, 1986). The SCL-90

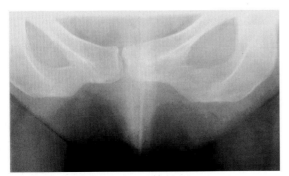

Fig. 21.4 Radiograph of patient standing on the right leg with the left leg hanging. The left pubic bone is 2 mm lower than the right.

results showed Maree scored high on depression, feelings of insufficiency and sleep disturbance. In addition, the overall score for psychoneuroticism was high.

Pain, disability, and energy level

The Visual Analogue Scale (VAS) pain score, a valid self-report measure of pain intensity (Downie et al., 1978), was 89 mm, indicating an intense sensation of pain. The McGill Pain Questionnaire, Dutch Language Version (MPQ-DLV) (van der Kloot et al., 1995), which is a reliable and valid version of the McGill Pain Questionnaire, was used to measure pain further. It comprises questions related to the location of pain, course of pain, influence of pain on the quality of daily life, a VAS pain rating, and a list of 20 groups of adjectives that are used to describe the sensory,

affective and evaluative dimensions of pain. Maree's MPQ-DLV pain rating index was 29, which suggests that the pain had a strong impact on her quality of life.

The degree of disability was measured with the Dutch version of the Quebec Back Pain Disability Scale (QBPDS; Schoppink et al., 1996). This self-reported scale was originally developed to measure the disability of patients with non-specific low back pain, but it has also proved suitable for patients with PPP. Twenty items are scored on a six-point scale ranging from 'not difficult' to 'impossible to perform'. Maree's score was 89, suggesting that she felt markedly limited in all aspects of her daily life.

The VAS for energy level was 90, indicating a major reduction in energy capacity.

REASONING DISCUSSION AND CLINICAL REASONING COMMENTARY

1 What significance did you place on the radiological findings?

Clinicians' answer

The radiographs of Maree showed increased mobility of the left ilium in an anterior direction (counter-nutation), as indicated by the asymmetries between the pubic bones and between the femoral heads. These findings were consistent with the working hypothesis (insufficient and inadequate use of muscles, associated with fear of movement and fear of pain) and with the results of the active SLR test.

2 What was your judgment of Maree's muscle control (awareness and function)?

Clinicians' answer

Maree demonstrated a rigid posture caused by tense muscles related to improper load transfer and because of defensive emotional patterns. She felt unaccepted, not taken seriously and disconnected. She was unable to express her emotions and displayed minimal sensory–motor awareness as if 'she lived out of her body'. It was also striking that Maree was completely preoccupied with the appearance of her own body and

at the same time was completely out of touch with it. These factors demonstrated that Maree's physical disability was not merely a consquence of tissue damage.

Maree could not adequately contract the muscles of the trunk and hip in order to achieve an adequate load transfer. Furthermore, achievement of relaxation and correct tension does not occur at the time at which these changes in muscle tension are required. Physical examination findings from the Isostation B-200 testing, video analysis and functional tests of load transfer are all consistent with this hypothesis.

3 Maree's clinical presentation appears to be quite complex. What pathobiological mechanisms did you hypothesize were underpinning her problems?

Clinicians' answer

Mechanisms related to pain and tissues can be identified.

Pathobiological mechanisms related to pain. From the clinical findings, some patterns emerged that were suggestive of central sensitization of pain responses, that is a change in the sensitivity state of the central nervous system (Gifford and Butler, 1997). These included persistent and inconsistent pain patterns, pain responses to inputs that would not normally provoke pain, and a reactive latent pain response to certain activities.

Pathobiological mechanisms related to tissues. The persistant ongoing pelvic pain of this patient was not simply a result of mechanical SIJ dysfunction. The tissues of the lumbopelvic region probably remained in a hypersensitive state through lack of use caused by movement anxiety, rather than because of significant tissue damage (Gifford, 1998). It is very likely that this excessive sensitivity helped to maintain the tissues in a weakened state.

4 What physical impairments and patient perspectives (with respect to potential unhelpful psychosocial issues) did you think were of particular clinical significance? Could you establish a diagnosis?

Clinicians' answer

The following impairments were of particular clinical significance:

In terms of physical impairment, the diagnosis of PPP (Mens et al., 1996) was established based on the following typical assessment findings (and based on the load transfer model):

- the pain began during pregnancy
- the pain was located in two of the joints of the pelvic girdle
- ability to perform activities of daily living was reduced
- there was no major pathology
- there was disturbed pelvic load transfer shown by:
  — reduced active muscular stabilization of the lumbopelvic region
  — positive active SLR test on the left side
  — the PPPP test and palpation of the LDL were positive
- significant radiological findings.

The occurrence of psychosocial impairment was indicated because the description of the complaints and the extent of the activity restrictions could not be explained by disturbed load transfer alone. From a biopsychosocial perspective, it is known that the factors maintaining pain can differ from the initiating factors (Vlaeyen et al., 1998). In view of the particularly high psychosocial test results, this patient could be described as being emotionally 'out of balance' and no longer with

control over her body or—even worse—over her own life. Problems of adaptation to the new situation and acceptance of things 'as they are' existed in relation to the pain, which originated during pregnancy. They were manifested as anger, fear, disappointment and feelings of frustration. Although there was no question of serious psychopathology, the scores on the psychosocial scales indicated the marked emotional impact of her present situation. The pathobiological mechanisms related to pain cause additional anxiety because she was unable to fathom her own disease process. Moreover, she felt entangled in maladaptive thoughts and emotions as a result of the persisting pain. It has been demonstrated that positive or 'helpful' psychological states have a healthy biological effect at many physiological levels (Butler, 1998). It is probable that the depressed mood and other maladaptive alterations in psychological function were largely the result of her pain state having a direct effect on her behaviour.

5 Could you please discuss the stabilizing mechanisms that you considered were of importance in understanding this patient's problems and in determining appropriate physical management?

Clinicians' answer

Under postural load, specific ligament and muscle forces are intrinsically necessary to stabilize the pelvis. Load transfer from spine to leg passes through the SIJs, helping to stabilize these joints effectively. This can be explained by a model of load transfer of the pelvis (Vleeming et al., 1993). Effective force transfer that withstands the shear forces of the SIJ is provided by a combination of specific anatomical features of the SIJ (form closure), such as the wedge-like and propeller-like form of the joint surfaces and the high friction coefficient (Pool-Goudzwaard et al., 1998; Vleeming et al., 1993). Orchestrated forces generated by muscles, ligaments and fascia also prevent shear forces by means of compression, which can be adjusted to the specific loading situation (force closure) (Vleeming et al., 1995). This model has been validated (Sturesson et al., 2000) and is frequently used to investigate impaired lumbopelvic function. It can be helpful in identifying abnormal movement patterns in the pelvic girdle and in establishing their clinical consequences. For instance, the model predicts that when the pelvis is loaded in a standing position, the pelvis generally becomes self-locked with a small rotation of the sacrum nodding anteriorly relative to the ilia (nutation). Laxity of pelvic ligaments and a painful pubic symphysis leads to an avoidance of nutation (especially during pregnancy), with Maree 'choosing' a counter-nutated position of the SIJ that disengages the self-locking mechanism of the pelvis (Vleeming et al., 1995).

New information has been reported on the stability of the lumbopelvic region and disturbances of motor control, notably affecting the segmental supporting capacity of the deep muscles of the abdomen and back (Jull et al., 1998). There is evidence that a particular exercise programme aimed at re-educating patients with chronic low back pain to activate the deep muscles specifically can influence the motor control strategies of these muscles (Jull et al., 1998).

■ Clinical reasoning commentary

The recognition of the relationship between this patient's physical presentation and psychological presentation, as manifest in her posture, movement patterns and her sensory–motor awareness, illustrates the biopsychosocial reasoning needed in contemporary manual therapy. Such breadth of information and understanding is difficult to capture simply by giving an account of examination

findings; it also requires skilled narrative and diagnostic reasoning strategies, as discussed in Chapter 1.

This discussion of the complex inter-relationships of physical and psychosocial factors in Maree's presentation provides evidence of the ability of the expert clinician to think simultaneously at the micro and macro levels, and across several hypothesis categories (e.g. patients' perspectives of their experience, physical impairments and associated sources, contributing factors, pathobiological mechanisms, etc.). While collecting and synthesizing specific clinical data (micro information), the clinician needs to interpret these data in the light of the larger biopsychosocial picture, particularly the patient's activity and participation restrictions (macro information).

It is also apparent that the clinical reasoning in this case has been largely driven by the recognition of familiar clinical patterns, that is, by a pattern recognition process. Key physical and psychosocial features of PPP have been identified in Maree's clinical presentation by relating clinical findings to a prototype stored in the clinician's memory. This has occurred for both the diagnostic syndrome of PPP and the associated pathobiological mechanisms/factors contributing to the maintenance of the patient's problems.

m ❘ Management

Maree met the inclusion criteria for admission to the SJC rehabilitation programme. After considering information from a range of sources (e.g. patient interview, physical examination, test results, published literature, and 'gut feeling'), specific physical dysfunctions and emotional influences were identified, as were the social consequences (Butler, 1998). To address these factors, it was clear that a comprehensive management approach needed to be implemented. Accordingly, the goals of management were to enable Maree to:

■ improve her pelvic force closure in order to facilitate self-bracing of the pelvic girdle, through appropriate exercises and re-education of movement patterns
■ improve her general cardiovascular condition so as to prevent further deconditioning
■ enhance her ability to manage and cope with her pain and related problems

■ resume a normal functional life, including returning to work
■ take control of her life
■ reduce or better use of health-care services.

At the SJC, physical therapists, manual therapists (physical therapists who have undertaken further education in manual therapy), psychologists and physicians collaborate to deliver a comprehensive programme via group therapy for 3 hours twice a week for 8 weeks. Initially, the patient is provided with pain and sleep medication to ensure that pain complaints are reduced to an extent that enables effective participation in the programme. The programme initially commences with restoration of the self-bracing mechanism for the SIJ and, therefore, the development of stability for the lumbopelvic region. Self-bracing of the SIJ is achieved by developing optimal biomechanics for this joint (Vlaeyen et al., 1998). Diminished nutation, or relative counter-nutation of the sacrum, reduces self-bracing of the SIJ and may lead to instability. It may also produce additional tension in the LDL and an altered load-bearing capacity of the joint surfaces, and hence dysfunction. It is known that articular dysfunction rapidly leads to inhibition of slow-twitch muscle fibres, which may result in reduced ability of muscles to sustain a contraction (Lee, 1997; Vlaeyen et al., 1998). It is also known that exercises alone will not bring about a successful resolution if the SIJ has become chronically compressed in a counter-nutated position. In these patients, a specific mobilization technique is first applied and the muscular system then utilized to maintain optimal joint mechanics (Don Tigny, 1997).

Initially in Maree's rehabilitation programme, articular dysfunctions were mobilized. In this technique, the SIJ dysfunction can be corrected by mobilizing the innominate bone posteriorly and downward on the sacrum, by using the leg as a lever, by grasping the innominate bone directly and rotating, or even by using a strong isometric hip extension contraction against a belt (Fig. 21.5). Following the mobilization, strength and endurance of the weakened muscles was addressed. The aim was to reactivate the stabilizing muscles, particularly to retrain their holding capacity and their ability to contract appropriately with other synergists, in order to support and protect the lumbo-pelvic girdle under various functional loads. The

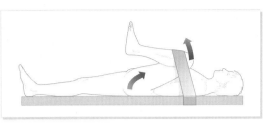

Fig. 21.5 Mobilization of the left sacroiliac joint using isometric hip extension contraction against a belt.

four-stage stabilization programme developed by Richardson and Jull (Jull et al., 1998; Richardson and Jull, 1995) was applied. Retraining of the posterior oblique, anterior oblique, and longitudinal muscle systems, as described by Vleeming et al. (1995), was integrated into this programme. Maree was also severely incapacitated, physically deconditioned and functioning at a low activity level (Shorland, 1998) with inefficient use of energy. To improve her overall condition and cardiovascular fitness, aerobic exercising was applied at each treatment session. The relevance of improved fitness and physical functioning with respect to pain was not entirely clear to Maree. However, the fact that improvement in her overall physical function was linked to improvement of her psychosocial function was clearly evident to Maree.

REASONING DISCUSSION AND CLINICAL REASONING COMMENTARY

1 Assisting patients to transform their understanding of their problems, and the various contributing factors, is clearly an important aspect of your management. Could you please comment on how this was specifically addressed in Maree's case?

■ Clinicians' answer

Another aspect of the integrated multifactorial approach is to make patients aware of the importance of their own 'empowerment'. In the case of Maree, we used educational lessons, enhancing her knowledge and understanding of her condition, thus enabling her to deal with her own pain and disability better and to cope with stress. Maree required specific and relevant information to assist her in making choices, overcoming negative beliefs and modifying her behaviour (e.g. increasing her activity). Fifteen sessions of

30 minutes each were reserved for this aspect of management. They included lessons dealing with the anatomy and function of the back, ergonomics, advice about activities of daily living, pelvic floor training and sexuality.

There is little evidence to suggest a long-term advantage of any particular psychological approach to disability (Waddell, 1998). A combination of cognitive, behavioural and psychophysiological techniques are used to manage pain. The aim is not to reduce pain per se but rather to develop the patient's responsibility for their own pain and to help them to control and manage it (Gatchel and Turk, 1996; Waddell, 1998). This is mainly achieved by changing the patient's beliefs and misunderstandings about chronic pain. Clinically, it proved helpful to explain to Maree that the excessive sensitivity of her lumbopelvic region was a problem in its own right, and that her pain was not caused by tissue damage alone. It was important to ensure that Maree did not only equate pain with damage and fear of movement (Mens et al., 1996). Maree demonstrated a particular behavioural pattern as a result of maladaptive thoughts and emotions centred around her pain. To address this issue, she was informed that general immobility leads to a loss of muscle strength, coordination, stability and muscular and physical endurance (Main and Spanswick, 1998).

In the management programme, the principle of 'movement for enjoyment' was stressed (McIndoe, 1995). To help to motivate Maree, the essential principles of traditional yoga were explained, including daily practice. Maree received a home-based exercise programme, combining daily practice and enjoyment of movement with stabilization, breathing, stretching and strengthening exercises. These exercises were checked each visit and it was stressed that her role was as important (or even more so) as that of the therapist. In one of the last sessions, the importance of maintaining a training programme in a suitable fitness or yoga centre was explained. Maree was also advised on a plan of action in case of exacerbations. It was emphasized that an exacerbation should never be seen as a failure or as evidence of her inability to manage the condition; it is merely a challenge of self-management, not the end of it.

Clinical reasoning commentary

Where management of physical impairment requires 'instrumental action' (e.g. mobilization and motor retraining), management of patient's perspectives judged to be potential obstacles to their recovery such as unhelpful beliefs and feelings requires 'communicative action' directed toward working with the patient to change their perspectives. As discussed in Chapter 1, changing these perspectives is not easy and necessitates skilled interaction to assist the patient to reflect on the basis of their beliefs. Simple, one-off explanations are rarely sufficient, as evidenced in this case by the time and effort the clinicians devoted to addressing the patient's understandings and beliefs. However, when successful learning does occur, patients' perspectives are transformed, allowing them to make better decisions. Critically, this dimension of reasoning and management is most successful when conducted collaboratively. The clinicians' reference here to helping 'to assist her in making choices' illustrates their collaborative reasoning approach.

Outcome

At the end of the therapeutic programme, Maree still experienced some pelvic pain; however, her coping mechanisms were greatly improved. She felt less restricted in her daily activities and had more control over her life. She was motivated to continue training in a fitness centre until she felt like 'her old self' again.

The TSK score was now 36, indicating that there was markedly less fear of movement, and the score on the QBPDS was 28, suggesting that she no longer had any major limitations in different aspects of her daily life. The VAS pain score was 22, indicating only a mild sensation of pain, and the VAS energy level score had greatly improved to 34.

By means of this multifactorial approach, the goals for this patient were achieved. She presented to the clinic with lumbopelvic pain that had become 'out of control'. A relatively minor load transfer problem had exploded into a serious pain and disability problem through a combination of biopsychosocial factors. This complexity is not usually well recognized in routine clinical practice. Partially as a result of single-modality treatment in the past, Maree felt that she had lost control over her body, the pain and her own life.

During the therapy, she started to see herself as changing from a patient with chronic pelvic pain to a whole person again. She realized the futility of waiting for someone else to make things better for her. The management programme helped her to discover the underlying complexities of pain and its physical, emotional and psychosocial implications. This information also prompted personal development for Maree. She is now able to view herself as a whole and connected being. After the rehabilitation programme, she no longer expects a total cure, instead she has taken control of her life. She can now decide where she wants to go and what she wants to do: a clear sign of good health.

REASONING DISCUSSION AND CLINICAL REASONING COMMENTARY

1 You appear to attribute some of the responsibility for Maree's problems to previous practitioners who were arguably more narrow in their management approach. Clearly, however, most patients do not go on to develop chronic pain and related psychosocial problems. What warning signs might have alerted these practitioners to the likelihood of Maree failing to respond to their treatment or perhaps actually worsening because of it?

Clinicians' answer

Ineffectiveness of therapy, or a poor response to treatment, is probably the key indicator of potential long-term pain or psychosocial problems. The experienced clinician has an expectation as to how a patient with a typical presentation will respond to a particular therapy. If the problem does not respond as anticipated, then the 'good' clinician will recognize this as a 'flag' indicating the possibility of more serious or complex problems. It is important that clinical tests and evaluation instruments are suitably relevant and sensitive to facilitate the early identification of non-responsiveness to treatment. Reassessment following the application of an intervention is crucial, as is the recognition of the need to change treatment approaches when the outcome is less than desired.

Clinical reasoning commentary

The importance of relevant clinical experience in the recognition of atypical responses to treatment is evident in this answer. The expert clinician learns and builds a knowledge base by reflecting upon each case, such that over a period of time a prototypical template of a particular clinical syndrome is embedded within their memory, including the associated expected or usual responses to various interventions. Without this experiential non-propositional knowledge, there is the danger that inappropriate or ineffective treatment may be prolonged, potentially contributing to the development of chronic pain or illness perspectives and behaviours (e.g. passive coping with dependence on others to solve the problem, pain-centred maladaptive beliefs and behaviours, etc.) and the delaying of the implementation of more appropriate management. Non-expert clinicians often fall into the trap of persisting with interventions that are ineffective in the longer-term either because they lack the clinical experience or because they have failed to learn from their clinical experiences sufficient to recognize the atypical response.

Evidence-based practice provides important guidelines to practice, but not 'recipe' solutions. Skilled clinical reasoning is essential to apply those guidelines. Appropriate reassessment, as the clinicians have highlighted here, is the means by which the optimal manner and dosage of the intervention is determined and the clinical validation is made. Importantly, while reasoning and interventions directed toward physical impairments are reassessed through objective outcome measurement, communicative management directed toward patient perspectives, such as their beliefs and fears, must also be reassessed.

References

Arindell, W.A. and Ettema, H. (1986). SCL-90: Handleiding bij een Multidimensionele Psychopathologie Indicator. Lisse: Swets and Zeitlinger.

Berezin, D. (1954). Pelvic insufficiency during pregnancy and after parturition. Acta Obstetrica et Gynaecologica Scandinavica, 23, 1–130.

Berg, G., Hammar, M. and Möller-Nielsen, J. (1988). Low back pain during pregnancy. Obstetrics and Gynecology, 71, 71–75.

Butler, D. (1998). Introduction. Integrating pain awareness into physiotherapy: wise action for the future. In Topical Issues in Pain 1 Whiplash—Science and Management,

Fear-avoidance Beliefs and Behaviour (L.S. Gifford, ed.) pp. 1–23. Falmouth, UK: CNS Press.

Chamberlain, W.E. (1930). The symphysis pubis in the roentgen examination of the sacro-iliac joint. American Journal of Roentgenology, Radium Therapy and Nuclear Medicine, 24, 621–625.

Don Tigny, R.L. (1997). Mechanics and treatment of the sacroiliac joint. In Movement Stability and Low Back Pain (A. Vleeming, V. Mooney, T. Dorman, C. Snijders and R. Stoekart, eds.) pp. 461–477. Edinburgh: Churchill Livingstone.

Downie, W.W., Leatham, P.A., Rhind, V.M. et al. (1978). Studies with pain rating scales. Annals of the Rheumatic Diseases, 37, 378–381.

Fast, A., Shapiro, D., Ducommun, E.J. et al. (1987). Low back pain in pregnancy. Spine, 12, 368–371.

Gatchel, R.J. and Turk, D.C. (1996). Psychological Approaches to Pain Management. New York: Guilford Publications.

Gifford, L.S. (1998). Tissue and input related mechanisms. In Topical Issues in Pain 1 Whiplash—Science and Management, Fear-avoidance Beliefs and Behaviour (L.S. Gifford, ed.) pp. 57–65. Falmouth, UK: CNS Press.

Gifford, L.S. and Butler, D.S. (1997). The integration of pain sciences into clinical practice. Hand Therapy, 4, 86–95.

Gomez, T., Beach, G., Cooke, C. et al. (1991). Normative data for trunk range of motion, strength, velocity and endurance with the isostation B-200 lumbar dynamometer. Spine, 16, 15–21.

Jull, G.A., Scott, Q., Richardson, C. et al. (1998). New concepts for the control of pain in the lumbopelvic region. In Third Interdisciplinary World Congress on Low Back and Pelvic Pain (A. Vleeming, V. Mooney, H. Tilscher et al., eds.) pp. 128–132. Rotterdam ECO.

Kori, S.H., Miller, R.P. and Todd, D.D. (1990). Kinesiophobia: a new view of chronic pain behaviour. Pain Management, 1, 35–43.

Lee, D.G. (1997). Treatment of pelvic instability. In Movement Stability and Low Back Pain (A. Vleeming, V. Mooney, T. Dorman, C. Snijders and R. Stoekart, eds.) pp. 445–460. Edinburgh: Churchill Livingstone.

Main, C.J. and Spanswick, C.C. (1998). Textbook on Interdisciplinary Pain Management. Edinburgh: Churchill Livingstone.

McIndoe, R. (1995). Moving out of pain: hands-on or hands-off. In Moving in on Pain (M.O. Shacklock, ed.) pp. 153–160. Oxford: Butterworth-Heinemann.

Mens, J.M.A., Vleeming, A., Stoeckart, R. et al. (1996). Understanding peripartum pelvic pain: implications of a patient survey. Spine, 21, 1363–1370.

Mens, J.M.A., Vleeming, A., Snijders, C.J. et al. (1997). Active straight leg raising test: a clinical approach to the load transfer function of the pelvic girdle. In Movement, Stability and Low Back Pain (A. Vleeming, V. Mooney, T. Dorman et al., eds.) pp. 425–433. Edinburgh: Churchill Livingstone.

Mens, J.M.A., Vleeming, A., Snijders, C.J. et al. (1999). The active straight leg raising test and mobility of the pelvic joints. European Spine Journal, 8, 468–473.

Mens, J.M.A., Vleeming, A., Snijders, C.J. et al. (2001). Validity and reliability of the active straight leg raise test in posterior pelvic pain since pregnancy. Spine, 26, 1167–1171.

Östgaard, H.C., Andersson, G.B.J. and Karlsson, K. (1991). Prevalence of back pain in pregnancy. Spine, 16, 549–552.

Östgaard, H.C., Zetherström, G.B.J. and Roos-Hansson, E. (1994). The posterior pelvic pain provocation test in pregnant women. European Spine Journal, 3, 258–260.

Pool-Goudzwaard, A.L., Vleeming, A., Stoeckart, R. et al. (1998). Insufficient lumbopelvic stability: a clinical, anatomical and biomechanical approach to 'a specific' low back pain. Manual Therapy, 3, 12–20.

Potter, N.A. and Rothstein, J.M. (1985). Intertester reliability for selected clinical tests of the sacroiliac joint. Physical Therapy, 65, 1671–1675.

Richardson, C.A. and Jull, G.A. (1995). Muscle control—pain control. What exercise would you prescribe? Manual Therapy, 1, 2–10.

Schoppink, L.E.M., van Tulder, M.W., Koes, B.W. et al. (1996). Reliability and validity of the Dutch adaptation of the Quebec Back Pain Disability Scale. Physical Therapy, 76, 268–275.

Shorland, S. (1998). Management of chronic pain following whiplash injuries. In Topical Issues in Pain 1 Whiplash—Science and Management,

Fear-avoidance Beliefs and Behaviour (L.S. Gifford, ed.) pp. 115–134. Falmouth, UK: CNS Press.

Sturesson, B., Udén, A. and Vleeming, A. (2000). A radiostereometric analysis of movements of the sacroiliac joints during the standard hip flexion test. Spine 25, 364–368.

Svensson, H.O., Andersson, G.B.J., Hagstad, A. et al. (1990). The relationship of low-back pain to pregnancy and gynecologic factors. Spine, 5, 371–375.

van der Kloot, W.A., Oostendorp, R.A.B., van der Meij, J. et al. (1995). De Nederlandse versie van de McGill Pain Questionnaire: een betrouwbare vragenlijst. Nederlands Tijdschrift voor Geneeskunde, 139, 669–673.

van Meeteren, J., Mens J.M.A. and Stam, H.J. (1997). Reliability of strength measurement of the hip with a hand-held dynamometer in healthy women. European Journal of Physical Medicine and Rehabilitation, 7, 17–20.

van Wingerden, J.P., Vleeming, A., Stam, H.J. et al. (1995). Interaction of spine and legs: influence of hamstring tension on lumbo-pelvic rhythm. In Second Interdisciplinary World Congress on Low Back Pain and its Relation to the SI Joint (A. Vleeming, V. Mooney, T. Dorman and C.J. Snijders, eds) pp. 109–123, Rotterdam ECO.

van Wingerden, J.P., Vleeming, A., Kleinrensink G.J. and Stoeckart, R. (1997). The role of the hamstrings in pelvic and spinal function. In Movement, Stability and Low Back Pain (A. Vleeming, V. Mooney, T. Dorman et al., eds.) pp. 207–210, Edinburgh: Churchill Livingstone.

Vlaeyen, J.W.S., Kole-Snijders, A.M.J., Boeren, R.G.B. et al. (1995). Fear of movement/(re)injury in chronic low back pain and its relation to behavioural performance. Pain, 62, 363–372.

Vlaeyen, W.S., Kole-Snijders, A.M.J., Heuts, P.H.T.G. et al. (1998). Behavioral analysis, fear of movement (re)injury and behavioral rehabilitation in chronic low back pain. In Third Interdisciplinary World Congress on Low Back and Pelvic Pain (A. Vleeming, V. Mooney, H. Tilscher et al., eds.) pp. 57–69, Rotterdam: ECO.

Vleeming, A. (1998). Introduction. In Third Interdisciplinary World Congress on Low Back and Pelvic Pain (A. Vleeming, V. Mooney, H. Tilscher et al., eds.) pp. iii–iv. Rotterdam: ECO.

Vleeming, A., Pool-Goudzwaard, A.L., Stoeckart, R. et al. (1993). Towards a better understanding of the etiology of low back pain.In First Interdisciplinary World Congress on Low Back Pain and its Relation to the SI Joint (A. Vleeming, V. Mooney, H. Tilscher et al., eds.) pp.545–553. Rotterdam: ECO.

Vleeming, A., Snijders, C.J., Stoeckart, R. et al. (1995). A new light on low back pain. In Second Interdisciplinary World Congress on Low Back Pain and its Relation to the SI Joint (A. Vleeming et al., eds.) pp. 123–131. Rotterdam: ECO.

Vleeming, A., Mens, J.M.A., de Vries, H. et al. (1998). Possible role of the long dorsal sacroiliac ligament in peripartum pelvic pain. In Third Interdisciplinary World Congress on Low Back and Pelvic Pain (A. Vleeming, V. Mooney, H. Tilscher et al., eds.) pp. 149–157. Rotterdam: ECO.

Waddell, G. (1998). The Back Pain Revolution. Edinburgh: Churchill Livingstone.

22

Acute on chronic low back pain

Richard Walsh and Stanley Paris

 SUBJECTIVE EXAMINATION

Tony is a 42-year-old male who works as a systems administrator for a newspaper company. He attended our clinic complaining of back pain, 'back spasms', and pain and tingling into the left posterolateral mid-thigh and the lateral plantar aspect of the left foot. During the last 3 months he had noted a gradual worsening of his symptoms, with a decreasing ability to perform gym workouts and recreational cycling as a result of the low back pain (LBP). Tony had a 10-year history of LBP with no initial precipitating incident. Seven years ago he attended approximately seven physical therapy sessions, which he reported consisted of heat, electrotherapeutic modalities and a 'gym-based' exercise programme, with minimal change in his symptoms. His other medical history included fractures of the right clavicle, forearm and left jaw, none of which occurred in the last 5 years, and atrial fibrillation and depression.

One month previously Tony had been evaluated by orthopaedic and physical medicine physicians at a specialty spine centre. The work-up included magnetic resonance imaging (MRI), bloodwork, nerve conduction studies and a physical therapy assessment. The blood work and nerve conduction studies were unremarkable. He was referred for physical therapy at our facility with a diagnosis of 'spondylolysis L5–S1, degenerative disc disease L4–L5'. The referring physician (physiatrist) recommended the avoidance of extension exercises.

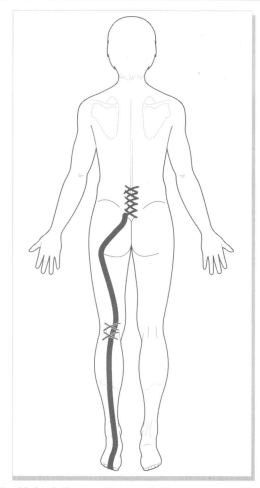

Fig. 22.1 Self-reported areas of pain.

Self-reporting forms

At our clinic, the standard intake forms include a body chart for pain, the McGill pain questionnaire (MPQ) (Melzack, 1975) and the Roland Morris Disability Questionnaire (Roland and Morris, 1983) in a modified form (mRMDQ) (Walsh, 1999). Tony marked his body chart (Fig. 22.1) with crosses in the region of the central lumbar spine, left popliteal fossa, and the plantar aspect of the heel and first metatarsal on the left side. He also indicated pain radiating from the lumbar spine down the posterior aspect of the left lower extremity. He rated his pain as 5/10 where 0 is no pain and 10 is excruciating pain. One week prior, while playing golf, his pain was 7–8/10.

The mRMDQ that was administered is based on the formatting and wording proposed by Patrick et al. (1995). It has demonstrated good reliability (test–retest reliability and internal consistency) and sensitivity to change (Walsh, 1999). The initial mean score on this scale for patients attending our clinic approximates 13/24. This patient's mRMDQ score was comparatively high (20/24). On the MPQ he marked 18 items in eight categories, with six of the marked items in categories 11 through 16.

Because of Tony's history of depression, a modified Zung Depression Index (ZDI) was also administered (Main and Waddell, 1984; Zung, 1965). The screening cut-off for depression with this tool has been reported as 33/69, the higher the score the greater the depression. This patient scored 53/69, an extremely high score.

REASONING DISCUSSION AND CLINICAL REASONING COMMENTARY

1 Could you identify any potential patterns in Tony's presentation at this early stage? What findings prompted your thoughts in this regard?

■ Clinicians' answer

It appeared that the symptoms were a result of lumbar spine pathology. At this stage, there was nothing definitive to indicate pathology of one particular lumbar tissue over another (for example, disc versus facet joint versus ligament). This is hardly surprising because the majority of the time it is not possible to identify a specific tissue as the cause of LBP (Deyo et al., 1992). The pain radiating below the knee may be indicative of a discogenic problem with neural tissue compromise. However, because muscles, ligaments and the facet joints are capable of producing pain with a similar distribution (Inman and Saunders, 1944; Kellgren, 1938; Mooney and Robertson, 1976) it is best to avoid jumping to hasty conclusions, particularly this early in the evaluation. Nonetheless, the provided radiological finding of a spondylolysis (L5–S1) meant that continued consideration of impairment (for example, hypermobility or hypomobility) at this level was warranted.

2 What was your interpretation of the results of the questionnaires? In particular, what ramifications did the findings have for your management and prognosis?

■ Clinicians' answer

Roland and Morris (1983) suggested patients with scores of 14 or greater (when using the original scale) on the disability questionnaire are more likely to have a poor outcome. It was, therefore, anticipated that this would be a potentially challenging case. For the MPQ, it has been suggested that category scores greater than 16, or the marking of items in categories 11 through 16, may represent severe or excessive emotional reaction to pain (Paris, 1980). On that basis, Tony's pain questionnaire indicated heightened emotional overlay.

Patients with LBP whose ZDI scores are greater than 33/69 have been categorized as 'depressed-distressed' in the distress and risk assessment model (Main et al., 1992). These patients are three to four times more likely to have a poor outcome compared with those who score less than 17/69 (classified as normal) on the ZDI. Because depression is a key indicator for poor outcome in patients with LBP (Burton et al., 1995), Tony was encouraged to follow-up with the medical professional who was overseeing this aspect of his health care. Following this recommendation Tony arranged to see his psychiatrist, with the referring physician informed of these developments.

The benefits of a holistic approach to the treatment of LBP were emphasized to Tony and he was agreeable to alerting the psychiatrist to his LBP.

It was planned to track the ZDI scores as Tony progressed through treatment. We hypothesized that a decrease in the depression score would correspond with an improvement in Tony's LBP and a reduction in his mRMDQ score. As we will later elaborate, we typically present the findings from these questionnaires to the patient on completion of the evaluation and this serves as part of the education process regarding the emotional component of their pain presentation and the patient's functional status. However, in instances such as here, when the scores are particularly elevated, we spend extra time with the patient explaining the physical reasons for their pain. We feel this helps the patient to rationalize their problem and, therefore, potentially reduces the emotional component of their presentation. It has been our experience that counselling the patient in this manner can bring about an immediate reduction in a patient's MPQ score. Furthermore, self-reporting questionnaires may later serve as useful adjuncts to the physical findings and functional goals in demonstrating improving status of the patient.

◼ Clinical reasoning commentary

Despite the note of caution about 'jumping to hasty conclusions', it is apparent the clinicians have recognized early cues and formed some tentative diagnostic hypotheses (e.g. discogenic problem with neural tissue compromise). Indeed, it would be unusual if they had not. Research has demonstrated that expert manual therapists normally generate hypotheses from the outset of the clinical encounter (Rivett and Higgs, 1997). These initial hypotheses are not accepted until they have been adequately tested with data from further examination, particularly in cases such as this where several pathologies are capable of producing similar patterns of symptoms. To do otherwise would invite errors in clinical reasoning resulting from biased thinking and incomplete data collection.

Manual therapists today are required to be multifaceted in their clinical reasoning in order to ensure they offer an effective and holistic approach to management. In this case, in addition to considering physical impairments, long the traditional domain of manual therapists, the expert clinicians have identified an important need to consider psychosocial impairments (e.g. depression). It is clear that they consider that dysfunctional/impaired and counterproductive beliefs and feelings must first be addressed through education and reassurance so as to enhance the likelihood of a favourable outcome.

It is of interest to note that the information obtained from the questionnaires has been used to inform clinical reasoning in a number of hypothesis categories, including activity/participation restrictions, physical and psychosocial impairments, management and prognosis. This makes the time spent on their administration and interpretation well justified.

Patient interview

It is often helpful to question a patient about the precise location of the onset of their pain because this site can help to indicate the possible source of the pain. In response to the question, 'Precisely where did your pain begin?', Tony reported three sites: both posterior superior iliac spines and the lateral aspect of the left thigh, at the junction of the proximal two-thirds of the thigh and the distal third of the thigh. Subsequently, he also noted tingling and numbness on the lateral aspect of the left foot.

When questioned about his present sleeping pattern, Tony volunteered that his life was in a period of turmoil, primarily through domestic conflict, and that this was reducing his sleep to only 3–4 hours each night. Moreover, whenever he fell asleep on his stomach his back and leg symptoms worsened and his sleep was further disrupted by the pain. If he did not sleep on his stomach, he reported awaking in the morning with less LBP and leg pain than at any other time of the day. The 24 hour pain pattern was one of gradual deterioration throughout the day, which appeared to be related to the amount of time he was up. Apart from resting in a supine-lying position, Tony was not aware of anything that reduced his symptoms. He had not self-administered ice or heat and he had not filled a prescription for celecoxib (anti-inflammatory medication) provided by the referring physician. He verbalized a dislike of medications as the basis for his non-compliance. His primary goal was a return to function, specifically 'working out at the gym and cycling'.

The patient denied any altered sensation, pain or numbness in the 'saddle' distribution, and any changes in bowel or bladder function. The patient had also not experienced any recent changes in body temperature or body weight.

REASONING DISCUSSION AND CLINICAL REASONING COMMENTARY

1 Did you directly or indirectly ascertain Tony's understanding of his condition and management to date?

Clinicians' answer

Up to this point, Tony had not undertaken any independent exercise programme or self-management for his LBP. In our experience, some patients prefer to be the recipients of passive care rather than being active participants in their rehabilitation. Perhaps this patient had not been afforded an opportunity to be actively involved in addressing his LBP or, alternatively, he had declined to do so. We believe that all LBP patients must be active participants in their care if recovery is to progress optimally. Initially it was felt that this patient had come to physical therapy to be passively 'fixed'.

Consequently, it was expected that the importance of accepting an active role in the treatment programme would need to be emphasized to Tony. He demonstrated some degree of understanding of his diagnosis but was unclear as to why he was not a surgical candidate for rectification of the spondylolysis at this time. We have found that many patients attending our clinic for their first visit frequently require further education regarding their problem. This particular patient was by no means ignorant of his diagnosis, but it was felt that he would benefit from a clear explanation of his diagnosis, his problem list and the projected plan of care, following the completion of his evaluation.

2 Given Tony's long history and apparent psychosocial impairment, did you at this stage think that his symptoms were dominantly nociceptive (i.e. emanating from peripheral somatic and/or neurogenic tissues) or did you hypothesize a central pain mechanism (i.e. altered processing or sensitivity of the central nervous system) as a further possibility?

Clinicians' answer

From the information gleaned thus far in the evaluation, we believed that to some degree this patient's symptoms emanated from mechanical compromise of peripheral somatic and/or neurogenic tissues. Mechanical and inflammatory nociceptive input from a variety of lumbar tissues was suspected. In support of this was the finding that Tony's symptoms were relieved in certain positions (supine lying) and made worse in other positions (prone lying). At this stage it was felt that a spondylolysis with accompanying instability could be responsible for such a pain presentation.

Given Tony's long history of LBP it was conceivable that there was also a central mechanism contributing to the pain. The chronic nature of the condition would sensitize the central nervous system (CNS) and the peripheral nociceptors, relatively reducing Tony's pain threshold, thus prolonging and amplifying the pain. This change in sensitivity of the CNS is sometimes referred to as 'wind-up'.

The third and possibly most important mechanism contributing to this patient's pain presentation was the psychosocial impairment. The history of depression, the results of the self-reporting measures and the discord present in his home setting suggested an affective pain mechanism was present and responsible for some of Tony's pain.

Clinical reasoning commentary

The clinicians are clearly attempting to gain an understanding of the patient as a person, that is the context of his problem. This includes both the patient's perspective of the problem (e.g. just a passive 'fix' is needed) and factors potentially contributing to the maintenance of the problem (e.g. stressful home situation). This requires a clinical reasoning strategy, referred to as narrative reasoning (see Ch. 1). The greater insight afforded by narrative reasoning is required to understand the patient and effectively interact with them to facilitate change in their behaviour, such as active participation in their management. Dysfunctional/impaired and counterproductive (to recovery) behaviours can often be positively addressed through education, as illustrated in this case (e.g. a clear explanation of his diagnosis, his problem list and the projected plan of care), and fostering the patient's insight into their own beliefs, feelings and behaviours. Consequently, effective narrative reasoning requires sound interpersonal and inquiry skills, relevant knowledge, and management strategies and referral pathways to other health professionals, particularly in the field of mental health.

PHYSICAL EXAMINATION

Increased thoracic kyphosis and lumbar lordosis were noted on examination (Tony is an ectomorphic Caucasian). In standing, there also appeared to be increased tone in the mid-lumbar paraspinal muscles in a 'band'. Palpation did not reveal any obvious tenderness or 'step' in the lumbar interspinous spaces. When patients have a spondylolisthesis, a 'step' may be apparent at that level if it is degenerative or dysplastic, and at the level above if it is isthmic (lytic, elongated but intact pars interarticularis, or traumatic) (Fig. 22.2). This difference occurs because in the isthmic states the posterior elements do not slip forward (Weinstein, 1995).

Active range of motion was recorded using the modified-modified Schöber method (Williams et al., 1993). This method involves measuring from the level of the posterior superior iliac spines to a point 15 cm superiorly and then noting the approximation between the two points with lumbar extension and the amount of skin distraction between the two points with lumbar flexion. Flexion was +2 cm (approximately 30% of normal range) and extension was within normal limits (−2 cm). Side bending was estimated as 50% of normal range to the right and 75% of normal range to the left, with LBP limiting both motions. All movements appeared to occur primarily in the mid-lumbar spine in a fulcrum-like manner.

Neurological assessment revealed normal strength, reflexes and light touch sensation in the lower extremities. Straight leg raise (SLR) was 50 degrees on the left and 60 degrees on the right with a muscle end-feel and Tony reported feeling a stretch in each

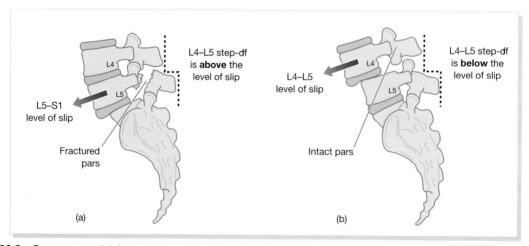

Fig. 22.2 Fracture spondylolisthesis (a) can be differentiated from degenerative spondylolisthesis (b) by the 'spinous process sign'. In the former, the forward slippage of the anterior portion of the vertebra creates a palpable step-off of the spinous processes at the interspace above the level of the slip. In the latter, the intact vertebra slips forward as a unit, creating a step-off at the interspace below the level of the slip. (From McKinnis, 1996, p. 198 as adapted from Greenspan, 1992, p. 10–42. Reproduced with kind permission of the publishers.)

hamstring. The addition of passive dorsiflexion at the ankle did not change the patient's report. Femoral nerve tension testing was unremarkable.

Examination of the sacroiliac joints using pain provocation tests (compression and gapping) was asymptomatic. A battery of tests were used to examine the hips including passive motion testing, the FABER test, the scour test and Trendelenburg's test, all of which were unremarkable. The sign of the buttock test was performed with Tony in supine lying and was normal. During this procedure, the clinician raises the patient's leg with the knee extended until the motion is limited or painful, which equates to a SLR test. At that point the knee is flexed and further hip flexion is attempted. If the patient tolerates continued hip movement then neither the hip nor the structures spanning the hip alone are likely to be responsible for the initial limitation. If, however, the patient cannot tolerate further movement then the hip may be implicated. Magee (1992) suggests that a positive test may indicate serious hip pathology in the form of osteomyelitis or sacral fracture.

Muscle length tests for the psoas and rectus femoris muscles (Thomas test), as well as Ober's test for the length of the iliotibial band, were within normal limits bilaterally.

When Tony was positioned in prone lying, the lumbar paraspinal muscle activity was less noticeable and again no 'step' was palpable. Passive physiological intervertebral movement (PPIVM) testing of the lumbar spine revealed diffuse, slight hypomobility (ranging from 2/6 to 2+/6; Gonella et al., 1982). A slump test was then performed as described by Butler (1991), which demonstrated a limitation in knee extension of 15 degrees on the right and 10 degrees on the left, with Tony reporting a stretch feeling in each hamstring but no reproduction of symptoms. This limitation was considered unremarkable.

Because of the elevated MPQ score and the possibility of non-organic pain, tests for Waddell's signs were performed (Waddell et al., 1979). These tests are used to identify if there are what Waddell terms 'behavioural signs' (Waddell, 1998; see Ch. 5 for a description and assessment of the significance of these signs in manual therapy). A positive response is occurrence of LBP with very mild axial loading of the spine, simulated trunk rotation or superficial skin rolling at the lumbar spine. Other Waddell signs are a marked difference in SLR in sitting versus supine lying, sensory change beyond the normal innervation field and dermatome distribution (for example, decreased light touch sensation in a 'stocking' distribution) and non-myotomal motor weakness (for example, weakness of the entire lower extremity). These tests were unremarkable (0/5 where a score of 3/5 or greater is suggestive of non-organic pain).

At this time the diagnostic imaging films were reviewed and the L5–S1 spondylolysis was confirmed, with the MRI also indicating the presence of a grade I spondylolisthesis at this level.

REASONING DISCUSSION

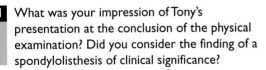

1 What was your impression of Tony's presentation at the conclusion of the physical examination? Did you consider the finding of a spondylolisthesis of clinical significance?

Clinicians' answer

The results of the physical examination suggested that Tony was demonstrating clinical signs of physical impairment and pathology as well as being depressed. Importantly, the examination did not reveal any strong evidence of 'red flags' for neurological compromise or systemic disease. The impression of Tony's presentation at this stage was of lumbar joint and soft tissue (hamstring) hypomobility, with a heightened emotional component. Lumbar instability was hypothesized as the underlying cause of the muscular guarding and consequent spinal hypomobility. Ideally, passive motion testing involves the clinician undertaking testing with the patient entirely relaxed. However, when the patient's resting muscle tone is higher than normal, for whatever reason (for example, muscle guarding because of pain), this may result in decreased passive joint mobility despite the fact that the tested joint(s) may actually be hypermobile. The hypothesis of lumbar instability was based on the 'banding' of muscle noted in the mid-lumbar spine, the worsening of symptoms as the day progressed

(Paris, 1985), caused by increasing tissue creep, and the fact that lying on his stomach aggravated the symptoms. The finding of a spondylolisthesis on imaging was also supportive as it can potentially cause spinal instability.

Instability has been defined primarily by the degree of vertebral translation or angulation seen on radiographs. While there is no absolute value, figures have been suggested for the lumbar spine of greater than 4.5 mm sagittal plane displacement or 22 degrees relative sagittal plane angulation between segments (White et al., 1999). It would have been desirable to have had flexion–extension films of this patient to help to determine the amount of vertebral translation

and angulation. This is despite the fact that our spines do not typically function in such extremes of motion (Paris, 1985).

It is possible that an individual without a spondylolisthesis could present in a similar fashion to this patient. Conversely, one might argue that another individual with grade I spondylolisthesis could be entirely asymptomatic. Therefore, it is more useful to reference a combination of signs and symptoms when making a judgment of instability, as a single definitive measure continues to be elusive at this time. While acknowledging these shortcomings, we feel justified in provisionally diagnosing Tony as having 'clinical instability' of the lumbar spine.

m Management

Visit 1

At the end of the assessment, the findings and working hypothesis were explained to Tony with the use of a model of the spine. A positive prognosis was conveyed to Tony, with eight to ten treatment sessions projected before discharge on a home and gym based exercise programme.

Part of our clinical approach often entails postponing treatment until the patient's second visit. This is because the evaluation stresses a variety of tissues and has the potential to aggravate the patient's condition. Therefore Tony was warned of the possibility of increased discomfort following the evaluation. Nothing further was undertaken on the first visit apart from education and advice about using ice at home for analgesic and anti-inflammatory purposes. Because Tony always felt improvement in his symptoms following periods of rest, he was encouraged to rest several times per day in the recumbent semi-Fowler position to facilitate disc nutrition. The rationale for this is the fact that the majority of disc rehydration occurs during the first hour of rest. He was also encouraged to avoid sleeping in prone lying as his symptoms appeared to be better when he did not sleep in this position. We have found that advising patients to sleep with a pillow between their legs, in addition to taping a bottle cap to their sternum, to be quite useful in discouraging them from sleeping on their stomachs. Following the evaluation Tony was also advised to initiate his celecoxib prescription as directed by the referring physician.

Visit 2

Tony reported no change in his symptoms. He had consulted with his psychiatrist who prescribed paroxetine for his depression.

The first actual treatment occurred at the second visit. Transversus abdominis (TA) spine stabilization exercises were initiated with Tony in supine lying (Jull and Richardson, 1994). TA contractions were held for 10 seconds for ten repetitions. This exercise was prescribed for the home setting and was to be performed five times per day. Single knee flexion exercises (30 seconds) and double knee flexion exercises (60 seconds) were also performed twice. These flexion exercises were to be carried out three times daily as a home exercise. Electrical stimulation and heat were also administered for analgesic purposes.

A back school education video was viewed that outlined the basics of spinal anatomy and the performance of sound body mechanics throughout the day. A call was also placed to the psychiatrist concerning Tony's high ZDI score and specifically his 'some or little of the time' response to the question 'Do you feel others would be better off if you were dead?'. The purpose of this call was to alert the psychiatrist to what may be considered a 'red-flag' response in the depression index. The psychiatrist appreciated this input and the call helped to facilitate a team approach to Tony's health care.

Visit 3

Tony reported no difficulties with the exercises and he was no longer having leg symptoms. However, since the last visit Tony had worked all weekend in the yard and now complained of 'low back muscle soreness' and left-sided superomedial scapula pain. He also reported continued non-compliance with taking his medications. He was again advised to initiate these medications. It was explained to him that his lack of sleep and persistent pain may both rapidly improve upon initiating the medications and that there was no real concern with addiction developing from taking these medications. It was also pointed out to Tony that there was some recent evidence to support the use of antidepressants even in non-depressed patients with LBP (Hampton Atkinson et al., 1998). Theoretically, these medications would help to address several of the hypothesized pain mechanisms (inflammatory nociceptive pain, increased central nervous system sensitivity and the affective contribution), so persuading Tony to take his medication was of real importance.

Treatment for this session involved advancing the spine stabilization exercises to include raising the leg from the bed with the knee flexed until the thigh approximated the vertical position, while simultaneously contracting the TA as previously instructed. Ten repetitions were performed on each side with maintenance of good control throughout. Two further stabilization exercises were added; alternate raising of each arm while in the four-point kneeling position (maintaining a neutral spine and a low grade TA contraction, 20 repetitions) and alternate raising of the knee from the ground when similarly positioned (10 repetitions). The patient was also instructed in hamstring stretches for both legs. These were to be performed at home twice daily for two repetitions and sustained for 60 seconds to increase the muscle length (Bandy et al., 1997). In addition, to help to counter the 'domestic stress' Tony was experiencing, he was instructed in diaphragmatic breathing in conjunction with progressive relaxation exercises (Jacobsen, 1938).

At this time it was decided not to treat the thoracic pain as this was not the primary reason for the initial referral and it was felt that this pain was probably the result of working in the yard and would subside with time.

Visit 4

Tony was now being seen for the second week and he reported that he had initiated his medications. The thoracic pain was now the primary complaint and it radiated around to the anterior chest. No positional

abnormality was detected with palpation of the thoracic spine. PPIVM assessment revealed hypomobility on right rotation at T3–T4 (graded as 2/6). Posteroanterior accessory movement of T3 reproduced the anteriorly radiating pain.

Traction of the thoracic spine in supine lying using a belt (Mulligan, 1992) decreased the symptoms and, therefore, this technique was performed for several minutes. Posteroanterior accessory movement of T3 was then found to be asymptomatic but the hypomobility with right rotation persisted. This was followed by a set of 10 oscillations into right rotation at the T3–T4 segment, progressing from mid-range initially to the end of available range by the final oscillation (Paris and Loubert, 1990). The patient was instructed to ice the thoracic spine region for 12–15 minutes following his home exercise programme. Although the thoracic spine pain appeared to be mechanical, Tony was advised to see a physician if the pain worsened because it had not been medically evaluated and the thoracic dysfunction had now been addressed. The TA exercise was also advanced to include alternate leg slides in the supine-lying position; however arm raises in four-point kneeling had to be temporarily ceased because of the thoracic spine pain.

Tony reported that he had been performing the progressive relaxation exercises, albeit rather intermittently, and they appeared to be helping with stress reduction. He was encouraged to continue to perform the activity on a daily basis and at times of heightened anxiety.

Visit 5

Five days later Tony reported the LBP continued to diminish, with the resting pain now 3/10 versus 5/10 on the initial evaluation. However, the thoracic pain continued to persist although it was less intense. The T3–T4 intervertebral joints were treated with pulsed ultrasound for 5 minutes. The spinal stabilization exercises were progressed with the addition of leg extension in prone lying. The mRMDQ and the ZDI were administered again. The score for the mRMDQ was 5/24 and the ZDI score was 39/69, both indicating substantial progress since the evaluation. This was explained to Tony who was delighted with this illustration of his progress. The improved scores may have been a result of our interventions, as well as from the pain-relieving and beneficial psychological effects of the medications. It is likely that improvements

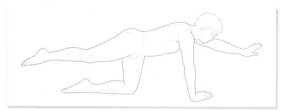

Fig. 22.3 Lumbar stabilization exercise in the four-point kneeling position, simultaneously raising the opposite arm and leg. (From Paris, 1997, p. 22. Reproduced with kind permission of the publisher.)

in both physical and psychological status combined to produce the changes in these measures.

Visit 6

The thoracic spine pain continued to lessen and the resting LBP was still rated at 3/10. The TA exercises were progressed to sitting (contraction held for 10 seconds and performed 10 times) and by simultaneously raising the opposite arm and leg while in the four-point kneeling position (Fig. 22.3). Alternate leg lifts in sitting were later added (30 repetitions). Again, Tony reported difficulty in disciplining himself to perform the relaxation exercises regularly.

Visit 7

One week later, Tony reported he had had no complaints of LBP or thoracic spine pain. He recorded that he was 'quite a bit better' on a Global Rating Scale (GRS) between −7 and +7 (Stratford et al., 1994). This equates to a numerical score of +5 on the GRS, which has been suggested as the cut-off for clinically important change in patients with LBP (Stratford et al., 1998). The ZDI score was down to 33/69 and the mRMDQ score was 3/24. A Modified Somatic Perceptions Questionnaire (MSPQ; Main, 1983) was administered and produced a score of 3. LBP patients with ZDI scores between 17/69 and 33/69 and who score greater than 12 on the MSPQ have a three- to fourfold increased risk of a poor outcome (Main et al.,

1992). Those who have ZDI scores between 17/69 and 33/69 and record less than 12 on the MSPQ have twice the likelihood of a poor outcome. Consequently, we felt that this patient was still at risk. Treatment continued with progression of the TA exercise to standing (10 repetitions with contraction held for 10 seconds), as well as the addition of gentle cardiovascular exercise for 5 minutes and knee extension (50 repetitions) and heel raise (40 repetitions) gym exercises. Arm raises in four-point kneeling were also recommended.

Visit 8

Tony's home exercises were reviewed. To address Tony's goal of returning to a gym-based programme, the following exercises were added: latissimus dorsi pulldowns; cable pulls for the trunk rotator muscles; seated rowing for the scapular retractor muscles; military presses for the shoulder musculature, including latissimus dorsi and serratus anterior; and modified squats for the hip and knee extensor muscles. Each of these exercises strengthen muscles that potentially help to stabilize the lumbopelvic region. Triceps muscle push downs were also added for variety. The recommended number of repetitions was 30 to 50 for each exercise, with the emphasis on good technique. Diagrams of each exercise were provided to Tony.

Visit 9

Tony was re-evaluated. He was now basically independent with a home-based exercise programme and had achieved his goals of returning to cycling and gym work-outs. Physical examination revealed that SLR was 80 degrees bilaterally. PPIVM was recorded as 3+ throughout the lumbar spine. Using the modified-modified Schöber method, flexion was recorded as +3.5 cm and extension as −2 cm, with minimal thoracic spine motion. Home exercises were again reviewed and the stabilization exercises progressed to include work with a Swiss ball. Tony had no further questions but was given the opportunity to contact the clinic if any concerns arose.

 ## REASONING DISCUSSION AND CLINICAL REASONING COMMENTARY

1 Your management at the end of the first consultation was primarily aimed at educating Tony to foster his understanding of the causes and management of his problem. What reasons did you have for adopting this approach?

Clinicians' answer

Pain can be described on the basis of three components: physical, emotional and rational (Paris, 1980). The explanation and prognosis provided the patient with a rational basis for understanding the physical component of his pain and thus help to diminish the emotional component of the pain (Paris, 1980) (Fig. 22.4). Extra emphasis was placed on education for this patient because his psychosocial presentation increased the likelihood that he would go on to have persistent pain. We believe that counselling patients in this manner helps to lay the foundation for successful physical treatment, especially if the patient has psychosocial dysfunction/impairment or is unclear of their expected role in the rehabilitation process. To date, Tony had been the recipient of 'passive' physical therapy interventions; therefore, clearly defining his involvement from the outset reduced the possibility of misunderstanding between the clinician and the patient. The intent of this approach is to maximize the chances of a positive outcome for the patient.

2 What was the rationale underlying the exercises you prescribed, including relevant clinical findings?

Clinicians' answer

The lumbar spinal stabilization regimen was initiated to counter the effects of mild instability and an intolerance to anterior shear forces. Patients with such a syndrome usually exhibit 'shaking' on forward bending, increased PPIVM range, increased muscle tone in standing, and an intolerance to static positioning,

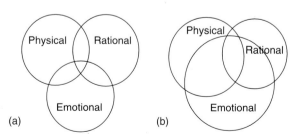

Fig. 22.4 The effects of pain (a) Three aspects of pain. (b) An overwhelming emotional concern can block out the physical component and reduce the rational component. (From Paris, 1980, p. 157. Reproduced with kind permission of the publisher.)

particularly at the end of the day or following prolonged activity when tissue creep may be at its greatest (Paris, 1985). Although this patient did not exhibit all of these signs, it is possible that the muscular guarding could have been responsible for masking any hypermobility during PPIVM testing. This was also the basis behind the decision not to provide mobilization or manipulation treatment. O'Sullivan et al. (1997) have demonstrated excellent results in a clinical trial using specific spinal stabilization exercises with such disorders. In this case, a similar exercise regimen was utilized, with the focus on correct technique and endurance training (gradually increased up to 3 minutes duration), in addition to progressing the level of difficulty and functional relevance of the exercises.

Concerning the prescription of flexion exercises, it is not uncommon for patients with a spondylolisthesis to experience aggravation of symptoms with exercises involving extension and relief with flexion exercises. This was exemplified by Tony experiencing increased symptoms when sleeping in a prone-lying position, thereby placing the lumbar spine in extension. The rationale for this hypothesis is the fact that extension of the lumbar spine produces anterior translation of the vertebral body, potentially exacerbating symptoms from the spondylolisthesis. Theoretically, flexion exercises should have the opposite effect by reducing anterior shear forces.

The prescription of hamstring stretches was based on the SLR testing and the slump test, which suggested that soft tissue restrictions of the hip extensor/knee flexor muscle groups existed. The aim of stretching these tissues was to address the dysfunction/impairment (decreased muscle length) and, therefore, optimize neuromuscular function across the involved joints, potentially reducing the patient's nociceptive pain. The progressive relaxation exercises were prescribed for pain control, stress and anxiety reduction, and to assist with the insomnia.

3 On reflection, how did the evident psychosocial issues influence your management of this patient?

Clinicians' answer

This patient was of particular interest because he presented with an array of symptoms and signs indicative of emotional overlay, that is, an excessive emotional component. Individuals with psychosocial distress have special requirements. For example, patients who are not sleeping well because of mental stress may continue to do poorly from a musculoskeletal standpoint unless the primary cause of their mental dysfunction/impairment is identified and addressed. In this instance, Tony required counselling by a mental health-care specialist regarding the stressful situation in his home setting. Patients receiving manual therapy are often seen more frequently by the treating therapist than by other members of the health-care team. This affords therapists an ideal opportunity for positively influencing psychological aspects of the patient's recovery, by explaining the physical, emotional and rational components of their pain on an ongoing basis.

The psychological component of this patient's presentation was also managed by the use of relaxation exercises. This was specifically intended to provide Tony with a self-management tool for his pain and stress. Treatment regimens that involve such an holistic approach are more likely to promote a rapid return to optimal functioning for the patient with LBP. In addition, by promptly communicating our concerns to the psychiatrist and the patient about the significant emotional component in the clinical presentation, recovery was facilitated by using a team approach. Finally, because of the psychosocial issues evidenced in this patient, a significantly greater amount of time was spent educating him regarding his pain than would be the case with a patient with pain of a predominantly nociceptive nature.

Despite reporting a gradual deterioration in his condition during recent years, Tony underwent clinically important changes during the period he attended the clinic. The self-reporting functional measure (mRMDQ) and depression index (ZDI) showed dramatic score reductions as Tony progressed through therapy. It is suggested that these tools are practical measures to track changes in the functional and psychological status of patients with LBP undergoing treatment. However, the precise reason for this patient's initially high ZDI and mRMDQ scores is unknown. Pain symptomatology could be a confounding factor for the ZDI score and depression could be a confounding factor for the mRMDQ score. While this patient was diagnosed with clinical depression, it could be that the LBP contributed to his originally high depression score and the subsequent decrease in

the score was at least in part a result of improvement in his LBP.

■ Clinical reasoning commentary

The importance of 'laying the foundation' for a successful outcome through addressing the patient's understanding of the problem (e.g. explaining the causes and prognosis) and expectations of treatment (i.e. passive versus active role) is very evident in the thinking of the expert clinicians. Such an approach should enhance the patient's ability to make informed choices regarding the proposed active programme of rehabilitation.

The explanation for the rationale underlying the exercises (Question 2) exemplifies the three types of knowledge that a manual therapist must access in successful management of patient problems. The use of propositional knowledge is evident in the rationale behind the prescription of the spinal stabilization exercises, with practice validated by clinical trials. Professional craft knowledge supported the implementation of the lumbar flexion and hamstring stretch exercises. Finally, personal knowledge facilitated a deep understanding of the clinical problem within the context of the patient's particular situation and was likely influential in the prescription of the progressive relaxation exercises (e.g. reducing stress resulting from domestic conflict). This overall awareness needed by manual therapists is best achieved in the context of real clinical problems.

The reflection about and learning from clinical experiences shown in the clinicians' discussion of the effect of psychosocial factors on management strategy is an essential part of developing a rich, well-organized knowledge base and clinical reasoning skill. However, the clinical expert takes reflective thinking to a higher level and employs metacognition, reflective appraisal of one's own thinking. Metacognition is evidenced in the clinicians' awareness of the quality and relevance of the information obtained through the self-report measures and their reasoning processes in utilizing these measures to understand the patient and his unique presentation and to achieve the goals of management. The development of clinical expertise requires a reasoning process that is reflective.

References

Bandy, W.D., Irion, J.M. and Briggler, M. (1997). The effect of time and frequency of static stretching on flexibility of the hamstring muscles. Physical Therapy, 77, 1090–1096.

Burton, A.K., Tillotson, K.M., Main, C.J. and Hollis, S. (1995). Psychosocial predictors of outcome in acute and subchronic low-back trouble. Spine, 20, 722–728.

Butler, D.S. (1991). Mobilisation of the Nervous System. Edinburgh: Churchill Livingstone.

Deyo, R.A., Rainville, J. and Kent, D.L. (1992). What can the history and physical examination tell us about low back pain? Journal of the American Medical Association, 268, 760–765.

Gonella, C., Paris, S. and Kutner, M. (1982). Reliability in evaluating passive intervertebral motion. Physical Therapy, 62, 436–444.

Greenspan, A. (1992). Orthopedic Radiology: A Practical Approach, 2nd edn. London: Lippincott–Raven.

Hampton Atkinson, J., Slater, M.A., Williams, R.A. et al. (1998). A placebo-controlled randomized trial of nortriptyline for chronic low back pain. Pain, 76, 287–296.

Inman, V.T. and Saunders, J.B. (1944). Referred pain from musculoskeletal structures. Journal of Nervous and Mental Disease, 90, 660–667.

Jacobsen, E. (1938). Progressive Relaxation, 2nd edn. Chicago, IL: University of Chicago Press.

Jull, G.A. and Richardson, C.A. (1994). Rehabilitation of active stabilization of the lumbar spine. In Physical Therapy of the Low Back, 2nd edn (L.T. Twomey and J.R. Taylor, eds.) pp. 251–274. Edinburgh: Churchill Livingstone.

Kellgren, J.H. (1938). Observations on referred pain arising from muscle. Clinical Science, 3, 175–190.

Magee, D.J. (1992). Orthopaedic Assessment, 2nd edn. London: Saunders.

Main, C.J. (1983). The Modified Somatic Perceptions Questionnaire (MSPQ).

Journal of Psychosomatic Research, 27, 503–514.

Main, C.J. and Waddell, G. (1984). The detection of psychological abnormality in chronic low back pain using four simple scales. Current Concepts in Pain, 2, 10–15.

Main, C.J., Wood, P.L.R., Hollis, S. et al. (1992). The Distress and Risk Assessment Method. A simple patient classification to identify distress and evaluate the risk of poor outcome. Spine, 17, 42–49.

McKinnis, L. (1996). Fundamentals of Orthopedic Radiology. Lansdale, PA: F.A. Davis.

Melzack, R. (1975). The McGill pain questionnaire: major properties and scoring methods. Pain, 3, 277–299.

Mooney, V. and Robertson, J. (1976). The facet syndrome. Clinical Orthopedics and Related Research, 115, 149–156.

Mulligan, B. (1992). Manual Therapy. 'NAGS', 'SNAGS', 'PRPS' etc. Wellington, New Zealand: Plane View Press.

O'Sullivan, P.B., Twomey, L.T. and Allison, G.T. (1997). Evaluation of specific stabilising exercises in the treatment of chronic low back pain with radiologic diagnosis of spondylolysis. Spine, 22, 2959–2967.

Paris, S.V. (1980). Manual therapy: Treat function not pain. In International Perspectives in Physical Therapy (T.H. Michel, ed.) pp. 152–167. Edinburgh: Churchill Livingstone.

Paris, S.V. (1985). Physical signs of instability. Spine, 10, 277–279.

Paris, S.V. (1997). Spinal Stabilization: Lumbar Spine. Understanding and Treatment. St Augustine, FL: University of St Augustine Institute Press.

Paris, S.V. and Loubert, P.V. (1990). Foundations of Clinical Orthopedics. St. Augustine, FL: University of St. Augustine Institute Press.

Patrick, D.L., Deyo, R.A., Atlas, S.J. et al. (1995). Assessing health-related quality of life in patients with sciatica. Spine, 20, 1899–1909.

Rivett, D.A. and Higgs, J. (1997). Hypothesis generation in the clinical reasoning behavior of manual therapists. Journal of Physical Therapy Education, 11, 40–45.

Roland, M. and Morris, R. (1983). A study of the natural history of low back pain. Part I: Development of a reliable and sensitive measure in low-back pain. Spine, 8, 141–144.

Stratford, P.W., Binkley, J., Solomon, P. et al. (1994). Assessing change over time in patients with low back pain. Physical Therapy, 74, 528–533.

Stratford, P.W., Binkley, J., Riddle, D.L. and Guyatt, G.H. (1998). Sensitivity to change of the Roland-Morris Back Pain Questionnaire Part 1. Physical Therapy, 78, 186–196.

Waddell, G. (1998). The Back Pain Revolution. Edinburgh: Churchill Livingstone.

Waddell, G., McCulloch, J.A., Kummel, E. and Venner, R.M. (1979). Nonorganic physical signs in low-back pain. Spine, 2, 117–125.

Walsh, R.M. (1999). Sensitivity of Three Modified Forms of the Roland Morris Disability Questionnaire. PhD Thesis, University of St Augustine, FL, USA.

Weinstein S.L. (1995). Deformities of the spine. In Essentials of the Spine (J.N. Weinstein, B.L. Rydevik and V.K.H. Sonntag, eds.) pp. 195–230. London: Raven.

White, A.A., Bernhadt, M. and Panjabi, M.M. (1999). Clinical biomechanics and lumbar spinal instability. In Lumbar Segmental Instability (M. Szpalski, R. Gunzburg and M.H. Pope, eds.) pp. 15–25. London: Lippincott Williams &Wilkins.

Williams, R., Binkley, J., Bolch, R. et al. (1993). Reliability of the modified-modified Schöber and double inclinometer methods for measuring lumbar flexion and extension. Physical Therapy, 73, 26–37.

Zung, W.W.K. (1965). A self-rating depression scale. Archives of General Psychiatry, 12, 63–70.

23

A non-musculoskeletal disorder masquerading as a musculoskeletal disorder

Peter E. Wells

SUBJECTIVE EXAMINATION

Steven is a 48-year-old self-employed graphic designer. He attended for a physiotherapy consultation regarding his low back and left leg pain. I met him first while he was sitting in the waiting room of the clinic and asked him to accompany me. He got to his feet with slight difficulty and carried a stick, which he used to walk and which he said helped if his back was bad. Steven was overweight but not obese and walked with a wide base. His right leg moved awkwardly (i.e. without normal rhythm) as he walked and he seemed unable to lift his right foot easily.

Steven said he tripped in the street 10 weeks previously and had fallen forwards with his hands in his pockets, more towards his right side. He had been unable to break his fall but he had not lost consciousness. He did not know why he had tripped but thought he may have stubbed his foot against a paving stone. At the time, he felt unharmed by the fall, but over the following 3 days he developed his symptoms (Fig. 23.1).

His main symptom was an intermittent left-sided mid-to-low lumbar deep aching, which when especially severe would spread across to include his right side. This pain would radiate bilaterally towards his outer hips, over the area of the greater trochanter. A further less-severe pain radiated posteriorly and down through his left buttock, posterior thigh and calf but did not extend into his foot. This was also intermittent and of a deep aching quality. The posterolateral aspect of his left calf felt 'extra sensitive' and the third and fourth toes of his left foot were perceived as slightly numb. Steven had had no pain at all in his right leg but commented he was dragging the leg as he walked, with

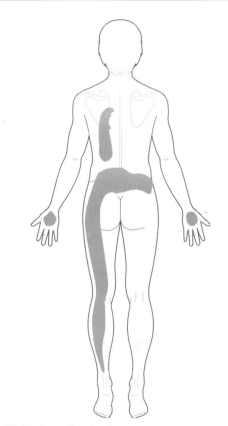

Fig. 23.1 Area of patient's symptoms.

his foot dropping towards the end of the day, and he had some difficulty in using his right leg.

In addition to the low back and leg symptoms, Steven reported that a band of left-sided thoracic 'electric sensitivity' occurred intermittently, extending from the lower border of his left scapula to his left thoracolumbar level. His arms had no symptoms except for a feeling of increasing weakness in his right hand and an intermittent ache over the dorsum of the hand. Because of these symptoms, he was finding it difficult to hold a pencil properly during his design work. He also reported some intermittent swelling and aching over the dorsum of his left hand. Finally, Steven had experienced aching across his upper thoracic region and the superior aspect of both scapulae, but this had improved with previous treatment. He had had no neck or head pain, nor throat, chest, or abdominal symptoms. The front of his legs and his feet were symptom-free, except for the two toes of his left foot.

Since the first week following his fall Steven's symptoms had remained fairly static, but varying somewhat. At present, all his symptoms were slightly easier. Initially he had sought help from an osteopath and received a series of treatments, which he described as 'cracking and crunching' of his neck and shoulder regions. This eased the pain he originally felt in this area but had not affected his other areas of symptoms.

The osteopath had recommended he consult a neurologist; therefore, he first went to his general practitioner (GP) to discuss the need for a referral. After Steven complained of unresolving low back pain, the doctor discussed his weight and general lack of fitness; however, no referral was provided. A friend had recommended he try physiotherapy treatment.

His low back and left leg pain were eased by lying supine but were aggravated by standing and walking, such that even after walking 100 m both his pains increased markedly and his right leg felt weaker. Working seated on the edge of his stool similarly increased his back and then leg pain.

When questioned about his general health, Steven reported having high blood pressure, which was controlled by medication. He suffered from gout for which he was prescribed allopurinol, and he had also taken ibuprofen occasionally over the previous weeks but with little effect. He was not diabetic and his weight was steady. No radiographs had been taken of his spine. Coughing and sneezing did not affect any of his symptoms and micturition was normal though slow. He had not suffered from any dizziness. The only reported numbness was of the toes of his left foot.

REASONING DISCUSSION AND CLINICAL REASONING COMMENTARY

1 What were your initial thoughts on meeting the patient? How did you interpret his symptoms and your early observations?

Clinician's answer

My initial thoughts on meeting the patient was that he was an intelligent, good-humoured man who, to some extent, made light of his problems and seemed to have no idea at all as to how serious his condition might be. I was beginning to suspect some form of tumour, the type and location of which I was not sure. The weakness of his right hand and his increasing difficulty holding a pencil led me to think that whatever pathological process was going on it must be below his mid-cervical spine. I also considered multiple sclerosis, remembering that pain, including backache, is occasionally an early symptom (Porth, 2002). Finally, I hypothesized that his back and left leg pain may have

been caused by a lumbar discal injury sustained at the time he tripped and fell.

2 You have spent considerable time mapping the patient's symptoms. What were your reasons for doing this? Did you have any thoughts regarding the pain mechanisms involved in this presentation?

Clinician's answer

I suppose that already, because of his gait pattern, I was entertaining the notion that there might be some upper motor neuron component to his disorder and I was initially looking for clues in the distribution and nature of his symptoms. Interestingly, the patient reported that there were no symptoms such as 'pins and needles' in the soles of his feet, which are often considered an early sign of cervical myelopathy

(Maitland et al., 2001). I thought that, whatever the underlying cause, there was a neurodynamic component to his disorder. This was suggested by the pain and paraesthesia extending through his left thoracic paraspinal area, left lumbosacral region and left leg. The weakness ('dragging') of his right leg and the weakness of his right hand were, to my mind however, more worrying aspects of his disorder.

3 What specific tests did you think were important to include in the physical examination and what were your reasons for planning to include them? Did you consider there were any precautions or contraindications to any part of the physical examination?

Clinician's answer

Since I was suspicious of a central neurological disorder from early on in the consultation, I proposed to 'cut corners' in the physical examination to focus on the central nervous system (CNS) in particular. However, I planned to be cautious with regard to his CNS and the forces I might impose upon it during examination. My suspicion of the possibility of a 'central lesion' without any knowledge of the underlying pathology caused me to worry. I planned to examine his CNS specifically, as well as his peripheral nervous system, using standard upper motor neuron clinical testing procedures (e.g. Babinski and clonus tests). The possibility of a cervical disc lesion, perhaps in the process of worsening, also meant I needed to be cautious with active cervical spinal mobility testing.

Other physical examination procedures to be performed included active lumbar spine flexion and extension, particularly but not exclusively as markers for a possible disc lesion. The addition of cervical flexion to lumbar flexion was to be used to test for any neurodynamic component to the disorder. Passive straight leg raise (SLR) and passive neck flexion tests were also to be employed, again to assess for possible neurodynamic components.

Clinical reasoning commentary

It is interesting to note that the clinician has from the outset focussed on the almost incidental finding of limb weakness, despite the patient's main complaint being that of back pain. He has recognized the potential significance of this finding and has immediately proceeded to test his primary hypothesis of a disorder affecting the conductivity of the CNS while mapping the patient's symptoms. This early recognition of 'red flags' is important because if his suspicion gains further supportive evidence then certain physical examination and treatment procedures are considered contraindicated for the time being until further medical investigation is undertaken, as they may worsen his condition or at the very least delay the implementation of appropriate treatment.

The clinician states that he intentionally plans to 'cut corners' in his physical examination. This may well sound to some as though he intends to undertake an incomplete physical examination, potentially increasing the risk of missing important information or biasing the examination toward his favoured hypothesis and, therefore, only paying 'lip service' to the aforementioned lower-ranked hypotheses (e.g. lumbar disc lesion). However, it is more than likely he will actually enhance his efficiency in conducting the physical examination by 'cutting corners', that is by employing 'maximizing principles', as he has ample clinical experience to recognize and avoid such errors of clinical reasoning. In fact, the use of maximizing principles is one of the hallmarks of expert clinicians and helps to promote efficiency and accuracy of their clinical reasoning. In this case, safety is foremost on the clinician's mind and while hypotheses in all categories (see Ch. 1) are, or could be, considered, the focussed physical examination is to be directed toward the testing of hypotheses regarding potential sinister pathology as the source of the symptoms, while bearing in mind the precautions and contraindications to physical examination and treatment.

PHYSICAL EXAMINATION

Analysis of Steven's gait showed he walked with a rather wide base of support and he reported feeling unsteady without his stick. His right leg looked

hypertonic in that the knee did not flex normally during the swing phase and he performed a circumduction movement. His foot likewise appeared not to dorsiflex during the lift off and swing phases. Steven appeared to be unable to lift his right foot clear of the ground with each step. His gait, therefore, suggested the presence of extensor spasm. Balancing on his left leg was steady, but he wobbled when attempting the same on the right leg.

Active spinal movements in standing were tested. Forward bending of the trunk was limited by increasing low back pain, with his fingertips just reaching his tibial tuberosities. Addition of cervical flexion to this movement produced some pain into the left buttock. Trunk extension was limited by stiffness at 20 degrees, with some central low back pain reproduced. Side bending to the left was restricted but painless, while moving to the right provoked right-sided low back pain and was limited.

In supine lying, passive neck flexion was approximately 70 degrees in range and was symptom-free.

Passive SLR was to 80 degrees on the left and produced no pain. However, upon the addition of ankle dorsiflexion, a stretching pain was provoked down the leg similar to Steven's familiar deep ache. His right-sided passive SLR was limited to 60 degrees by a marked feeling of hard resistance.

The neurological examination revealed bilateral moderate calf muscle weakness in standing. His right ankle dorsiflexors and evertors were also considerably weak. There was decreased sensation to light touch and pinprick throughout his left leg. Tendon reflexes at the ankle and knee were hyper-reflexic bilaterally. Ankle clonus was present on the right side and a positive Babinski reflex (upgoing big toe) was present bilaterally. At this stage the physical examination was concluded.

REASONING DISCUSSION

1 What was your interpretation of the SLR findings, particularly the end-feel?

Clinician's answer

My interpretation of the left SLR was in keeping with the hypothesis of increased neural sensitivity (mechanical or physiological). It was not, at a limitation of 80 degrees, typical of discal compression. The restriction on the right side was, if anything, more interesting. It was, in spite of the patient having no pain in the right leg and the fact that the back pain was worse on the left side, significantly more limited. The end-feel of the right SLR, a very hard resistance or block to movement, suggested a powerful guarding reaction.

2 What were your reasons for ceasing your examination at this time? Specifically, what

hypotheses were you entertaining and what findings supported and refuted each hypothesis?

Clinician's answer

The examination was stopped because of the significant responses elicited during my basic neurological examination. My primary hypothesis was that these upper motor neuron responses to testing were caused by a space-occupying lesion high in the spinal canal/cord. It had to be a cervical or cervicothoracic lesion to produce the weakness of the right hand. Alternatively, I thought that perhaps multiple sclerosis was a possible diagnosis/secondary hypothesis, particularly as it may present with low back pain as an initial symptom. Although the relief obtained in the supine-lying position might suggest a discogenic component to the disorder, it is of markedly lesser clinical significance. I cannot claim any greater insight than this.

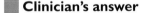

m Management

It was explained to Steven that the examination so far indicated that the weakness and numbness and the disturbance of gait were more important features to investigate than the back and the leg pain. In order

to not alarm him it was suggested to him that some 'nerve irritation' needed to be looked into before any further physiotherapy could be considered and the sooner this was done the better. The GP was telephoned at this point and the need for an urgent review of his presentation was discussed. An appointment was made for the patient to attend the doctor's surgery the next morning and the consultation was concluded.

Following this visit to his GP, Steven was urgently referred to a neurosurgical hospital. A magnetic resonance imaging scan revealed a major cervical disc prolapse at C5–C6 compressing the spinal cord. He underwent a cervical discectomy and fusion (Cloward procedure) a few days later and was subsequently placed in a firm collar.

REASONING DISCUSSION AND CLINICAL REASONING COMMENTARY

1 Communication was obviously a key part of your management at this stage. What were your main considerations in your conversations with the patient and the doctor, bearing in mind that the doctor had missed the neurological findings?

Clinician's answer

Mainly, I did not want to alarm the patient. This was because:

- there was no point since he was being seen by his doctor the following day
- there was nothing to be gained by alarming or worrying the patient, who might then have passed a distressing 24 hours before seeing his doctor
- I did not consider it within my remit as a physiotherapist to raise the possibility of various medical diagnoses, all of which were serious.

My only consideration in speaking to the doctor was to impress on him the urgency of the situation so that the patient could be diagnosed without delay and appropriate medical or surgical intervention instituted at the earliest point in time. I was very diplomatic, emphasizing that the patient appeared to have considerably worsened since his consultation with the doctor, and stating my findings of upper motor neuron signs.

The doctor, for whatever reason, did not appear to realise the urgency of the situation and I had to insist on the patient being seen the following day. I told him that my 'gut feeling' was that the patient had a very serious pathology that would brook no delay. The doctor never contacted me after he saw the patient.

2 On reflection, were you able to identify any factors that contributed to the development of this problem? What was your prognosis?

Clinician's answer

All symptom areas appeared within 3 days after the patient's fall, not having been present beforehand. His gait had worsened since, as had his right-hand weakness. It seems likely the fall had provoked or severely worsened the underlying cause of his problem. He was a heavy man and probably the violence of his fall, perhaps with a whiplash-like effect on his neck, caused the discal prolapse.

Once I knew the diagnosis and surgery had been performed, I thought full recovery of normal arm and leg function was unlikely, although I hoped residual paresis and spasticity would be minimal. The extent of neurological recovery is notoriously difficult to predict, especially in the long term, and I held out hope that even over several years any neurological deficit might improve further.

Clinical reasoning commentary

'Gut feeling' is a term commonly used by clinicians for describing a vague, nagging sense that a particular clinical impression or course of action is correct, despite incomplete or equivocal evidence. It is also sometimes referred to as 'clinical intuition' and is often dismissed as being an unscientific and subjective hunch. The expert clinician, however, has learnt to heed such feelings, as in this case. The clinician had discovered through reflection on his own clinical experiences that this 'inner prompting', perhaps caused by the subconscious recognition of a previously encountered clinical cue or pattern, should not be ignored and warranted closer attention.

Intuitive skills have been recognized as an important part of expert clinical reasoning and have been linked to clinical experience with specific patient cases.

Outcome

Five weeks after his spinal surgery, Steven was referred back for a physiotherapy assessment of his gait and general mobility problems. He was beginning to show improvement in his hand function but progress in the function of his legs was much slower. Rehabilitation was undertaken over the following 3 months to facilitate an improvement in his coordination and balance. At 6 months after surgery, his condition ceased to improve. His gait was less spastic but he continued to need a stick in order to walk. The strength and coordination of his hands had improved greatly. Nevertheless, Steven remained considerably disabled. He also continued to have low back stiffness and aching, with occasional aching down his left leg, for which he received treatment. His neural provocation tests, such as passive SLR, remained quite restricted, but at the time of his discharge were not associated with any ongoing symptoms.

References

Maitland, G., Hengeveld, E., Banks, K. and English K. (2001). Maitland's Vertebral Manipulation, 6th edn. Oxford: Butterworth-Heinemann.

Porth, C.M. (2002). Pathophysiology. Concepts of Altered Health States, 6th edn. London: Lippincott Williams &Wilkins.

CHAPTER 24

Forearm pain preventing leisure activities

Israel Zvulun

SUBJECTIVE EXAMINATION

Dan is a 51-year-old married man with three children who has been referred for physiotherapy by an orthopaedic surgeon who had diagnosed 'cervical discopathy at the C6–C7 level with radiculopathy'. Dan is the owner of a material factory specializing in exclusive cuttings for the clothing market. He has worked for 20 years as the manager of the factory and has been subjected to intensive and stressful working conditions because of market demands. His only leisure activity was during weekends, when he used to ride a Jet Ski for 2–4 hours. Since the onset of the recent problem he had stopped that activity.

Four years before the commencement of the presenting condition, he underwent open-heart surgery for coronary heart disease. There was no history of smoking or poor dietary habits and the heart disease

was mainly related to a genetic predisposition. Dan reported that since the surgery he had no time for regular exercise, although he was aware of the importance of cardiovascular fitness. His mother, aged 82, had suffered three myocardial infarctions and had a heart functioning at 35% of maximal capacity. His father died of lung cancer at a relatively young age. This was the first time Dan had suffered from any problem in the upper quadrant. In the past, he had experienced a backache and dealt with the pain by use of rest and analgesics. Dan had not received any physiotherapy treatment previously. The orthopaedic surgeon did not prescribe any medications but recommended a cervical collar, cervical mobilization, ultrasonic therapy and transcutaneous electrical nerve stimulation (TENS).

REASONING DISCUSSION AND CLINICAL REASONING COMMENTARY

1 What were your initial thoughts based on the patient's profile?

■ Clinician's answer

Medical diagnoses for many musculoskeletal conditions are very often non-specific (e.g. neck pain, cervicobrachialgia). The medical diagnosis in this case described a very specific condition (clinical pattern)

that might include pain in the posterior neck area, radicular pain referred distally, paraesthesiae and other neurological signs and symptoms. However, other hypotheses related to the anatomical sources of the symptoms had to be considered. These included the extensor/supinator muscle group of the wrist, the radial nerve at the arcade of Froshe, the elbow and proximal radioulnar joints, referred pain from the shoulder, and the wrist joint.

Referred pain of visceral origin could also be a source of the symptoms (his father died of a lung cancer). Pancoast's tumour (tumor of the lung apex) can refer pain to the forearm and can mimic a C8–T1 nerve root lesion. Thyroid carcinoma or other site-occupying lesions of the neck and throat can also spread metastases to the brachial plexus and cause referred symptoms to the forearm. However, these usually manifest in a non-dermatomal distribution as opposed to nerve root syndrome.

The heart disease might have served as a visceral origin for the forearm pain. This may have occurred through the sensitization of nociceptive afferents of the heart by ischaemia and the trauma of surgery, which may, in turn, irritate convergent afferent neurons from the upper limb and initiate the onset of referred pain to the forearm (Ness and Gebhart, 1990).

Surgery causes tissue damage (somatic, visceral and neural), which may disrupt nociceptive afferent fibres and postoperative pain could contribute to the development of central sensitization (Hayes and Molloy, 1997). Therefore, pain mechanisms might include a peripheral nociceptive and neuropathic pain mechanism with a central component. These mechanisms are also applicable to the 'orthopaedic' condition, notably the disc (and other somatic structures) and the nerve root. This necessitates more than just examining and directing treatment to specific structures in the neck; it is important also to look for the expression of central sensitization (e.g. increased receptive fields and motor phenomena) caused by intense stimulation of nociceptive afferent fibres. This requires a broader approach to physical examination and management.

Open-heart surgery may markedly stress the costovertebral joints and other anatomical structures attaching to the thoracic cage and cervical spine (for example the scalene muscles). This may predispose the cervical spine to muscular imbalance, but it can also cause an imbalance of the whole neuromusculoskeletal system. This muscular imbalance can increase the stress on anatomical structures of the cervical and thoracic spine. The contribution of muscular imbalance can lead to the development of a disc problem, compression of nerves of the brachial plexus by the scalenes muscles and problems in the shoulder girdle as a result of weakening or tightening of shoulder girdle tissues (such as pectoralis major tightness and rhomboid weakness). In addition, the original anatomical alignment may not be reestablished when the sternum is sutured at the end of the operation. From my own clinical experience, most patients undergoing open-heart surgery develop pain and limited mobility of one shoulder (usually the left) and often pain in the pelvic/buttock area (usually the right). The 'new' anatomical alignment may cause a permanent imbalance between pelvic, trunk and upper limb structures, and in particular between ipsilateral latissimus dorsi and contralateral gluteus maximus (Vleeming et al., 1997). This 'new' anatomical alignment may have contributed to the development of the forearm pain.

Recurrent lower back pain may point to a postural problem, poor ergonomics and/or poor body mechanics during work and other functional activities as contributing factors to the onset of the recent problem.

The patient's stress during work may have been a possible contributing factor to the amplification of pain (and of course to the heart problem). However, Dan 'had no time to be sick and wanted to get rid of the problem as quickly as possible'. At this stage, it was reasonable to hypothesize that stress may not be a significant contributing factor; on the contrary, the fact that Dan wanted to get well quickly may be a positive factor that may have enhanced the improvement of his condition. This hypothesis remained to be proven during the assessment and management of that disorder.

Anticoagulant therapy and the fact that Dan had a disc protrusion are contraindications to manipulation (high-velocity low-amplitude thrust), particularly rotatory manipulation that might stress the disc material and cause further protrusion.

Positive factors related to prognosis were the facts that this was the first time Dan had suffered an upper limb problem, he had not received physiotherapy treatment previously and he was relatively young. In contrast, potential negative prognostic factors included poor compliance with physical exercise ('he complained he had no time for regular exercise'), the open-heart surgery, a 20-year history of stressful work and the fact that his leisure activity (jet skiing) potentially involved sustained cervical extension, vibration and compression.

▪ Clinical reasoning commentary

Some manual therapists believe that specific judgments about a patient's problem should be avoided until the examination is completed. The answer to Question 1 nicely highlights the breadth and depth of reasoning that can and does occur even in the opening moments of a patient interview. In the midst of a patient exchange, when the clinician is focussed on listening to and understanding the patient's answers, the thoughts elicited are often tacit. However, when questioned, as evident here, expert manual therapists are doing much more than just listening. Even in these opening moments with the patient, the clinician is beginning to formulate an impression of the patient as a person and the scope of the patient's problem. Here the clinician has reflected on a broad range of thoughts from possible sources of the patient's symptoms to contributing factors, pain mechanisms, precautions and prognosis. When viewed as 'hypotheses', this initial problem formulation is not set, rather it provides a framework by which these early thoughts can be further tested throughout the patient interview, physical examination and ongoing management.

Area and type of symptoms

A week prior to his referral, Dan experienced a spontaneous onset of a deep, sharp pain in the dorsolateral aspect of the left forearm with pins and needles in the distal palmar aspect of the second and third fingers. He reported that the forearm pain was present at rest, while the pins and needles appeared mainly with extension of the cervical spine. Dan's posture during work included long periods of sustained neck flexion. Riding the Jet Ski involved generally cervical extension with some lower cervical flexion and mid to upper cervical extension; vibrations and shocks were transmitted from the machine while in motion. Dan could not recall any recent or past trauma that could explain the onset of the symptoms. In-depth questioning for further areas of symptoms revealed no other complaints or symptoms, except for a dull ache in the lower back that had been present for years with no recent exacerbation. Dan's presenting symptoms are depicted in Figure 24.1.

Disability and pain behaviour

During daily activities, Dan reported mild forearm pain but could work cutting materials while his neck was flexed. The movements of the upper limbs during work included a combination of shoulder horizontal adduction and internal rotation, elbow flexion, forearm pronation, and wrist and finger flexion of both hands. The right hand was used to cut the material in a movement of horizontal adduction, while the left hand

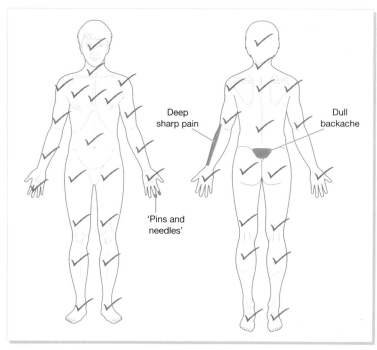

Deep
sharp pain

Dull
backache

'Pins and
needles'

Fig. 24.1 Area and types of symptom.

stabilized the material. If Dan attempted to extend his neck, pain in the forearm and paraesthesiae would immediately increase in intensity. When returning to the flexed position, the level of pain decreased within a few seconds, but the pins and needles remained for a minute or two. Isolated upper limbs and trunk positions or movements did not aggravate his symptoms.

Before the problem started Dan used to sleep in the prone-lying position with his head rotated to the left. At present, he could only sleep in the supine-lying position with two pillows and he woke up occasionally when rolling over in bed as a result of forearm pain. Pain subsided quickly when the supine position was readopted. He would wake up in the morning with a feeling of stiffness in the neck that disappeared after taking a hot shower. Initially, Dan was worried that his symptoms were related to his previous heart disease. His cardiologist had ruled this out, which alleviated those concerns. His main concern at this stage was 'to get rid of this problem as soon as possible'. Dan expressed that he did not have time to be sick and he also wanted to get back to his Jet Ski riding as soon as possible. He was worried about the anatomical origin of the problem and did not know what the consequences of a disc bulge were and how this could be treated by physiotherapy. He was also anxious about the possibility of being paralysed.

Medical and hereditary history

Dan underwent open-heart surgery four years prior to referral for physiotherapy. During the postoperative time he experienced an event of atrial fibrillation that was treated by electric shock therapy. Pain control during the postoperative period was adequate according to Dan's report. During the months following cardiac surgery he had two additional events of atrial fibrillation treated in a similar way. At present, his cardiac condition was being managed by medications, with regular follow-up visits to his cardiologist.

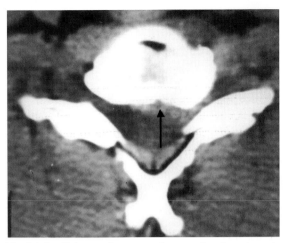

Fig. 24.2 Computed tomography scan showing a lateral disc herniation at the C6–C7 level.

Investigations

The findings from computed tomography (CT) scanning of the cervical spine were intervertebral disc bulges at C3–C6, hypertrophic and spondylotic changes from C1–C6 with narrowing of the neuroforamina on the left, and a lateral disc herniation at the C6–C7 level with compression of the spinal cord (Fig. 24.2). Magnetic resonance imaging studies were recommended by the radiologist; however, Dan was not referred. The nature of the disc herniation was not defined by the radiologist.

Medications

At present, Dan took medications for his heart problems, which included 50 mg atenolol for the control of blood pressure, 150 mg propafenone for the control of the heart pace and 100 mg aspirin as an anticoagulant. No medications were prescribed by the orthopaedic surgeon for his presenting problem, and Dan did not take non-prescription drugs.

REASONING DISCUSSION AND CLINICAL REASONING COMMENTARY

1 Given the onset and behaviour of symptoms, what were your hypotheses regarding the dominant pain mechanisms contributing to his problem(s) (physical and/or psychosocial)?

Clinician's answer

The dominant pain mechanisms present in this patient appeared to be a combination of peripheral neurogenic and nociceptive mechanisms. Looking simplistically at the clinical presentation, Dan demonstrated a clinical pattern consistent with compromise of the C7 nerve root. His symptoms were increased by extending his neck. It is common to think that extension of the neck compromises the nerve root or dorsal root ganglion mechanically, especially if neurological symptoms are present. If this is the case, a peripheral neurogenic mechanism is likely to be the dominant pain mechanism because of primary neural structure involvement. Recently, it has been suggested that inflammation, and not mechanical pressure alone, may be the primary cause of nerve root pain (Hasue, 1993). In such conditions, pain is severe, excruciating, burning in nature, experienced mainly at rest and referred distally to the relevant dermatome. Dan's presentation did not appear to have a major inflammatory component, although moderate pain was present at rest. His symptoms were made worse by a mechanical trigger (neck extension). Extension of the cervical spine can also compress or impinge somatic structures, including joint capsules, discs, muscles and ligaments. In this case, a concurrent pain mechanism could be a peripheral nociceptive mechanism.

Although the clinical presentation pointed to a peripherally mediated pain (neurogenic and nociceptive), an underlying central pain mechanism had to be considered. It is reasonable to think that the involved neural structures were compromised long before the symptoms started. The symptoms may have started as a result of inflammation or a lowering of nociceptive threshold. This means that nociceptive activity (without pain at this stage) occurred in the neural and somatic structures before the symptoms started. The visceral component of heart ischaemia and surgery would also have been potent sources for the development of central sensitization. The impact of neurogenic pain on the central nervous system is much greater than the input from nociceptive pain (Dubner, 1997). The primary neural involvement and the somatic and visceral components of the disorder may, therefore, have enhanced the development of central sensitization.

An affective and cognitive component may also have been present. However, a negative affective component did not appear to be dominant in this case. Dan expressed that 'he wanted to get rid of the problem as soon as possible' and that 'he had no time to be sick'. He was the owner of the factory and this position required him to cope with the problem and resolve it rapidly. He was eager to go back to his normal activities. In spite of that, his personal interpretation of the problem may have been a source of anxiety and

might have contributed to the maintenance or aggravation of his symptoms. This could be dealt with by explaining the benign course and self-limiting nature of the disorder and emphasizing the limited relevance of imaging studies.

> **2** Had you identified any other potential contributing factors to the onset and maintenance of his activity and participation restrictions and symptoms at this stage?

Clinician's answer

Several factors might have contributed to the onset and maintenance of his activity and participation restrictions and symptoms.

- Working for 20 years in poor ergonomic conditions (with the neck flexed and, asymmetrical use of the upper limbs against resistance) may have stressed somatic structures such as the C6–C7 disc, which in turn had compressed the spinal nerve root.
- Dan's heart disease and surgery are likely to have played a central role in this problem. The sympathetic innervation of the heart may begin as high as C3 but mainly comes from the T5 segment; sympathetic innervation of the upper limb may reach as far as T9 (Grieve, 1994). It is known that inflammation and ischaemia of cardiac tissue cause sensitization of visceral nociceptors and an increase of afferent input; excitation of central neurons leading to the persistence of pain (Cervero, 1995). Pain sensitivity can also be increased by intense stimulation of visceral structures. It might be that the neural and somatic structures involved were already sensitized by previous visceral input. The fact that visceral afferents converge with somatic afferents onto the central nervous system may partly serve as an explanation for the somatic component of Dan's disorder. Furthermore, plastic changes in the central nervous system induced by intense afferent input (from the heart surgery or ischaemia) play a role in the development and maintenance of hyperalgesia (Cervero, 1995; Zermann et al., 1998).
- A complementary hypothesis may be a sympathetic impairment caused by the heart disease. Abnormal sympathetic activity may have induced trophic changes at the disc and other somatic structures of the spine and extremities through convergent input from visceral to somatic neurons and vice versa and the occurrence of viscerosomatic and somatovisceral reflexes.

- Riding a Jet Ski once a week for 2–4 hours may have been a mechanical factor that contributed to the onset of the problem. Vibrations and shocks transmitted from the machine while the cervical spine is mainly held in extension could potentially produce disc damage and injure other tissues as well.
- The lower back pain may reflect a previously mechanically disadvantaged spine. The likely origin of the lower back pain appears to be a combination of poor posture and alignment of the whole spine and possibly inadequate muscular control. Initial observation of Dan's posture supported this hypothesis.
- Dan's interpretation of his problem might be another contributing factor. Developing structure-oriented beliefs may lead to fear of movement and contribute to the amplification and maintenance of the symptoms and activity or participation restrictions.
- Dan's sleeping position appears to be important as a contributing factor. Sleeping for a reasonable period of time mainly in prone lying with the neck rotated to the left may have induced changes in somatic tissues of the cervical spine. Bony changes are likely to have occurred mainly on the left side as the joints and other tissues are compressed. This may gradually have caused narrowing of the foramina, compromising the pain-sensitive nerve root or dorsal root ganglion.

3 What significance did you place on Dan's concerns regarding the anatomical origin of his problem and the consequences of the disc bulge (e.g. potential paralysis) he had been told was the source of his symptoms?

Clinician's answer

Dan's understanding and concerns regarding the diagnosis and potential outcome of paralysis were likely to be unhelpful to his recovery. Therefore I felt that, while the recent onset of the problem was a positive prognostic factor that diminished the likelihood of fixation of abnormal illness behaviours, explanations regarding the natural course of such a usually benign problem were of primary importance in order to avoid structure-oriented beliefs and fear-avoidance behaviour. Pathoanatomy, pathoneurobiology and pathobiomechanics were areas of knowledge that provided a basis for these explanations. Dan was highly motivated to resolve his problem. He felt he had to get back to maximal functioning quickly because he was the owner of a factory. Through a process of explanation and sharing my own reasoning with Dan in relation to pathological aspects of the problem, pain mechanisms and the limited validity of imaging findings, he was able to develop a revised and more productive understanding.

4 At another level of your thinking, would you comment on any clues regarding potential precautions and contraindications to either the physical examination or the management that you would have picked up by this stage in the patient interview?

Clinician's answer

There were several points:

- flexion of the cervical spine was contraindicated in order to avoid causing further damage to the disc and related neural structures
- manipulation was contraindicated because of the potential involvement of the disc and nerve root and the use of anticoagulants
- exercising against forced resistance (especially of the upper limbs), if relevant, would require obtaining approval from his cardiologist.

Clinical reasoning commentary

The clinician's organization of knowledge into clinical patterns is clearly evident. The patterns are not limited to the underlying diagnosis or pathology. Rather he speaks of evidence emerging across a range of hypothesis categories. While novices commonly make premature conclusions based on one or two dominant features in a presentation, experts should be able to recognize evidence for competing hypotheses and overlapping patterns. This is apparent in the clinician's answers here, where the evidence for different pain mechanisms is discussed.

The breadth of consideration associated with expert reasoning is also well demonstrated in this clinician's thoughts regarding potential contributing factors. Ergonomic, biomechanical, endogenous physical and psychosocial (cognitive and behavioural) factors are all mentioned. It is also characteristic of expert reasoning that explanation is presented as being of primary importance and a central feature of the management rather than a simple routine 'this is your problem and this is what it needs' edict.

PHYSICAL EXAMINATION

Observation

Dan's posture in the upright position is depicted in Figure 24.3. Observing his posture in this position revealed a median sternal scar, a 'forward-head posture', bilateral shoulder protraction and concomitant lower cervical spine flexion. An attempt to straighten the whole trunk, including the cervical spine, increased the forearm pain and pins and needles, which subsided after a few seconds. Extending the trunk alone did not change the symptoms. During observation, it seemed that Dan's willingness to move the cervical spine was limited. A line of tightening of the inframandibular soft tissues was also apparent from the inferior part of the mandible down to the upper part of the sternum. His lower abdominal area appeared slightly distended. No signs of muscular atrophy or other trophic changes were observed.

Mobility testing

Cervical spine

Extension of the cervical spine in standing was approximately 5 degrees and increased the pain and pins and needles. The movement occurred primarily in the upper cervical spine, with no movement observable below the C5 level. Performing a gentle passive posterior translation of the lower cervical spine in the sitting position increased Dan's forearm pain and paraesthesia significantly. Returning to the resting position eased the symptoms within a few seconds. Active flexion was of normal range, but overpressure at the end of flexion range was avoided in the light of the radiological findings. Rotation in the sitting position was slightly restricted to the left, more so than to the right, with no reproduction of the symptoms. Lateral flexion was not tested as this movement is coupled with rotation and true side bending of a cervical vertebra is not possible because of the anatomical configuration of the cervical vertebrae (Bogduk, 1994). Testing of rotation in various positions of cervical flexion or extension was not necessary as the symptoms were already reproduced by cervical extension. Manual traction performed in sitting and in supine lying increased Dan's symptoms. Tightness of the infrahyoid muscles could also be felt during manual examination of the transverse mobilization of these muscles to the right.

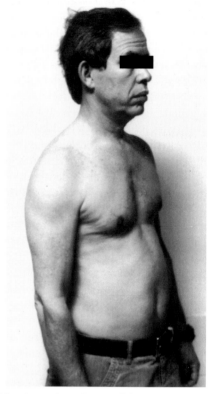

Fig. 24.3 Anterolateral view of the patient.

All other cervical region muscle length was considered normal, except for tight splenae on the left.

Thoracic spine

Rotation was 60 degrees to the right and 80 degrees to the left, with no symptoms reproduced during either movement. Extension and flexion of the thoracic spine appeared normal. Lateral flexion was not tested. Mobility of the thoracic cage in the cephalad direction was examined by asking the patient to inspire deeply and then mobilizing the lower part of the rib cage upwards. During this procedure, resistance could be felt and Dan reported remarkable tenderness of the lower part of the rib cage.

Lumbar spine

Extension of the lumbar spine tested in prone lying (while adding a manual posteroanterior force from L4 to S1) was limited by resistance at end range, with a feeling of stiffness experienced by Dan. The movement was only slightly limited and mainly in the lower lumbar segments. Flexion was tested in the long sitting position and lumbar spine movement was considered normal. Finger to toe reach was more significantly reduced with the knees fully extended than with both ankles fully dorsiflexed and with the knees slightly flexed. Neck flexion in long sitting did not have any effect on the overall movement.

Shoulder girdle

All signs and symptoms produced by the shoulder during examination were more pronounced on the left side than on the right. The symptoms were pain in the upper part of the deltoid and subacromial areas, and also tightness in the chest and shoulder anteriorly.

Shoulder flexion was limited by resistance, with slight discomfort in the subacromial area. The left shoulder was more restricted than the right in both flexion and internal rotation (in 90 degrees abduction). The end-feel of these movements was stiffer on the left as compared to the right. A mild resistance could be felt during the last 20 degrees of external rotation of the left shoulder and at the end range of flexion, and Dan reported tightness in the anterior aspect of the chest. Muscle length testing revealed tight pectorals, latissimus dorsi and teres major; again more marked on the left than on the right. Inferior and anteroposterior accessory movements of the left glenohumeral joint tested at the end range of flexion were also more restricted on the left than on the right. Subacromial pain was reproduced with the inferior glide performed also at the end of the flexion range. Other joint play movements of the shoulder were normal, with no symptoms reproduced during these movements.

Elbow region

Both active and passive flexion movements of the left elbow were normal. There was a limitation of 5 degrees at the end of extension range with a 'leathery' end-feel. Dan reported a dull ache and a feeling of tightness in the anterior aspect of the elbow during this movement. Supination was slightly limited at end range, as was pronation, but no symptoms were provoked during either movement. A combination of supination and elbow extension revealed an increase in resistance and an increase of the dull ache in the anterior elbow region. A combination of pronation and elbow extension with wrist palmar flexion produced discomfort over the dorsal aspect of the wrist. None of these movements reproduced Dan's symptoms. The same movements of the right elbow were normal.

Wrist

All physiological movements of the wrist were normal and free of symptoms.

Muscle control

Testing for rectus abdominis length produced a feeling of tightness in the upper abdominal area. When asked to perform an isometric contraction of transversus abdominis in the standing position, it took several attempts before Dan could perform the correct action. The contraction could only be held for a few seconds while performing the movements he uses at work, following which substitution with external oblique and rectus overactivity was apparent.

Neurological examination

Reduced muscle strength of the biceps and triceps muscles and a decreased triceps reflex were found on the left side. No cord signs were detected during examination. Sensation was considered normal.

Neurodynamic tests

Upper limb neurodynamic test 1 (median nerve bias). This upper limb neurodynamic test (ULNT) did not reproduce Dan's symptoms. However, all components showed restricted motion on the left side compared with the right side, with a dull ache felt from the wrist up to the axillary region. This ache was not present on testing the right side.

Upper limb neurodynamic test 2 (radial nerve bias). Except for a feeling of tightness in the lateral aspect and dorsum of the upper arm, forearm and wrist, no other symptoms could be reproduced and the range of movement was normal on the right side. This feeling of tightness was more marked on the left side, with a slight restriction of range evident.

Slump test. No significant symptoms could be reproduced with the slump test.

Palpation

A large area of allodynia (i.e. pain from a stimulus that does not normally provoke pain) was detected with firm palpation and mobilization of the skin over the posterior cervical area and the left side of the back down to the lumbar spine. Skin mobility was also restricted, especially in the left cervical and posterior shoulder girdle area. The skin in this area was thickened. Interestingly, pain and pins and needles in the forearm could be reproduced while palpating and mobilizing the skin of all the above areas and also with non-specific pressures applied to the deep structures of the cervical and thoracic regions. Dan had not reported any symptoms in these areas prior to palpation.

Tight bands of muscles on the left side could be felt during palpation of the deep muscles of the cervical spine, with remarkable tenderness elicited and forearm pain and pins and needles reproduced. The upper trapezius muscle on the left was thickened and tender. Deep palpation of the bony structures showed marked thickening over the articular pillar, most notably at the C6 level on the left side, and to a lesser degree at the C5 and C7 levels.

Pressure on the left forearm skin and muscles in the symptomatic area produced hyperalgesia (an increased response to a stimulus that is normally painful). On the right forearm, allodynia was present in an identical area as the left forearm (as the patient had not reported any symptoms in the right forearm, the response to palpation was defined as 'allodynia'). Significant tenderness was also found over the deltoid region, more on the left side than on the right side, and especially in the posterior part of the muscle. Palpation of the left radial nerve in the radial groove produced paraesthesiae in the dorsal forearm and wrist. This response was not elicited with the right radial nerve. Palpation of the abdominal area and the anterior chest detected large areas of allodynia, particularly over the surgical scar and the upper abdominal area. A marked restriction of mobility of the skin in these areas was also detected. During palpation and mobilization of rectus abdominis, dysaesthetic pain (i.e. a painful, unpleasant abnormal sensation) was produced in the left forearm and wrist regions, with an expansion of the pins and needles area to the whole upper limb and hand.

REASONING DISCUSSION AND CLINICAL REASONING COMMENTARY

1 Despite the emerging pattern of a C7 nerve root compromise from the examination of the spine and shoulder, you still proceeded to carry out quite an extensive physical examination of other areas at the first visit. Could you comment on your reasoning for this?

Clinician's answer

In spite of an emerging clinical pattern of C7 nerve root syndrome, the hypothesis put forward during data collection (interview and physical examination) was that this clinical presentation is the 'final common pathway' of a much more complex disorder. It has to be noted that C7 nerve root syndrome is a medical diagnosis or a medical clinical pattern that does not essentially contain the same chunks of information as a manual therapy clinical pattern. Although both descriptions should have in common the pathological background and cervical spine pathomechanics,

numerous presentations are possible within a C7 nerve root syndrome diagnosis. For the manual therapist's management to be successful, their understanding must be broader and include the full biopsychosocial picture. The picture emerging for this patient was one of a centrally mediated pain mechanism underlying the disorder, with pathokinesiology present as a result of poor body mechanics during work and possibly predisposed by his previous open-heart surgery.

Visceral pathologies such as heart ischaemia cause sensitization of primary afferents. The nervous system and tissue injury pain from surgery or nerve root compression may lead to a centrally mediated pain characterized by central sensitization, disinhibition and structural reorganization in the central nervous system (Woolf et al., 1998). Furthermore, pain in general, and more particularly following myocardial ischaemia, surgery and irritation of the nerve root and other somatic structures, may be accompanied by a whole body reaction (Wall, 1999). These reactions may include phenomena such as muscular contraction in many parts of the body and changes in blood flow and hormones in tissues of the body. This resembles the picture found in complex regional pain syndrome (type I) that has recently been considered a neurological disease (Janig, 2001). The mechanical component of heart surgery is another factor that may have altered cervical spine mechanics and posture. The cervical spine is the most mobile region of the entire spine and, consequently, may be particularly vulnerable to altered postural alignment and abnormal biomechanics of other parts of the body. Work ergonomics may have also led to the fixation of aberrant movement patterns, which had facilitated the development of 'whole body' abnormal mechanics.

The adoption of a traditional medical model would result in a diagnosis of C7 nerve root syndrome (i.e. a 'tissue-based' approach). Treatment would, therefore, aim at reducing pressure or inflammation of the nerve root, thereby alleviating the signs and symptoms. This would end clinical intervention. However, this model may not be applicable to many musculoskeletal conditions in general and more particularly to this situation. The impact of the patient's medical history, his occupation and the influences of tissue injury (neural and somatic) necessitate an alternative model for diagnosis and management. This model emphasizes the neurobiological aspect of the clinical problem and the fact that all parts of the movement system are anatomically and functionally related. Nevertheless, this model does not negate the consideration of specific mechanical causes and anatomical sources responsible for the patient's physical impairments and symptoms.

In the light of the above approach, it was expected that changes in many parts of the movement system would be present and an extensive examination to prove or negate these theories and hypotheses would be justified. It was considered that understanding, from the start, the presentation in terms of pain neurobiology and functional biomechanics was of primary importance and would have a significant impact on the management context of this clinical disorder.

---

2 Please discuss your rationale for undertaking such an extensive palpatory examination with this patient, particularly why you thought it was important to palpate and mobilize the skin and muscular tissue in regions such as the chest and abdomen.

Clinician's answer

The rationale behind the palpation examination was mechanical and neurobiological. Mechanically, skin mobility is of extreme importance to overall mobility and function as it is continuous to the deepest mucosae (Williams and Warwick, 1980). Considering the skin as a continuum, it may have adhered to subcutaneous tissues during healing and repair processes following surgery. Fluids (e.g. seroma) present at the site of operation may infiltrate through subcutaneous tissues to distant sites (such as the lumbar region), as is often seen, for example, in fractures of the humerus where haematoma is observed in the forearm and hand. The median sternotomy scar may have influenced movement of the thoracic spine, cervical spine, shoulder girdle and upper limbs. For instance, the scar may have contributed to restricted cervical extension and shoulder flexion/abduction.

The superficial abdominal muscles, especially rectus abdominis, appeared to be overactive, possibly reflecting a learned activation pattern secondary to postoperative guarding. Continued overactivation of the superficial abdominal muscles at the expense of the deeper stabilizers (such as transversus abdominis) (Richardson et al., 1999) is also often associated with learned or maladaptive cervical postures and movement patterns dominated by lower cervical flexion and upper cervical extension. This may overload lower cervical segments and contribute to the development of disorders or to the aggravation of already existing pathologies.

Thoracic segments (T1–T12) that have convergent input from the viscera innervate the chest and abdomen (for example the heart is innervated by T5–T6). This convergent input may cause segmental facilitation, which renders the target tissues and organs sensitive to pain. A similar logic based upon neurophysiological principles can also be found in the technique of connective tissue manipulation (Ebner, 1985), whereby the aim of the technique is to influence the function of visceral organs via specific connective tissue zones located in the back of the trunk area.

One of the features of centrally mediated pain is increased receptive fields. The receptive fields may spread segmentally and also multisegmentally. A massive nociceptive input from the viscera or from somatic or neural tissue may contribute to a centrally mediated pain. Therefore, an extensive palpation examination was justified in order to detect possible areas of tenderness (i.e. allodynia and hyperalgesia), which are features of central sensitization. In addition, stress from myocardial infarction and cardiac surgery produces adrenaline and noradrenaline and activates the hypothalamic–pituitary–adrenal axis to increase corticosteroids. The neurohormones cause an increase in sympathetic activity, which may, in turn, affect tissue trophism. Tissues can become tight and demonstrate poor compliance with mechanical loading as a result of trophic changes. Tissues may also become sensitive to pain.

Another explanation may be found in the innervation of latissimus dorsi. Latissimus dorsi is innervated partly by the C7 segment. Although it is hard to differentiate clinically between lumbar structures and latissimus dorsi, it is possible that the initial involvement of the C7 segment may have contributed to the sensitivity detected at the lumbar region with palpation. Muscles contain nociceptors and can be a potential source of pain (Mense, 1993).

3 Please comment on how the physical examination findings contributed to your understanding of this patient's problem(s), identifying, where possible, specific hypotheses that were or were not supported by particular findings.

Clinician's answer

A major observation that can be drawn from the physical examination is that the forearm symptoms had multiple sources. Physical examination findings indicate the inadequacy of the medical model for diagnosis and treatment in this patient. Searching for a single source to the symptoms would have been an error in spite of an obvious clinical presentation of nerve root syndrome. What could explain the allodynia in the right forearm? What is the basis for hyperalgesia and reproduction of the forearm symptoms by stretching the skin of the back? What could account for the increased sensitivity of the radial nerve to palpation? Symptomatic responses obtained during the physical examination pointed to major involvement of the central nervous system. If there were a single anatomical source to the symptoms, stretching the abdominal skin, for example, would not reproduce the forearm symptoms. Nevertheless, abnormal mechanics of the C6–C7 functional spinal unit was clearly primarily responsible for Dan's functional problems

and symptoms. This sensitive physical impairment constituted a peripheral mechanism for the symptoms. Therefore, it was hypothesized that a centrally mediated pain was present in combination with a peripherally mediated pain.

Regarding other involved structures and mechanisms, it was demonstrated during the physical examination that altered body mechanics was of significance. The restricted movements of the left upper limb, the limited range of motion of the thorax to the right, the upper abdominal tightness and the lower abdominal weakness were all part of a general physical impairment, probably caused by poor body mechanics during daily activities and by the cardiac surgery. These pathoanatomical aspects of the problem may also have impaired neural tissue.

Paradoxically, the responses obtained during the upper limb neurodynamic tests did not show a major neurogenic component. It was hypothesized that if a nerve root was involved in this syndrome it was likely that the ULNTs should reproduce the symptoms. Elvey (1998) has suggested that neural tissue treatment should be considered when a neurogenic pathology is present. However, it is still not clear yet what the features of such a neurogenic pathology are (Elvey 1998). Butler (1998, 2000) states that producing or reproducing symptoms during an ULNT simply means that the specific movement is sensitive. This sensitivity may be a result of peripheral as well as central nervous system input. It was expected that the ULNTs would reliably reproduce Dan's symptoms if there were a major neural involvement. The major finding in both ULNTs was a limitation of movement. It would not be plausible to correlate this limitation of movement solely with neural structures. Therefore, the findings of the ULNTs did not support the hypothesis of altered neurodynamics. The response obtained in applying the ULNT (radial nerve) to the left side pointed to a tissue restriction component (not necessarily neural in origin), which may have developed as a result of surgery or from sympathetic dysfunction leading to a poor trophic condition of these tissues. A similar rationale may be applied to the response to the slump test. Nevertheless, it is possible that conventional ULNTs were not sufficient to reproduce neural symptoms. In addition, considering that this disorder was mostly non-inflammatory, mechanosensitivity was relatively low.

Traction increased the symptoms when performed in the sitting and the supine-lying positions. A generally accepted notion is that, in the presence of nerve root compression in the cervical spine (or lumbar spine), traction should relieve the pressure on the nerve and as a result symptoms should be eased. This assumption may be wrong for several reasons. First, traction has little effect on vertebral separation in the lumbar spine (Bogduk, 1997). It is possible that similar mechanics are applicable to the cervical spine. Secondly, the nerve root is connected to the vertebra and longitudinal movement of the vertebra may also affect the nerve. It should also be noted that intradural connections exist between the dorsal rootlets of C5, C6 and C7 (Tanaka et al., 2000), an anatomical fact that might be a source of confusion in the interpretation of clinical findings. Finally, movement of sensitive somatic tissues or tensioning of the dura mater in the cervical spine may reproduce the symptoms. Traction as a clinical test, therefore, does not support nor negate the involvement of nerve root pathology.

The findings of the neurological examination may have different interpretations. Weakness of the triceps and biceps muscles could be explained by compromise of the C6–C7 nerve root. However, weakness of these muscles can also be explained by the phenomenon of peripheral pseudoparesis, involving a central nervous system inhibition of the muscles as a result of osteoarticular or neural pathology (Janda, 1988). Consequently, the neurological examination does not definitively support or negate nerve root pathology.

The palpation examination revealed interesting findings that negated the likelihood of a single source and mechanism for the symptoms. The increased sensitivity of many tissues and the reproduction of the symptoms from remote structures supports the hypothesis of a central nervous system contribution to the symptoms. This contribution was expressed in the expansion of sensitivity throughout the musculoskeletal system and in the trophic changes induced by sympathetic dysfunction or the healing process following surgery.

■ Clinical reasoning commentary

The key feature of expert reasoning evident in the philosophy expressed in this answer is the recognition of the inter-relationship of the body's systems (i.e. neural, articular, myofascial, visceral and endocrine). The significance of this appreciation for the clinical reasoning used by manual therapists is that specific foci of reasoning, such as the source of the patient's symptoms, must be entertained with full consideration of other components of the problem such as pain mechanisms (see Ch. 1). Without consideration of the likelihood of central pain mechanisms contributing to this patient's presentation, including the probability of false-positive signs of somatic and neurogenic impairment in multiple areas, the less-experienced source-focussed therapist would either proceed to treat each region as a separate problem or simply write the patient off as being 'psychogenic'. Similarly, the clinician here has not reached the premature judgment of labelling the whole presentation as being 'central' and, therefore, potentially not appropriate for hands-on therapy. Rather, his hypotheses remain open, with recognition that peripheral and central pathological pain mechanisms can coexist.

Also evident in the clinician's reasoning is his ability and willingness to consider different interpretations for the clinical findings. For example, he discussed clinical (experience-based) and biomedical (research-based) evidence for a neurogenic hypothesis, which at this stage was not confirmed given the competing interpretations he outlined. He does not ignore findings that do not fit with a likely explanation (e.g. effect of traction when considering nerve compression) nor does he overemphasize findings that support this particular explanation (e.g. neurological). Such open-minded, critical and flexible thinking typifies an expert. Further differentiation of the relative contribution of each mechanism and the different sources being considered can only come from strategic and reflective intervention.

m Management

At the end of the examination, Dan was given a detailed explanation of the assessment findings and their clinical significance. The relevant clinical hypotheses regarding the possible sources, causes, pain mechanisms and biomechanical issues were outlined. The general management plan and estimated treatment outcomes were also discussed.

REASONING DISCUSSION AND CLINICAL REASONING COMMENTARY

1 Patient understanding is clearly important to your management. Could you comment on this in general and also its specific relevance to this patient? How do you balance the patient's desire to have a 'physical' explanation for his problem with the risk of overmedicalizing and promoting pathology-focussed beliefs?

Clinician's answer

The patient's own knowledge, beliefs and reasoning are a key factor in my management. Dan was concerned by the fact that he had a disc compressing his nerve. The picture he had in his mind (on the basis of viewing CT findings) was that a mass was compressing the nerve and causing his symptoms and functional problems. It was important to broaden his understanding of the problem by elaborating about the mechanisms of his physical impairments and pain, by supplying 'new' knowledge, and by assisting him to adopt a new perspective about the validity of this information. The aim was to draw his attention towards factors other than the disc that were responsible for the onset of the disorder and that might have contributed to his ongoing problem. My explanation focussed on the limited validity of imaging findings and on the importance of ergonomic factors and pain mechanisms (in particular the central component). Dan was not hard to convince, as he trusted my explanations. In his case, since he was able to conceptualize and accept this explanation, his beliefs did not interfere with his cooperation during management.

Clinical reasoning commentary

As discussed in Chapter 1, narrative reasoning that aims to understand the individual's 'pain or illness experience' leads to communicative management. In communicative management, as illustrated in this case, the therapist works collaboratively to help the patient understand their activity/participation restrictions, physical impairments and pain. Assisting patients to change their perspectives when these have been judged to be unhelpful or counterproductive to their recovery requires exploring the basis of those perspectives and then providing the patient with new information to improve their understanding of their problems and pain state. When successful, the patient is then able to transform their previously unhelpful perspective to a new way of seeing and understanding, ideally with better appreciation of their role in the management required.

Treatment 1

The first treatment included a posteroanterior mobilization of the deep posterior cervical muscles and skin mobilization to the posterior thoracic and lumbar areas in the supine-lying position. During treatment, pain and a pins and needles sensation were reproduced in the left forearm when using both techniques. On reassessment, an improvement of approximately 5 degrees of active cervical spine extension was achieved. Neurological examination and palpation findings remained unchanged. Other physical examination findings were not reassessed at this stage as the neurological examination and palpation findings were considered of primary importance in relation to pain and neural compromise. Dan was advised to avoid working with sustained neck flexion and to modify his position during work, such as sitting instead of standing. No specific exercises were given at this stage.

Treatment 2

Dan reported no treatment soreness following the first treatment and a significant decrease in the intensity of the symptoms after 24 hours. Extension of the cervical spine remained at 10 degrees, as it was at the end of treatment 1. The second treatment focussed mainly on improving posterior translation at the C6–C7 level in the sitting position, while provoking the symptoms to a tolerable level. The symptoms subsided immediately when the technique was ceased.

Posterior translation is one of the movements occurring during extension of a cervical vertebra (the other movements being posterior sagittal rotation and compression of the posterior elements). The technique used to improve posterior translation involved fixation of the C7 vertebra while extending the lower cervical spine and emphasizing the translation component of C6. The aim of this technique was to restore normal extension, as restriction of this movement was clearly contributing to Dan's symptoms. Because of the limited inflammatory component of the disorder, it was considered reasonable to reproduce the symptoms to a certain extent without risking aggravating the condition. The soft tissue technique applied to the left cervical deep muscles was combined with the posterior translation mobilization of the C6–C7 articulation. Active neck retraction was also added simultaneously in order to enhance the translation movement of the lower cervical segments and to facilitate contraction of the deep anterior cervical muscles and lower cervical extensors, while lengthening the middle cervical extensors. This technique yielded 30 degrees of cervical extension, with forearm symptoms reproduced at end range. The skin-stretching technique was also repeated, yielding a decrease in the intensity of the forearm symptoms at end range of cervical extension. Following these techniques, the range of movement of both ULNTs was improved, with symptom reproduction remaining the same. Neurological examination findings were still unchanged. Dan was advised to start neck retraction exercises while mildly reproducing the symptoms and sustaining the movement for approximately 10 seconds for 10 repetitions twice a day.

Treatment 3

Dan reported a significant functional and symptomatic improvement. Since the last treatment, he had not felt any pain or other symptoms in the forearm and hand. However, he reported a dull pain in the lateral upper third of the left arm at rest. This pain had not been reported previously. On examination, cervical extension range of movement was maintained, while symptoms in the upper arm, forearm and hand were reproduced at end range of cervical extension. The arm pain remained unchanged with cervical extension. The posterior translation movement of the C6–C7 level was almost full range, with mild resistance evident at end range. Allodynia was reduced in area to the left upper quarter of the thoracic region and was associated with reproduction of pins and needles in the upper arm, forearm and hand. Initially, allodynia had been present over the whole of Dan's back on the left side but had only reproduced the forearm pain and pins and needles.

The treatment techniques used in the second treatment were repeated. On reassessment, a dull ache in the forearm was reproduced with active full-range cervical extension without overpressure. Dan was advised to continue cervical retraction exercises. As pelvic and lumbar spine alignment was considered to be a contributing factor to Dan's problem, straight leg raise and lumbar extension exercises were also added in order to enhance postural alignment.

Treatments 4 to 6

Since the previous treatment, Dan had not felt any pain or paraesthesiae in the forearm and hand. However, a dull ache was present in the lateral upper third of the forearm and lower third of the upper arm. This ache was not initially present. Cervical extension range of movement was maintained, with the symptoms in the upper arm, forearm and hand still reproduced at the end range. The posterior translation movement of C6–C7 was full range, with normal resistance detected. Allodynia remained reduced in the left upper quarter of the thoracic area, with reproduction of pins and needles in the upper arm, forearm and hand during skin mobilization.

The therapeutic techniques used during treatments 4 to 6 included stretching of the sternohyoid muscles, performed with simultaneous guided active posterior translation of the C6–C7 segments. Simultaneously, mobilization of the scar tissue and skin over the chest and upper abdominal areas and stretching of the upper part of the rectus abdominis with transverse mobilization of the muscle to the right were applied. Stretching of left pectoralis major combined with ULNT 1 (median nerve bias) was performed, adding sustained end-range elbow extension with wrist extension. In this position, rotation of the pelvis to the right (i.e. relative thoracic rotation to the left) was also added and increased the forearm and upper arm symptoms remarkably (Fig. 24.4). This technique was also directed to latissimus dorsi. These interventions led to an improvement of the shoulder signs and symptoms. Application of wrist palmar flexion with shoulder internal rotation in ULNT 2 (radial nerve bias) was followed by an improvement in the symptomatic response and range of movement of both neurodynamic tests.

Stretching of the rectus abdominis was performed on a gym ball (Fig. 24.5). An interesting response was obtained during this abdominal soft tissue technique. Dan reported a very intense feeling of pins and needles in the whole left upper limb. This was consistently

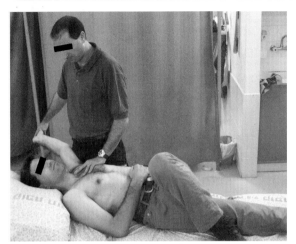

Fig. 24.4 Stretching of left pectoralis major combined with the upper limb neurodynamic test 1 and rotation of the pelvis to the right.

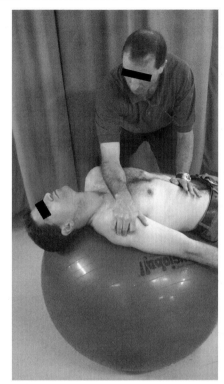

Fig. 24.5 Stretching rectus abdominis performed on a gym ball.

produced only with this technique and changing the position of other structures (including the cervical spine) did not influence the response. Furthermore, while performing the technique with Dan in supine lying (and with all other components at rest), a similar symptom response occurred. During the abdominal technique on the gym ball, an isometric contraction of transversus abdominis was added, simultaneous with stretching of rectus abdominis.

Following treatments 4 to 5, an improvement in muscle strength in the neurological examination was noticed. Pain in the forearm was occasionally present, but with minimal and tolerable intensity. Pins and needles were not present at rest. Range of movement of cervical extension was full, with a dull ache reproduced in the forearm on overpressure. Palpation of the anterior chest and abdominal areas reproduced pins and needles in the posterolateral aspect of the forearm.

REASONING DISCUSSION

1 What mechanisms might account for the 'interesting response' you highlighted where upper limb pins and needles were consistently reproduced during the abdominal soft tissue technique? How did your treatment address these mechanisms?

Clinician's answer

Possible neuroanatomical links may explain this phenomenon. The innervation of the treated abdominal area is from anterior and lateral cutaneous branches of T6–T8. The intercostal nerves communicate with each other in the posterior parts of the intercostal spaces (Williams and Warwick. 1980). Links also exist between the lower five intercostal nerves as they communicate while traversing the abdominal wall. The intercostobrachial nerve communicates with the posterior brachial cutaneous branch of the radial nerve. If the intercostal nerves are connected to each other, then a reasonable hypothesis would be that a stimulus (for example the abdominal soft tissue technique) applied to one or some of these nerves may be transmitted to other parts. In this case, stimulation of the T6–T8 nerves may have elicited a response in the intercosto-brachial nerve and subsequently at the lower posterior branch of the radial nerve. This response would have been possible only if the nervous system was in an already sensitized state. This theoretical basis might also account for the responses obtained during palpation of the posterior trunk area, as posterior branches of the fifth and sixth thoracic nerves supply the skin over the scapula and latissimus dorsi.

The abdominal soft tissue technique was aimed at improving flexibility of the tissues, decreasing muscle shortening, lowering excitability of alpha motor neurons, releasing pressure on intercostal nerves caused by fibrosis and tightening of the soft tissues, and improving blood supply to the nerves and somatic tissues. These procedures were all intended to normalize nervous system activity and influence motor patterns related to the rib cage and cervical spine. Besides the significant peripheral and local effects of this soft tissue technique, such manual manipulation of soft tissues, muscles and joints may alter information processing within the central nervous system by modifying the quality and quantity of its neural input (Vujnovich, 1995).

At treatment 6, Dan did not complain of any activity restrictions or symptoms. Neurological examination remained unchanged and all other movements in all considered areas maintained their improvement, including the range of motion of the ULNTs and shoulder. On the right side, sensitivity to pressure applied to the forearm was reduced, although all other findings remained unchanged.

The home programme was revisited, combining cervical spine extension and trunk extension in prone lying. Pectoralis major stretching in the ULNT 1 position with wrist extension and right pelvic rotation was added. The plan was to review the patient 2 weeks later.

■ Treatment 7

Dan was re-examined after 19 days. During this period, lateral forearm pain reappeared slightly. Cervical spine extension was slightly restricted with overpressure and reproduced a dull pain in the forearm. All previously detected areas of allodynia were free of symptoms during palpation, except for an area in the posterolateral part of the arm. Assisted active cervical posterior translation was repeated concurrently with the soft tissue technique to the deep cervical muscles. Skin mobilization techniques were performed to the sensitive area of the arm. Following these techniques, range of movement of the cervical spine was normal with no symptoms produced on overpressure.

■ Treatment 8

The forearm ache recurred after 3 days, but was very low in intensity. Similar treatment techniques were repeated and the outcomes were similar to those obtained at the previous treatment session. Dan kept progressing with the home programme and was asked to call whenever he could not control his problem and symptoms.

■ Treatment 9

More than a month after the last treatment, Dan asked for assistance. He had spontaneous paraesthesiae in the left upper limb not related to any particular movement or activity. Cervical spine extension was normal. Examination of the soft tissues of the arm and forearm revealed tenderness and reproduction of pins and needles on palpation of the triceps and dorsal forearm muscles. Palpation of the radial nerve in the posterior part of the arm also reproduced pins and needles in the posterior aspect of the forearm and hand. Treatment focussed on desensitizing the involved tissues, including friction massage of the radial nerve. Following treatment Dan reported no complaints.

■ Outcome

Dan kept up with the home programme. In general, Dan returned to maximal function and symptoms were minimal. However, it was expected that there could be occasional bouts of symptoms. Dan was discharged with the option of returning for 'on-call' treatment whenever required.

REASONING DISCUSSION AND CLINICAL REASONING COMMENTARY

1 There appears to have been a number of different specific physical impairments that you judged were contributing to this patient's presentation and hence addressed in your management. Could you discuss your thoughts on the relevance and interplay of these physical impairments in this case?

Clinician's answer

Managing specific (e.g. a restricted cervical segment), general (e.g. inability to sleep in prone lying) and mental (i.e. patient's feelings or cognitive interpretations) dysfunctions in manual therapy requires considering the human body as an integrated functioning system where all of its parts are linked and function as a whole: referred to by Butler (2000) as a 'big picture' approach. This was the approach adopted in the management of this patient (and should be a fundamental principle in manual therapy practice). The employment of lateral thinking strategies (i.e. looking for multiple alternatives, even those that seem to be unlikely or even ridiculous) had guided the process of hypothesis generation from the start. From the beginning of the patient encounter, the aim was to work out what could have led to Dan's impairment and functional problems. As mentioned above, it would have been naive and simplistic to think that the nerve root (or dorsal root ganglion) and intervertebral disc were the only structures responsible for Dan's symptoms and dysfunction. If this had been the case, treatment would have been directed solely to these structures. However, the multiple sources and components responsible for Dan's symptoms and dysfunction would have been missed, and treatment would have been incomplete or even ineffective. All the impairments that were addressed during treatment were all pieces of a larger puzzle.

The various impairments addressed during treatment were obviously related to each other and individually contributed to the neck problem. The cervical spine is the most mobile area of the spine; however, local problems or physical impairments distant to the cervical spine may have a significant impact on cervical spine movement. The rib cage and thorax played a major role in this case. As observed during the physical examination, thoracic rotation was more limited to the right than to the left. Tightening and stiffening of the tissues on the left side of the trunk and upper limb may explain the restriction of thoracic rotation to the right. These tissues include pectoralis major and minor, latissimus dorsi, the left cervical muscles and soft tissues, the left abdominal muscles, and the left erector spinae. Consequently, relative rotation of the trunk to the left may have occurred, explaining the relative limitation of left cervical rotation, restriction of thoracic rotation to the right and the restricted mobility of the left shoulder.

Considering the position of protraction and elevation of the scapula and the tight pectorals, the elbow might have been affected through involvement of the biceps muscle. In addition, scapular protraction encourages lower cervical flexion, perhaps adding to the already restricted segmental mobility in the direction of extension. This could explain the limited range of movement at the elbow and may have also led to a pattern of internal rotation of the whole upper limb. An internally rotated upper limb can lead to a general restriction of external rotation and may cause impingement-like shoulder symptoms. This could also cause a secondary impairment of the nerves of the upper limb and contribute to altered neurodynamics.

Rectus abdominis inserts onto the sternum. Any interference with the anatomy of the sternum (such as cardiac surgery) may influence muscle alignment and mechanics. Rectus abdominis is considered a 'white' muscle with the tendency to shorten. Shortening of this muscle may lead to impaired mobility of the rib cage and consequently to restriction of cervical spine movements, notably extension and rotation considering possible asymmetry obtained or reinforced following suturing of the sternum during the surgical procedure. This may have contributed to the degenerative process of the disc through impaired nutrition and metabolism.

Furthermore, a loss of lumbar spine extension along with shortened hamstrings could cause a posterior pelvic tilt and a concurrent thoracic kyphosis, leading to lower cervical flexion and mid-to-upper cervical extension.

All these related impairments are orchestrated through the central nervous system, which may provoke abnormal movement patterns, sensory abnormalities, abnormal sympathetic function and behavioural influences.

2 How would you manage your stated plan for further 'on-call' treatment for this patient without increasing the risk of dependency on yourself and passive treatment?

■ Clinician's answer

It was hypothesized during the clinical assessment of this patient that the risk of dependency on the system was low for Dan. Nevertheless, my plan was for Dan to be independent of others in managing future symptoms. On the one hand he was used to responsibility in that he had to keep his business going and could not rely on anyone else to replace him or to do his job. The fact that he was the owner of the factory was important. On the other hand, he did not pay much attention to his physical condition because of that very fact. This could have been a negative factor in cooperation and it was my impression that this attitude was initially an obstacle for him that had to be removed. During the course of management, these issues were discussed at length; in time I became confident that he was cooperating with the home programme, on the basis of maintenance of the improvement and by checking each treatment session how he was performing the exercises and applying my instructions.

In addition, Dan's active participation during treatment (for example active neck retraction while performing posterior translation, as well as contractions of transversuse abdominis and stretching rectus) conveyed an important message. The fact that he had to be active during treatment showed him that active movement was possible (even if reproducing the symptoms) and that it had a healing potential. Dan understood that it was worthwhile performing movements because doing so may improve his condition. This is an extremely important message. The aim in almost every clinical intervention should be to achieve active participation of the patient during management and decision making by adopting a patient-centred approach in clinical reasoning (Higgs and Jones, 2000). First, forces exerted by the patient can sometimes be greater than forces applied manually (such as when mobilizing an ankle in weight bearing while the patient performs dorsiflexion) and, secondly, it has a psychological impact and may reduce fear-avoidance behaviours.

3 You mention that you expected there could be occasional bouts of symptoms in the future for this patient. Could you comment on the key supporting evidence for this prognostic hypothesis?

■ Clinician's answer

Every physical intervention (or injury) leads to a 'learning process' in the nervous system. As the problem was initially hypothesized to be an acute manifestation of a chronic disorder, it was expected that until the nervous system was fully reset there might still be occasional bouts. It is not clear how long it can take for the nervous system to return to its initial state and whether this occurs at all. The behaviour of the disorder during the physical examination and treatment demonstrated an increased sensitivity of the nervous system. During treatment, Dan had spontaneous relapses of symptoms with no obvious cause and which were non-specific in nature and distribution.

Centrally mediated pain and symptoms provide the best explanation for the fact that many areas in the body reproduced the symptoms of forearm pain or pins and needles even though they were not anatomically related to the arm. Centrally mediated pain (and other symptoms) may leave a 'memory of pain' in the central nervous system (Basbaum, 1996), a phenomenon called neuronal plasticity. Neuronal plasticity refers to functional and plastic changes in the nervous system as a result of pain or other peripheral input (Dubner, 1997). It has been shown that central sensitization also occurs as a result of 'wind-up' (Li et al., 1999). Wind-up refers to the repetitive stimulation of C fibres, leading to a progressive increase in the magnitude of C fibre-evoked responses of dorsal horn neurons. These theoretical explanations might explain the phenomena observed in this case. As a result, it was expected that 'resetting' the nervous system might take longer because of the gradual 'relearning' of the system.

■ Clinical reasoning commentary

Manual therapists are often accused of overservicing. In the absence of level 1 evidence (randomized controlled trials) for many of our interventions, especially as they are often applied in combination, our best safeguard against unsubstantiated excessive treatment is our own reflective reasoning. This requires a holistic and critical biopsychosocial perspective that draws on what is understood in pain science (while recognizing much is still not understood about pain and its complex interplay with the different body systems), and which is guided by an open-minded yet cautious systematic approach of intervention and reassessment. The reasoning evident in this case illustrates just such a broad and questioning approach to manual therapy, and one that involves an active partnership between patient and therapist in the management of chronic clinical problems.

Acknowledgments

I wish to express my gratitude to my wife Nurit for being my other half.

I would also like to thank Yossi Sadovnik for taking the photographs and Illan Shaoul, student of physiotherapy, for serving as a model in Figures 24.4 and 24.5.

References

Basbaum, A.I. (1996). Memories of pain. Science and Medicine, 3, 22–31.

Bogduk, N. (1994). Biomechanics of the cervical spine. In Physical Therapy of the Cervical and Thoracic Spine (Grant, R. ed.) pp. 27–45. Edinburgh: Churchill Livingstone.

Bogduk, N. (1997). Clinical Anatomy of the Lumbar Spine and Sacrum. Edinburgh: Churchill Livingstone.

Butler, D. (1998). Adverse mechanical tension in the nervous system: a model for assessment and treatment (commentary). [In 'Adverse Neural Tension' Reconsidered (Maher, C. ed.)] Australian Journal of Physiotherapy Monograph, 3, 33–35.

Butler, D.S. (2000). The Sensitive Nervous System. Adelaide, Australia: Noigroup Press.

Cervero, F. (1995). Mechanisms of visceral pain. In Visceral Pain (Gebhart, G.F. ed.) pp. 25–40. Seattle, WA: IASP Press.

Dubner, R. (1997). Neural basis of persistent pain: sensory specialization, sensory modulation and neuronal plasticity. In Proccedings of the Eighth World Congress on Pain (Jensen, T.S., Turner, J.A. and Wiesenfeld, Z. eds.) pp. 243–257, Seattle, WA: IASP Press.

Ebner, M. (1985). Connective Tissue Manipulation. Malabar: Robert E. Krieger.

Elvey, R. (1998). Treatment of arm pain associated with abnormal brachial plexus tension (commentary). [In 'Adverse neural tension' reconsidered (Maher, C. ed.)] Australian Journal of Physiotherapy Monograph, 3, 13–17.

Grieve, G.P. (1994). The autonomic nervous system in vertebral pain syndromes. In Grieve's Modern Manual Therapy: The Vertebral Column (Boyling, J.D. and Palastanga, N. eds.) pp. 259–269. Edinburgh: Churchill Livingstone.

Hasue, M. (1993). Pain and the nerve root. An interdisciplinary approach. Spine, 18, 2053–2058.

Hayes, C. and Molloy, A.R. (1997). Neuropathic pain in the perioperative period. International Anesthesiology Clinics, 35, 67–81.

Higgs, J. and Jones, M. (2000). Clinical Reasoning in the Health Professions. Oxford: Butterworth-Heinemann.

Janda, V. (1988). Muscle weakness and inhibition (pseudoparesis) in back pain syndromes. In Modern Manual Therapy of the Vertebral Column (Grieve, G.P. ed.) pp. 197–201. Edinburgh: Churchill Livingstone.

Janig, W. (2001). CRPS-I and CRPS-II: a strategic view. In Complex Regional Pain Syndrome (Norman Harden, R., Baron, R. and Janig, W. eds.) pp. 3–15. Seattle, WA: IASP Press.

Li, J., Simone, D.A. and Larson, A.A. (1999). Windup leads to characteristics of central sensitization. Pain, 79, 75–82.

Mense, S. (1993). Nociception from skeletal muscle in relation to clinical muscle pain. Pain, 54, 241–289.

Ness, T.J. and Gebhart, G.F. (1990). Visceral pain: a review of experimental studies. Pain, 41, 167–234.

Richardson, C., Jull, G., Hodges, P. and Hides, J. (1999). Therapeutic Exercise for Spinal Segmental Stabilization in Low Back Pain. Edinburgh: Churchill Livingstone.

Tanaka, N., Fujimoto, Y., An, H.S., Ikuta, Y. and Yasuda, M. (2000). The anatomic relation among the nerve roots, intervertebral foramina, and intervertebral discs of the cervical spine. Spine, 25, 286–291.

Vleeming, A., Mooney, V., Dorman, T., Snijders, C. and Stoekart, R. (1997). Movement Stability and Low Back Pain: The Essential Role of the Pelvis. Edinburgh: Churchill Livingstone.

Vujnovich, A.L. (1995). Neural plasticity, muscle spasm and tissue manipulation: a review of the literature. Journal of Manual and Manipulative Therapy, 3, 152–156.

Wall, P. (1999). Pain—The Science of Suffering. London: Weindenfeld and Nicolson.

Williams, P.L. and Warwick, R. (1980). Gray's Anatomy, 36th edn. Edinburgh: Churchill Livingstone.

Woolf, C.J., Bennett, G.J., Doherty, M. et al. (1998). Towards a mechanism-based classification of pain? Pain, 77, 227–229.

Zermann, D.H., Ishigooka, M., Doggweiler, R. and Shmidt, R.A. (1998). Postoperative chronic pain and bladder dysfunction: windup and neuronal plasticity: do we need a more neurourological approach in pelvic surgery? Journal of Urology, 160, 102–105.

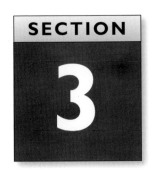

Theory and development

Educational theory and principles related to learning clinical reasoning

Joy Higgs

Introduction

This book is primarily addressed to practitioners such as physiotherapists, chiropractors and other health professionals working in the field of manual therapy. Some readers will be teachers, some mentors of junior colleagues and some will be learners. The task of this chapter is to explore educational discourse, theory and principles relevant to teaching and learning clinical reasoning. The practical applications of this theory to learning clinical reasoning poses an interesting challenge and a number of questions, which reflect the starting point of any educational endeavour. What is the topic or subject of the teaching exercise? What assumptions can be made about the readers? What goals do they have, compared with the goals of the teachers? What is the scope and depth of the topic that can reasonably be covered to address these goals? What language and style of 'teaching' (or writing) are appropriate for the audience, goals and content?

One of the purposes of educational theory and its application is to articulate and make transparent the answers to these very questions. In this way, education is similar to clinical practice, in that our stakeholders expect professionals (educators and clinicians) to be accountable for their practice and to be able to articulate the rationales, decisions and strategies which form the basis of this practice. When an adult learning approach is adopted, the common elements of awareness of thinking and cognitive strategies, responsibility and articulation of thinking are reflected in both the learning process and the learning content, creating a powerful synergy between the two. This matching of the process and content of learning programmes is typical of process-inclusive learning programmes (Everingham and Bandaranayake, 1999), which deliberately target, exemplify and depict the processes of thinking and reasoning as core values, goals and learning outcomes.

This chapter is written not for novice teachers and learners but rather for experienced practitioners who have practical experience of teaching and learning, who are actively engaged in their own learning and in facilitating the learning of others. The goal of this chapter is to extend or consolidate readers' knowledge of educational theory and discourse and to promote reflection on the use of educational knowledge as a tool to facilitate self-directed learning or to help others to learn. The chapter is also a bridge between Chapter 1, which dealt with clinical reasoning itself in manual therapy, and Chapter 26, which considers ways of facilitating clinical reasoning development.

What is expected of health science graduates?

The goal of most curricula today is to produce autonomous, competent professionals who can demonstrate discipline-specific technical competencies and who act professionally. There has been an increasing emphasis recently on adding to curricular expectations the acquisition of generic competencies, including interpersonal skills, problem-solving skills, cultural competence and competence in information technology (Hunt and Higgs, 1999). Health professionals are expected to demonstrate social responsibility (Prosser, 1995), accountability and the capacity to recognize their limitations (Sultz et al., 1984), to practise with integrity and personal tolerance, and to communicate effectively across language, cultural and situational barriers (Josebury et al., 1990).

The capacity to act as autonomous professionals is a central concept in professional practice. Professional autonomy implies independence in decision making and action, acceptance of responsibility for actions taken, and the demonstration of accountability towards those who receive the services of the professional. The capacity to make defensible clinical decisions relies on a sound knowledge base, skills in clinical reasoning and metacognition, and the capacity to interact effectively with other participants (especially the client) in the decision-making process. Competent clinicians need not only to be able to make autonomous decisions but also to be able to take 'wise' action, meaning taking the best-judged action in a specific context (Cervero, 1988; Harris, 1993). Alongside the privilege and the obligation to work autonomously, professionals need to be able to make sound, independent, accountable decisions and to implement them in a spirit of critical appraisal. Today, more than ever, professionals are facing a climate of challenge and contestation, where professional judgment is subject to increased public scrutiny, where there is lack of consensus on what expertise comprises and where authority-based claims are undermined (Frost, 2001). These factors, along with unquestioning support of narrow views of evidence-based practice, challenge the autonomy of professional decision making and increase the need for professionals to have justifiable confidence in the soundness and defensibility of their reasoning; sound reasoning is more important than ever.

Educational theory

So, how can we achieve these teaching and learning goals? Educational theory provides the framework (the goals, rationale, context, philosophical basis and guidelines) for the facilitation of learning. In any particular situation, the task facing the educator or the self-directed learner who is planning learning activities is to choose educational theory and related strategies appropriate to the topic (in this case, learning clinical reasoning) and the situation. This chapter pursues a number of key questions facing people designing learning programmes, whether to facilitate their own learning or that of others, and provides a range of educational theories and issues arising from research, theorizing and experience that addresses these questions. Some of these theories (e.g. adult learning) could be discussed under a number of headings and there are many areas of overlap and compatibility among these theories and principles. Figure 25.1

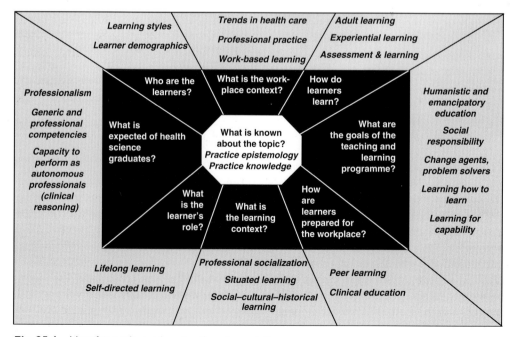

Fig. 25.1 Identifying relevant learning theories and discourse.

illustrates this process and framework. The next chapter deals with strategies utilizing these theories to promote the learning of clinical reasoning.

What is known and understood about the phenomenon being taught?

To understand the phenomenon being taught, we need to reflect on the available knowledge in the field in question (i.e. clinical reasoning). What types of knowledge have been generated about this topic? How do we come to know about this phenomenon? An understanding of four key factors addresses these questions:

- clinical reasoning
- metacognition
- the process of generating knowledge/practice epistemology
- practice knowledge.

Since Chapter 1 examined clinical reasoning and metacognition in depth, those topics are not repeated here. In seeking practice knowledge, the teacher recognizes the value of the educational principle that calls for teachers to have (or to have access to) content knowledge, as well as knowledge and skills in the processes of teaching. Similarly, for learners, there is a need to know what it is they are seeking to know.

Practice epistemology

Practice epistemology refers to the nature of knowledge and knowledge generation that underlies practice (see Higgs et al., 2002). The questions of practice epistemology are of fundamental importance for the quality and understanding of practice. The current climate of accountability and public scrutiny in the health and social care professions requires the adoption of a high level of responsibility by health professionals in terms of understanding, scrutinizing, generating, updating and credibly using their professional knowledge. To achieve this, health professionals need to acknowledge the wide variety of sources from which their knowledge is generated, to understand the knowledge that underpins their practice, to justify their practice through this knowledge, and to recognize practice epistemology as a necessary dimension of professional responsibility. The implications for clinical reasoning of these arguments for learning programmes are relatively transparent. As clinical

reasoners, practitioners clearly use knowledge as an essential reasoning tool. They need to be able to trust (through testing, learning and critical self-appraisal) this knowledge, and they need to be able to articulate the sound reasoning behind their clinical decisions. To demonstrate accountability for their practice, clinicians need to understand the nature of their dynamic knowledge base, so that they can explore its complexity, apply it appropriately and participate in the never-ending process of critical appraisal, extension and review of the profession's knowledge base (Titchen and Higgs, 2001).

Forms of practice knowledge

What types of knowledge do practitioners need? Health professionals seek to make sense of clients' or patients' problems by drawing on their knowledge. The knowledge that clinicians bring to the clinical encounter is a key aspect of the therapeutic intervention (Jensen et al., 1992). This knowledge can be categorized (Higgs and Titchen, 1995a,b) as:

- propositional, theoretical or scientific knowledge
- professional craft knowledge, or knowing how to do something
- personal knowledge about oneself as a person and in relationship with others.

Propositional knowledge is derived through research and/or scholarship. It is formal and explicit knowledge that is expressed in propositional statements, which enunciate, for example, relationships between concepts or causes and effects and which identify the generalizability or transferability of research knowledge to populations and settings. Theoretical knowledge may be developed from arguments of principle, from dialogue and logic, and through use of existing empirical and theoretical knowledge.

Professional craft knowledge and personal knowledge are collectively called non-propositional knowledge. They are derived from the processing (e.g. through reflection) of professional and personal experiences, respectively, and may be tacit and embedded in practice or in the personal identity and lives of the knowers. Cervero (1992, p. 98) described professional craft knowledge as a 'repertoire of examples, images, practical principles, scenarios or rules of thumb that have been developed through prior experience'. Professional craft knowledge comprises general knowledge gained from practice experience (e.g. knowledge about how a population of patients respond to disease or disability) and specific knowledge about a particular patient, in a particular situation and context at a particular time. Professional craft knowledge can be expressed in propositional statements, but here no attempt is made to generalize beyond the practice of the individual or group who have generated that knowledge.

Personal knowledge is accrued from life experiences, such as relationships and cultural influences that contribute to shaping individual perspectives; as such, it influences personal interactions, personal values and beliefs. This knowledge, in its general form, can be gained, as with professional craft knowledge, through socialization into a society, group or professional community. In its particular form, personal knowledge is perhaps acquired more consciously by reflecting upon one's knowing, being, doing and feeling in each unique situation.

Practitioners use all three forms of knowledge in practice. Propositional knowledge can provide the basis for understanding the medical, psychosocial and cultural context and the physical and psychosocial nature of the client's needs and problems. In relation to clinical reasoning, practitioners need to accumulate and update carefully a rich and dependable knowledge base, to appraise critically the salience and applicability of such knowledge to a particular case, and to be vigilant in checking for potential errors in the currency and use of this knowledge, particularly when making important decisions of diagnosis, treatment and prognosis. Professional craft knowledge enables practitioners to tailor clinical decision making in recognition of the individual client's needs (Rew and Barrow, 1987). Such knowledge enables clinicians to plan, modify and critique their treatments to consolidate their understanding of the particular clinical problem (Jensen et al., 1992) and to implement sound, efficient and timely decision making. Research has demonstrated that it is the ability of experienced professionals to integrate propositional knowledge with professional craft knowledge that enables them to assess the relevance of clinical data and to distinguish and comprehend the significance of crucial cues (Dreyfus and Dreyfus, 1986; Elstein et al., 1990; Larkin et al., 1980; Payton, 1985). Health professionals draw on their professional craft knowledge and their personal knowledge to interact effectively with patients and carers. Such knowledge, combined with skills in communication, listening and problem solving, facilitates interpersonal interactions and enables

practitioners to relate well to their clients as individuals with unique needs, fears, hopes and expectations. Carper (1978, p. 20) argued that personal knowledge 'promotes wholeness and integrity in the personal encounter, the achievement of engagement rather than detachment'. The ability to place the clinical problem within the patient's world and to design personalized care and interventions that take the patient's experience into account is recognized across the health sciences as a key element of expertise that develops from clinical practice experience (Benner, 1984; Burke and DePoy, 1991; Crepeau, 1991; Jensen et al., 1992; Jones et al., 2002).

An important consideration in understanding practice knowledge is to recognize its changing context. Beyond long-understood ideas of the knowledge explosion, we now face knowledge issues linked to global recasting of the boundaries of many aspects of life, including the state, employment, practice and the nature of knowledge itself. Edwards and Usher (1998) considered the role played by globalization in reshaping knowledge, and the implications for adult learning. They argued that globalization brings about a heightened sense of the world as one place with universal knowledge, but paradoxically it also enhances the sense of the local, the relative and the particular in our understanding. These observations have implications both for the nature of the knowledge we would seek to learn and for the learning experiences that are needed to gain both global and local understanding. This same globalization is occurring within the health professions and within the specialized world of manual therapy. The cases presented in Section 2, by authors from around the world, reflect the growing challenge facing today's practitioners to critique and broaden their perspectives.

What is the context of learning?

The education of health professionals occurs within a broad context of professional socialization. In specific terms, the context of learning is the particular learning situation, with its cultural, historical, social and task dimensions.

Professional socialization

Health professional education occurs before and after graduation as part of the process of socialization or induction into the profession. In this process, the individual gains a professional identity, develops professional values/behaviours and gains the capacity to perform effectively as a member of the profession. Socialization into a profession brings with it the privilege and responsibility of autonomy (or independent decision making and action), a sense of dedication or calling to the professional field, the practice of using the professional organization or community as a reference, belief in the indispensability of the profession, belief in collegial control, community rather than self-interest, recognition by the public, involvement in professional culture and membership in the professional association (Hall, 1968; Ritzer, 1971). The capacity to reason effectively and professionally is the key to drawing together all these areas of responsibility and privilege. Manual therapists occupy professional subgroups within their respective professions. While their approaches and practice philosophies differ across these groups, as is evident in Section 2, clinical reasoning is a common denominator bridging the more superficial differences in viewpoint and linking the broader professional responsibility, identity and practice of manual therapy.

Situated learning

The theory of situated learning (arising from the work of Brown et al. (1989), Lave and Wenger (1991), Vygotsky (1978) and others) assumes that knowledge is embedded within the context where it is used. Learning is a function of the activity, context and culture in which it is situated. Situated learning is commonly incidental and unintentional rather than deliberate (Lave, 1996). Activities that facilitate situated learning (McLellan, 1996) include stories, reflection, cognitive apprenticeship, collaboration, coaching, multiple practice, articulation of learning skills and the use of technologies or tools to enhance learning.

The learning principles underpinning this theory (Lave, 1996) are:

- knowledge needs to be presented and learned in an authentic context (i.e. in settings and applications that would normally involve that knowledge)
- learning requires social interaction and collaboration.

Cope et al. (2000, p. 851) drew attention to the connection between situated learning and professional development. They noted that there is wide acceptance of the finding (Berliner, 1988; Dreyfus and Dreyfus, 1986) 'that experts do not operate by following rules derived from higher-order knowledge but rather, by using complex situational understanding, a mature and practised dexterity which comes from their breadth and depth of experience'. Relating this insight to the previous discussion of knowledge, it is evident that experts use a combination of both propositional and non-propositional knowledge.

Situated theorists propose that learning is socially constructed. Such learning (by practitioners and patients alike) is facilitated through shared interaction, common language, shared sociocultural context, collaboration and negotiation of meanings or perspectives. The situated learning environment can be described as a community of practice (Lave and Wenger, 1991) in which learners are cognitive apprentices (Brown et al., 1989). Learners benefit from 'imitation and practice in cooperative, authentic activity' (Gieselman et al., 2000, p. 263). According to Resnick (1989, cited in Gieselman et al., 2000), this process enables learners to:

- gain motivational support
- participate in shared thinking and expertise
- engage in conflicts stimulating further debate
- be exposed to different models of thinking and learning strategies.

Within clinical practice settings, practitioners should endeavour to maximize their learning of clinical reasoning skills and associated knowledge by creating practice environments and pursuing situated learning activities, as described in Chapter 26.

What are the goals of teaching and learning programmes?

Formal health science learning programmes and informal professional development activities are influenced by trends in education and by professional education goals. Five key areas of learning theory and discourse can be seen to articulate the goals of health sciences education:

- humanistic
- emancipatory and student-centred education
- social responsibility
- becoming agents for change and problem solvers
- learning how to learn and learning for capability.

■ Humanistic, emancipatory and student-centred education

Fundamentally, humanist psychology (which is the basis for humanistic education) is concerned with the humanity, individuality and worth of each person (Spencer et al., 1992). Humanistic education begins with the assumption that teaching is first and foremost a relationship between teacher and student, which includes human behaviour, human meanings, and human understandings that grow out of uniquely human experiences (Read and Simon, 1975). Humanistic education is built around the principle that individuals grow through positive relationships (Rogers, 1983). Rogers' assumptions about learning can be summarized as follows:

■ human beings have a natural capacity and desire for learning
■ significant or meaningful learning takes place when the subject matter is perceived by students as relevant to their needs, aspirations and goals
■ learning is acquired and retained best in an environment free from threat
■ learning is facilitated when, as far as possible, it is self-initiated and self-directed
■ learning that involves the whole person (feelings as well as intellect) is more lasting and pervasive.
■ self-evaluation is valuable as it promotes creativity, independence and self-reliance
■ the most socially useful learning is learning about the process of learning.

A significant contribution to humanistic education is the concept of a hierarchy of needs (Maslow, 1970). These needs, in ascending order, are physiological or survival needs; safety needs; love, affection and belonging needs; esteem needs; and need for self-actualization. Maslow proposed a number of principles of operation for these needs. Gratifying needs at each level (starting with the lowest) frees a person for gratification at higher levels; where a need has been satisfied, a person is best able to deal with deprivations of that need in the future; healthy persons have had their basic needs met and are principally motivated by their needs to actualize their highest possibilities. In harmony with these arguments, the adult educator's role (within the context of the learning situation) is to help individuals to meet their more basic needs (e.g. safety, belonging) and then to help them to achieve their fullest potential. This process could be described as helping learners to achieve the freedom of self-actualization by controlling, or helping them to control, the elements in the learning environment that relate to their needs.

In humanistic education, learners are granted responsible freedom and are encouraged and expected to become responsible for their learning within the framework for learning provided by the teacher and the learning programme (Table 25.1). Such education promotes the role of teachers as facilitators of learning and supports the goal of helping students to learn how to learn and to become fully functioning people. This theme of empowerment of the individual is inherent in the teaching philosophy and practice of critical pedagogy espoused by Freire (1972). Freire advocated learning as a process of becoming aware of one's social and political situation through problem posing and dialogue between teachers and students in situations that reduce the power imbalance between them (Burnard, 1995). Such education seeks to liberate people both socially and politically.

Critical pedagogy is a mode of teaching often pursued in contemporary education, in which students are given the opportunity to think critically about the limitations to their freedom, thereby helping them to learn to be free. The importance of critical awareness has also been emphasized by Torbert (1978) and Mezirow (1985a). Torbert (1978, p. 109) argued that increased awareness is the key to liberating education. It involves 'a higher quality of attention than we ordinarily bring to bear on our affairs'. Such attention is necessary for the search for shared purpose, self-direction and high-quality work, which 'create the possibility for adult relatedness, integrity, and generativity and therefore represent the essence of genuinely liberating higher education' (Torbet, 1978, p. 110). Torbert's goals can be related to the goals in the health-care industry of achieving effective teamwork, autonomous professional behaviour and self-direction, and quality assurance.

According to Mezirow (1985a), the promotion of 'critical awareness' should be aimed at helping students to direct their own learning, to learn how to make meaning out of their experience, and to identify values in their lives. Mezirow's (1985b) critical theory of adult learning and education draws on the ideas of the philosopher–sociologist Jürgen Habermas (1970, 1971). Habermas' critical learning theory identifies three domains in which human interest generates knowledge. These are the technical, the

Table 25.1 Characteristics of humanistic, learner-centred learning programmes

Maslow	Knowles	Rogers
Empathic listening	Learning involves collaboration	A climate of trust in which curiosity
Students share responsibility with	between a facilitator and student	and the natural desire to learn can be
the facilitator for the content	Learners move from a position of	nourished and enhanced
and direction of the course	dependency upon the teacher	A participatory mode of decision
The ability to self-evaluate is an	to one of self-direction	making in all aspects of learning, in
important part of education	The increasing store of experience	which students, teachers and
Differences among students are	held by adult learners provides a	administrators each have a part
expected and respected	profound resource for learning for	Helping students to prize themselves,
Instructor criticism must be	themselves and others	to build their confidence and
constructive and meaningful	The need to cope with real-life	self-esteem
	situations provides the stimulus for	Uncovering the excitement of
	learning	intellectual and emotional discovery,
	Teachers are responsible for creating	which leads learners to become
	conditions and providing tools to	lifelong learners
	help students to discover their need	Developing in teachers the attitudes
	to know	that research has shown to be most
	Education programmes should be	effective in facilitating learning
	designed according to students'	Helping teachers to grow as people,
	abilities and needs	finding rich satisfaction in their
	The goal of education is to build	interaction with learners
	increased competence for students so	An awareness that the good life is
	they can reach their fullest potential	within, not something that is
	in life	dependent on outside sources

Derived from Knowles (1980), Maslow (1970), Rogers (1983).

practical and the emancipatory domains. These three 'ways of knowing' can be described as the 'empirical-analytic (sciences) approach', with the goal of establishing causality; the 'communicative action' or 'historical-hermeneutic (sciences) approach', which seeks interpretation and explanation of individual experiences and perspectives; and the 'emancipatory action approach', which involves an interest in self-knowledge. Such emancipation frees us from forces (e.g. environmental forces) that limit our options and control over our lives. Identification of these three ways of knowing supports the contention that manual therapists must be able to draw on the full spectrum of available evidence (research and experience based) to guide their clinical decisions and actions.

Student-centred learning is linked to humanism, emancipatory and adult learning. This approach to learning focusses on the human resources potential of learners, seeking to provide learners with the tools needed to learn throughout life, to be able to adapt to new circumstances and to be proactive in addressing their needs for learning, change and action. The learner is the centre of the learning programme, not only as the principal focus of the learning but also as an active participant in shaping the learning programme through setting goals and planning learning activities and assessment. The teacher acts as a facilitator and guide rather than an instructor. Table 25.1 illustrates this approach.

Social responsibility

The changes in health-care and professional practice (including manual therapy) have a number of implications for the education of beginning practitioners (Higgs et al., 1999). These include the need to:

- educate health science students for their role in the political arena of health and health care, remembering that knowledge of the political system is important if people are to be effective in influencing policy resource allocation (Gardner, 1995)
- convince students that it is relevant to their education to learn 'how the world works'; this involves

notions of how politics, economy and environment interact, notions that for many years were thought to be outside the purview of professional education related to health

- socialize students for a new approach to professionalism; for doctors, nurses and allied health professionals, the changing view of health 'asks whether health care is something we do for people or something we do *with* them' (Lawson et al., 1996, p. 11; italics added).
- prepare students for a broader role than simply that of the competent beginning practitioner in a clinical sense: we need to educate them for social responsibility.

Prosser (1995) contended that learners should learn something about their future responsibility to the community at large. He argued that learning is influenced in many ways by the teacher's choices and actions. These impact on health science education programmes in several ways: students observe their (positive and negative) role models; learning goals, content and assessment can focus simply on technical aspects of the professional role or can more broadly encompass discussion about issues of community interest; more comprehensive interpretation and debate of ethical practices can include not just the individual client's medical needs but also matters of responsibility to society. Hill (1994) further contended that education must embrace and promote social justice as a principal educational imperative, reminiscent of Freire's vision of humanity and social improvement. In the context of manual therapy, as discussed in Chapter 1, clinical reasoning is not limited to decisions regarding pathology and technical management. Contemporary manual therapists must be able to make both diagnostic and non-diagnostic decisions. Through skilled narrative reasoning they can acquire an understanding of the patient's individual experience and the basis for the patient's perspectives. This understanding enables therapists to act as effective advocates for social justice in a health system where attention to justice and rights of individuals often suffer at the expense of economic rationalism.

Becoming agents for change and problem solvers

To meet current and future expectations of the professional workplace, practitioners need the ability to interact with and change the context of practice. That is, they need to be able to be problem solvers and agents for

change. In order to produce convincing and successful change agents, educational programmes need to help students to work within the reality of the workplace, not trampling blindly, naively or arrogantly on existing hard-won progress or tilting futilely at the windmills of intransigent bureaucracy, becoming disillusioned in the process. Instead, change agents work with people and systems to understand the status quo and facilitate achievable shared goals and actions for change.

Engel (2000) argued that the health professions should take the lead in preparing future graduates to adapt to the impending changes of the 21st century and to participate in the management of change. A model of health practitioners as 'interactional professionals' (Higgs and Hunt, 1999) has been developed to address these expectations. It is located within a model of social ecology. Social ecology deals with interactivity among people and between people and their environment; it acknowledges the importance of basing behaviour on promoting optimal, supportive relationships between humanity, community and the environment. The characteristics of interactional professionals are given in Table 25.2. These capacities will enable practitioners to act in a competent professional manner and to engage in effective reasoning, collaborative problem solving, critical self-evaluation, lifelong learning and professional review and development.

Learning how to learn

Helping students learn how to learn is an important goal in health sciences education. The literature presents a range of approaches for this. These include individual study guides, individual tuition, special teaching skills subjects and integrated curriculum 'actions' aimed at improving students' learning. Such programmes increasingly recognize the importance of enhancing students' awareness of and control over their learning processes, rather than just teaching them learning skills (Martin and Ramsden, 1986). It is desirable for students to become aware of their learning style/approach options, to develop their ability to use effective learning strategies, and to take responsibility for managing their approaches to learning. Gibbs (2000) argued that one way of improving the ability to learn is to understand the learning process. Approaches to learning are presented below. In addition to learning to learn, however, it is important not to lose sight of the main purpose of learning, as articulated by Ramsden (1986), which is to learn or change one's conceptions about the content at a

Table 25.2 Characteristics of interactional professionals

Feature	Characteristics
Competence	Technical competence (discipline-specific) and generic skills (including skills in communication, evaluation and investigation, self-directed learning, interpersonal interaction and cultural competence)
Reflection	Competence in reflective practice and critical self-evaluation
Problem solving	Competence in problem solving and clinical reasoning
Professionalism	Demonstrated characteristics and behaviours of members of professions, including professionalism and responsibility for one's professional decisions and actions
Social responsibility	The capacity to demonstrate responsibility in serving and enhancing society
Interactivity and change agency	The ability to interact effectively with people and environment and to change the context of practice
Situational leadership	The capacity to provide situationally relevant leadership

Based on Higgs and Hunt (1999).

relevant level (e.g. learning that is oriented to graduate practice-based matters) within the context in which one is learning (e.g. health care, manual therapy).

Learning for capability

Health professionals are expected to demonstrate competence. Capability is a broader concept than competence and is concerned with the ability to perform effectively, particularly in the here-and-now (Stephenson, 1998, p. 3): 'Capability embraces competence but is also forward-looking, concerned with the realization of potential. A capability approach focusses on the capacity of individuals to participate in the formulation of their own developmental needs and those of the context in which they work and live'. A capability approach is developmental, self-directed and involves learners managing their own learning. Capability implies being able to look ahead and act accordingly in a changing world. Capability exists (Stephenson, 1992) when people, with justified confidence, are able to:

- take effective and appropriate action
- explain what they are about
- live and work effectively with other people
- continue to learn from their individual experience and their experiences with others in a diverse and changing society.

These actions require self-knowledge, self-awareness, self-confidence, self-critique and the capacity to work effectively with others. These are characteristics that are inherent in skilled clinical reasoning and expected of capable, autonomous health professionals.

Who are the learners? What difference does it make?

Learner characteristics and styles are important considerations in the design and implementation of learning programmes.

Learning styles

'The quality of student learning depends on the student's approach to learning' (Ramsden, 1985, p. 52). Research concerning learning styles has emphasized the finding that learners' responses vary with the ways in which learning is offered and the learning environment is created. Students' learning styles are also strongly influenced by their past learning experience and their perceptions of their learning situation (Prosser and Trigwell, 1998). Teachers, therefore, need to consider the effects that the teaching method and setting have on their students' learning. Knowledge and effective use of learning styles are also important in that teachers can facilitate students' adoption of more effective learning styles (e.g. deep learning) and of learning approaches more suited to the task. Further, discussion of learners' approaches to learning can result in students developing more effective strategies for lifelong learning and acquiring greater success in the use of metacognitive learning or learning that actively involves critical self-appraisal. For self-directed learners (e.g. manual therapy practitioners), it is useful to know how to learn and how to learn more effectively.

Three of these learning styles models are described in Table 25.3.

Table 25.3 Learning styles

Model	Style	Characteristics
Honey and Mumford (1982)	Activist	Open minded, concerned with the here and now, enthusiastic about new things, filled with activity, likes crises, likes brainstorming, thrives on challenge, gregarious, likes new experiences
	Reflector	Likes to ponder on things, likes to stand back and view events, cautious and thorough, likes to 'sleep on it', takes a back seat, keeps a low profile
	Theorist	Logical, step-by-step approach, rational, concerned with basic concepts, detached and analytical, likes to analyse and synthesize
	Pragmatist	Practical, likes to try out theories and ideas, acts quickly, likes problem solving, likes new ideas, likes to get on with things
Kolb (1984)	Converger	Relies primarily on active experimentation and abstract conceptualization. Strength lies in problem solving, decision making and the practical application of ideas. Knowledge organization favours hypothetical deductive reasoning. Prefer dealing with tasks and problems rather than social and interpersonal issues
	Diverger	Relies primarily on concrete experience and reflective observation. Strength lies in imaginative ability and awareness of meaning and values. Concrete situations are viewed from many perspectives organized into a meaningful 'gestalt'. Performs best in situations calling for generation of alternative ideas and implications. Interested in people and tends to be imaginative and feeling oriented
	Assimilator	Relies primarily on abstract conceptualization and reflective observation. Strength lies in inductive reasoning and the ability to create theoretical models, assimilating disparate observations into an integrated explanation. Less focussed on people and more concerned with ideas and abstract concepts
	Accommodator	Relies primarily on concrete experience and active experimentation. Strength lies in doing things, carrying out plans and becoming involved in new experiences. Best able to adapt to changing circumstances as opportunity seekers and risk takers. Tends to solve problems in an intuitive, trial-and-error manner, relying heavily on other people for information rather than their own analytical ability. At ease with people
Entwistle and Ramsden (1983)	Meaning orientation	Active, deep learning approach to constructing personal meaning, which involves intrinsic motivation
	Reproducing orientation	Similar to surface learning, with an emphasis on rote learning and responding to extrinsic motivation
	Strategic orientation	Aiming at good results; similar to Biggs (1987) concept of achieving dimension
	Non-academic orientation	Lack of interest in or concern for academic results

■ Honey and Mumford (1982) identified four learning styles, activist, reflector, theorist and pragmatist, and found that people commonly have elements of all four styles.

■ Kolb (1984, p. 38) regarded learning as 'a process whereby knowledge is created through the transformation of experience'. He described four basic forms of knowing, divergence, assimilation, convergence and accommodation, and argued that a major influence on individual learning styles is the underlying structure of the learning process. He demonstrated that effective and skilled learning encompasses elements of these four approaches.

■ Entwistle and Ramsden (1983) examined general tendencies/approaches to learning and attitudes to studying and identified four study orientations: meaning orientation, reproducing orientation, strategic orientation and non-academic orientation.

Ramsden (1988, p. 20) described the deep (or meaning orientation) and surface (or reproducing orientation) approaches to learning as follows:

Deep approaches exemplify the type of learning that employers and teachers expect students to demonstrate. Only through using these approaches can students gain mastery of concepts and a firm hold on detailed factual knowledge in a given subject area. Such approaches embody the imaginative and adaptive skills and wide sphere of interests that are increasingly demanded in the world of work. In acute contrast surface approaches epitomise low-quality learning, are geared to short-term requirements, and focus on the need faithfully to reproduce fragments of information presented in class or textbooks ... surface approaches are concerned with 'getting the right answer' to the exclusion of knowing how to get it and of what it means when it has been obtained.

The deep learning approach reflects the goals of health science education, including a commitment to lifelong learning, accountability of practice and critical self-evaluation. These outcomes are preferable to outcomes that reflect surface learning approaches, such as a preference for following rules, responding only to direct supervision, and reliance on evaluation by others. Health care is an inexact science, and deep approaches to learning are entwined with other practices of the health professional, including exercising professional judgment and making clinical decisions in an arena often characterized by uncertainty, complexity and multiple alternative action choices.

Learner demographics

If we are aiming to facilitate learner-centred adult learning, we need to know who our learners are. This knowledge enables teachers to match planned learning goals with learner characteristics. Factors that could be considered in seeking to understand a learning group include, first, contextual factors, such as programme level, location and mode; these give guidance as to learner motivations and expectations. Secondly, teachers can assess student profile factors, including enrollment numbers, age, gender, educational background, socioeconomic characteristics and cultural situation. To create an optimal learning environment to encourage adult, deep, and self-directed learning requires consideration of learners' task maturity (Higgs, 1993), which encompasses their preparation for and readiness to engage in the current learning task, and the creation of programmes that liberate self-directedness and learner responsibility.

How do learners learn?

Learners learn in many ways. However, it is most useful to look at several key learning theories or movements, which can help us to understand both how different learners learn and how we could help learners to learn more effectively, and be better learners ourselves. This section focusses on adult learning, experiential learning, and the interaction between assessment and learning. It is important to remember that adult learning is an approach to learning. Adults, particularly those strongly schooled in rote learning approaches, may need to learn to become adult learners. They may need to learn how to be self-directed, to be responsible partners in learning programmes, to be self-evaluative and to set and pursue their own learning goals.

Adult learning

Adult learning is a common and popular aspect of teaching and learning today. The foundations of adult learning theory are key assumptions (supported by subsequent research) made about adult learners (as cited in Knowles et al., 1998):

- adults become ready to learn the things they need to know and be able to do in order to cope effectively with their real-life situations; therefore, these are the appropriate starting points for organizing adult learning activities
- in contrast to childrens' subject-centred orientation to learning, adults are life-centred (or task/problem-centred) in their learning orientation; therefore, the appropriate units for organizing adult learning are life situations, not subjects
- adults come into an educational activity with a greater volume and a different quality of experience than young people; experience is the richest resource for adults' learning and, therefore, the core methodology of adult education is the analysis of experience
- adults have a deep need to be self-directing; therefore, the role of the teacher is to engage in a process of mutual inquiry with them rather than to transmit knowledge to them and then evaluate their conformity to it
- individual differences among people increase with age; therefore, adult education must make optimal provision for differences in style, time, place and pace of learning
- adults need to know why they need to learn something before undertaking to learn it
- adults have a self-concept of being responsible for their own decisions and lives
- while adults are responsive to some external motivators (e.g. jobs), the most potent motivators are internal pressures (e.g. the desire for increased self-esteem, job satisfaction such as success in patient management, quality of life).

The philosophy and practice of adult learning has been influenced by numerous individuals and groups. Boud (1987) categorized adult learning into four traditions.

Training and efficiency in learning: freedom from distraction in learning. This approach regards teaching and learning as a technology. 'Once a learner has decided to study a particular topic or to learn new skills, the aim of practitioners of this approach is to make this task as straightforward as possible and to ensure that all learning is directed efficiently towards this end' (Boud, 1987, p. 223). This approach arises out of the programmed learning tradition.

Self-directed learning and the adult learning (or andragogy) school: freedom from the restrictions of teachers/freedom as learners. 'This approach places the unique goals of individual learners as central in the learning process and provides a structure to assist learners to achieve their own ends' (Boud, 1987, p. 224). According to Boud, this approach is most suitable for situations where learners are able to identify and articulate their learning needs and goals and where appropriate resources are available. The learning contract approach of Knowles et al. (1998) is typical of this tradition.

Learner-centred education and the humanistic educators: freedom to learn. This approach focusses on the facilitation of learning by a non-directive facilitator within a highly supportive, accepting and respectful environment. This is typical of the tradition of Carl Rogers (1969). Learning is seen to be an activity that should involve the whole person, including attitudes, values, and emotions as well as cognitive and psychomotor aspects. There is also the recognition that learners may be inhibited from learning by past experiences and emotions, and that part of the teacher's role is to liberate learners from such inhibiting factors, thereby providing them with freedom to learn.

Critical pedagogy and social action: freedom through learning. While the previous three approaches position learning as an individual phenomenon, according to this approach learning is a social phenomenon in which learners not only learn in a group but have responsibility for other learners. Supporters of this approach (e.g. Freire, 1972, 1973) see learning as a means of freeing people, using learning as a way of removing the limits that lack of knowledge places upon people, and encouraging them to take part in shaping the society in which they live.

Boud (1987, p. 228) contended that each of these approaches 'may be a valid response to a given adult learning need'. Each approach has strengths and weaknesses, but all four have two common elements: respect for learners and their experience and the need to commence with the learner's present understanding. A most interesting aspect of Boud's categorization is the strong theme of freedom used to highlight each approach.

Numerous authors have reported their experiences and hypotheses concerning conditions that facilitate

Table 25.4 Adult learning conditions and behaviours

Environmental conditions	Decision-making/management factors	Adult learning behaviours
Motivation	Shared goals	Problem-solving
Acceptance of learner as person	Shared management	Interaction with teacher and other learners
Freedom/autonomy	Mutual decision making/planning	Active participation in learning
Individuality	Shared resource acquisition	Experiential learning
Emphasis on abilities/experience	Learner involvement in learning,	Self-correction
Student-centred learning	needs diagnosis, and evaluation	Interdependence
Resource-rich environment	Learner direction in posing questions/	Critical reflection
Mutual respect/trust	seeking answers	Progressive mastery
Teacher support/facilitation	Effective communication	Active seeking of meaning
Learning via experience relevant	Choice in participation	Individual pacing
to learner	Collaborative facilitation	Empowered self-direction practice
Praxis: integrating reflection,	Ongoing review by teacher and	Enthusiasm for learning
theory, experience	learners	Reciprocal learning
Interaction between learners	Learner identification of community	Internal drive/motivation
Effective/appropriate group	goals and needs as part of own	
dynamics	learning context	
Security/support	Learner acceptance of responsibility	
	for learning	

From Terry and Higgs (1993).

adult learning. These include 'principles of teaching' (Knowles, 1980), 'major generalizations' (Knox, 1977) about how teachers can facilitate adult learning, principles of effective adult learning (Bagnall, 1978) and the 'charter for andragogy' (Mezirow, 1981, 1985a,b), which is based on the theories of Habermas (1971). Mezirow proposed that teachers in adult learning need to make important decisions and operate according to values that give priority to the learner's developing autonomy. The work of these authors supports the following two propositions. First, a number of accepted conditions for learning can be identified and these can be subdivided into environmental conditions and conditions related to the decision-making and management strategies employed in the programme (Table 25.4). Secondly, the role of the teacher in adult learning programmes is to create these conditions (with the learners) through management of the learning programmes.

Experiential learning

How do learners experience their learning and make sense of it? The essence of experiential learning was characterized by Boud and Pascoe (1978; cited in Burnard, 1995) as:

- the involvement of individual learners in their learning, engaging their full attention
- the correspondence of the learning activity to the outside world, emphasizing the quality of the learning experience rather than its location
- allowing learners to have control over the learning experience so that they can integrate it with their own mode of operation in the world and can experience the results of their decisions.

This list has parallels with adult and humanistic education. In addition, there is a need, as Michelson (1998) emphasized, to remember that learning through experience involves embodied knowing as well as being an experience of the mind and a social experience. This is particularly pertinent to fields such as manual therapy, which involve high levels of physical interaction in data collection and treatment, and where manual therapists often come to 'know through their fingertips'.

Boud and colleagues (Boud et al., 1985; Boud and Walker, 1990) developed a model for experience-based learning that focussed on helping students and staff to attend to salient features of the learner, to understand opportunities and constraints provided by the setting and learning activities, and to operate effectively in challenging and complex real-world learning environments. The model emphasized three stages of engagement in a learning event: activities and experiences prior to the event, during the event and and after the event. Learners engage in noticing, intervening and reflection-in-action, as well as reflection after the event (without the distractions of the setting), in order to make sense of and learn from their experiences. Reflection after the event essentially involves feelings and emotions, as well as intellectual work. Three elements are return to experience, attending to feelings and re-evaluation of experience (Fig. 25.2). The basic assumption underlying this model (Boud and Edwards, 1999) is that learning is always grounded in prior experience and that attempts to promote new learning must in some way take account of that experience. Since learning builds on existing perceptions and frameworks of understanding, links must be made between new learning and what is known if learners are to make sense of what is happening or has happened to them. This is particularly pertinent for clinical fieldwork, which involves affective as well as cognitive learning, and which situates learners (clinicians and patients) in the social, psychological, cultural and material environments of professional practice (Boud and Edwards, 1999). As discussed in Chapter 1, practitioners often need to assist patients to reflect on their perspectives regarding their pain experience and health beliefs, including the bases to those perspectives. Such communicative management requires the practitioner's understanding and skill in working with the patient to reflect on the patient's perspectives and associated feelings.

Hagar (1998) emphasized the connection between experience and reflection. He explored the various connotations of reflection through the works of different authors. Dewey (1966), for example, required that education gives learners the lifelong capacity to grow and to readjust themselves continually to their environments through reflective thinking, enquiry, democracy, problem solving, active learning and experiential learning. Dewey's reflective thinking is 'holistic, incorporating social, moral and political aspects of the contexts' (Hagar, 1998, p. 37). Schön's (1983, 1987) notion of the reflective practitioner emphasized the practices of reflection in action: a spontaneous practice of noticing, seeing or feeling features of their learning and actions. Marsick and Watkins (1990) linked experience and reflection in their exploration of informal and incidental learning. Both of these are modes of learning particularly relevant to learning in the complexity and bustle of clinical practice. From the various theories explored, Hagar (1998, p. 42) concluded that two major assumptions underpinned effective workplace/experience-based learning: 'that learning from experience is fundamental to individual personal growth and development' and 'that in a rapidly

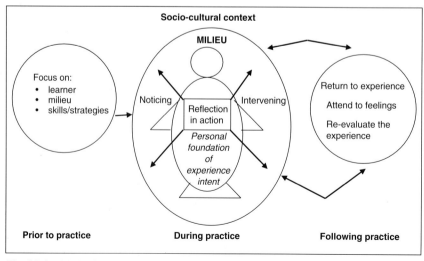

Fig. 25.2 Model for promoting learning from experience. (From Boud and Edwards, 1999, based on Boud and Walker, 1990.)

changing world successful and competitive enterprises require workers who have certain broad generic skills'.

Assessment and learning

Assessment facilitates, indeed shapes, learning, because students' responses to assessment govern what they learn. Studies by Marton and Säljö (1976) and Ramsden (1979, 1984), for instance, have demonstrated that assessment methods can profoundly influence students' approaches to learning, in particular their use of deep and surface approaches to learning. Assessment is not, and should not be seen to be, an independent factor added on to learning programmes to accredit learning. This perspective is increasingly recognized in learning programme design and implementation. A new 'holistic' view of assessment is needed (Boud and Higgs, 1999) in which (good) assessment closely reflects desired learning outcomes and demonstrates a directly beneficial influence on the learning process. Assessment needs to be reframed as part of the total package of learning and assessment, focussing clearly on the assessment profile *as students see it*, in relation to the total learning experience. Students need greater opportunities to practise and gain feedback, and greater time for self- and peer-assessment.

What are the roles of learners?

The learners' roles in higher education and professional development largely centre around self-directedness and lifelong learning. As professionals (actual or prospective), they have the responsibility to participate in ongoing learning and to use their learning and self-evaluation skills to maintain and enhance their capabilities.

Self-directed learning

Wilcox (1996, p. 166) argued that 'self-directed learning's emphasis on personal autonomy, personal responsibility, and personal growth embodies some of the most fundamental principles of higher education'. Self-directed learning is an approach to learning that is a derivative of adult learning and humanistic education. It implies internal motivation for learning, rather than learning in isolation. Learners may elect to learn by themselves; however, many authors argue strongly that effective learning involves interaction with others. Griffith (1987), for instance, discussed the concept of independence versus interdependence in learning programmes. She stressed the importance of learners valuing the contributions each can make to others' learning.

Self-direction in learning is widely acknowledged as a fundamental educational goal. Harris (1989, p. 112) regarded the aim of self-directed learning as, 'to assist individuals to take increasing control over their learning processes and content. In this way, they will develop the realization that they have the power to alter their individual and social environment and to create their own reality. This is the "empowerment view" of adult education.'

Self-directed learning embodies a number of key elements: autonomy, the pursuit of competence/excellence, the variability and development in a learner's capability as a self-directed learner over time, the variability between different learners' independent learning abilities, the idea of learner responsibility for the learning process and outcome, and the notion that independent learning can occur as an individual or group activity. In self-directed learning programmes, the learner's behaviour demonstrates:

- responsibility for and critical awareness of his or her learning process and outcome
- a high level of self-direction in performing learning activities and solving problems that are associated with the learning task
- active input to decision making regarding the learning task
- the use of the teacher as a resource person
- effective interaction with other learners and the teacher in a collaborative learning manner.

Practitioners, such as manual therapists, are (ideally) constantly engaged in self-directed learning as they critique their knowledge, skills and abilities and seek to enhance them.

Lifelong learning

Lifelong learning is a central concept in the theory and practice of self-directed learning. For example, Knowles (1970) identified the main characteristics of self-directed learners as an increasing self-directedness, a readiness to learn in relation to life tasks and roles, a rich background of experience that serves as a resource for learning, and an orientation to learning that is problem-centred rather than subject-centred. A principal goal of in helping students to become self-directed learners is to promote the transfer of self-directed learning into life and work situations. Such transfer can be facilitated, for instance, through the analysis of the real patient cases, as presented in this book.

Bateson (1987; cited in Rawson, 2000) argued that learning to learn is a level of learning rather than purely a skill set. Bateson proposed three levels of learning to learn.

Learning I.   This involves change in the specificity of responses. At this stage, learners learn to arrive at a correct choice of problem or issue solution. They are not focussing on conceptualization of the problem or issue.

Learning II.   Here, change in the process of learning I occurs. At this stage, learners are learning about learning, not just about learning to solve problems. A higher level of critical thinking and problem conceptualization is involved.

Learning III.   The final stage involves change in the process of learning II. Here learners become conscious of their conceptions of the world, how they are formed and how they are changed. Learners become involved in self-reflexive learning processes (that is, learning that is reflective about self as learner and person).

Beyond this level of learning, it is argued, lies another level in which not only does the philosophical perspective of the learner becomes a conscious act and a development goal but also the capacity to create as well as acquire new knowledge is preeminent. In the earlier section on practice epistemology, this level of learning was introduced as a conscious, learning-as-knowledge-generation process, informed by critical and reflexive incorporation of the learners' epistemological perspective and goals into practice. This point is also relevant to some current views of evidence-based practice, which limit acceptable evidence to propositional knowledge acquired through quantitative research (Higgs et al., 2001; Jones and Higgs, 2000). Such a restriction would limit the discovery of new ideas, as the cutting edge of practice is frequently in advance of empirical research and evidence.

A number of authors have considered the value of the learning environment in promoting and facilitating lifelong learning. Senge (1990), for instance, advocated the development of learning organizations that integrate learning with work and actively encourage employees to learn from the problems, challenges and successes inherent in everyday activities. 'By working in this climate of priority for learning, individuals will become more aware of the need to learn, and will be helped and encouraged in the process of learning how to learn' (Gibbs, 2000, p. 234). Billett (2001) cautioned that, while lifelong learning in the workplace is more important than ever, individuals, however well motivated to pursue their professional development, may be restricted in this goal if the workplace constrains rather than supports learning opportunities.

Battersby (1999) argued that ongoing learning in the workplace (or continuing professional development), can be enhanced by adopting the humanistic and transformative imperatives associated with learning organizations. Ward and McCormack (2000) placed adult learning at the centre of practice development as a means of creating a learning culture to respond to the desired learning and organizational outcomes. Rawson (2000) concluded that a learning society requires a society of self-determining learners, not just a society of self-managed learners; that is, individuals who have the ability to challenge the status quo along with the skills to make their voices heard within the context of a dialectical process between developing individuals and developing societies.

What sort of work environment will graduates enter and influence?

For students, educators and graduates of professional entry educational programmes, the nature of the work environment is an important issue in shaping curricula and professional development goals and strategies. Teachers and learners, therefore, need to be familiar with trends in health care, with the nature and expectations of professional practice, and with the opportunities provided by work-based learning.

Trends in health care

Health professionals need to understand the continually changing world of work and prepare themselves for its demands. Changes in the health-care arena include:

- the changing view of health (as wellness and as a commodity, rather than as absence of illness)

- a re-evaluation of the concept of health care (with increasing emphasis on health promotion and community and managed care)
- changes in methods of measuring health (reflecting broader issues of lifestyle and society, e.g. socioeconomic status, rather than measures of ill health)
- local health-care developments (linked to economic rationalism and managed care)
- global health management developments (in particular, changing patterns of employment and health-care management associated with globalized economies).

These changes have been accompanied by a growing dissatisfaction with the medical model as a complete or relevant strategy for emergent health-care needs. One response is the adoption of managerial modes of health care, while a counterresponse seeks to reposition people, not managment, at the centre of our health-care system. Hancock (1985, p. 1) argued that 'the emphasis has shifted from a simplistic, reductionist cause-and-effect view of the medical model to a complex, holistic, interactive hierarchical systems view known as an ecological model'. This model focussed on the interactivity among people, human society and the environment and on the intersection between environment and culture, integrating the natural and social sciences (Hancock, 1985). Health care does not and cannot operate in isolation from the many local and global forces impacting on people's lives and environments.

The medical model of health care is often applied in a reductionist systematic manner rather than a holistic systemic manner. Adopting a social ecological perspective in the management of health care creates a more holistic approach, which places people at the centre of the system and ensures that the relationship between health care and costs focusses on the health care of people not on the operation and self-perpetuation of the health-care system. At a more individual level, clinicians, whether considering the cases in this book or reasoning in their own practice environments, need to go beyond traditional diagnostic reasoning and more overtly develop their practice knowledge and skills in non-diagnostic reasoning. Manual therapists of today must be able to conduct narrative and collaborative reasoning and practise communicative (not just instrumental) management (i.e. they need to develop skills of psychosocial assessment and management). This analysis also includes consideration of the broader effectiveness and efficiency of the patient's health-care management, particularly with respect to appropriate collaboration across the health professions.

Professional practice

Schön (1987) called the field of professional practice a 'swampy' area, because many of the decisions made in managing practice problems are based on data and knowledge that are often uncertain, ambiguous or hidden. Situations to which professionals apply their practice knowledge and skills are often complex because they involve people. People bring to the situation their own perceptions, needs and experience. These features influence the nature of the health problem. Problem clarification and management decisions, then, cannot be made without reference to the person concerned. The nature of professional practice requires health professionals to develop knowledge from their practice about the variety of contexts in which they practise and to develop advanced skills in clinical reasoning.

Work-based learning

'There has been a dramatic shift in recent years away from viewing educational institutions as the principal places in which learning occurs towards a recognition of the power and importance of the workplace as a site of learning. The nature of work is changing and this has given rise to changing demands for learning' (Boud, 1998, p. 1). These arguments are highly applicable to undergraduate education in the health sciences, where clinical education (in the field) forms a major avenue for students to learn in the workplace setting about the expectations of the workplace and its stakeholders and the development of a professional identity. For graduates, learning in and through their work is a vital element of professional development.

New trends in viewing and using workplace learning illustrate a collapse in the differences between practice and theory, between body and mind, and between learning and work (Boud, 1998). Learning in the workplace is increasingly gaining a value of its own, replacing the old view of the workplace as somewhere to practise the knowledge and skills learned in academia. The value of the workplace as a key site for learning is evident when we consider the nature of this workplace and the learning opportunities it provides. In particular, learning in the workplace is contextualized and consequential, rather than isolated from the reality or impact of practising similar professional skills or developing professional knowledge in the classroom. The context of the workplace changes rapidly, both locally and in response to the dynamics of external forces (e.g. government policy and economic changes). Clients bring their own complex and unique situations, cultures, needs and expectations to the professional–client interaction. Further, the workplace engages directly with employer, government and client expectations of quality standards of service delivery and interpersonal interaction. Each of these factors makes the workplace (particularly for health-care professionals engaged directly with the quality of people's lives) an essential and invaluable forum for learning and professional development.

Also of importance has been a change in the way people need to learn and a sharpening of the concept of lifelong learning, which should imply continuous learning that is responsive to continual environmental changes, not just learning throughout the duration of a working life. In work-based learning, learning is a student-centred continuous process grounded in experience (Sangster et al., 2000). Work-based learning adopts 'a structured and learner-managed approach to maximizing opportunities for learning and professional development in the workplace' (Flanagan et al., 2000, p. 360). Characteristics of work-based learning (based on Foster, 1996 (as cited in Flanagan et al., 2000); Sangster and Marshall, 2000) are:

- student centred
- autonomously managed
- team-based and cooperative, relying on partnerships
- interdisciplinary
- concerned with performance enhancement and upgrading experience
- process oriented, activity based and performance related
- problem based; focussing on complex work-based problems
- capable of producing new theoretical insights
- encompassing both education and training
- lifelong learning
- innovative, focussing on new approaches to gain experience and manage change.

The value of work-based learning is supported by a range of learning theories, including theories that present learning as deep, discovery, problem-based, autonomous, experiential, action and work-based (Johnson, 2000). In dealing with a real workplace problem, Johnson (2000) argued that learners responsible for solving the problem will become part of their own research (Watson, 1994), adopting an action learning approach. 'Action learning seeks to provide both a formalized learning opportunity and a means of developing the individual's learning abilities' (Johnson, 2000, p. 131).

How can learners be prepared for the reality of the workplace?

To face the real world of work and to continue to maintain and enhance competence in the face of the knowledge explosion, advancing technology and the changing work contexts in the health and social services arenas, students must be effective and committed lifelong learners. Professional socialization is the framework for developing these skills and commitment, along with a confident yet evolving professional identity and broader technical and generic competencies. Two valuable strategies for facilitating the professional socialization process are fieldwork education and peer learning. Fieldwork (or clinical) education provides the real-world context that most closely reflects the complexities and contingencies of the various social service contexts where health professionals work.

Clinical/fieldwork education

The education of health professionals is distinguished by their exposure to real-life practice through fieldwork education. Whereas clinical education traditionally involved the supervised practice of professional skills, fieldwork and clinical education today are becoming more commonly recognized as opportunities for learning and professional socialization, not just for practice. Apart from developing their professional identity and preparing for the complexities of real-world practice in clinical settings, students and graduates particularly need to employ these settings to develop their clinical reasoning skills and management skills. The goals of clinical education (Higgs et al., 1991) include:

- contributing to the development of the student's understanding of health, illness and the health-care system

- awareness of own attitudes, values and responses to health and illness
- ability to cope effectively with the demands of the professional role
- understanding of the inter-related roles in the health-care team
- clinical competencies relevant to the student's discipline, including clinical reasoning skills, psychomotor competencies, interpersonal and communication skills
- ability to provide a sound rationale for intervention/actions
- skills in the education of relevant people, e.g. patients, clients, the community, staff
- self-management skills, e.g. time and workload management
- ability to process, record and use data effectively
- ability to evaluate critically and develop one's own performance
- ability to review and investigate the quality of clinical practice
- professional accountability, commitment to clients/self/employers
- commitment to maintaining and developing professional competence
- skills necessary for lifelong professional learning
- ability to respond to changing community health-care needs.

Clinical education can be considered as a mode of work-based learning, defined as 'student learning for credit designed to occur either in the workplace or in on-campus settings that emulate key aspects of the workplace' (Reeders, 2000, p. 205).

Peer learning

Learning with peers is a useful strategy for the development of complex cognitive skills such as clinical reasoning. Working with peers on collaborative decision making and receiving feedback from peers helps practitioners to develop their reasoning in many ways: they become more aware of how they reason, they learn to be more critical of their reasoning, they learn reasoning alternatives through listening to others' reasoning, they recognize the limits of their reasoning ability/knowledge by receiving feedback from others, and they gain competence in articulation of their reasoning. Through reasoning aloud with peers and critiquing their reasoning, practitioners can gain valuable insights into the (largely) unobservable process of decision making. For a successful peer-learning experience to take place, interdependence, individual accountability and group-processing ability need to be present (Johnson, 1981). Peer learning can involve novice practitioners learning alongside their peers. This can enhance professional competence and reasoning skills (Ladyshewsky et al., 2000), foster peer discussion in the workplace setting to promote exposure of the learner's thoughts and arguments, and allow discussion and restructuring of knowledge (Regehr and Norman, 1996).

Summary

Which learning theory to follow

How do we, as teachers and learners, know which learning theories to choose? Figure 25.3 illustrates the factors to consider in the ranges of choices we can make in seeking to plan and implement relevant learning programmes. The educational strategy of choice depends on thoughtful application of available theory and knowledge/evidence to the given situation (including needs, preferences, etc.). First, teachers (and learners designing their own learning programmes) need to be familiar with theories and contexts of learning. Secondly, a number of factors must be considered, such as consumer/participant differences (e.g. needs and goals), variables specific to the situation (e.g. the professional context and topic to be learned), and broader context or 'big picture' issues (e.g. community expectations and trends in education). Teachers and learners bring to the learning process a number of skills and capabilities, including their skill in using different learning styles/approaches, reflexivity, creativity and the capacity to explain and understand concepts and phenomena. In drawing these factors together, a number of teaching and learning principles can be employed, such as identification of salient factors, the pursuit of authenticity in matching espoused and practised principles and strategies, and the creation of learning environments that promote mutual respect among learners and teachers. Readers are invited to reflect on the parallels between educational decision making presented in Figure 25.3 and clinical decision making using collaborative decision making within a broad evidence-based and patient/client-centred framework.

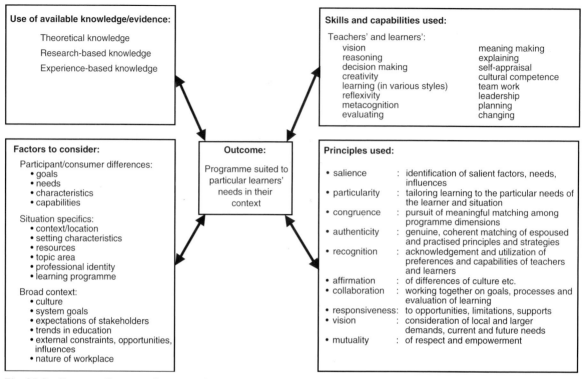

Fig. 25.3 Factors influencing planning and implementation of learning programmes.

Putting it all together

Figure 25.4 illustrates one way of putting these many ideas together. It places learning at the core with a focus on the four core learning capabilities or approaches proposed by Kolb (1984). Informing decision making about teaching are learning theories, the teacher's and learner's experience, a commitment to learning with others, being enriched by their experience and aspirations, and the particular aspects of the learning task and situation. These factors occur within a multifaceted context where realities, expectations and visions interact to produce rich and complex environments for learning.

Teaching as art, craft and science

Teaching is a blend of art, craft and science. The educational discourse, principles and theories relevant to clinical reasoning have been described, emphasizing the parallels between reasoning and learning in the imprecise worlds of teaching, learning and professional practice. These principles and theories have arisen from research (the science of teaching), from

theory (conceptualizations and visions of practice) and from experience (reflection on practice, giving rise to professional craft knowledge). At the core of all the forms of knowledge underpinning practice lies practice epistemology. That is, understanding how knowledge is generated, knowing its sources, understanding the need for rigour and ongoing critical reflection in the constant appraisal and evolution of practice knowledge, and recognizing the situatedness and salience of this knowledge allows the knowledge user (teacher, practitioner, learner) to use knowledge wisely. Herein lies the essence of practice wisdom, which provides the foundation for professional artistry in practice. We need, in our learning and teaching (of clinical reasoning), to recognize that principles and theories of learning, and other educational tools such as 'evidence-based teaching practice', are simply guidelines that the teacher and learner can use to facilitate learning. The optimal learning strategy for a given situation depends on many factors as discussed above. Advanced skills in learning (e.g. varying learning styles, self-directed learning) and teaching need to be developed. Advanced skills in teaching can include metacognitive teaching (i.e. choosing an educational

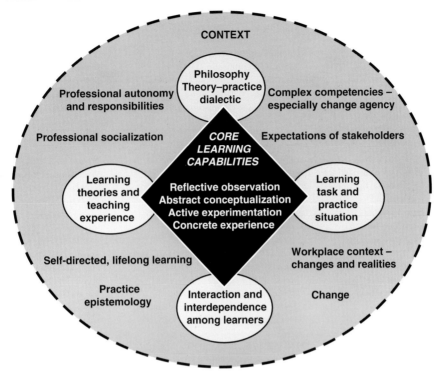

Fig. 25.4   Summary.

and philosophical stance, utilizing a rich knowledge base of the subject area; Higgs, 2001) and the creation of liberating learning frameworks (i.e. learning situations characterized by controlled freedom that provides sufficient and appropriate structure to match the learner's readiness for the task; Higgs, 1993). This is expanded in Chapter 26, which deals with ways of enhancing clinical reasoning.

References

Bagnall, R.G. (1978). Principles of adult education in the design and management of instruction. Australian Journal of Adult Education, 28, 19–27.

Bateson, G. (1987). Steps to an Ecology of Mind: Collected Essays Anthropology, Psychiatry, Evolution and Epistemology. Northvale, NJ: Aronson.

Battersby, D. (1999). The learning organization and CPE: some philosophical considerations. Learning Organization, 6, 58–62.

Benner, P. (1984). From Novice to Expert: Excellence and Power in Clinical Nursing Practice. London: Addison-Wesley.

Berliner, D. (1988). The Development of Expertise in Pedagogy. Washington, DC: American Association of Colleges for Teacher Education.

Biggs, J.B. (1987). Student Approaches to Learning and Studying. Melbourne: Australian Council for Educational Research.

Billett, S. (2001). Learning throughout working life: interdependencies at work. Studies in Continuing Education, 23, 19–35.

Boud, D. (1987). A facilitator's view of adult learning. In Appreciating Adults Learning: From the Learners' Perspective (D. Boud and V. Griffin, eds.) pp. 222–239. London: Kogan Page.

Boud, D. (1998). A new focus on workplace learning research. In Current Issues and New Agendas in Workplace Learning (D. Boud, ed.) pp.1–8. Leabrook, South Australia: National Centre for Vocational Education Research.

Boud, D. and Edwards, H. (1999). Learning for practice: promoting learning in clinical and community settings. In Educating Beginning Practitioners: Challenges for Health Professional Education (J. Higgs and H. Edwards, eds.) pp. 173–179. Oxford: Butterworth-Heinemann.

Boud, D. and Higgs, J. (1999). Assessment and learning. In Educating Beginning Practitioners: Challenges for Health Professional Education, (J. Higgs and H. Edwards, eds.) pp. 221–227. Oxford: Butterworth-Heinemann.

Boud, D. and Pascoe, J. (1978). Experiential Learning: Developments in Australian Post-secondary Education. Sydney: Australian Consortium on Experiential Learning.

Boud, D. and Walker, D. (1990). Making the most of experience. Studies in Continuing Education, 12, 61–80.

Boud, D., Keogh, R. and Walker, D. (1985). Reflection: Turning Experience into Learning. London: Kogan Page.

Brown, J.S., Collins, A. and Duiguid, P. (1989). Situated cognition and the culture of learning. Educational Researcher, 18, 32–42.

Burke, J.P. and DePoy, E. (1991). An emerging view of mastery, excellence, and leadership in occupational therapy practice. American Journal of Occupational Therapy, 45, 1027–1032.

Burnard, P. (1995). Learning Human Skills: An Experiential and Reflective Guide for Nurses. Oxford: Butterworth-Heinemann.

Carper, B.A. (1978). Fundamental patterns of knowing. Advances in Nursing Science, 1, 13–23.

Cervero, R.M. (1988). Effective Continuing Education for Professionals. San Francisco, CA: Jossey-Bass.

Cervero, R.M. (1992). Professional practice, learning, and continuing education: an integrated perspective. International Journal of Lifelong Education, 10, 91–101.

Cope, P., Cuthbertson, P. and Stoddart, B. (2000). Situated learning in the practice placement. Journal of Advanced Nursing, 31, 850–856.

Crepeau, E.B. (1991). Achieving intersubjective understanding: examples from an occupational therapy treatment session. American Journal of Occupational Therapy, 45, 1016–1025.

Dewey, J. (1966). Democracy and Education. New York: Free Press.

Dreyfus, H.L. and Dreyfus, S.E. (1986). Mind over Machine: The Power of Human Intuition and Expertise in the Era of the Computer. Oxford: Basil Blackwell.

Edwards, R. and Usher, R. (1998). 'Moving' experiences: globalisation, pedagogy and experiential learning. Studies in Continuing Education, 20, 159–174.

Elstein, A.S., Shulman, L. and Sprafka, S. (1990). Medical problem-solving: a ten year retrospective. Evaluation and the Health Professions, 13, 5–36.

Engel, C.E. (2000). Health professions education for adapting to change and for participating in managing change.

Education for Health: Change in Training and Practice, 13, 37–43.

Entwistle, N.J. and Ramsden, P. (1983). Understanding Student Learning. London: Croom Helm.

Everingham, F. and Bandaranayake, R. (1999). Teacher education programs for health science educators. In Educating Beginning Practitioners: Challenges for Health Professional Education, (J. Higgs and H. Edwards, eds.) pp. 263–270. Oxford: Butterworth-Heinemann.

Flanagan, J., Baldwin, S. and Clarke, D. (2000). Work-based learning as a means of developing and assessing nursing competence. Journal of Clinical Nursing, 9, 360–368.

Foster, E. (1996). Comparable but Different: Work Based Learning for a Learning Society. WBL Project, Final Report 1994–1996, University of Leeds.

Freire, P. (1972). The Pedagogy of the Oppressed, Harmondsworth, UK: Penguin.

Freire, P. (1973). Education for Critical Consciousness. London: Sheed and Ward.

Frost, N. (2001). Professionalism, change and the politics of lifelong learning. Studies in Continuing Education, 23, 5–17.

Gardner, H. (ed.) (1995). The Politics of Health: The Australian Experience, 2nd edn. Melbourne, Australia: Churchill Livingstone.

Gibbs, V. (2000). Learning how to learn: a selective review of the literature. Radiography, 6, 231–235.

Gieselman, J.A., Stark, N. and Farruggia, M.J. (2000). Implications of the situated learning model for teaching and learning nursing research. Journal of Continuing Education in Nursing, 31, 263–268.

Griffith, G. (1987). Images of interdependence: authority and power in teaching/learning. In Appreciating Adults Learning: From the Learners' Perspective (D. Boud and V. Griffin, eds.) pp. 51–63. London: Kogan Page.

Habermas, J. (1970). Toward a Rational Society. Boston, MA: Beacon Press.

Habermas, J. (1971). Knowledge and Human Interests. Boston, MA: Beacon Press.

Hagar, P. (1998). Understanding workplace learning: general perspectives. In Current Issues and New Agendas in Workplace Learning

(D. Boud, ed.) pp. 31–46. Leabrook, South Australia: National Centre for Vocational Education Research.

Hall, R. (1968). Professionalization and bureaucratization. American Sociological Review, 33, 92–104.

Hancock, T. (1985). The mandala of health: a model of the human ecosystem. Family and Community Health, 8, 1–10.

Harris, I.B. (1993). New expectations for professional competence. In Educating Professionals: Responding to New Expectations for Competence and Accountability (L. Curry and J. Wergin, eds.) pp. 17–52. San Francisco, CA: Jossey-Bass.

Harris, R. (1989). Reflections on self-directed adult learning: some implications for educators of adults. Studies in Continuing Education, 11, 102–116.

Higgs, J. (1993). The teacher in self-directed learning: manager or co-manager? In Learner Managed Learning: Practice, Theory and Policy (N.J. Graves, ed.) pp. 122–131. London: World Education Fellowship.

Higgs, J. (2001). How can I lecture that topic?. In Lecturing: Case Studies, Experience and Practice (H. Edwards, B. Smith and G. Webb, eds.) pp. 137–145. London: Kogan Page.

Higgs, J., Glendenning, M., Dunsford, F. and Panter, J. (1991) Goals and Components of Clinical Education in the Allied Health Professions; Proceedings of the 11th World Conference for Physical Therapy pp. 305–307.

Higgs, J. and Hunt, A. (1999). Rethinking the beginning practitioner: 'the interactional professional'. In Educating Beginning Practitioners: Challenges for Health Professional Education, (J. Higgs and H. Edwards, eds.) pp. 10–18. Oxford: Butterworth-Heinemann.

Higgs, J. and Titchen, A. (1995a). Propositional, professional and personal knowledge in clinical reasoning. In Clinical Reasoning in the Health Professions (J. Higgs and M. Jones, eds.) pp. 129–146. Oxford: Butterworth-Heinemann.

Higgs, J. and Titchen, A. (1995b). The nature, generation and verification of knowledge. Physiotherapy, 81, 521–530.

Higgs, C., Neubauer, D. and Higgs, J. (1999). The changing health care context: globalization and social ecology. In Educating Beginning Practitioners: Challenges for Health Professional Education, (J. Higgs and H. Edwards, eds.) pp. 30–37. Oxford: Butterworth-Heinemann.

Higgs, J., Titchen, A. and Neville, V. (2001). Professional practice and knowledge. In Practice Knowledge and Expertise in the Health Professions (J. Higgs and A. Titchen, eds.) pp. 3–9. Oxford: Butterworth-Heinemann.

Higgs, J., Richardson, B. and Abrandt Dahlgren, M. eds. (2002). Understanding Practice Knowledge in the Health Sciences. Oxford: Butterworth-Heinemann.

Hill, D. (1994). In Freire's footsteps: neo-liberal hegemony and the domestication of education. New Zealand Journal of Adult Learning, 26, 48–55.

Honey, P. and Mumford, A. (1982). The Manual of Learning Styles, Maidenhead, UK: Peter Mumford.

Hunt, A. and Higgs, J. (1999). Learning generic skills. In Educating Beginning Practitioners: Challenges for Health Professional Education, (J. Higgs and H. Edwards, eds.) pp. 166–172. Oxford: Butterworth-Heinemann.

Jensen, G.M., Shepard, K.F., Gwyer, J. and Hack, L.M. (1992). Attribute dimensions that distinguish master and novice physical therapy clinicians in orthopedic settings. Physical Therapy, 72, 711–722.

Johnson, D. (1981). Student–student interaction: the neglected variable in education. Educational Researcher, 1, 5–10.

Johnson, D. (2000). The use of learning theories in the design of a work-based learning course at masters level. Innovations in Education and Training International, 37, 129–133.

Jones, M. and Higgs, J. (2000). Will evidence-based practice take the reasoning out of practice? In Clinical Reasoning in the Health Professions, 2nd edn (J. Higgs and M. Jones. eds.) pp. 307–315. Oxford: Butterworth-Heinemann.

Jones, M., Edwards, I. and Gifford, L. (2002). Conceptual models for implementing biopsychosocial theory in clinical practice. Manual Therapy, 7, 2–9.

Josebury, H.E., Bax, N.D.S. and Hannay, D.R. (1990). Communication skills and clinical methods: a new introductory course. Medical Education, 24, 433–437.

Knowles, M.S. (1970). The Modern Practice of Adult Education: Andragogy versus Pedagogy. Chicago, IL: Follett.

Knowles, M.S. (1980). The Modern Practice of Adult Education: From Pedagogy to Andragogy. New York: Adult Education Company.

Knowles, M.S., Holton, E.F. and Swanson, R.A. (1998). The Adult Learner, 5th edn. Woburn, MA: Butterworth-Heinemann.

Knox, A.B. (1977). Adult Development and Learning. San Francisco, CA: Jossey-Bass.

Kolb, D.A. (1984). Experiential Learning: Experience as the Source of Learning and Development. Englewood Cliffs, NJ: Prentice-Hall.

Ladyshewsky, R., Baker, R. and Jones, M. (2000). Peer coaching to generate clinical-reasoning skills. In Clinical Reasoning in the Health Professions, 2nd edn (J. Higgs and M. Jones, eds.) pp. 283–289. Oxford: Butterworth-Heinemann.

Larkin, J., McDermot, J., Simon, D.P. and Simon, H. (1980). Expert and novice performance in solving physics problems. Science, 208, 1135–1142.

Lave, J. (1996). Learning Techniques: Situated Learning. Available online (8 October 2001): http://www.educationau.edu.au/archives/cp/04k.htm.

Lave, J, and Wenger. E. (1991). Situated Learning: Legitimate Peripheral Participation. New York: Cambridge University Press.

Lawson, J.S., Rotem, A. and Bates, P.W. (1996). From Clinician to Manager: An Introduction to Hospital and Health Services Management, Sydney, Australia: McGraw Hill.

Marsick, V. and Watkins, K. (1990). Informal and Incidental Learning in the Workplace. London: Routledge.

Martin, E. and Ramsden, P. (1986). Do learning skills courses improve student learning. In Student Learning: Research into Practice; The Marysville Symposium (J.A. Bowden, ed.) pp. 149–166. Parkville, South Australia: The University of Melbourne Centre for the Study of Higher Education.

Marton, F. and Säljö, R. (1976). On qualitative differences in learning. II: outcome as a function of the learner's conception of the task. British Journal of Educational Psychology 46, 115–127.

Maslow, A.H. (1970). Motivation and Personality. New York: Harper and Row.

McLellan, H. (1996). Situated learning: multiple perspectives. In Situated Learning Perspectives (H. McLellan, ed.) pp. 5–17. Englewood Cliffs, NJ: Educational Technology Publications.

Mezirow, J. (1981). A critical theory of adult learning and education. Adult Education, 32, 3–24.

Mezirow, J. (1985a). A critical theory of self-directed learning. In Self-Directed Learning: From Theory to Practice (S. Brookfield, ed.) pp. 17–30. San Francisco, CA: Jossey-Bass.

Mezirow, J. (1985b). Concept and action in adult education. Adult Education Quarterly, 35, 142–151.

Michelson, E. (1998). Re-membering: the return of the body to experiential learning. Studies in Continuing Education, 20, 217–233.

Payton, O.D. (1985). Clinical reasoning process in physical therapy. Physical Therapy, 65, 924–928.

Prosser, A. (1995). Teaching and Learning Social Responsibility. Canberra, Australia: Higher Education Research and Development Society of Australasia.

Prosser, M. and Trigwell, K. (1998). Understanding Learning and Teaching: The Experience in Higher Education. Buckingham, UK: Open University Press.

Ramsden, P. (1979). Student learning and perceptions of the academic environment. Higher Education, 8, 411–428.

Ramsden, P. (1984). The context of learning. In The Experience of Learning (F. Marton, D. Hounsell and N. Entwistle, eds.) pp. 144–164. Scottish Academic Press. Edinburgh.

Ramsden, P. (1985). Student learning research: Retrospect and prospect. Higher Education Research and Development, 4, 51–70.

Ramsden, P. (1986). ANZAME Conference 1985 Special interest session: Implications of research into how students learn for medical education. Bulletin, Australasian and New Zealand Association for Medical Education, 13, 11–13.

Ramsden, P. (1988). Studying learning: Improving teaching. In Improving

Learning: New Perspectives.
(P. Ramsden, ed.) pp. 13–31.
London: Kogan Page.

Rawson, M. (2000). Learning to learn:
more than a skill set. Studies in
Higher Education, 25, 225–238.

Read, D.A. and Simon, S.B. (1975).
Humanistic Education Sourcebook.
Englewood Cliffs, NJ: Prentice Hall.

Reeders, E. (2000). Scholarly practice in
work-based learning: fitting the glass
slipper. Higher Education Research
and Design, 19, 205–220.

Regehr, G. and Norman, G. (1996). Issues
in cognitive psychology: implications
for professional education. Academic
Medicine, 71, 988–1000.

Resnick, L.B. (ed.) (1989). Knowing,
Learning and Instruction: Essays in
Honor of Robert Glaser. Hillsdale, NJ:
Erlbaum.

Rew, L. and Barrow, E. (1987). Intuition:
a neglected hallmark of nursing
knowledge. Advances in Nursing
Science, 10, 1, 49–62.

Ritzer, G. (1971). Professionalism and
the individual. In The Professions and
Their Prospects (E. Friedson, ed.)
pp. 59–73. Beverly Hills, CA: Sage.

Rogers, C.R. (1969). Freedom to Learn.
Columbus, OH: Charles E. Merrill.

Rogers, C.R. (1983). Freedom to Learn
for the 80s. Columbus, OH: Charles E.
Merrill.

Sangster, A., Maclaran, P. and Marshall,
S. (2000). Translating theory into
practice: facilitating work-based

learning through IT. Innovations in
Education and Training International,
37, 1, 50–58.

Schön, D.A. (1983). The Reflective
Practitioner: How Professionals Think
in Action. London: Temple Smith.

Schön, D.A. (1987). Educating the
Reflective Practitioner: Towards a
New Design for Teaching and Learning
in Professions. San Francisco, CA:
Jossey-Bass.

Senge, P. (1990). The Fifth Discipline:
The Art and Practice of the Learning
Organization. Sydney, Australia:
Random House.

Spencer, J.D., Connor, P., Maxwell, T.W.
and Nesbitt, V. (1992). Humanism in
Education: Perceptions and Dilemmas,
pp. 45–51. Armidale, NSW: University
of New England.

Stephenson, J. (1992). Capability and
quality in higher education. In Quality
in Learning: A Capability Approach in
Higher Education (J. Stephenson and
S. Weil, eds.) pp. 1–9. London: Kogan
Page.

Stephenson, J. (1998). The concept of
capability and its importance in higher
education. In Capability and Quality in
Higher Education. (J. Stephenson and
S. Weil, eds.) pp. 1–13. London: Kogan
Page.

Sultz, H.A., Sawner, K.A. and Sherwin,
F.S. (1984). Determining and
maintaining competence: an
obligation of allied health education.
Journal of Allied Health, 13, 272–279.

Terry, W. and Higgs, J. (1993).
Educational programmes to develop
clinical reasoning skills, Australian
Journal of Physiotherapy, vol. 39,
1, 47–51.

Titchen, A. and Higgs, J. (2001). A
dynamic framework for the
enhancement of health professional
practice in an uncertain world: the
practice-knowledge interface. In
Practice Knowledge and Expertise
in the Health Professions (J. Higgs
and A. Titchen, eds.) pp. 215–225.
Oxford: Butterworth-Heinemann.

Torbert, W.R. (1978). Educating toward
shared purpose, self-direction and
quality work: the theory and
practice of liberating structure.
Journal of Higher Education, 49,
109–135.

Vygotsky, L. (1978). Mind in Society.
Cambridge, MA: Harvard University
Press.

Ward, C. and McCormack, A. (2000).
Creating an adult learning culture
through practice development.
Nurse Education Today, 20,
259–266.

Watson, T.J. (1994). Managing, crafting
and researching words, skills and
imagination in shaping management
research. British Journal of
Management, 51, 577–587.

Wilcox, S. (1996). Fostering self-directed
learning in the university setting.
Studies in Higher Education, 21,
165–176.

CHAPTER 26

Improving clinical reasoning in manual therapy

Darren A. Rivett and Mark A. Jones

Clinical expertise in manual therapy is dependent on the development of a high level of skill in many aspects of professional practice. Superior technical skills, advanced communication skills and a substantial store of knowledge are features commonly regarded as core components of clinical expertise. However, these components of clinical performance are also often identifiable in the 'average' manual therapist, who, while competent in their field, is not recognized as a leading practitioner. The missing factor, which differentiates the expert from other clinicians, could well be cognitive or clinical reasoning skill—a performance component that is not as readily apparent to casual observers. Although sound technical and communication skills (and associated knowledge) are needed to elicit optimal clinical data, the information obtained is only as useful as the clinician's reasoning skill allows. That is, it is the thinking or reasoning processes that guide the collection of clinical data and extract the value of the data for making clinical decisions.

Whilst most manual therapists are diligent in undertaking continuing education to develop new manual skills and acquire knowledge pertaining to clinical theory and research, there is a tendency to neglect the development of clinical reasoning skills. Newly acquired facts and techniques are often initially employed with enthusiasm but soon fall by the wayside as results fall short of expectation (Rivett, 1999). This is commonly because short continuing education courses in manual therapy often fail to address the necessary associated clinical reasoning skills. The integration of new information with existing categories of clinical knowledge will generally be limited without

the reasoning ability to recognize the clinical value and relevance of information, and the capacity to access it efficiently in the clinical context. Similarly, technical skills must be associated with 'if/then' rules of action; otherwise their application may be inappropriate and their value unrecognized. Therefore, good skills in clinical reasoning are needed to make the most of new procedural information and avoid 'information overload' from the ever increasing amount of professional knowledge. Without them, the clinician is at risk of unquestioningly accepting 'fashionable' practices and manual therapy becomes merely a technical operation.

As discussed in Chapter 25, interacting professionals can be characterized by skills in problem solving, clinical reasoning, reflective practice and critical self-evaluation, in addition to self-directed learning (see Table 25.2). The role of the health professional as a learner was similarly identified as comprising self-direction, lifelong learning and the generation of new knowledge. Accordingly, it is important that the manual therapist, both as an autonomous health professional and as an adult learner, takes responsibility for improving their clinical reasoning ability. Similarly, there is a responsibility for teachers of manual therapy to teach skills in clinical reasoning. There are many factors that should motivate clinicians or learners to strive for greater expertise in their thinking skills. These include external factors, such as the increasing demands of funding agencies and patients to bring about a quick and effective resolution to the patient's problem, and internal factors, such as work satisfaction and the respect of peers. Although these are strong motivational factors, frequently clinicians are unaware of the importance of reasoning skills in developing clinical expertise or do not know how to go about improving their cognitive skills. It is the aim of this chapter to address both these issues.

The expert clinician

Clinical expertise is of interest to all concerned in manual therapy: clinicians want to be able to solve problems encountered in clinical practice; patients want to be treated by manual therapists who are highly competent (Jensen et al., 1999); and funding agencies wish to ensure that patient management is both efficient and effective. Traditionally, colleagues and patients have revered practitioners who had accumulated many years of experience at the clinical 'coal face', commonly granting them 'expert' status. However, there is now a consensus amongst researchers studying expertise in professional practice that clinical experience, although essential, is only one component, and, in fact, many experienced clinicians never truly become experts. This begs the question as to 'what defines clinical expertise and how can it be attained?'

Research into expert behaviour in a number of fields (e.g. physics, mathematics, medicine, chess playing) have identified characteristics of expertise that appear to be generic (Glaser and Chi, 1988). Experts:

- excel mainly in their own domain
- perceive large meaningful patterns in their domain
- are faster than novices at performing the skills of their domain, and solve problems with greater accuracy and less effort
- have superior short-term and long-term memory
- see and represent a problem in their domain at a deeper and more principled level than novices (i.e. novices tend to represent a problem at a superficial level)
- spend a great deal of time analysing a problem qualitatively
- have strong self-monitoring skills and employ high levels of metacognition in their clinical reasoning
- possess the affective dispositions (e.g. inquisitiveness, self-confidence, open-mindedness, flexibility, honesty, diligence, reasonableness, empathy and humility) necessary to reflect on and learn from their experiences.

In addition to these generic skills, clinical expertise in the health professions needs to satisfy additional criteria. Clinical expertise, of which clinical reasoning is a critical component, can be viewed as a continuum along multiple dimensions (Higgs and Jones, 2000), including clinical outcomes, personal attributes such as professional judgment and empathy, technical clinical skills, communication and interpersonal skills (needed to involve the patient and others in decision making and to consider the patient's perspectives), sound knowledge base, and cognitive and metacognitive proficiency (i.e. clinical reasoning skills). Therefore, additional characteristics of manual therapy experts (Higgs and Jones, 2000) would include:

- recognizing the value of different forms of knowledge in their reasoning and using this knowledge critically
- sharing their expertise to help to cultivate expertise in others
- communicating their reasoning well and in a manner appropriate for the audience
- demonstrating cultural competence in their reasoning and communication
- employing lateral thinking to generate new hypotheses, redesign treatment when progress is poor, and adapt treatment when resources are limited
- possessing a patient-centred view, understanding and responding appropriately to patients' experiences, perspectives and expectations
- valuing the participation of relevant others (patients, caregivers, members of the health-care team) in the decision-making process.

The last two characteristics merit closer examination. Whilst experts are expected to demonstrate superior clinical performance, this is often only viewed with respect to diagnostic accuracy and treatment outcomes (Higgs and Jones, 2000). However, the description of clinical expertise requires a broader perspective that includes the patient's unique experience and perception of their problem. That is, it is inadequate simply to judge clinical performance and the associated clinical reasoning on the basis of clinical results, such as whether the surgery or therapeutic intervention worked. Recipients of health care may have regained their health or function yet still feel the clinician's performance was inadequate. Shared decision making between patient and clinician is important if 'success' is to be realized from the patient's perspective. Therefore, clinical expertise requires the clinician to be attuned to the patient's pain or illness experience.

Expert reasoning processes

It has been suggested (Simon, 1980) that it takes at least 10 years of experience to obtain proficiency in any profession. While experience is obviously necessary to obtain expert status, it is equally recognized that individuals with comparable years of experience can have markedly different levels of expertise. The development of clinical expertise, particularly expertise in reasoning, requires much more than just 'clocking up' years of clinical experience.

It is important to understand the reasoning processes used by clinical experts because this facilitates critical evaluation and enhancement of our own clinical reasoning skills. Research has determined that experts typically use inductive or forward reasoning (i.e. problem cues elicit understanding and recognition of the solution strategies without any specific hypothesis testing) when dealing with a familiar problem; this is an efficient process that enables them to solve problems quickly with little error. This form of clinical reasoning has low demand on cognitive capacity and thus frees up the remaining capacity for other tasks. However, when confronted with an unfamiliar or complex problem, experts will revert to the slower and more cognitively demanding deductive or backward reasoning (i.e. hypotheses elicit a return to the data for either re-interpretation or collection of further confirming or negating evidence) (Elstein, 1995); this is the process typically used by novices. In addition, it should be noted, as discussed in Chapter 1, that judgments directed toward understanding patients' pain experience from their perspective are reached through consensus validation between patient and therapist, as opposed to the more instrumental process of hypothesis testing used to validate diagnostic judgments pertaining to pathology and physical impairment.

Expertise is largely domain specific and requires extensive exposure to a variety of clinical presentations and problems. The prompt retrieval of a well-structured association of data is necessary for inductive reasoning. This process of pattern recognition is dependent on the possession of, and the ability to use, a deep and highly organized knowledge base built mainly on a wealth of clinical experience (Elstein, 1995; Jensen et al., 1999; Jones, 1999). The process of recognizing relevant cues and perceiving patterns amongst these cues requires accessing pertinent information from the databank of previous cases. Consequently, pattern recognition is an extremely specific knowledge-based problem-solving strategy (i.e. it is case specific) and constitutes a form of 'knowing-in-action' (Schön, 1983).

It is, therefore, apparent that a superior organization of knowledge (propositional and non-propositional) is a key feature differentiating the expert from the novice clinician, and this helps to explain why expertise is domain specific and does not readily transfer across fields. A well-structured knowledge base enables efficient and accurate clinical reasoning by facilitating ease of information retrieval. Also, by having a greater ability to recognize relevant information and organize it into meaningful chunks or patterns, experts save space in their working memory for other cognitive processes (e.g. metacognition). However, ready access to their knowledge base requires that experts acquire their knowledge in the context in which it will be used, that is in the clinical context. Indeed, learning theory contends that optimal learning occurs when knowledge is presented and learned in an authentic context (i.e. in settings and applications that would normally involve that knowledge) (Lave, 1996). This principle applies to the development of clinical reasoning skills both in the undergraduate student during clinical/fieldwork education and the experienced manual therapist in their own practice (see p. 396).

An expert's professional craft knowledge evolves as they continually learn from their clinical experiences, ideally critiqued through continual review of research-validated evidence. This is principally achieved through reflective enquiry during (reflection-in-action) and after (reflection-about-action) the patient encounter (Jensen et al., 1999; Jones et al., 2000; Schön, 1983, 1987). Both forms of reflection allow for self-correction and adaptation of practice (including on-the-spot experimentation with reflection-in-action) and help clinicians to make sense of their combined research and experienced-based knowledge to find, with the patient, an effective approach to the problem. For this, reflection must include critical consideration of the reliability and validity of information obtained, the patterns recognized and their level of substantiation, and recognition of the limitations in the clinician's own knowledge and skills. In this way, reflective reasoning also leads to confirmation or refinement of old patterns and acquisition of new patterns, which may be hidden within the ambiguity of a clinical presentation. Experts become experts, in part, because they know their own limitations and this drives them continually to broaden and deepen their understanding of people and their problems. Importantly, for meaningful changes in knowledge structure to occur, the learner must relate the new learning experience (academic, clinical or personal) to their prior understanding, which, in turn, will lead to changes in reasoning. There is an obvious analogy between this reasoning process and that of experiential learning (described in Ch. 25) as involving reflection-in-action and reflection after the learning event.

Although professional craft or procedural knowledge is particularly highly developed in expert clinicians (Higgs and Bithell, 2001; Jensen et al., 1999), it seems that biomedical knowledge is not explicitly utilized by expert practitioners when diagnosing a familiar problem. Boshuizen and Schmidt (2000) have proposed that this is because biomedical knowledge has been integrated into, or subsumed under, the expert's clinical knowledge during clinical exposure. Biomedical knowledge appears only to be explicitly accessed if the expert is dealing with a difficult or unfamiliar problem for which their domain knowledge is inadequate, generally as part of a backward-directed causal reasoning strategy within the hypothetico-deductive process (Boshuizen and Schmidt, 2000) or when communicating their reasoning to others (Patel and Kaufman, 2000).

The clinical patterns or illness scripts used by expert clinicians contain an association of clinically relevant and easily retrieved information that aids accurate and rapid reasoning (Sefton et al., 2000). Boshuizen and Schmidt (2000) have identified three main components of illness scripts:

- enabling conditions of the problem, e.g. hereditary, social and other factors affecting health and the course of the condition
- the fault or pathophysiological process in an 'encapsulated' form
- consequences of the fault, that is the signs and symptoms of the disorder.

Illness scripts or clinical patterns are matched to the information provided by the patient and generate expectations about other signs and symptoms, thus guiding the enquiry process. There is a risk, however, that uncritical use of this cognitive process can habituate the expert's thinking to the detriment of flexible, open-minded and innovative thinking. Accordingly, experts employ strong metacognitive skills to self-monitor and self-evaluate their thinking processes. It is generally accepted that the ability to be cognitively self-aware and self-critical is essential for skilled clinical reasoning

(Brookfield, 1989; Higgs and Jones, 2000; Jensen et al., 1999). Without metacognition, reasoning is less responsive to the dynamics of problem-solving contexts and less capable of effectively dealing with the complexity of clinical problems and the diversity of people and circumstances within which they occur. Because advanced clinical reasoning requires metacognitive as well as cognitive skills, the manual therapist must learn to develop the ability to think on two levels simultaneously. Skilled reflective metacognitive clinical reasoning can, therefore, be seen to be analogous to Bateson's third level of learning (Learning III: self-reflexive learning) (Bateson, 1987 as cited in Rawson, 2000; see Ch. 25).

■ Clinical 'intuition'

Expert clinicians sometimes explain their clinical decisions on the basis of a 'gut feeling' or 'hunch', which can be described as a strong feeling or perception about a patient or an anticipated outcome sensed without obviously undertaking an analytical reasoning process. This could be thought of as a refined or subtle form of professional judgment; in some fields (particularly nursing), it is referred to as 'intuitive' reasoning. Experts often have difficulty articulating how they interpret incomplete and ambiguous data, draw inferences and identify implications that are not directly deducible from explicit data (Higgs and Titchen, 2000). However, tacit knowledge can be linked to past experience of specific patient cases in similar contexts (i.e. it is experiential knowledge), and is therefore probably the result of an unconscious and automatic form of inductive reasoning (Higgs and Jones, 2000). It appears that substantial clinical experience, combined with and related to prior learning, is required for the development of tacit knowledge and such advanced reasoning. Clinical 'intuition' can, therefore, be viewed as a form of learned awareness, principally involving the process of pattern recognition, in which decisions and actions are largely a function of tacit knowledge.

While a significant component of experts' knowledge is tacit (Fleming and Mattingly, 2000), this knowledge also carries with it a real potential for error because, by virtue of its subconscious existence, it can escape the critical review from self-reflection to which more conscious knowledge structures are subjected. If clinicians can learn to externalize this tacit knowledge and intuitive thinking through clinical reasoning activities, as described below, errors that may be present are more likely to be recognized and corrected. In particular, the use of peer learning or coaching has been advocated to enhance reasoning skills (Ladyshewsky et al., 2000) through articulation of the clinician's or learner's thoughts and decisions, thus facilitating restructuring of knowledge (Regehr and Norman, 1996; see Ch. 25).

Similarly, some of the enquiry strategies that the expert clinician employs may seem to be no more than unsubstantiated 'short-cuts' or 'rules of thumb', giving the appearance that experts' clinical reasoning is less than thorough, even sloppy (Barrows and Tamblyn, 1980). However, in such cases, it is more than likely the expert is applying *maximizing principles*—strategies that reduce the number of questions or actions necessary to understand a problem (Kleinmuntz, 1968)—to avoid wasting time exploring every conceivable pathway. The use of such strategies enables the best quality of information to be obtained in the most efficient manner, radically reducing the problem environment with each question or procedure. Maximizing principles can, therefore, be viewed as maximizing the benefits (i.e. accuracy and efficiency of decision making) and minimizing the costs (i.e. the effort involved in gathering and analysing information) required in solving a clinical problem. The use of these principles is the privilege of the expert clinician because the associated forward reasoning is based on domain knowledge and is, therefore, highly error-prone in the absence of an adequate knowledge base (Mechanic and Parson, 1975; Patel and Kaufman, 2000) and continual critical reflection on that knowledge (i.e. metacognition). Maximizing principles are, therefore, continually devised and revised in the light of this critical reflection on research- and experience-based evidence (Boud, 1988; Rivett and Higgs, 1995). Examples of maximizing principles are highlighted in the experts' case reasoning in Section 2.

Clinical reasoning errors

Whilst clinical reasoning is conceptually relatively simple, in practice it is quite difficult to perform efficiently and effectively and it can be fraught with errors. An essential element in learning to be a better clinical reasoner, and developing expertise in manual therapy, is to understand and avoid errors in reasoning. Awareness of potential errors in the reasoning process helps to promote critical reasoning. Errors may occur at any stage of the clinical reasoning process: perception, enquiry, interpretation, synthesis, planning, and reflection (Jones, 1992). Scott (2000) highlights three main causes of clinical reasoning errors:

- faulty elicitation or perception of clinical cues (deficient clinical skills)
- inadequate knowledge, for example about a clinical condition (deficient propositional or professional craft knowledge)
- misapplication of knowledge to a specific problem (deficient reasoning strategies).

These three causes of error may well be inter-related. For instance, faulty elicitation or perception and interpretation of cues can be related to inadequate knowledge (both experimental and experience based) of the relevant clinical cues or to underdeveloped professional craft knowledge in recognizing those cues. Similarly, misapplication of known facts to a specific clinical problem relates to incorrect use of heuristics, an example of poor procedural knowledge.

Following from these causes, Scott (2000) identifies three main categories of common reasoning errors.

Forming a wrong initial concept of the problem (framing error).   If clinicians fail to attend to or correctly interpret initial or critical cues, they can form an incorrect initial concept of the clinical problem. This can result in flawed or inadequate diagnostic or management decisions being formulated, significant time wasted in pursuing erroneous lines of inquiry, and the implementation of inappropriate (e.g. harmful, wasteful or useless) treatments. This type of error can be avoided by spending time carefully checking and interpreting cues (e.g. not overemphasizing previous diagnoses or investigation results), questioning the validity of the emerging picture of the clinical problem and clarifying rather than assuming patient responses (e.g. not accepting patients' use of medical terms such as migraine on face value).

Failure to generate plausible hypotheses and to test them adequately.   Clinicians can miss cues, misinterpret clinical data (e.g. overinterpreting cues that have little relevance, such as normal variations) or fail to take sufficient information into consideration (e.g. ignoring the importance of normal or absent findings); as a result, they can fail to generate sound diagnostic or management hypotheses. This problem is further compounded if the error is not detected or the process of testing hypotheses is also faulty (e.g. clinicians may seek to confirm inadequate or

Table 26.1 Categories of clinical reasoning errors

Category	Characteristics
Vagueness	The purpose of evaluation or treatment is unclear, and there is insufficient information to judge the wisdom of clinical decisions
Narrowness	Familiar approaches that seem effective are used without consideration of alternative methods
Rigidity	Standardized regimens of evaluation and treatment are used routinely with little or no consideration of important differences in individual patient needs and responses. In addition, treatment reactions are not monitored to detect unexpected results. Such practice may be appropriate for a preprofessional technician but not for a manual therapist
Irrationality	Clinical choices are based on convenience, habit, subjective impressions and the word of 'gurus' advocating specific techniques, rather than on sound evidence
Wastefulness	Investigations are extensive, but their results have little influence on treatment selection. Costly treatment techniques are used without considering whether more economical interventions might be equally effective. Critical reflective reasoning about clinical experience and available research evidence should minimize this error
Insensitivity	Patients' and families' personal values and psychosocial concerns are ignored, and physical performance improvement is given higher priority than enhanced quality of life. This is basically not using narrative reasoning and associated communicative management to attend to patients' pain experiences (Ch. 1)
Mystery	The clinician's process of decision making cannot be explained in terms patients and colleagues can understand, and so others cannot question and contribute to this process

From Watts (1995).

erroneous hypotheses or may test hypotheses insufficiently). Attending to both supporting and negating evidence and disproving hypotheses—rather than assuming that evidence supporting one hypothesis implies that competing hypotheses are not valid—will assist in avoiding this type of error. Conversely, clinicians may overutilize hypothesis testing, making judgments on their own, when consensus validation with the patient is called for, as with narrative reasoning judgments regarding the patient's personal perspective of their pain experience.

Inadequate testing and premature acceptance of hypotheses. Problems can arise when clinicians prematurely accept hypotheses (e.g. they may adopt favoured, common or obvious hypotheses) and then during the testing process fail to detect that an error in reasoning has occurred because they are expecting the hypothesis to be confirmed. In addition, confirmation bias can result when clinical cues are selectively chosen or interpreted as validating favoured hypotheses. Critical evaluation of hypothesis testing processes and consequent clinical findings is important to prevent this type of reasoning fault.

Common clinical reasoning errors have been further categorized by Watts (1995) (Table 26.1).

It is clearly important for clinicians to avoid clinical reasoning errors during clinical practice. Critical self-evaluation by the clinician and constructive and accurate feedback by a peer or mentor are essential to prevent reasoning errors becoming habit. Without this cognitive vigilance, reasoning errors can remain undetected for some time and result in ineffective, or even hazardous, clinical interventions.

To avoid reasoning errors in your own clinical practice, it is important to take 'time-out' to reflect on your clinical reasoning and seek any evidence of errors in your decision making. Past clinical experience may provide you with specific examples where you have committed an error, as described above. Consider how the error was detected (i.e. by you or by someone else) and what consequences arose because of the error. In particular, look out for the specific errors in your own clinical reasoning (Christensen et al., 2002; Jones, 1992) as outlined in Table 26.2. As can be seen in the table, errors in clinical reasoning are frequently related to errors in cognition, including analysis and synthesis of data and use of enquiry skills. These errors will also likely contribute to the development of poorly organized knowledge, thus compounding the problem.

Creative, lateral thinking

Historically, the new ideas and significant contributions in manual therapy have generally come from a small

Table 26.2 Common clinical reasoning errors

Activity	Errors
Information collection	Neglecting important information or failing to sample enough information
	Misinterpreting information or making assumptions without clarifying
	Basing decisions on insufficient evidence
	Overemphasizing either biomedical (propositional) or clinical (non-propositional) knowledge and evidence
	Failing to detect inconsistencies in the clinical presentation
Hypothesis formation	Focussing too much on favourite (or obvious) hypotheses
	Only attending to, or overemphasizing, those features of a presentation that support a favourite hypothesis, while neglecting negating features (confirmation bias)
	Considering too few hypotheses or not testing competing hypotheses
	Prematurely limiting the hypotheses considered
	Formulating non-specific hypotheses
	Not considering hypotheses in other categories (see 'hypothesis categories' in Ch. 1)
	Misinterpreting non-contributory information as confirming an existing hypothesis
	Reaching firm decisions prematurely
Identifying vital cues (flags)	Missing contraindications or precautions to examination or treatment
	Failing to detect cues indicative of serious pathology or link the cues to hypotheses
Diagnosis	Overemphasizing clinical findings that are minor in the context of the whole patient presentation
	Misdiagnosing
	Missing a relationship between symptoms or confusing a relationship between symptoms as confirming cause and effect
	Confusing and inappropriately applying deductive and inductive logic, leading to incorrect interpretations
Treatment	Taking unwarranted action
	Failing to monitor your own reasoning (metacognition)
	Using clinical 'recipes', not clinical reasoning (i.e. blindly following treatment protocols)
	Failing to involve the patient in decision making
	Not taking into account the context of the patient's problem or its impact on their life

number of individuals and often more than one significant contribution has come from the same individual. Clearly, there are many reasons for this, including previous education and experience, external work constraints and genetically influenced levels of intelligence and thinking styles. While these factors may be largely out of our control, Edward De Bono (1977, 1993), a prolific writer on the topic of thinking and lateral thinking, argues that creative, lateral thinking can be promoted by making people aware of their current thinking processes and encouraging the practice of looking at old patterns in new ways.

De Bono distinguishes between 'vertical' and 'lateral' thinking, with vertical thinking being characterized by logical, sequential, predictable and what might be called conventional thinking. Lateral thinking, by comparison, involves restructuring and escape from old patterns and creation of new ones. It is concerned with the generation of new ideas and looking at things in a different way; vertical thinking is then concerned with proving or developing these new ideas. While vertical thinking is hindered by the necessity to be right or 'logical' at each stage of the thought process, lateral thinking maintains that premature formalization and expression of an idea may inhibit its natural development. In vertical thinking, one selects out only that information considered relevant; however, in lateral thinking one may deliberately seek out irrelevant information because this information may assist in viewing a problem from a different perspective and as such contribute to promoting a different view.

The clinical reasoning literature across the health professions, including manual therapy, has highlighted the expert's ability to recognize patterns. This can be attributed to superior organization of knowledge in their particular area of practice. Efforts to facilitate learners' organization of knowledge in manual therapy education have arguably contributed to this pattern recognition skill by teaching learners the classic clinical patterns of presentation. It is worth considering whether encouraging learners to identify clinical patterns might not lead to a narrow form of reasoning, whereby problems are forced into discrete sets of 'black and white' patterns, a situation that rarely occurs in actual clinical practice. Such an overly focussed view of clinical patterns can tend to make these rigidly established, since it is the patterns that control our attention. Other disadvantages of overattending to patterns include:

- difficulty in changing patterns once they have become established
- restricting cognitively the availability of information: information arranged as part of one pattern cannot easily be used as part of a completely different pattern
- tendency towards 'centring', whereby anything that has any resemblance to a standard pattern will be perceived as part of that pattern
- creating patterns by divisions that are more or less arbitrary (i.e. dividing what is continuous into distinct units); once such divisions are created they become self-perpetuating.

One way to gain the benefits of pattern recognition while controlling for these risks is to ensure that teaching facilitates learners' acquisition and organization of knowledge with equal and simultaneous attention to a reasoning process that enables knowledge to be challenged and tested. In this way, learners acquire not only the classic presentation of common problems but also an appreciation of the typical overlap that exists between many clinical patterns. In addition, they develop critical and reflective thinking habits, which ensure that patterns are continually tested and new patterns sought.

Nevertheless, this critical, hypothetico-deductive mode of reasoning will not necessarily contribute to the development of truly novel, creative ideas. For this, we support De Bono's view that learners should be exposed to lateral thinking strategies. Some of De Bono's strategies to promote creative, lateral thinking are:

- instead of stopping when a promising approach to a problem has been found, continue to generate as many alternatives as possible
- instead of always moving usefully in one direction, play around with no specific purpose other than to see its effect, which may, in turn, be a stimulus to a different idea
- welcome outside, seemingly irrelevant, information as a potential stimulus for altering a pattern; if

only things that appear to be relevant are considered, the current pattern will be perpetuated
- explore the least likely paths
- challenge the assumptions of current thinking; sometimes a problem cannot be solved by trying different arrangements of the given parts but only by re-examination of the parts themselves
- suspend judgment; do not be too quick to dismiss a seemingly incorrect idea as its exploration may lead to the correct idea
- perhaps most importantly, recognize the dominant idea/approach.

To promote your own creative, lateral thinking you must first be able to recognize the dominant idea or approach you are presently taking toward a problem. Without this, any new idea you trial will only be a variation on the same theme. Once you recognize the dominant theme to how you have approached a problem, you can then look outside that to discover alternative ideas or solutions. The dominant idea does not reside in the situation itself but in the way you look at it.

Activities to improve clinical reasoning

There are many learning activities and related tools that the manual therapist can use to enhance the development of clinical reasoning skills. Ideally, these should encompass the interdependent components of knowledge, reasoning ability and metacognition (Refshauge and Higgs, 2000). Indeed, studies of experts have shown that domain knowledge and the associated skills to use this knowledge develop simultaneously (Boshuizen and Schmidt, 2000). Learning experiences should, therefore, promote active integration of cognitive processes and knowledge derived from clinical experiences into the clinician's or learner's existing knowledge structures, consistent with learning theory (Shepard and Jensen, 2002; see Ch. 25). Newly acquired knowledge should be tested for its consistency and connectedness and used to fill any identified gaps in pre-existing knowledge. To achieve this, the practitioner must try to find the time to learn from cases, whether it be in clinical practice or in clinical simulations, and carefully reflect upon these experiences. As was argued in Chapter 25, experience and reflection must be connected for learning to occur in the complex and busy clinical situation.

Clinicians seeking to promote the development of their own clinical reasoning skill need to be cognizant of the adult learning principles discussed in Chapter 25. It is imperative that clinicians do not adopt a passive, 'spoon-feeding' approach to learning; they should be actively engaged in the management of their learning experience, as well as the learning process itself. Deep, meaningful learning should be fostered, and this can only be brought about by the employment of higher or adult learning skills, including self-direction and critical self-appraisal, and by seeking appropriate knowledge, feedback and help, consistent with the previously espoused principles of humanistic education. Clinicians must accept responsibility for managing their own learning and learning outcomes, in addition to self-monitoring their learning. It is important to recognize that all these key elements of self-directed learning (see 'Self-directed learning' in Ch. 25) are facilitated through skilled clinical reasoning, as similar cognitive processes and behaviours are required for both self-directed (adult) learning and clinical reasoning.

Skills in clinical reasoning can be fostered through the use of adult learning principles, which heighten awareness of cognitive errors and knowledge gaps. The application of these principles includes:

- relating new clinical concepts and experiences to previous knowledge
- relating the clinical and research evidence to the decisions made
- critically examining the logic of reasoning processes
- understanding the deeper principles and concepts underlying manual therapy assessment and management
- developing skills in lifelong professional learning
- communicating reasoning and justifying clinical decisions
- undertaking regular reflection (both during and after the learning or clinical experience)
- developing awareness of one's cognitive processes, including self-monitoring, self-evaluation and control (metacognition)
- seeking and acting on feedback about clinical performance.

In addition, the development of expertise in clinical reasoning can be promoted through the use of the following strategies:

- increasing awareness of reasoning processes and reasoning errors, which helps to make the clinician's internal cognitive processes more accessible

- using a broadened perspective beyond diagnostic reasoning (i.e. hypothesis categories, as discussed in Ch. 1)
- identifying relevant cues and their significance at the beginning of the patient encounter, thus facilitating accuracy in hypothesis generation and reaping maximal benefit from related inquiry strategies
- making greater use of enquiry strategies to prove or disprove hypotheses (i.e. hypothesis testing)
- making more explicit attempts to understand each patient's unique pain experience (i.e. narrative reasoning), with impressions validated through patient–clinician consensus
- improving the depth and organization of knowledge; attending to broader models of health and disability (Ch. 1) and using hypothesis categories may assist clinicians' development of contemporary and clinically applicable knowledge
- reflecting regularly about clinical experiences; clinical experience without reflection will not facilitate the application of available evidence or the development of professional craft knowledge and reasoning expertise.

Reflection should include thinking about:

- the reliability and validity of information obtained
- patients' personal perspectives or pain experiences, including their basis
- any specific interpretations and judgments (hypotheses) made
- any supporting/negating evidence for decisions
- the different focus of decision making required (see discussion of clinical reasoning strategies in Ch. 1)
- whether your knowledge (propositional and non-propositional) is sufficient to understand and to help the patient and problem in question.

Much of this reflection is inherent in the clinicians' answers to the reasoning questions posed throughout Section 2 and should also be used by readers attempting to answer the questions themselves when working through a case.

Ideally, the clinician should undertake a long-term formal postgraduate course in manual therapy that has a strong emphasis on supervised clinical practice and clinical reasoning. Where this is not feasible, there are a variety of activities that the clinician can undertake to promote the development of their reasoning skill and which actively engage the learner in thinking and doing. Learning activities should preferably provide an opportunity for feedback and reflection and encourage critical debate, experimentation, open-mindedness and intellectual curiosity. During these activities, manual therapists should consciously strive to identify any deficiencies in their knowledge structures and increase their awareness of their cognitive processes (metacognition). Experts not only know a good deal in their area of special interest, they also recognize what they do not know and are ever ready to seek further knowledge and evidence from the literature and through consultation with colleagues.

In selecting an activity that fosters deep learning, manual therapists should take into consideration their individual learning styles, the learning setting and their stage of reasoning development. Readers are encouraged to review the descriptions of learning styles from the different learning theories presented in Chapter 25 and attempt to identify characteristics they feel best describe themselves. Commonly, individuals have strengths in some learning styles while being weaker in others. Such self-reflection can assist readers to become more aware of their 'weaknesses', which may partly underlie any reasoning bias they have; such self-knowledge assists in broadening personal learning style and hence potential to learn.

◼ Clinical practice

As described in Chapter 25, it is desirable to employ learning activities that facilitate situated learning: that is, learning undertaken in the context where it will be used. Patients are the best resource for learning and developing reasoning expertise; however, the clinician needs to be open-minded and willing to think about the clinical encounter. Importantly, the use of a mentor or critical companion (Titchen, 2001) in the learning process has been shown to be instrumental in the development of clinical expertise (Jensen et al., 1999; Jones, 1999; Martin et al., 1999; Titchen, 2001). Indeed, research by Jensen et al. (1999) has demonstrated the value of practising in the presence of other clinicians, who help to guide and refine thinking and reasoning processes; this is the 'cognitive apprenticeship' approach referred to in Chapter 25. Similarly, Ladyshewsky et al. (2000) referred to reciprocal peer coaching, which involves demonstration, observation, collaborative practice, feedback and discussion, and problem solving with a peer. Consistent with taking responsibility for their own learning, clinicians may

need to be proactive in seeking out an appropriate manual therapist to act as their mentor(s). Mentors should not only possess attributes of clinical expertise and be good role models but should also be tolerant of mistakes, capable of openly communicating their own thinking and willing to provide constructive feedback and direction (i.e. not necessarily all the answers). In addition, consistent with the aims of humanistic education discussed in Chapter 25, mentors should strive to create (or help the learner create) a highly supportive and accepting learning environment, which is conducive to the individual learning and applying clinical reasoning. The clinician seeking mentorship must, by the same token, be willing to express their professional craft knowledge and clinical reasoning, as well as readily accept feedback. That is, learners must be willing and able to take a responsible and self-directed role in their own learning.

Knowledge is made particularly meaningful and accessible when it is acquired in the context in which it will be utilized (see 'Situated learning' in Ch. 25). Initially in learning activities, clinicians should be exposed to typical cases (i.e. textbook presentations), with atypical presentations introduced as their level of expertise warrants (Hayes and Adams, 2000). In addition to a colleague (mentor or peer) making comment upon the clinician's decision making, it should be borne in mind that the patient can also provide invaluable feedback. There are several activities to improve clinical reasoning that can be undertaken with a mentor or peer using real patients.

Demonstrating an assessment of a patient. The clinician assesses and treats a patient while being observed by a mentor; alternatively, the mentor can assess and treat a patient while being observed by the clinician. Two peers of equal rank can also be involved (reciprocal peer coaching). In all instances, discussion can occur either throughout the patient encounter, in the form of evolving thoughts, or as soon as possible after the patient encounter.

Collaborative assessment. Shared and collaborative assessment and treatment involves explicit discussion of plans and thoughts; open-ended questions are regularly asked of one another. Optimal learning requires such social interaction and collaboration (Lave, 1996).

The use of a reflective diary of clinical patterns. This facilitates skills in pattern recognition by recording typical pattern features (including associated management principles) and by comparing similar patterns (see Appendix 1 for an example). In particular, features that are shared by several patterns and features that may vary within a specific pattern can be highlighted. This learning tool also primes the practitioner to look for information to add to their evolving diary, for example during clinical practice, and provides a stimulus for independent study, such as reviewing available evidence to substantiate or challenge the clinical patterns identified (Carr et al., 2000; Sackett et al., 2000).

The thoughts of the clinician or the mentor/peer can be made explicit and accessible to the other in several ways:

■ 'thinking aloud' (i.e. real-time articulation of their thoughts) while solving the patient problem
■ using verbal stimulus questions to help access reasoning processes, but this must be done in a manner that does not erode either the credibility of the clinician in the eyes of the patient or the clinician's confidence
■ using strategically placed pauses at key stages of the examination and treatment to encourage the clinician to interpret findings, formulate and justify hypotheses, identify enquiry strategies to validate hypotheses, and to consider interventions
■ interrupting by the mentor if the clinician follows an incorrect or unsubstantiated line of enquiry; this should be balanced with the need for the clinician to experience the results of his/her own enquiries and reasoning
■ continuing discussion about the clinician's reasoning after the patient encounter, which can further help in facilitating reflective learning.

It is important that an informal contract is negotiated beforehand to delineate the extent and method of such discussion (Carr et al., 2000), particularly if the mentor is going to interrupt. The many benefits of peer learning that involves collaborative decision making and feedback from peers are discussed in Chapter 25 in the section on 'Peer learning'.

Clinical learning activities involving a mentor offer several important benefits to clinicians striving to improve their reasoning expertise. The modelling of exemplary decision making by mentors, in which their thinking processes are articulated and their interpretation of the problem is explicated, provides a framework for comparison with the clinician's reasoning. The relevance, depth and complexity of expert knowledge

and reasoning is thus clearly demonstrated to the clinician. In addition, by receiving immediate, specific and constructive feedback on their evolving thoughts and decisions, clinicians are able to modify their reasoning during the case consistent with that of the expert, rather than simply being 'corrected' in hindsight (Prion, 2000). Finally, by having to communicate their thoughts, arguments and rationale for clinical decisions, clinicians are required to clearly understand and organize their own knowledge and its use, and to recognize the adequacy of their knowledge base (Refshauge and Higgs, 2000).

Self-reflection worksheets, such as the Clinical Reasoning Reflection Form (Appendix 2), can also be used to prompt and record the clinician's thinking processes. Relevant sections of the form are completed at key points, such as after taking the history or just prior to the first treatment. These periods of 'time-out' encourage the clinician to review and reflect on the clinical data, as well as plan for future action. The form may also be checked for accuracy and completeness by the mentor. Initially, completion of the entire form is helpful to identify areas of enquiry, reasoning and associated knowledge where the learner could improve. Then, as the learner demonstrates consistent competence with different sections, they can be requested to only complete those sections where further practice with additional patients and varying presentations is considered beneficial. In addition, the mentor can provide general written feedback throughout the patient encounter for later consideration, particularly when it is undesirable to interrupt the clinician's reasoning. It should be noted that the example form in Appendix 2 will not suit all learners and, therefore, students and practitioners are encouraged to develop their own form to meet their own clinical reasoning (reflection) needs and learning situation.

Analogous to self-reflection worksheets, computer software for patient information recording is now available with reflection prompts to stimulate the clinician's reasoning (e.g. Adoc Services Llc., 2002).

Learning from one's clinical practice, that is work-based learning, requires real effort on the part of the clinician to integrate the immediate, practical demands of work with the need to learn from the daily experiences involving patients and their problems. The reader is referred to the section on 'Lifelong learning' in Chapter 25 regarding the importance of cultivating a work environment that encourages ongoing learning.

Clinical simulations

Real or hypothetical clinical problems can be presented in a variety of formats that simulate the clinical situation. Clinical simulations can provide a realistic and less-threatening forum for the identification and correction of reasoning errors and the development of metacognitive skills. Clinical reasoning activities that involve clinical simulations can be undertaken independently or with a mentor or peer. Resources for clinical simulations include:

- videotapes
- interactive computer programmes
- simulated patients
- paper-based and oral cases

Videotapes

Videotapes are recordings of real or simulated patients being interviewed, assessed and treated. They are commercially available (e.g. Maitland, 1999) or can be produced by clinicians in the workplace. Videotaped cases lend themselves to both group activities and independent study and have the obvious advantage of providing visual and auditory cues. The tape can also be replayed for clarification and close examination of critical parts of the patient encounter.

Interactive computer programmes

Self-instructional computer programmes can present real-life or hypothetical clinical scenarios by using text and video and audio clips. Clinical reasoning questions designed to elicit the clinician's thinking, and explore their understanding and knowledge, may also be included. Varying forms of feedback and resource direction facilitate the integration of new information into existing knowledge structures (Christie et al., 2000; Schneiders and Rivett, 2000).

Simulated patients

A simulated patient is a healthy person trained to portray the historical, physical, social and emotional features of an actual patient. The ability to take unlimited 'time out' for discussion with peers and self-reflection is an important advantage of using simulated patients. In addition, the simulated patient can provide specific feedback on the clinician's performance from the perspective of the patient. While it may be difficult to access a properly trained simulated patient outside the tertiary education sector, it is quite feasible for a peer or mentor to role play the clinical presentation of one of their patients.

Paper-based and oral cases

Case reports are available in many professional journals (e.g. Manual Therapy) and books (e.g. Section 2 of the present text) and are often presented by clinicians at in-service or other professional meetings. Better case reports describe the clinical reasoning utilized by the reporting practitioner. They also attempt to engage the reader or listener actively by interspersing questions throughout the clinical findings to stimulate the reader/listener's knowledge and reasoning processes. Story telling by clinical experts is another form of oral case presentation in which they reflect on and interpret their own experiences, with the opportunity provided for questions from others. While there is no best formula for how to conduct these case reports, valuable discussion can emerge by presenting chunks of the unfolding patient information followed by discussion of what is considered key information (perception of relevant information represents one of the earliest cognitive tasks in clinical reasoning), including how different individuals in the discussion would interpret or synthesize that information. The hypothesis categories presented in Chapter 1 provide one means of directing the focus of these discussions of interpretation. Importantly, such discussions should also explore the clinicians' evidence for their interpretations, be it clinical or research based.

The written case report (as in Section 2) is an effective tool for building cognitive schemata, which are directly transferable to the real clinical context (Prion, 2000). Some possible activities for independent or group learning using case reports include:

- read a section of a case report (e.g. the history) and identify any information that was 'missed' and justify why this information might be helpful
- from an actual photograph of a patient or the patient's first comments from the interview, attempt to identify the relevant clinical cues and possible interpretations (i.e. your initial perceptions and hypotheses)
- using the main findings from the patient examination, decide upon a treatment and provide the reasons behind the decision
- read the physical examination findings of a case and hypothesize about the likely history that might

be expected with such a presentation, then compare your expectations to the actual case history

- consider the assessment and management decisions made in the case against your own clinical experience and against the available research evidence (Herbert et al., 2001); when differences are identified, do not simply assume you or they are correct, rather, explore the basis of your thoughts and decisions with an open mind to adjusting your perspective.

At the undergraduate level of education, Carr et al. (2000) have described a small group problem-based tutorial approach to the preliminary learning of reasoning skills that is conducted over two tutorial sessions. The activities involved require the students to draw on their lay (or limited health professional) knowledge and to identify their learning needs as they work through an unfolding simple simulated case. Following an initial trigger, usually a brief video clip of a patient rich in cues, the students' learning is facilitated by a tutor, whose primary role is to keep the learning process 'on track' rather than provide the answers. The tutor progressively provides patient information as they role play the patient during the interview and for physical examination procedures. At various stages during the problem-solving process, the students undertake tasks, which include listing cues and related inferences, summarizing the problem(s) and what is known about it, generating hypotheses accompanied by supporting/ negating evidence, obtaining patient information (i.e. data collection), developing learning goals, and identifying further information (e.g. bioscience knowledge, clinical assessment skills) required to solve the problem(s). As well as fostering the development of skills in clinical reasoning, such a problem-based learning activity (Barrows and Tamblyn, 1980) also encourages self-responsibility in learning.

Learning activities involving simulated clinical scenarios offer many advantages. These include diminished ethical and safety risks compared with learning activities with real patients, and the opportunity to explore alternative evaluation and treatment decisions in the absence of time constraints and potential negative effects on the patient. Clinicians can safely learn from their mistakes, change their minds, explore options, critique alternative explanations and identify assumptions and biases in their thinking. Furthermore, simulated case scenarios provide control over problem type, consistency and complexity, allowing the case to

be matched to the clinician's level of expertise. For example, a novice clinician might commence with more straightforward and shorter case scenarios and progress to more complex and time-consuming scenarios as their expertise develops. If needed, longer learning sessions are possible with clinical simulations, a situation that may be neither ethical or practical with a real patient. Alternatively, if time is limited, or if the learning goals dictate, then just a part of the patient encounter (e.g. the history) can be used in the simulation. In addition, some forms of simulation allow clinicians to learn at their own pace and at a time and place of their choosing, consistent with adult learning principles. It should be recognized, however, that clinical simulations are unable to approximate fully the dynamics of a real patient encounter, nor the unpredictability and variability inherent in dealing with real patients.

The case reports presented in Section 2 attempt to simulate the natural temporal sequence of a patient encounter by providing real clinical data in stages, thus allowing responses to the associated clinical reasoning questions to be based on limited data. The judicious placement of reasoning questions, interspersed amongst the unfolding clinical findings but often at natural 'breaks' in the information flow, is designed to stimulate the reader's cognitive processes. The stimulus questions are open ended and, therefore, require explanation, justification and extrapolation. The provision of the expert clinicians' responses to the questions enables the clinician to compare their thinking with that of the expert and obtain immediate feedback. An awareness of clinical reasoning theory is also facilitated through the use of the clinical reasoning commentaries, which highlight the reasoning processes evident in the experts' responses.

■ Further activities

Cognitive/mind maps

An excellent way to facilitate the exploration of a clinician's knowledge base and reasoning processes is through the use of cognitive maps, or mind maps (Cahill and Fonteyn, 2000; Higgs, 1992). Mapping externalizes a clinician's organization of knowledge on a given topic (e.g. a clinical syndrome) in a way that allows new knowledge to be added. It is a graphical representation of associated knowledge, revealing preconceptions, assumptions, biases and scope of perception.

Relationships and connections between concepts and ideas are clarified by the mapping, and the formation of new relationships and meanings is facilitated by fostering of creative and divergent thinking. It is, therefore, a powerful learning tool that primarily uses critical self-reflection to promote the development of metacognitive skills and the positive reconstruction of knowledge networks.

The process of completing a cognitive map commonly involves three stages.

1. Brainstorming and thinking of anything to do with the topic in question
2. Grouping the brainstormed items in a logical manner, with consideration given to the relationships between individual items
3. Relating the groupings of items to one another showing the connections with lines or arrows, accompanied by a brief description as to how they are related (e.g. 'leads to' or 'is needed for').

A (pre-) cognitive map may be completed before a particular reflective learning activity, and another (post-) cognitive map completed afterwards. Completing the map before the learning activity (e.g. lecture, continuing education course, etc) activates the individual's existing knowledge on the topic, something recommended in experiential learning (Kolb, 1984). Completing a second post-learning map serves as both a review of the information obtained (now hopefully integrated into the prior knowledge on the topic) and a means of evaluating what was learned and the learning activity itself. If the learning activity was successful, you would expect to see significant changes (e.g. more inter-relationships of greater complexity) in the post-learning cognitive map.

Panel discussion or 'fish-bowl' groups

Small group learning activities are also feasible for classes in manual therapy and for manual therapy professional groups. In particular, actual or hypothetical case reports can be explored in depth using a 'fish-bowl' or panel discussion group format (Carr et al., 2000). An approach to this style of learning has been described (Higgs, 1990) as follows. Participants are seated before an audience in a semicircular arrangement with three panels and the chairperson. The first panel of two or three participants represents the patient and is responsible for preparing the case report (if necessary, with the assistance of a more senior practitioner)

and presenting it by the use of role playing and overhead transparencies. Following the provision of introductory cues, subsequent case information is only released on request in a piecemeal fashion. The second panel of two or three participants are the novice clinicians, whose role it is to work through and solve the clinical problem. The final panel consists of one or two expert manual therapists and possibly an expert in a related field (e.g. orthopaedic surgery). Their role is to pose stimulus questions to the novice clinician panel in order to challenge their knowledge and reasoning processes, in addition to providing feedback to the novice clinicians. The reasoning of the novice clinicians is explored via questions such as 'What information do you next need?', 'Why do you want to know that?' and 'How do you interpret these findings and how do they relate to your working hypotheses?'. The chairperson is in overall control of the learning activity, guiding the general direction of the discussion (including promoting discussion on the nature of clinical reasoning) and managing time. At the end of the session, feedback from peers in the audience is encouraged through general debate about the case.

The aims of the 'fish-bowl' format are to increase the novice clinician's awareness of the nature of clinical reasoning and their own reasoning processes (including the relevance and breadth of their own knowledge base) and to promote the development of skills in metacognition and communication of reasoning (Carr et al., 2000). Questions posed by the expert clinicians prompt the novice clinicians to evaluate the validity of their knowledge and to review their clinical reasoning strategies critically, thus enhancing self-awareness and facilitating reflection and metacognition. Novice clinicians are required to express and critique their thoughts verbally, including the formulation of hypotheses and provision of justification for requesting further patient data. Furthermore, key progress findings can be withheld until the learner has committed to a working hypothesis, decided what additional information they require and why and developed criteria for ruling-in or ruling-out hypotheses (Scott, 2000). This approach accelerates the acquisition of the pattern-rich, situation-specific and readily recallable heuristic knowledge typical of expert clinicians (Scott, 2000), that is clinical patterns and associated 'if/then' guides to action. It also impels novice clinicians to assess and revise their knowledge base in terms of accuracy, comprehensiveness and organization (Carr et al., 2000).

Rethinking a patient presentation

To foster skills in creative or lateral thinking, a clinician can choose a patient from their current list and attempt to re-approach the problem by thinking laterally using the previously discussed strategies of re-examining the parts or re-analysing previous interpretations (i.e. looking outside the approach that is presently being taken). While the re-analysis of previous interpretations can be done in one session, the clinician should use their own discretion as to how long to follow through with any change in the treatment itself. After completing the exercise, a brief (one page) account of the results of the re-analysis and change in treatment can include any new insights or re-confirmations of previous interpretations. This will not necessarily produce any new breakthroughs in manual therapy, or even a definite improvement in the patient's status from what was previously being achieved, rather it is an exercise in facilitating looking outside one's own patterns. New ideas and approaches are not discovered in every attempt at lateral thinking. However, if clinicians never re-examine their existing patterns or attempt something outside their usual approach, then any ideas that do emerge will simply be variations of existing ideas rather than genuine new approaches.

Electronic media

Finally, electronic media and communication have provided forums in recent years where clinicians can seek input and feedback from their international peers on patient problems or contribute their own thoughts about clinical problems raised by others. Interactive web-based forums, including e-mail lists, news groups, electronic discussion groups and real-time chat sessions can facilitate the sharing of clinical experiences and exchanging of ideas.

Conclusion

Clinical reasoning underpins all types of manual therapy practice and is the foundation of clinical success. Expertise in manual therapy requires highly organized knowledge structures built on reflective clinical experience, in addition to advanced cognitive and metacognitive skills. An awareness of clinical reasoning processes, especially expert decision making and common reasoning errors, is also essential for the development of clinical expertise. Clinicians wishing to enhance their clinical reasoning skill and advance along the continuum of expertise need to adopt adult learning principles and actively engage in clinical practice learning and professional development. Learning undertaken in the clinical context with real patients provides the optimal opportunity for progress. However, there are also a variety of other activities that simulate the clinical situation and promote reasoning proficiency. Case reports, such as those in Section 2, provide a particularly rich resource for improving clinical reasoning. No matter which learning activities are used, collaborative interaction with a mentor or peer in this process is crucial for building the extensive body of clinically relevant and clinically accessible propositional, craft and personal knowledge typical of expert practitioners.

References

Adoc Services Llc (2002). Physiosphere. Available online: http://www.physiosphere.com

Barrows, H.S. and Tamblyn, R.M. (1980). Problem-Based Learning. An Approach to Medical Education. Stuttgart: Springer.

Bateson, G. (1987). Steps to an Ecology of Mind: Collected Essays in Anthropology, Psychiatry, Evolution and Epistemology. Northvale, NJ: Aronson.

Boshuizen, H.P.A. and Schmidt, H.G. (2000). The development of clinical reasoning expertise. In Clinical Reasoning in the Health Professions, 2nd edn (J. Higgs and M. Jones, eds.) pp. 15–22. Oxford: Butterworth-Heinemann.

Boud, D. (1988). How to help students learn from experience. In The Medical Teacher, 2nd edn (D. Cox and C. Ewan, eds.) pp. 68–73. Edinburgh: Churchill Livingstone.

Brookfield, S.D. (1989). Developing Critical Thinkers. Challenging Adults to Explore Alternative Ways of Thinking and Acting. San Francisco, CA: Jossey-Bass.

Cahill, M. and Fonteyn, M. (2000). Using mind mapping to improve students' metacognition. In Clinical Reasoning in the Health Professions, 2nd edn (J. Higgs and M. Jones, eds.) pp. 214–221. Oxford: Butterworth-Heinemann.

Carr, J., Jones, M. and Higgs, J. (2000). Learning reasoning in physiotherapy programs. In Clinical Reasoning in the Health Professions, 2nd edn (J. Higgs and M. Jones, eds.) pp. 198–204. Oxford: Butterworth-Heinemann.

Christensen, N., Jones, M. and Carr, J. (2002). Clinical reasoning in orthopaedic manual therapy. In Physical Therapy of the Cervical and Thoracic Spine, 3rd edn

(R. Grant, ed.) pp. 85–104. Edinburgh: Churchill Livingstone.

Christie, A., Worley, P. and Jones, M. (2000). The Internet and clinical reasoning. In Clinical Reasoning in the Health Professions, 2nd edn (J. Higgs and M. Jones, eds.) pp. 148–155. Oxford: Butterworth-Heinemann.

De Bono, E. (1977). Lateral Thinking. London: Penguin Books.

De Bono, E. (1993). Serious Creativity: Using the Power of Lateral Thinking to Create New Ideas. New York: HarperCollins.

Elstein, A.S. (1995). Clinical reasoning in medicine. In Clinical Reasoning in the Health Professions (J. Higgs and M. Jones, eds.) pp. 49–59. Oxford: Butterworth-Heinemann.

Fleming, M.H. and Mattingly, C. (2000). Action and narrative: two dynamics of clinical reasoning. In Clinical Reasoning in the Health Professions, 2nd edn (J. Higgs and M. Jones, eds.) pp. 54–61. Oxford: Butterworth-Heinemann.

Glaser, R. and Chi, M.T.H. (1988). Overview. In The Nature of Expertise (M.T.H. Chi, R. Glaser and M.J. Farr, eds.) pp. xvii–xx. Hillsdale, NJ: Erlbaum.

Hayes, B. and Adams, R. (2000). Parallels between clinical reasoning and categorization. In Clinical Reasoning in the Health Professions, 2nd edn (J. Higgs and M. Jones, eds.) pp. 45–53. Oxford: Butterworth-Heinemann.

Herbert, R.D., Sherrington, C., Maher, C. and Moseley, A.M. (2001). Evidence-based practice: imperfect but necessary. Physiotherapy Theory and Practice, 17, 201–211.

Higgs, J. (1990). Fostering the acquisition of clinical reasoning skills. New Zealand Journal of Physiotherapy, 18, 13–17.

Higgs, J. (1992). Developing knowledge: a process of construction, mapping and review. New Zealand Journal of Physiotherapy, 20, 23–30.

Higgs, J. and Bithell, C. (2001). Professional expertise. In Practice Knowledge and Expertise in the Health Professions (J. Higgs and A. Titchen, eds.) pp. 59–68. Oxford: Butterworth-Heinemann.

Higgs, J. and Jones, M. (2000). Clinical reasoning in the health professions.

In Clinical Reasoning in the Health Professions, 2nd edn (J. Higgs and M. Jones, eds.) pp. 3–14. Oxford: Butterworth-Heinemann.

Higgs, J. and Titchen, A. (2000). Knowledge and reasoning. In Clinical Reasoning in the Health Professions, 2nd edn (J. Higgs and M. Jones, eds.) pp. 23–32. Oxford: Butterworth-Heinemann.

Jensen, G.M., Gwyer, J., Hack, L.M. and Shepard, K.F. (1999). Expertise in Physical Therapy Practice. Oxford: Butterworth-Heinemann.

Jones, M.A. (1992). Clinical reasoning in manual therapy. Physical Therapy, 72, 875–884.

Jones, M.A. (1999). Orthopedic expert practice. In Expertise in Physical Therapy Practice (G.M. Jensen, J. Gwyer, L.M. Hack and K.F. Shepard, eds.) pp. 264–270. Oxford: Butterworth-Heinemann.

Jones, M., Jensen, G. and Edwards, I. (2000). Clinical reasoning in physiotherapy. In Clinical Reasoning in the Health Professions, 2nd edn (J. Higgs and M. Jones, eds.) pp. 117–127. Oxford: Butterworth-Heinemann.

Kleinmuntz, B. (1968). The processing of clinical information by man and machine. In The Formal Representation of Human Judgement (B. Kleinmuntz, ed.) pp. 149–186. Chichester, UK: Wiley.

Kolb, D.A. (1984). Experiential Learning: Experience as the Source of Learning and Development. Englewood Cliffs, NJ: Prentice-Hall.

Ladyshewsky, R., Baker, R. and Jones, M. (2000). Peer coaching to generate clinical-reasoning skills. In Clinical Reasoning in the Health Professions, 2nd edn (J. Higgs and M. Jones, eds.) pp. 283–289. Oxford: Butterworth-Heinemann.

Lave, J. (1996). Learning Theories: Situated Learning. Available online (2 August 2002): http://www.educationau.edu.au/archives/cp/04k.htm

Maitland, G.D. (1999). Vertebral Manipulation: A Case Study in Low Back Pain. [Video] Oxford: Butterworth-Heinemann.

Martin, C., Siösteen, A. and Shepard, K.F. (1999). The professional development of expert physical therapists in four areas of clinical practice. In Expertise

in Physical Therapy Practice (G.M. Jensen, J. Gwyer, L.M. Hack and K.F. Shepard, eds.) pp. 231–244. Oxford: Butterworth-Heinemann.

Mechanic, D. and Parson, W. (1975). Editorial: shortcuts are not necessarily bad. Journal of Medical Education, 50, 638–639.

Patel, V.L. and Kaufman, D.R. (2000). Clinical reasoning and biomedical knowledge: implications for teaching. In Clinical Reasoning in the Health Professions, 2nd edn (J. Higgs and M. Jones, eds.) pp. 33–44. Oxford: Butterworth-Heinemann.

Prion, S. (2000). The case study as an instructional method to teach clinical reasoning. In Clinical Reasoning in the Health Professions, 2nd edn (J. Higgs and M. Jones, eds.) pp. 174–183. Oxford: Butterworth-Heinemann.

Rawson, M. (2000). Learning to learn: more than a skill set. Studies in Higher Education, 25, 225–238.

Refshauge, K. and Higgs, J. (2000). Teaching clinical reasoning. In Clinical Reasoning in the Health Professions, 2nd edn (J. Higgs and M. Jones, eds.) pp. 141–147. Oxford: Butterworth-Heinemann.

Regehr, G. and Norman, G. (1996). Issues in cognitive psychology: implications for professional education. Academic Medicine, 71, 988–1000.

Rivett, D.A. (1999). Manual therapy cults. [Editorial] Manual Therapy, 4, 125–126.

Rivett, D. and Higgs, J. (1995). Experience and expertise in clinical reasoning. New Zealand Journal of Physiotherapy, 23, 16–21.

Sackett, D.L., Straus, S.E., Richardson, W.S. et al. (2000). Evidence-Based Medicine: How to Practise and Teach EBM, 2nd edn. Edinburgh: Churchill Livingstone.

Schneiders, A.G. and Rivett, D. (2000). Evaluation of a computer assisted learning (CAL) program for clinical reasoning in manipulative physiotherapy. In Proceedings of the International Federation of Orthopaedic and Manipulative Therapists Conference (K.P. Singer, ed.) pp. 395–399. Perth, Australia: International Federation of Orthopaedic and Manipulative Therapists.

Schön, D.A. (1983). The Reflective Practitioner: How Professionals Think in Action. London: Temple Smith.

Schön, D.A. (1987). Educating the Reflective Practitioner. San Francisco, CA: Jossey-Bass.

Scott, I. (2000). Teaching clinical reasoning: a case-based approach. In Clinical Reasoning in the Health Professions, 2nd edn (J. Higgs and M. Jones, eds.) pp. 290–297. Oxford: Butterworth-Heinemann.

Sefton, A., Gordon, J. and Field, M. (2000). Teaching clinical reasoning to medical students. In Clinical Reasoning in the Health Professions, 2nd edn (J. Higgs and M. Jones, eds.) pp. 184–190. Oxford: Butterworth-Heinemann.

Shepard, K.F. and Jensen, G.M. (2002). Handbook of Teaching for Physical Therapists, 2nd edn. Oxford: Butterworth-Heinemann.

Simon, H.A. (1980). Problem solving and education. In Problem Solving and Education: Issues in Teaching and Research (D.T. Tuma and F. Reif, eds.) pp. 81–96. Hillsdale, NJ: Erlbaum.

Titchen, A. (2001). Critical companionship: a conceptual framework for developing expertise. In Practice Knowledge and Expertise in the Health Professions (J. Higgs and A. Titchen, eds.) pp. 80–90. Oxford: Butterworth-Heinemann.

Watts, N.T. (1995). Teaching the components of clinical decision analysis in the classroom and clinic. In Clinical Reasoning in the Health Professions (J. Higgs and M. Jones, eds.) pp. 204–212. Oxford: Butterworth-Heinemann.

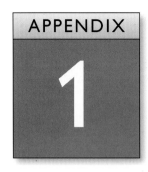

Reflective diary

An example of a reflective diary of clinical patterns used to facilitate skills in pattern recognition by recording typical pattern features and comparing similar, competing patterns. This diary, from the University of South Australia, is designed to facilitate thinking about biomedical features of nociceptive patterns.

Comparative patterns

Area:

Source	Behaviour	Precautions/Contraindications	History

Area:

Source	Contributing factors	Physical examination	Management

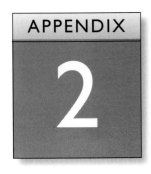

Self-reflection worksheet

Self-reflection worksheets, such as this Clinical Reasoning Reflection Form from the University of South Australia, can be used to prompt and record the clinician's thinking processes.

Clinical Reasoning Reflection Form

NAME.................................. DATE........................ PATIENT'S NAME..

Perceptions/interpretations on completion of the subjective examination

It is important to recognize that the patient's presentation and factors affecting it (e.g. physical, environmental, psychosocial and health management via physiotherapy or other means) can be characterized in pain language/mechanisms by the dominant Input, Processing or Output pain mechanisms that appear to be affected. This should be considered when forming judgments regarding the other hypothesis categories, as interpretations of the patient's symptoms, psychosocial status and signs will vary with the dominance of pain mechanisms present.

1 Activity and participation capabilities/restrictions

1.1 Identify the key abilities and restrictions the patient has in executing activities.
Abilities: ....
Restrictions: ....
....

1.2 Identify the key abilities and restrictions the patient has with involvement in life situations (work, family, sport, leisure).
Abilities: ....
Restrictions: ....
....

2 Patient's perspectives on their experience

Identify the patient's perspectives (positive and negative) on their experience (e.g. *cognitive* – patient understanding, beliefs, attributions, and *affective* – patient feelings/emotions regarding the problem and its management
....
....

3 Pathobiological mechanisms

3.1 Tissue mechanisms

At what stage of the inflammatory/healing process would you judge the principal disorder to be (e.g. acute inflammatory phase 0–72 h, proliferation phase 72 h to 6 weeks, remodelling and maturation phase 6 weeks–several months)?

....

....

....

If the disorder is past the remodelling and maturation phase, what do you think may be maintaining the symptoms/activity-participation restrictions? (e.g. unhelpful perspectives/psychosocial factors, physical/biomechanical impairment, systemic disease, environmental/ergonomic factors, behavioural factors, central processing factors, etc.)? ....

....

....

3.2 Pain mechanisms

3.2.1 List the subjective evidence which supports each specific mechanism of symptoms. Remember that all mechanisms are operating in every presentation but in different ways. The key is to identify the dominant mechanism and potential risk factors for normal mechanism involvement to become pathological (i.e. counterproductive to recovery):

Input Mechanisms			Processing Mechanisms		Output Mechanisms
Nociceptive symptoms	**Peripheral evoked neurogenic symptoms**	**Centrally evoked neurogenic symptoms**	**Patient's perspectives (cognitive/affective influences)**		**Motor and autonomic mechanisms**

3.2.1 Draw a 'pie chart' on the diagram below that reflects the proportional involvement of the pain mechanisms apparent after completing the subjective examination.

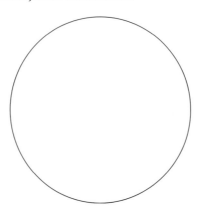

3.3   Identify any potential risk factors (e.g. yellow, blue and black flags) for normal mechanism involvement to become maladaptive (i.e. counterproductive to recovery):

....

....

....

3.4   From your subjective examination, identify any features in the patient's presentation that may reflect impairment in the neuroendocrine and neuroimmune systems:

Neuroendocrine: ....

....

Neuroimmune: ....

....

4   The source(s) of the symptoms

4.1   List in order of likelihood all possible structures at fault for each area/component of symptoms.

Source	Area 1:	Area 2:	Area 3:	Area 4:
Somatic local				
Somatic referred				
Neurogenic (peripheral and/or central)				
Vascular				
Visceral				

Highlight with * those structures which must be examined DAY 1

4.2   Do the symptoms appear to fit those .commonly associated with a particular physical syndrome/disorder/pathology?

....

....

If not, does this suggest the need to examine other factors (e.g. yellow flags, sinister pathology)?

....

....

5   Contributing factors

5.1   Are there any contributing factors associated with the patient's symptoms? Specify:

Physical (e.g. biomechanical, muscle length/strength/control, joint mobility, neural mobility, posture, etc.).

....

Environmental/ergonomic...

Psychosocial (e.g. patient's perspectives/understanding of problem and requirements for recovery/management, feelings regarding problem and its management, attributions, health beliefs, etc..

....

6 The behaviour of the symptoms

6.1 Give your interpretation for each of the following:

Severity |——————|——————|
                        low   high

Irritability symptom 1 |——————|——————|
             non-irritable   very irritable

Irritability symptom 2 |——————|——————|
             non-irritable   very irritable

Give example of irritability: ....
....

What are the implications of this answer to your physical examination? (see 8.3, 8.4)
....
....

Relationship of patient's activity/participation restrictions and/or symptoms to each other
Behavioural (e.g. can symptoms occur alone or are they linked via aggravating and easing factors) ....
....
....

Historical (e.g. what is the relationship of the symptoms over time—biomechanically, motor control, patho-physiological processes?)...
....

Precautionary questions (e.g. general health, red flags (e.g. spinal cord, vertebrobasilar insufficiency, cauda equina, weight loss), medications, investigations, yellow flags and psychosocial factors, etc.).........................
....
....

6.2 Give your interpretation of the contribution of mechanical and/or inflammatory features to the nociceptive component.

Inflammatory |——————|——————|
               0   10

Mechanical |——————|——————|
               0   10

List those factors that support your decision.

Factor	Supporting evidence
Inflammatory	
Mechanical	

What are the implications of this answer to your physical examination? (see 8.3, 8.4)..............................
....
....

7   History of the symptoms

7.1   Give your *interpretation* of the history (present and past) for each of the following:
Nature of the onset (e.g. is it consistent with a particular syndrome or suggest a dominant pain mechanism?)..
....

Extent of impairment and associated tissue damage/change (e.g. mild versus severe and supporting evidence). Also does this fit with a predominantly peripherally evoked or centrally mediated process?..............
....
....

What are the implications for the physical examination (specifically, how do your priorities change for day 1 physical examination)?..
....

Progression since onset (including stage and rate of impairment and stability of the disorder)...................
....
....

Are the patient's symptoms consistent with the history?...
Explain if not, why not: ....
....

8   Precautions and contraindications to physical examination and management

8.1   Does the subjective examination indicate caution (e.g. highly irritable condition, rapidly worsening, progressive neurologically, general health, potential vertebrobasilar or spinal cord impairment, weight loss, medications, investigations, etc.). Explain..
....
....
....

8.2   Do the symptoms indicate the need for specific testing as a day 1 priority (e.g. instability tests, peripheral or central nervous system neurological, vertebral artery tests, further medical investigations, etc.)?
Explain...
....

8.3   At which points under the following headings will you limit your physical examination? Circle the relevant description.

Local symptoms (consider each component)	Referred symptoms (consider each component)	Dysthesias	Symptoms of vertebrobasilar insufficiency	Visceral symptoms
	Short of P1	Short of production		
Point of onset/ increase in resting symptoms	Point of onset/ increase in resting symptoms	Point of onset/ increase in resting symptoms	Point of onset/ increase in resting symptoms	Point of onset/ increase in resting symptoms
Partial reproduction	Partial reproduction	Partial reproduction	Partial reproduction	Partial reproduction
Total reproduction	Total reproduction	Total reproduction		Total reproduction

8.4 Considering your answers to Question 8.1, and in addition to your answer to Question 8.3, at which point will you limit the extent of your physical examination? Tick the relevant description.

Active examination	Passive examination
Active movement short of limit	Passive movement short of R1
Active limit	Passive movement into moderate resistance
Active limit plus overpressure	Passive movement to full over-pressure
Additional tests	

If the dominance of the presentation with this patient is hypothesised to be central as opposed to peripherally evoked, provide an example of how you will attend to this in this particular patient's physical examination..........
....
....

What would your priorities be for day 1?...
....
....
....

8.5 Is a peripheral or central nervous system neurological examination necessary?
Why?...
....
Is it a day 1 priority?...
....

8.6 If relevant, do you expect a comparable sign(s) to be easy/hard to find?
Explain...
....
....

8.7 What are the clues (if any) in the subjective examination to management and specific treatment techniques that may be used?..
....
....

Perceptions, interpretations, implications following the physical examination and first treatment

9   Concept of the patient's illness/pain experience

9.1 What is your assessment of the patient's understanding of his/her problem (Have you asked the patient?...
....
....
....
....

9.2 What is your assessment of the patient's feelings about his/her problem, its affect on his/her life and how it has been managed to date?..
....
....
....

9.3 What does the patient expect/want from you/your management (i.e. patient's goals)?........................

....

Are the patient's goals appropriate? Explain...

....

....

Have you and the patient been able to agree on modified goals? Explain...

....

9.4 What effect do you anticipate the patient's understanding and feelings regarding his/her problem may have on your management or the prognosis?...

....

....

....

10 Physical impairments

Identify the key physical impairments from the physical examination that may require management/ re-assessment (e.g. posture, movement patterns/motor control, soft tissue/muscle/joint/neural mobility/sensitivity, etc.).

1..

2..

3..

4..

5..

etc.

11 Sources and pathobiological mechanisms of the patient's symptoms

11.1 List the components of symptoms and pathobiological mechanisms identified in Section 4.0 and 3.0 and number in order of likelihood the possible structure(s) at fault for each apparent component.

Then identify supporting and negating evidence from the **physical examination** for each structure and pathobiological mechanism

Component	Possible structure(s) at fault	Physical examination supporting evidence	Physical examination negating evidence

Pain mechanisms	Supporting evidence	Negating evidence
Input mechanisms: ■ Nociceptive ■ Peripherally evoked neurogenic		
Processing mechanisms: ■ Centrally evoked neurogenic ■ Cognitive and affective		
Output mechanisms: ■ Motor ■ Autonomic		

Tissue mechanisms	Supporting evidence	Negating evidence
Acute inflammatory phase		
Proliferation phase		
Remodelling and maturation phase		

11.2   Indicate your principal hypothesis regarding the primary syndrome/disorder and the dominant pathobiological mechanism(s)...
....
....

11.3   Tissue mechanisms—healing mechanisms
Do your findings on **physical examination** change your interpretation related to Question 3.1 regarding the stage of the inflammatory/healing process? Explain..
....
....
....

11.4   Based on your understanding of the nature of the disorder (e.g. inflammatory, degree of irritability, worsening, rate of impairment, and other indicators of the need for caution), the pathobiological mechanisms operating, the patient's perceptions (i.e. cognitive/affective status) and possible contributing factors, list the favourable and unfavourable prognostic indicators:

Favourable	Unfavourable

Implications of perceptions and interpretations on ongoing management

12   Management

12.1   Do the physical signs fit with the symptoms? If not, how might this influence your management and treatment prognosis..
....
....

12.2   Is there anything about your physical examination findings which would indicate the need for caution in your management?...
Explain..
....

12.3   Does your interpretation of the physical examination change the emphasis of treatment as outlined?...
....
....

12.4   What was your management on day 1 (e.g. advice, exercise, passive mobilisation, referral for further investigations, etc.)?...
Why was this chosen over the other options? ....
....
If passive treatment was used, what was your principle treatment technique(s)?...
....
What physical examination findings support your choice? (Include in your answer a movement diagram of the most comparable passive sign). ....
....
....

Movement diagram

12.5   If you used an active or passive treatment or advice on day 1, what was its effect? ....
....
....
....

What is your expectation of the patient's response over the next 24 hours?
....
....

12.6 What is your plan and justification of management for this patient (rate of progression; addressing other problems/components)?..
....
....

12.7 Do you envisage a need to refer the patient to another health provider (e.g. physician, orthopaedic surgeon, neurologist/neurosurgeon, vascular surgeon, endocrinologist, psychologist/psychiatrist, anaesthetist, dietician, feldenkrais practitioner, etc.)?..
....

Reflection on source(s), contributing factors(s) and prognosis

13 After third visit

13.1 How has your understanding of the patient's problem changed from your interpretations made following the first session? ....
How has the patient's perceptions of his/her problem and management changed since the first session?...........
....
Are the patient's needs being met?..
....

13.2 On reflection, what clues (if any) can you now recognize that you initially missed, misinterpreted, under- or overweighted?
....
....
What would you do differently next time?..
....

14 After sixth visit

14.1 How has your understanding of the patient's problem changed from your interpretations made following the third session?...
....
How has the patient's perceptions of his/her problem and management changed since the third session?
....
....

14.2 On reflection, what clues (if any) can you now recognize that you initially missed, misinterpreted, under- or over-weighted?..
....
What would you do differently next time?..

14.3 If the outcome is to be short of 100% ('cured'), at what point will you cease management and why?..
....

15 After discharge

15.1 How has your understanding of the patient's problem changed from your interpretations made following the sixth session? ....
....

How has the patient's perceptions of his/her problem and management changed since the sixth session?

....

....

15.2   In hindsight, what were the principal source(s) and pathobiological mechanisms of the patient's symptoms? ....

....

Identify the key subjective and physical features (i.e. clinical pattern) that would help you to recognize this presentation in the future.

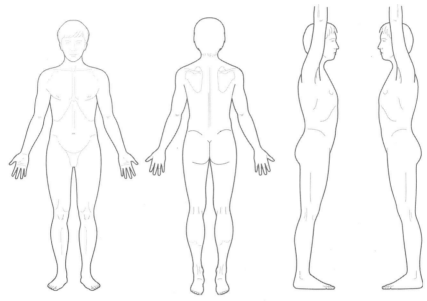

Subjective	Physical

Index

Also available...

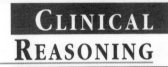

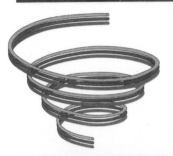

Edited by Joy Higgs Mark Jones

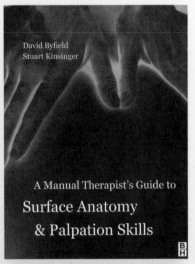

David Byfield
Stuart Kinsinger

A Manual Therapist's Guide to
Surface Anatomy
& Palpation Skills

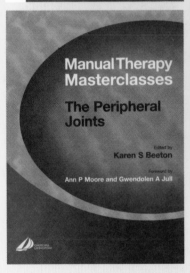

Manual Therapy
Masterclasses

The Peripheral
Joints

Edited by
Karen S Beeton

Foreword by
Ann P Moore and Gwendolen A Jull

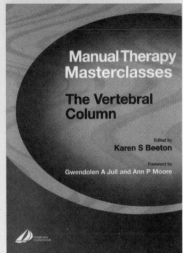

Manual Therapy
Masterclasses

The Vertebral
Column

Edited by
Karen S Beeton

Foreword by
Gwendolen A Jull and Ann P Moore

You can order these, or any other Elsevier Science title (Churchill Livingstone, Saunders,
Mosby, Baillière Tindall, Butterworth-Heinemann), from your local bookshop,
or, in case of difficulty, direct from us on:

EUROPE, MIDDLE EAST & AFRICA
Tel: +44 (0) 20 8308 5710
www.elsevierhealth.com

CANADA
Tel: +1 866 276 5533
www.elsevier.ca

AUSTRALIA
Tel: +61 (0) 2 9517 8999
www.elsevierhealth.com

USA
Tel: +1 800 545 2522
www.us.elsevierhealth.com

**ELSEVIER
SCIENCE**

Coventry University